T0202510

Statistical Literacy for Clinical Practitioners

William H. Holmes • William C. Rinaman

Statistical Literacy for Clinical Practitioners

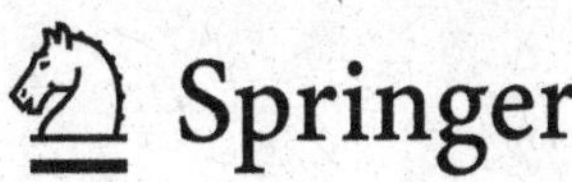

William H. Holmes
Le Moyne College
Syracuse
New York
USA

William C. Rinaman
Pinehurst
North Carolina
USA

ISBN 978-3-319-34583-3 ISBN 978-3-319-12550-3 (eBook)
DOI 10.1007/978-3-319-12550-3
Springer Cham Heidelberg New York Dordrecht London

Printed on acid-free paper

Springer is part of Springer Science+Business Media (www.springer.com)

Preface

We wrote this book for readers who wish to acquire a basic understanding of statistical analysis and the various functions that statistics perform in clinical research. Our intended audience includes practitioners of evidence-based medicine, practitioners-in-training, students working on research projects under the supervision of their faculty, and clinicians collaborating with professional researchers. Members of this audience are, of course, highly accomplished, but they are often short on time and sometimes uncertain of their mathematical skills. Consequently, our goal was to provide a representative and accessible cross-section of statistical techniques while respecting the readers' intelligence and avoiding being simplistic.

To instantiate many of the statistical concepts we discuss, we include output generated by IBM® SPSS® statistics software, and explain how to interpret it. SPSS is frequently used in clinical research, so for readers who want hands-on experience in analyzing data with it, we give an overview of SPSS in Chap. 2 (*Introduction to SPSS*), and in each chapter thereafter, we explain how to use SPSS to conduct the analyses of that chapter on data sets taken from actual studies. SPSS is updated periodically, each update identified by a version number. The book is based on version 22, but most of our instructions should apply to other versions as well. Permission to use reprinted SPSS dialogs and output is courtesy of International Business Machines Corporation, © International Business Machines Corporation. SPSS Inc. was acquired by IBM in October 2009. IBM, the IBM logo, ibm.com, and SPSS are trademarks or registered trademarks of International Business Machines Corporation.

To allow readers to test their understanding of the material on the fly, we quiz them throughout each chapter. With the exception of Chap. 2, readers should be able to respond without having access to SPSS. So that readers can further test themselves, we conclude each chapter with a set of exercise questions. To meet the needs of readers wishing to learn SPSS, most exercises from Chaps. 2–17 require access to SPSS.

We obtained most of the data sets from either published primary or secondary sources. A handful of data sets are from unpublished master's projects conducted by physician assistant students under the supervision of one of the author's of this book (WHH). The sources of the data sets of a given chapter are listed at the end of the chapter. The data sets themselves can be found at http://www.springer.com/978-3-319-12549-7, as can the answers to the in-chapter questions and end-of-chapter exercises. On the assumption that course instructors might wish to assign the end-of-chapter exercises as homework, their solutions are available only to instructors on the Springer page for the book (http://www.springer.com/978-3-319-12549-7).

We would like to thank the publishing houses and researchers who granted us permission to use their data, and IBM for permission to use screenshots of SPSS dialogs and output. We also thank Marc Strauss, Editorial Director, Mathematics Department, and Hannah Bracken, Associate Editor, Springer Science+Business Media, for their advice and encouragement. Earlier drafts of the book were reviewed by the faculty and students of the Department of Physician Assistant Studies of Le Moyne College. We are grateful for their feedback and support. Finally, WHH would like to thank his wife, Joan Dalton for her endless patience and unflagging support.

William H. Holmes, PhD
Le Moyne College
Syracuse, NY

William C. Rinaman, PhD
Pinehurst, NC

Contents

1 Introduction 1
1.1 Functions of Statistics 1
1.2 Common Study Designs in Clinical Medicine 2
1.3 Categories of Research 16
1.4 Looking Ahead 18
1.5 Exercise Questions 20
References 22

2 Introduction to SPSS 25
2.1 Overview 25
2.2 Opening SPSS Data Files 26
2.3 Structure of SPSS Data Files: Data and Variable Views 27
2.4 Saving SPSS Data Files 38
2.5 Selecting Cases for an SPSS Analysis 40
2.6 Sorting a Dialog Box' Variables List 51
2.7 Labeling SPSS Output 51
2.8 Printing and Pasting SPSS Output 52
2.9 Saving and Exporting SPSS Output Files 55
2.10 Exercise Questions 57
Data Set and Reference 57

3 Describing the Distribution of a Categorical Variable 59
3.1 Overview 59
3.2 Frequency Tables 60
3.3 Bar Charts and Pie Charts 64
3.4 Transforming Variables 70
3.5 Copying SPSS Charts into MS Word Documents 73
3.6 Exercise Questions 84
Data Set and Reference 86

4 Describing the Distribution of a Quantitative Variable 87
4.1 Overview 87

4.2 Describing the Distribution of a Sample ... 88
4.3 The Standard Error of the Mean ... 96
4.4 Comparing Distributions Across Values of a Categorical Variable ... 98
4.5 Transforming a Quantitative Variable ... 104
4.6 Exercise Questions ... 117
Data Sets and References ... 125

5 Introduction to Statistical Inference ... 127
5.1 Overview ... 127
5.2 Confidence Intervals for a Population Mean ... 128
5.3 Test of Hypotheses ... 132
5.4 Test of Normality ... 136
5.5 Nonparametric Test of Hypotheses: Testing a Population Median ... 140
5.6 Statistical Power ... 142
5.7 Clinical Versus Statistical Significance ... 143
5.8 Exercise Questions ... 144
Data Sets and References ... 147

6 Inference for Proportions ... 149
6.1 Overview ... 149
6.2 CIs for Population Proportions ... 150
6.3 Testing a Single Proportion ... 153
6.4 CIs for the Difference Between Two Population Proportions ... 155
6.5 Testing Two Proportions ... 158
6.6 Relative Risk and Odds Ratios ... 161
6.7 Exercise Questions ... 174
Data Sets and References ... 177

7 Relationships in Categorical Data ... 179
7.1 Overview ... 179
7.2 Contingency Tables ... 180
7.3 Clustered Bar Charts ... 184
7.4 Testing Hypotheses About Whether Two Categorical Variables are Related ... 185
7.5 Measuring the Strength of the Relationship: Cramér's *V* ... 193
7.6 Measuring the Strength of the Relationship: Gamma ... 199
7.7 Exercise Questions ... 200
Data Set and Reference ... 204

8 Assessing Screening and Diagnostic Tests ... 205
8.1 Overview ... 205
8.2 Positive and Negative Predictive Values ... 206

8.3 True Positives, True Negatives, False Positives, and False Negatives ... 208
8.4 Sensitivity and Specificity ... 211
8.5 Prior Odds, Posterior Odds, and the Likelihood Ratio ... 212
8.6 The Receiver Operating Characteristic (ROC) Curve ... 217
8.7 Exercise Questions ... 226
Data Sets and References ... 231

9 Relationships in Quantitative Data ... 233
9.1 Overview ... 233
9.2 Scatter Plots ... 234
9.3 Pearson Correlation Coefficient ... 238
9.4 Spearman's Rho Coefficient ... 244
9.5 Exercise Questions ... 247
Data Sets and References ... 250

10 Comparing Means of Independent Samples ... 251
10.1 Overview ... 251
10.2 Comparing Two Means: The Independent-Samples t-Test ... 253
10.3 Comparing Two Means: One-way Analysis of Variance ... 259
10.4 Effect Size ... 263
10.5 Comparing More than Two Means ... 268
10.6 Exercise Questions ... 277
Data Sets and References ... 281

11 Comparing Means of Related Samples ... 283
11.1 Overview ... 283
11.2 Paired-Samples T-Test ... 285
11.3 Repeated Measures Analysis of Variance ... 288
11.4 Exercise Questions ... 298
Data Sets and References ... 302

12 Analysis of Variance with Two Factors ... 303
12.1 Overview ... 303
12.2 ANOVA with One Independent Groups Factor ... 304
12.3 ANOVA with Two Independent Groups Factors ... 308
12.4 ANOVA with Two Repeated Measures Factors ... 318
12.5 ANOVA with One Independent Groups and One Repeated Measure Factor ... 327
12.6 Exercise Questions ... 336
Data Sets and References ... 339

13 Simple Linear Regression ... 341
13.1 Overview ... 341

13.2 Describing the Best Fitting Straight Line 342
13.3 The Coefficient of Determination 348
13.4 Estimating and Testing Population Coefficients 351
13.5 Prediction Intervals 355
13.6 Residual Analysis 359
13.7 Exercise Questions 362
Data Sets and References 366

14 Multiple Linear Regression 367
14.1 Overview 367
14.2 Assessing the Impact of a Single Predictor on Prediction Accuracy 369
14.3 Improving Prediction by Adding a Second Predictor 373
14.4 Interpreting Standardized and Unstandardized Slope Coefficients 378
14.5 Using Categorical Predictors 382
14.6 Testing Model Coefficients 385
14.7 Interaction Effects 389
14.8 Exercise Questions 393
Data Sets and References 396

15 Logistic Regression 397
15.1 Overview 397
15.2 Logistic Regression with One Predictor 399
15.3 Logistic Regression with Two Categorical Predictors 405
15.4 Logistic Regression with Quantitative and Categorical Predictors 413
15.5 Adjusted Odds Ratios 418
15.6 Testing for an Interaction Effect 419
15.7 Exercise Questions 420
Data Sets and References 421

16 Survival Analysis 423
16.1 Overview 423
16.2 Kaplan–Meier Estimator of the Survival Function 424
16.3 Comparing Two Survival Functions 432
16.4 Hazard Functions, the Proportional Hazards Model, and Relative Risk 436
16.5 Cox Regression with One Covariate 439
16.6 Cox Regression with Two Covariates 444
16.7 Interaction Effects 446
16.8 Exercise Questions 449
Data Sets and References 450

17 Regression Analysis of Count Data 451
17.1 Overview 451
17.2 Negative Binomial Regression with One Predictor 452
17.3 Testing Two or More Predictors 462
17.4 Testing for an Interaction Effect 469
17.5 Regression with Unequal Follow-up Times 471
17.6 Exercise Questions 475
Data Sets and References 478

Index 481

Chapter 1
Introduction

Abstract This chapter summarizes the various functions of statistics in clinical research, reviews study designs that guide how data are typically collected and analyzed, and provides examples of statistical procedures frequently used in clinical studies. The designs include the case study, case-control study, the survey, prospective and retrospective cohort studies, parallel group and crossover trials, and systematic reviews and meta-analyses. The ability of each design to draw confident causal conclusions is also discussed. The chapter concludes with an overview of the content of the book.

1.1 Functions of Statistics

The practice of medicine is continuously informed by clinical research into health and disease. The research is empirical, generated by observational procedures that are grounded in physical reality and which can be clearly communicated to and repeated by anyone with sufficient training and ability. Often these observations or *data* are numerical and are of various chemical and biological processes related to health and disease. It goes without saying that in order to grasp the findings of clinical studies, medical practitioners need to be literate in chemistry and biology. But clinical research documents probabilities, tendencies or what is true on average. It determines, for example, whether people who have been exposed to a suspected carcinogen are more likely to contract cancer, not about whether exposure to the carcinogen always leads to cancer, or whether on average a particular cancer treatment helps patients, not whether the treatment always works or works equally well for all patients. Because of the probabilistic nature of clinical data, researchers must use statistical analysis to uncover patterns within those data. Consequently, to understand clinical studies, practitioners need to have a working knowledge of statistics as well.

An analysis of a set of data can involve the use of a wide range of statistics that perform a variety of functions. Usually, investigators begin an analysis by summarizing their observations with *descriptive statistics*. Descriptive statistics include percentages, means and standard deviations, among many others. Researchers also use various graphical techniques such as *bar charts* and *histograms*. Investigators

W. H. Holmes, W. C. Rinaman, *Statistical Literacy for Clinical Practitioners*,
DOI 10.1007/978-3-319-12550-3_1

then use *measures of association* to determine whether two variables are related and if so, how strongly, and in what direction. Examples include the *odds ratio* (*OR*), *relative risk*, the *hazard ratio*, and the *rate ratio*. Other measures of association include *Cramér's V* and *gamma*, the *Pearson correlation coefficient*, *Spearman's Rho* coefficient, and the difference between the means of two or more groups.

In addition to summarizing observations and documenting associations between variables, investigators use certain statistical procedures to assess the degree of relationship between two variables after controlling for the presence of a third variable with which the two variables are related. This *statistical control* of potential *confounding variables* is often achieved through some form of *regression analysis*. Researchers also use regression for the purpose of *prediction* or *estimation*, that is, to predict or estimate health-related outcomes of patients with various characteristics. For example, a regression analysis might be used to estimate the *mortality rate* of cardiac patients of a given gender, age, and health history.

In most clinical studies, participants constitute a *sample* that is drawn from a larger *population*. Due to a phenomenon known as *random sampling variability*, researchers use *inferential statistics* to help them decide whether their sample results should be attributed to chance or can be used to make inferences about the populations from which they drew their participants. Inferential statistics make use of various *test statistics* that generate *confidence intervals* and *p-values* that help researchers make this decision.

Identify each of the following as an example of a descriptive statistic, a measure of association, an inferential statistic, statistical control or prediction.

1.1.1 The probability of recurrence of breast cancer over the next 10 years for a postmenopausal woman who does not smoke

1.1.2 The proportion of a sample of Americans who are prehypertensive

1.1.3 A 95% confidence interval for the proportion of Americans who are prehypertensive

1.1.4 The correlation between the body mass index (BMI) of anorexics and their preferred BMI

1.1.5 Using regression to take into account gender in a study of the relationship between forced expiratory volume and age in a sample of children

1.2 Common Study Designs in Clinical Medicine

At the level of procedural detail, research studies can be very different from one another. In fact, it is safe to say that no two studies are exactly the same in terms of their specifics. However, at a global level, many clinical studies can be classified in terms of a relatively small number of *study designs*. These designs serve as a kind of blueprint that researchers follow as they collect their data. For example, a study design stipulates whether the investigator will observe the impact of a factor by systematically exposing volunteers to it or by observing patients who during the course of their lives had already been exposed, whether patients are to be observed on a single occasion or followed over a period of time, and whether follow-up data are to be obtained directly from patients until the study ends at some point in the future, or extracted from preexisting medical records that extend from the present to some point in the past. Because study designs guide how data are to be collected, they influence how the data are to be analyzed. An analysis that would be appropriate for one study design might not work for another. Consequently, in this section, we shall review some of the more common designs in clinical research, and give examples of the statistical analyses that are associated with them.

Although clinical research tries to pin down the causes of disease, researchers often use study designs that fall short of generating strong evidence of causality. This is because practical and ethical limitations can prevent researchers from using designs that convincingly establish the conditions for demonstrating causality. One of these conditions is *covariation.* To show that one variable causes another, researchers must first show that the two variables covary, that is, that they are correlated with one another. For example, if a researcher believes that lack of exercise is a cause of overweight, then he or she must show that people who do not exercise tend to be heavier than people who do, other things being equal. This is not to say that the researcher will not find thin people who do not exercise or that there are not any overweight people who work out. Weight is a result of many causes after all. But if lack of exercise is to be considered one of them, then the researcher will have to show that the *likelihood* of being overweight is greater for people who do not exercise regularly.

Causes not only covary with their effects, but they also come before their effects. So a second condition researchers must demonstrate is the *correct time order* between the two variables. Researchers must show that the hypothesized causal variable precedes in time its hypothesized effect. For example, to show only that lack of exercise and BMI are correlated would not reveal the direction of causality between exercise and weight. We would be left wondering whether people who do not exercise *become* heavy, or whether people do not exercise *because* they are heavy.

Sometimes a researcher will find that a factor covaries with a health-related outcome when in fact the factor has no impact on patients. This can happen because of *random sampling variability* or because of *confounding*. In the former instance, the association between the factor and the medical outcome is a chance coincidence. In the latter instance, the association is genuine but is due to the factor's correlation with a causal variable, not because it is itself a cause. For example, if a researcher were to find that lack of exercise and BMI are correlated, we might wonder if the observed relationship was just a fluke. If we were to be persuaded that chance was not responsible, then we might wonder if people who do not exercise are overweight not because they are sedentary but because they have poor eating habits. Consequently, before researchers can point to the correlation between the factor and the medical outcome as strong evidence of a causal relationship between the two, they must rule out both random sampling variability and confounding as *plausible alternative explanations* of that relationship.

1.2.1 List three conditions that must be established in clinical research in order to demonstrate cause and effect.

1.2.2 Which of these three conditions cannot be established when confounding is present?

Study designs vary in their ability to establish covariation and the correct time order, and to rule out random sampling variability and confounding as alternative explanations. As a result, study designs not only influence the choice of statistical analysis, but they also affect the confidence that can be placed in any causal conclusions drawn from that analysis. As we review some of the most common designs, we shall see why this is so.

Case Reports and Case Series In a case report, the investigator details the experience of a single patient (called a case). In a case series, the investigator reports the experiences of several individual patients. These designs are frequently used to document highly unusual medical conditions. For example, Newsom-Davis et al. [1] presented the case of an 82-year-old woman who had been referred because she had experienced postmenopausal bleeding during the past month. She died about 18 months later from postoperative complications. In the report, the authors discuss the challenges of diagnosing and treating uterine teratoma, a rare tumor.

Case reports and case series are also used to get a sense of the effectiveness of new interventions. For example, de Paleville et al. [2] noticed that the benefits of aerobic exercise on breast cancer patients undergoing chemotherapy had been studied only when exercise had been introduced during therapy. Curious about the effects of exercise if it were begun prior to chemotherapy, they documented the fatigue and functional abilities of a breast cancer patient who was about to participate in a supervised home-based walking program 1 week prior to as well as throughout an 8-week course of chemotherapy. The investigators found that at the end of the 9-week period, the patient experienced less fatigue and improved functional abilities, suggested that these outcomes were due to her having begun her exercise program before chemotherapy was initiated, and recommended that further research on "prehabilitation" should be conducted.

Case reports and case series struggle to establish the three conditions of causality that must be met in order to establish a causal conclusion. Consequently, they are used to document cases rather than to demonstrate causality. For example, it is often impossible to evaluate the effectiveness of a new treatment with a case report because the report did not establish covariation. Notice that the case report reported by de Paleville et al. did not include a patient who did not participate in the prechemotherapy exercise regimen. Consequently, the investigators could not show that variation in the supposed causal factor (being or not being prehabilitated) was associated with variation in the supposed effect (having higher or lower levels of energy or functional ability).

Even if a case report had included a patient who had not been given the treatment and even if this patient had shown less improvement than the patient who had been treated, we would not be able to rule out plausible alternative explanations for why the treated patient showed more improvement than the untreated one. Recall that one possibility could be random sampling variability. The apparent effect of the treatment could have been due not to the treatment but to one or more factors that were present by chance at the time the treatment was administered. For example, most if not all measurement in clinical research is influenced at least to some extent by random factors. A blood pressure reading, a laboratory test result or a patient's self-report are all likely to be affected by factors that occur by chance at the time the blood pressure reading is taken, the lab test conducted, or the self-report given. This *random measurement error* is one source of random variability. A problem with a case report is that it is difficult to determine to what extent the patient's observed improvement was genuine, that is, due to the treatment, and to what extent it was due to random factors such as measurement error. Combining several cases into a case series can be helpful in this regard, since if the effect of the treatment is genuine, it should help other patients as well, but the resulting number of cases in a case series is usually too small to allow researchers to confidently rule out the possibility that chance was the sole cause of the observed change in the patients' condition.

Another possible explanation for improvement observed in a treated patient is that the improvement was not due to chance but to confounding, that is, to a factor that is reliably associated with the treatment and with the medical outcome under investigation. A factor that is consistently associated with both the treatment and the outcome is referred to as a *confounding factor* or a *confounder*. To convincingly show that a treatment is effective, a researcher must demonstrate that although there may have been random factors at work in the study, there were no *systematic* differences between the patient who was treated and the one who was not other than the treatment itself. There are techniques that researchers can use to take into account or *control* confounding factors, but to be effective they require a large number of patients.

Despite their shortcomings as evidence of causality, information reported in a case report or a case series can alert practitioners to diagnoses and treatments that they might not have otherwise considered. Moreover, a case report or series can lead to additional research that uses study designs better suited to establishing causal connections. One such design is the *case-control study*.

Is each of the following statements true or false?

1.2.3 In general, case reports can provide strong evidence of covariation.

1.2.4 Case reports have little or no role to play in clinical research.

Case-Control Studies Case-control studies compare people (called cases) who already have a specific condition or disease with people (called controls) who do not. The logic of this type of study is to work backward from the disease to identify a factor that distinguishes between the two groups. The factor might be a demographic, physical or psychological characteristic, or a life experience of some kind. Case-control studies often rely on preexisting records such as medical charts or on participant self-report to identify these factors. Rarely if ever does the identified factor perfectly distinguish between cases and controls. Although none of the controls will have the illness, it is likely that some will have been exposed to the factor, and while all of the cases suffer from the disease, it is likely that some will not have been exposed to the factor. So case-control studies compare the *likelihood* that those who have been exposed to the factor have the disease to the *likelihood* that those who have not been exposed have the disease. These likelihoods are expressed in terms of *odds*. A *risk factor* is associated with an increase in the likelihood or odds of disease, while a *protective factor* is associated with a decrease in odds. The extent to which a factor increases or decreases the odds of disease is calculated by dividing the odds of the exposed group by the odds of the unexposed group. The result is called an *odds ratio* (OR). A risk factor generates an OR greater than 1.0; a protective factor generates an OR less than 1.0. An OR equal to 1.0 indicates that the factor has no impact on disease.

As an example of research on a protective factor, consider a study conducted by Kim et al. [3] in Korea. They asked 358 breast cancer patients and 360 women with no known history of malignant neoplasm to complete a food intake frequency questionnaire. The investigators found that the odds of having breast cancer were lower for women who reported that they consumed relatively large amounts of fish high in omega-3 fatty acid. In fact, dividing the odds of having breast cancer for women whose diets were greatest in omega-3 fatty acid by the odds for women whose diets were lowest in omega-3 generated an OR of 0.47. This means that diets highest in fatty acid were associated with odds of breast cancer that were less than half the odds of diets lowest in omega-3. The investigators concluded that a diet high in fatty fish is a protective factor for breast cancer.

The exact value of a statistic obtained in any given study is subject to random sampling variability. If the study were to be repeated many times, we would not obtain the exact same value each time. Instead, we would see a range of values. Consequently, researchers often report an estimate of that range known as the *95% confidence interval* (95% CI). If the sample statistic is an OR, and if the interval does not include the value of 1.0, then random factors can be confidently ruled out as an explanation for the finding. For example, in the Kim et al. study, the OR of 0.47 has a 95% CI that ranges from 0.27 to 0.80. This range does not include 1.0, so we can be confident that the observed difference in odds of contracting breast cancer between the people in the study who consumed a lot of omega-3 acid and those in the study who consumed very little of it was not due just to random sampling variability.

Case-control studies have at least three advantages over case reports and case series. First, by including a group of patients that are free of disease, that is, by including the controls, case-control studies can demonstrate covariation. For example, in the study of diet and breast cancer conducted by Kim et al., the point was not that the cases did not eat fatty fish. The point was that the cases ate less fatty fish than did the controls. By including the controls in their study, they were able to show covariation between fish consumption and breast cancer.

The second and third advantages have to do with the fact that the number of cases and controls observed in a case-control study is usually large. Collecting observations from a large sample of cases and controls helps to compensate for the random measurement error associated with each observation, and so allows researchers to have more confidence in their findings. For example, Kim et al. based their conclusions on their assessment of the dietary habits of over 700 patients. In contrast, de Paleville et al. based their conclusions on a single case. In addition, using a large sample allows researchers to employ inferential statistics. These procedures help researchers to decide whether covariation was due solely to chance or to a systematic difference between their cases and controls. One way they do this is by generating 95 % CIs. For instance, by generating a 95 % CI, Kim et al. were able to conclude that that the covariation they observed between levels of fish consumption and the odds of having breast cancer was not due solely to random factors.

Although case-control studies can demonstrate covariation between exposure to a risk or protective factor on the one hand and the odds of having a disease on the other, exposure may be associated or confounded with one or more other factors. Consequently, researchers assess the degree of relationship between the factor and the disease after they have first controlled for confounders. Several methods exist for controlling confounding. For example, Kim et al. collected information about each patient's age, BMI, breast cancer family history, smoking status, physical activity, and many other factors that might have something to do with the etiology of breast cancer and be correlated with dietary habits. Then using a statistical procedure known as *logistic regression* to take these confounders into account, they found that the odds of having breast cancer were lower for women whose diet was high in fatty fish.

Other methods for controlling confounding are *stratification* and *matching*. Stratification refers to the procedure of first computing the OR at each value of a confounder. For each comparison, the confounder is held constant, so any difference between the cases and controls in their odds of having been exposed to the factor under investigation cannot be due to the confounding variable. Then the ORs across the levels of the confounder are combined to give a representative estimate of the size of the difference in odds between cases and controls when the confounder has been held constant. Matching involves recruiting controls that are similar to the cases in terms of a subset of confounders. When matching is used in a case-control study, the research design is called a *matched case-control study*. Often in matched case-control studies, logistic regression is used to control for additional confounders, in which case the regression is called *conditional logistic regression*.

A study by Rajaraman et al. [4] is an example of all three of these methods of controlling confounding. These researchers investigated whether exposure to diagnostic radiation in utero or in early infancy or to ultrasound scans in early infancy is associated with childhood cancer. Cases were 2656 children 14 years of age or younger living in the UK who had been diagnosed between 1992 and 1996 as having leukemia, lymphoma, or a tumor of the central nervous system. The investigators wished to control for each child's sex, age, birth weight, mother's age, the geographical region in which the child lived, and whether the child's cancer was diagnosed before or after the age of five. To control these six confounders, the investigators first identified a control who was of the same sex, had within 1 month the same date of birth, and came from the same geographical area as the case to which he or she was to be matched. Obtaining data from medical records, the investigators then compared the extent to which each case and his or her matched control had been exposed to radiation or ultrasound scans in utero or up to 100 days following birth. They made these comparisons while using conditional logistic regression to control for the mother's age and the child's birth weight, and stratified the analysis by the age at which the child's cancer was diagnosed. In general, the investigators found a "slight" increase in risk associated with exposure to X-rays in utero or in early infancy, but the increases could have been due to random variability. For example, across all cancers, the OR was 1.14, but the 95% CI ranged from 0.90 to 1.45. No adverse effects associated with ultrasounds were found.

Although case-control studies are an improvement over case reports, they have their weaknesses. Medical charts may not always be accurate, complete or even available, and patient self-reports can be unreliable. These problems can make it difficult to identify a risk or protective factor, to be certain that the cases were exposed to the factor more often than the controls or to be sure that the exposure occurred before the onset of the disease. Our next study design addresses these problems. In addition, in a case-control study, only confounding factors that are known to exist and which are measured can be controlled. This leaves open the possibility of *residual confounding*. For example, say that Rajaraman et al. had found an association between exposure to X-rays and lymphoma. This association would not appear to be explainable in terms of the six confounders that the investigators controlled. However, controlling six confounders does not guarantee that all confounders had been taken into account, so while we could have been confident that lymphoma is associated with X-ray exposure, and that this association is probably not due, for example, to the age at which the diagnosis was made, we would have to be cautious about concluding that X-ray exposure causes lymphoma.

1.2.5 A regression analysis is one method of controlling confounding in a case-control study. Name two others.

1.2.6 Although researchers can use a number of techniques to control confounding in a case-control study, some confounders may be overlooked. This produces ________________ confounding.

Cohort Studies In a *cohort study*, a group (called a cohort) of people who have not yet experienced the outcome of interest is observed over time. Whether or not the outcome is experienced by each member of the cohort during the lifetime of the study is recorded, and differences between those who experience the outcome

Table 1.1 Death rate ratios (95% CI) by age started smoking for men and women current versus never Japanese smokers born between 1920 and 1945. (Adapted from BMJ Publishing Group Limited [5])

Age started smoking	Men	Women
<20	2.21 (1.97–2.48)	2.61 (1.98–3.44)
20–29	1.71 (1.53–1.91)	2.01 (1.79–2.25)
≥30	1.48 (1.07–2.05)	1.40 (1.22–1.62)

and those who do not are identified. Often two or more cohorts are studied and the outcome of interest is whether one cohort is more likely to experience some event than another. For example, two cohorts known to vary in their degree of exposure to a suspected risk or protective factor might be followed to determine whether they differ in their incidences of disease or death. The extent to which exposure affects the probability of disease onset or of death is assessed after confounders have been taken into account, and inferential statistical tests are used to see if random sampling variability can be ruled out as an explanation of the findings. Often the probability of disease or death of the exposed group is compared to the probability of disease or death of the unexposed group by taking the ratio of the former to the latter. This ratio is called *relative risk, hazard ratio*, or *rate ratio*. Risk factors are associated with relative risks, hazard ratios, and rate ratios that are greater than 1.0, protective factors less than 1.0.

An example of a cohort study of a risk factor for death can be seen in the work of Sakata et al. [5] who examined the relationship between cigarette smoking and mortality due to all causes among nearly 68,000 Japanese men and women born before August 1945. The cohort was followed for an average of about 23 years. Using *Poisson regression*, Sakata et al. compared the death rates of current smokers and of former smokers to never smokers for people who were born before 1920 and again for people born between 1920 and 1945. Table 1.1 displays the death rate ratios for current smokers born between 1920 and 1945 as a function of the age at which they began smoking. Each ratio compares the death rate of current smokers to the death rate of respondents who never smoked. We can see from the table that the death rate for current smokers who started smoking before the age of 20 was more than twice the death rate of people who never smoked (rate ratio of 2.21 for men, 2.61 for women). We can also see that the death rate ratio was lowest for current smokers who did not start to smoke until they were at least in their thirties. However, even for these late starters, the death rate was still higher than for life-long nonsmokers (rate ratio of 1.48 for men, 1.40 for women).

As with case-control studies, cohort studies can show covariation between exposure to a risk or protective factor on the one hand and the presence or absence of disease or death on the other. However, by obtaining data from participants at the beginning of the study and again periodically over time, cohort studies are better at verifying that the factor preceded the outcome, and at tracking any changes that might have occurred in health status and exposure to the factor and to confounders. But, as in all research designs, cohort studies have disadvantages. For example, because they often take many years to complete, they can be expensive to conduct, and tracking and retaining patients can be difficult. Moreover, although cohort studies can employ techniques such as matching, stratification and regression to control confounders, they are subject to the problem of residual confounding.

True or false?

1.2.7 In a cohort study, a protective factor will have a relative risk greater than 1.

1.2.8 In order for a researcher to conclude that a factor is a risk to health, the 95% confidence interval of the hazard ratio must include the value of 1.

Randomized Controlled Trials A scientific experiment intended to assess the efficacy of an intervention is called a *randomized controlled trial* (RCT). In this study design, at least one group of people is exposed to an intervention and one is not. The effects of the intervention are then assessed. Sometimes the intervention is a treatment or therapy that is intended to restore health or at least control or slow the progression of disease. Other times the intervention is intended to maintain health or to prevent disease or some other adverse event. In either case, the safety of the intervention is often also assessed.

Not unlike a cohort study, an RCT establishes the correct time order by following participants over time after they have been exposed to the intervention and covariation by comparing the outcomes experienced by those were exposed to the intervention to the outcomes experienced by those who were not. However, an RCT has several advantages over a cohort study. One is that an RCT can give investigators more precise control over the administration of the intervention and the measurement of the outcomes so that both are more uniform across participants. This reduces random sampling variability which in turn makes it easier to rule out chance as an explanation of the results. Another is that investigators can have more control over *inclusion and exclusion eligibility criteria* by which participants are chosen for study. This allows investigators to reduce chance differences across participants in their demographic or other physical or psychological characteristics, which can also decrease random sampling variability. If the intervention is a drug therapy, the patients and the investigators can be *blinded* or *masked,* that is, kept unaware of whether the patient is receiving the drug under investigation or a standard treatment or placebo. But perhaps the single most important advantage of an RCT is that it uses *randomization* to control confounding.

There are two basic types of randomization procedures that are used in an RCT. The type depends on whether the participants in the group exposed to the intervention are the same or different from the participants in the group that is not exposed. In a *parallel group trial,* two or more different groups or *arms* are used. Randomization takes the form of *random assignment* of each participant to one of the arms. When random assignment is used, investigators let chance decide to which group a participant will be assigned. For example, if a treatment is to be compared against a placebo, the investigator would, in effect, flip a coin to decide whether a participant will be given the treatment or the placebo. By randomly assigning participants to groups, investigators can be highly confident that the arms on average will be similar with respect to all potential confounders that are related to participant characteristics such as age, health status, race, eating and exercise habits, and so on. Random assignment is a powerful tool for controlling confounders associated with participant characteristics. It controls confounders without needing to measure them, and more importantly, controls confounders of which investigators might be unaware.

An example of a parallel group design is an Australian study conducted by Clemson et al. [6] of the impact of exercise on the rate of falls among the elderly living at home. A total of 317 men and women aged 70 or older who within the past 12 months had experienced either at least two falls or one injurious fall were randomly assigned to one of three arms. One group of participants was asked to perform various physical movements that increase strength and balance but which can be easily integrated into daily activities. For example, participants were encouraged to bend from the knees instead of from the waist when picking up objects. A second group was asked to engage in a structured program of balance and strength exercises three times per week. The third arm served as the control group; these participants were asked to engage in 12 "gentle and flexibility exercises." The number of falls and other adverse events reported by each participant was recorded for up to 1 year, or until the participant left the study or died. In addition, various measures of balance and strength were taken at the beginning of the study to establish baselines, and again at 6- and 12-month follow-up. Using *negative binomial regression,* Clemson et al. compared the fall rates of the integrated and structured exercise groups to the fall rate of the control group, and found that the rate ratio for the integrated program group was 0.69, with a 95 % CI of 0.48 to 0.99, while the rate ratio for the structured program group was 0.81 (95 % CI, 0.56–1.17). Using *analysis of variance* and *pairwise comparisons*, Clemson et al. then compared the average balance and strength scores of the three arms from baseline to 12-month follow-up, and found on several measures that the integrated exercise group experienced greater increases in balance and strength compared either to the structured program or to the control group, increases that were unlikely to be due to random variability alone. Regarding adverse events other than falls, one participant in the integrated program arm experienced a pelvic stress fracture but continued to participate, while one participant in the structured program arm experienced a groin strain and withdrew from the study. The investigators concluded that a program of physical activities designed to increase balance and strength can substantially reduce falls among the elderly if the program is incorporated into everyday living.

The second type of RCT is the *crossover trial.* In this study, the same group of people is exposed at different points in the study to the presence and absence of the intervention, or to two different interventions. Investigators then compare each participant's outcomes he or she experienced under the two conditions. This design is often used to assess the effects of a drug relative to a placebo or to an alternative remedy. If a drug is being tested, the administrations of the drug and placebo (or alternative remedy) may be separated by a fixed interval of time or *washout period.*

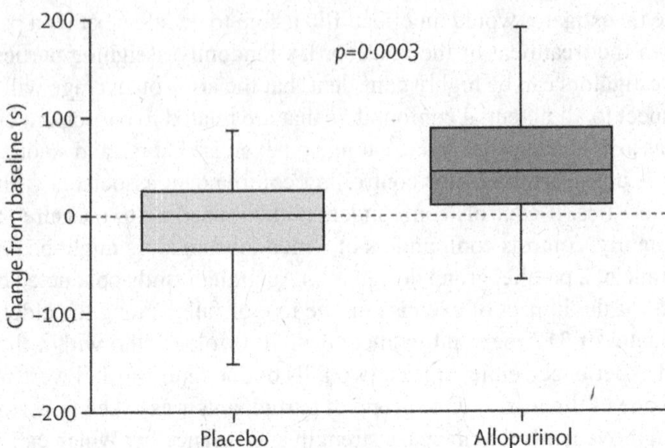

Fig. 1.1 Box plot of change in total exercise time from baseline. (Reproduced with permission from the Lancet Publishing Group [7])

The form of randomization used here is *random sequencing* of the two treatments. By using a random order for each participant, investigators control *carryover effects,* confounders related to the order of treatments.

An example of a crossover trial is a study reported by Noman et al. [7] who investigated the effects of high-dose allopurinol on exercise in patients with chronic stable angina. At the beginning of the study, 65 outpatients underwent exercise tolerance tests to provide baseline measurements of total exercise time, time to ST depression, and time until chest pains occurred. Then a 6-week course of allopurinol followed by a 6-week course of placebo was randomly assigned to 31 of the patients. The opposite sequence was assigned to the remaining 34. In other words, each patient began at random with either allopurinol or placebo and then 6 weeks later "crossed over" to the placebo or allopurinol. The investigators found that on average, allopurinol produced a reliable increase in all three performance measures. A *box plot* comparing the median changes from baseline in total exercise times of the placebo and allopurinol groups is displayed in Fig. 1.1. The median is represented by the horizontal line near the middle of each box. For the placebo group, the median change is close to zero. The *p*-value displayed in the figure tells us that the probability of obtaining a difference between two median exercise times equal to or greater than that observed in the sample is three in 10,000 if allopurinol in fact has no impact on exercise times. By convention, scientists rule out random sampling variability as a plausible alternative explanation if the *p*-value is equal to or less than 0.05. In this case, the probability that the observed difference between the two group medians was due solely to random sampling variability is much less than 0.05.

Despite their ability to make strong inferences about causality, RCTs have their share of weaknesses. One is the possibility of *differential attrition.* This refers to participants in one arm of the study being more likely to withdraw from the study than participants in another. An example would be patients who withdrew from a drug study because the medicine was not helping them. If by the end of the study only those who found the drug helpful remain, the efficacy of the drug could appear to be greater than it really is. A similar problem occurs when patients fail to follow their regimens appropriately, as might happen if they do not understand instructions, experience unpleasant side effects or find the regimen inconvenient. Noncompliance can make an intervention appear to be less efficacious than it really is. Another problem is a result of one of the strengths of an RCT. Its ability to tightly control and standardize various aspects of the study can raise questions about *generalizability,* that is, about whether the intervention would be effective in more natural settings. A therapy which may show *efficacy* in an RCT might demonstrate less *effectiveness* in clinical practice where, for example, administration of the drug may be more variable, patient compliance may be less prevalent, or patient populations may differ from those selected for the trial. Finally, while RCTs are valuable for determining the efficacy of treatments, ethical considerations prevent them from being used to establish the causes of disease.

Researchers have a number of methods for addressing at least some of the limitations of an RCT. For example, to get a truer sense of the effectiveness of the treatment, researchers would conduct an *intention-to-treat analysis*. This means that regardless of whether patients complied with the request of the researcher, the outcomes experienced by the patients assigned to the treatment condition are compared to the outcomes experienced by the patients who were not assigned to the treatment condition. For example, the outcomes experienced by patients in the treatment condition who were discovered to have failed to follow the treatment regimen correctly would be included with the outcomes experienced by treatment patients who were known to have followed the regimen as intended. Perhaps more importantly, researchers would conduct additional studies to see if trial results can be *replicated.* One study might be a larger trial conducted at a number of clinical sites distributed across a broad geographical area on patients with diverse demographic characteristics. Another might be a cohort study conducted in a setting that more closely approximates daily clinical practice. At some point, researchers would then draw conclusions about treatment effectiveness based on the accumulated evidence.

1.2.9 A randomized controlled trial has two basic types: the parallel group trial and the _____ trial.

1.2.10 Which of these two types of trials controls patient-related characteristics through random assignment?

1.2.11 A(n) _____ analysis assesses the effectiveness of a treatment by including all patients assigned to the treatment condition, even those who failed to follow the treatment regimen correctly.

Systematic Review and Meta-Analysis Assessing accumulated evidence is the goal of a *systematic review* or *meta-analysis*. Researchers conducting a systematic review begin by identifying a fairly specific research topic and methodically locating reports of research studies that meet explicitly stated inclusion and exclusion criteria. Next, they critically evaluate the findings of each study, compare and contrast them, and integrate their assessments into an overall conclusion. Finally, they make recommendations for clinical practice and identify issues to be explored in future research. The steps taken by authors of a meta-analysis are similar except that they focus on studies that are more homogeneous in various aspects of their methodology compared to studies in a systematic review. This allows authors of a meta-analysis not only to compare the size of the effect of a given treatment or intervention in each study, but also to combine these individual *effect sizes* into an overall quantitative measure of effect size. The pooled effect size is likely to be a more reliable estimate of impact than the effect size assessed in a single study.

As an example, Schulze-Rath et al. [8] conducted a systematic review of research on whether exposure to diagnostic X-rays is a risk factor for cancer in children. The reviewers restricted their review to cohort and case-control studies of children and adolescents who for diagnostic reasons had been exposed to low doses of prenatal or postnatal ionizing radiation. Each study had to have been published in English between 1990 and 2006, and to have reported risk estimates for leukemia, lymphomas, solid tumors or tumors of the central nervous system. To locate the studies, the reviewers first searched through the database, PubMed, using the following search key words, "(child or child preschool or infant) and neoplasms and (radiograph*/adverse effects) and (pregnancy or pregnant women or infant or fetus or embryo)." The reviewers also consulted six other databases, the reference lists of the studies they uncovered in the seven databases, and 2-yearly volumes of two important journals in the field. The search led the reviewers to 59 articles from the databases and another 88 from the reference lists of those 59. After sifting through the 147 studies, the authors identified 19 case-control and six cohort studies that met their eligibility criteria, although some of the studies included adults up to the age of 31 among their participants. Most of the case-control studies included 40–500 patients and each cohort study included 300–31,000 patients. Of the 25 studies, 12 were conducted in Europe, seven in the USA, four in Canada, and one each in Shanghai and Israel.

Schulze-Rath et al. discovered that the variability across the 25 studies in the type of design (case-control or cohort), the timing of the radiation (pre or postnatal) and the type of cancer studied limited their ability to draw meaningful conclusions. Nevertheless, they were able to identify nine studies that shared the same study design, risk factor, and outcome, so they decided to conduct a meta-analysis of them. These were case-control studies of prenatal exposure and leukemia. Using the OR as a measure of effect size, the reviewers pooled the data from the nine studies to generate an overall measure of risk associated with prenatal radiation. The results are presented in Fig. 1.2.

Figure 1.2 is often referred to as a *forest plot,* a visual display of the effect sizes of each study and the pooled effect size. The OR for each of the nine studies is represented by a small square. The size of each square represents the weight that

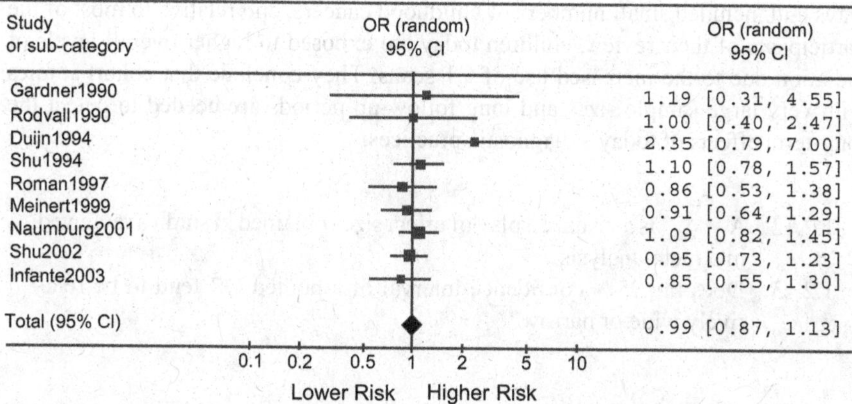

Fig. 1.2 Forest plot of odds ratios from nine case-control studies of prenatal diagnostic X-rays and leukemia. (Adapted with permission from Springer Science+Business Media [8])

was given to the OR of that study when the pooled OR was calculated: The greater the weight, the bigger is the square. The pooled OR is represented by the diamond beneath the nine squares. As we can see from the forest plot, the ORs of eight of the nine studies cluster around 1.0. One study found an OR substantially greater than 1 but this result clearly is not typical, and the pooled OR is 0.99. Because an OR of 1.0 means that the likelihood of disease is the same for both the exposed and unexposed groups, the reviewers concluded that this body of research has failed to show that prenatal exposure to radiation is a risk factor for leukemia.

The horizontal line going through each square of the forest plot is the 95 % CI of the OR. The width of the diamond represents the 95 % CI of the pooled OR. A measure of an effect size that has a narrow confidence interval is more reliable than a measure that has a wide confidence interval. Notice that the size of each square seems to be inversely related to the width of the confidence interval. This is because in a meta-analysis more reliable effect sizes are given more weight in the calculation of the pooled effect. Notice too that the confidence interval of the pooled OR is relatively narrow compared to most of the others. This demonstrates an advantage of a meta-analysis: It tends to generate conclusions that are more reliable than conclusions that are based on the findings of a single study.

Systematic reviews and especially meta-analyses are very useful tools for evaluating evidence to date for they help researchers to assess the reliability and generalizability of a given finding, to discern relationships among data that might not be apparent in any single study, and when the reviews include randomized controlled trials, generate highly confident causal conclusions. But conclusions from reviews and meta-analyses are often limited by the methodologies of the studies they review, and their conclusions should not be generalized beyond the conditions under which the reviewed studies were conducted. Recognizing these limitations, Schulze-Rath et al. caution that most of their studies were case-control studies, the few cohort studies that they were able to locate differed from one another in many ways and included small numbers of childhood cancers, and relative to most of the participants of their review, children today are exposed to higher overall levels of radiation due to the increased use of CT scans. They conclude that cohort studies with very large sample sizes and long follow-up periods are needed to detect the long-term effects of today's diagnostic practices.

1.2.12 A_____ is a visual display of effect sizes obtained in studies reviewed in a meta-analysis.

1.2.13 Does the 95 % confidence interval of a pooled OR tend to be relatively wide or narrow?

1.3 Categories of Research

Our review of study designs does not include every type of study design used in clinical research. Rather than try to present each of these additional types of studies, here we will give an overview of the various categories of research into which most clinical investigations fall. Knowing these categories will help you to understand designs that we have not covered and to interpret the statistics that they generate. The categories are *retrospective* versus *prospective* research, *experimental* versus *observational* research, and *cross-sectional* versus *longitudinal* research.

Retrospective Versus Prospective Research A *retrospective study* focuses on an outcome that study participants have already experienced. A *prospective study* investigates an outcome that participants have not yet experienced. Case-control studies are always retrospective. Randomized controlled trials are always prospective. Cohort studies can be either prospective or retrospective.

Recall that cohort studies track participants over an interval of time, and that at the beginning of the interval, none of the participants has experienced the outcome of interest. When a *prospective cohort study* is conducted, a cohort study is designed to answer specific research questions. Appropriate cohorts are identified, and procedures intended to measure relevant risk factors, protective factors, outcomes, and confounders are carefully planned. These measurements are then taken of the cohorts at the beginning of, during, and at the end of the time interval, and the resulting data are analyzed to answer the questions the study was designed to address. Sometimes data collection goes on indefinitely, in which case study findings are updated periodically. The study by Sakata et al. [5] on smoking and mortality that we reviewed earlier is a prospective cohort study.

When a *retrospective cohort study* is conducted, a research question is answered by consulting a data archive that contains information about groups that can serve as relevant cohorts and of whom observations were made before and after a time interval that serves the investigators' purpose. An example of a retrospective cohort study is an investigation conducted by Dosoretz et al. [9] who wished to know the effect of neoadjuvant hormone therapy (Lupron or Zoladex) on prostate cancer patients receiving brachytherapy. The outcome variable that interested them was mortality due to any cause. To answer their question, they sifted through the medical records of 20 oncology centers and selected 3744 men who had undergone brachytherapy for localized prostate cancer between May 1991 and September 2005, had not also received external-beam radiation, and had been followed after brachytherapy for at least 2 years. Using *Cox regression* to control confounding variables such as tumor classification and pretreatment PSA levels, the investigators obtained a hazard ratio (HR) of 1.24 (95 % CI, 1.01–1.53) among patients who had been 73 years old or older at the time of brachytherapy. The HR of 1.24 means that among men in this age group, those who had also received the hormone therapy were 24 % more likely to have died compared to men who had not received hormone therapy.

Retrospective and prospective cohort studies are similar in many ways. Both focus on groups that prior to a given time interval had not experienced the outcome of interest, both use the same statistical procedures to assess the role of random sampling variability and to control confounding, and both are subject to the problem of residual confounding. But because retrospective cohort studies are more problematic—for example they are more susceptible to bias when participants are selected and record keeping is more likely to be incomplete or inaccurate—prospective cohort studies are preferred.

Experimental Versus Observational Research In an *experimental study*, the investigator systematically exposes participants to a suspected causal factor after having controlled confounding variables by holding them constant or by using randomization. The investigator then measures an outcome variable and compares the measurements across the exposure conditions of the experiment. In an *observational study*, the investigator does not systematically expose participants to a causal factor. Instead the investigator observes people who have already been exposed. If possible, the investigator will also observe people who have not been exposed and compare the two sets of observations. In an observational study, the investigator cannot control confounding variables before the exposure occurs, and therefore is less confident that the exposure is the only systematic difference between the two groups. Consequently, experimental studies are superior to observational studies in establishing cause and effect. An RCT is an example of an experiment, but one in which the causal factor is an intervention. Case-control and cohort studies are examples of observational research.

Experimental and observational studies often employ the same statistical procedures. However, the ability to draw causal conclusions from the results of a statistical analysis is greater for experimental data. For example, we could use an *independent-samples t-test* to compare the average blood pressure of hypertensive patients who had been on a low sodium diet for a year to the average blood pressure of hypertensive patients who had not been on a low sodium diet for a year, regardless of whether the diet was randomly assigned to the patients (experiment) or self-selected (observational study). But if the data were observational, we would be particularly cautious about drawing causal conclusions, even if the average blood pressure of the low sodium group were lower than that of the second group, and the results of the *t*-test allowed us to rule out chance as the cause of the difference.

Cross-Sectional Versus Longitudinal Research A *cross-sectional study* is an observational study that takes measurements from a sample of people on a single occasion. It can document covariation between a suspected cause and its suspected effect, but is less able than the longitudinal study and the experiment to establish that a suspected cause preceded its suspected effect, and inferior to the experiment in controlling confounding. It is often used to provide a snap-shot of a population at the time the sample was taken, as when it is used to determine *disease prevalence*, the proportion of a population that has a given disease. A *survey* is often conducted as a relatively cost-effective method of collecting cross-sectional data. The annual telephone survey conducted by the Behavioral Risk Factor Surveillance System (BRFSS) [10] of the Centers for Disease Control and Prevention (CDC) is an example. Each survey allows the CDC to document the prevalence of various risk factors such as obesity within the USA and its territories.

A *longitudinal study* is an observational study that takes measurements from a sample of people on two or more occasions. A longitudinal study is useful for tracking changes in a given group over time, documenting how a disease progresses as times passes, and for determining *disease incidence*, the rate of new occurrences of a given disease. A longitudinal study can document covariation between a suspected cause and its suspected effect while also establishing the correct time order between the two variables. However, it lacks the ability of the experiment to control confounding. A cohort study is an example of a longitudinal study.

Cross-sectional and longitudinal studies employ somewhat different statistical procedures. This is because an analysis of longitudinal data must take into account the fact that the measurements were made of the same individuals. For example, if we wanted to compare the mean blood pressure of a group of hypertensive patients before they had decided to go on a low sodium diet to their average blood pressure 1 year later, we could not use the independent-samples *t*-test. Instead we would use a *paired-samples t-test* to compare the two sets of blood pressure readings.

True or false:

1.3.1 A cohort study is always prospective.

1.3.2 Disease prevalence is the proportion of a population that has a given disease.

1.3.3 Longitudinal studies are useful for measuring disease incidence.

1.4 Looking Ahead

Clinical investigators can call upon a very large number of statistical methods to help them understand their data, so our review of study designs provides only a sampling of the statistics that are used in clinical research. However, researchers tend to draw from the same set of study designs when they plan their research projects, so they tend to draw from the same set of statistical procedures when analyzing their data. As a result, the statistics that are typically used in clinical research are a subset of those that are available. However, that subset is still substantial, and includes some highly sophisticated techniques that require advanced training. Moreover, older methods are sometimes replaced with new ones. Consequently, we will not cover all of the methods that you are likely to encounter in clinical studies. But we will give you a representative sampling, and one that will help you to master more complex techniques and understand new ones as they come along.

Descriptive statistics and graphical techniques are the focus of our discussion in Chaps. 3 ("Describing the Distribution of a Categorical Variable") and 4 ("Describing the Distribution of a Quantitative Variable"). We also discuss graphing data throughout the book, including in Chap. 9 ("Relationships in Quantitative Data") where we describe *scatter plots*, Chap. 12 ("Analysis of Variance with Two Factors") where we discuss plots of *interaction effects*, and Chap. 16 ("Survival Analysis") where we describe *survival functions*.

As for measures of association, we discuss ORs and relative risk in Chap. 6 ("Inference for Proportions") and again in Chap. 15 ("Logistic Regression"), hazard ratios in Chap. 16, and rate ratios in Chap. 17 ("Regression Analysis of Count Data"). We explain using the difference between means as a measure of association in Chaps. 10 ("Comparing Means of Independent Samples"), 11 ("Comparing Means of Related Samples") and 12. In addition, we review the *Pearson correlation coefficient* and *Spearman's Rho coefficient*, measures of association between two quantitative variables, in Chap. 9, and *Cramér's V* and *gamma*, measures of association between two categorical variables, in Chap. 7 ("Relationships in Categorical Data"). Building on the concepts of *contingency tables*, and *row and column percentages* of Chap. 7, we explain in Chap. 8 ("Assessing Screening and Diagnostic Tests") how the degree of association between diagnostic test results and the presence of disease is determined.

We discuss regression analysis in five chapters. We review the analysis of the relationship between a *quantitative outcome variable* and either a single *predictor variable* or two or more predictor variables in Chaps. 13 ("Simple Linear Regression") and 14 ("Multiple Linear Regression"). We explain binary logistic regression in Chap. 15 where the outcome variable is categorical and binary, Cox regression in Chap. 16 where the outcome variable is *time to event* or *survival time*, and negative binomial regression in Chap. 17 where the outcome variable is a rate, such as a *mortality rate*.

Finally, we introduce basic concepts of inferential statistics, such as confidence intervals, *tests of hypotheses*, and *test statistics*, in Chap. 5 ("Introduction to Statistical Inference"). We then apply these concepts throughout the remainder of the book to a range of *population parameters*. Along the way, we review several test statistics, including the Z and t statistics, the *F-ratio*, *chi-square*, and the *Wald* statistic.

To help you understand the statistical concepts we discuss, we include in each chapter output generated by SPSS [11], and explain how to interpret it. SPSS is a statistics software package frequently used in clinical research. On the assumption that you will learn more if you are actively involved in the analyses, we will also explain how to generate the output and invite you to replicate the analysis. Most of the exercises at the end of each chapter will give you additional opportunities to use SPSS. If you do not want hands-on experience with data analysis or do not have access to SPSS, you can skip Chap. 2, which provides an overview of the software, and in subsequent chapters you can ignore our SPSS-related instructions. You will still be able to interpret the output we provide and tackle those exercise questions that can be answered independently of SPSS.

1.5 Exercise Questions

1. Bissonauth et al. [12] asked 280 French-Canadian women who had breast cancer and were nongene carriers of the mutated BRCA gene to complete a lifestyle questionnaire. For each of these women, a French-Canadian woman of the same age (within 10-year intervals) without any cancer and who also did not carry the gene was recruited and asked to complete the questionnaire. After statistically controlling confounders such as alcohol consumption and smoking status, the investigators compared the odds of having breast cancer among women who engaged in moderate physical activity for long periods of time each week to the odds of having breast cancer for women who engaged in moderate physical activity each week relatively infrequently. The resulting OR was 0.48 (95% CI, 0.31–0.74).

    a. Which of the following was used to control age?

        Matching
        Random assignment
        Statistical control
        Stratification

    b. According to this study, engagement in moderate physical activity is

        A protective factor
        A risk factor
        Unrelated to whether or not women have breast cancer

    c. Given their study design, can we conclude from their statistical analysis that moderate physical activity prevents breast cancer? Why or why not?

2. Franco et al. [13] reviewed the medical charts of 67 African-American patients with lupus nephritis and found that the odds of developing end stage renal disease (ESRD) requiring dialysis for patients with low glomerular filtration rates were about 15 times greater than the odds for patients with higher glomerular filtration rates (OR = 15.28; 95% CI, 3.18–73.38). The investigators concluded that low glomerular filtration rates are a risk factor for ESRD requiring dialysis for this patient population.

a. Was this study retrospective or prospective?
b. Why were the authors able to rule out chance as the explanation for their finding?

3. Srinivas-Shankar et al. [14] randomly assigned 274 intermediate-frail and frail elderly men living in the UK to a 6-month course of either transdermal testosterone or placebo gel treatment. The investigators concluded that testosterone treatment can have beneficial effects on muscle strength, quality of life and physical function.

   a. Was this study an experiment or an observational study?
   b. The title of this article implies that the authors documented a causal relationship between testosterone and a number of outcome variables. Does the study design justify drawing causal conclusions? Why or why not?

4. Shaikh et al. [15] tracked the acute and early-onset effects of anthracycline, a cardiotoxic chemotherapeutic agent, on the cardiac functioning of 110 pediatric cancer patients living in Pakistan. For each child, a number of echocardiographic parameters, including ejection fraction, were assessed at baseline, and then 1 month and 1 year after chemotherapy. The mean ejection fraction values at baseline, 1 month and 1 year were 69.9 %, 67.3 %, and 62.6 %, respectively, ($p < 0.001$).

   a. Was this study cross-sectional or longitudinal?
   b. Which of the following was most likely used to analyze the children's ejection fractions?

      Analysis of variance
      Independent-samples *t*-test
      Logistic regression
      Negative binomial regression

   c. Can the investigators rule out the possibility that chance was responsible for the observed differences among the three ejection fraction means? Why or why not?

5. Using the medical records of the U.S. Department of Veterans' Affairs (VA), Turakhia et al. [16] tracked over 122,000 patients who had been newly diagnosed with nonvalvular atrial fibrillation/flutter (AF) to determine whether risk of death was higher for those who had received digoxin in an outpatient care setting within 90 days of diagnosis. Risk of death was derived from survival time data, also extracted from VA records. Patients with no record of death were assumed to be alive as of September 30, 2011. After controlling for various confounders, the investigators reported a hazard ratio of 1.26 (95 % CI, 1.23–1.29). The investigators concluded that digoxin is associated with increased risk of mortality.

   a. Which of the following best describes the design of this study?

      Case-control
      Prospective cohort

Retrospect cohort
Randomized controlled trial

b. Which of the following was most likely used to analyze the survival times of the AF patients?
Analysis of variance
Cox regression
Logistic regression
Paired-samples *t*-test

c. Complete the following sentence: AF patients who had received digoxin were _____% more likely to die than AF patients who had not received digoxin.

References

General Reference Materials and Data Sources[1]

Bowerman, B.L., O'Connell, R.T.: Linear Statistical Models: An Applied Approach, 2nd ed. Duxbury, Pacific Grove (1990)
Cameron, C., Trivedi, P.K.: Regression Analysis of Count Data. Cambridge University Press, New York (1998)
Dupont, W.D.: Statistical Modeling for Biomedical Researchers. 2nd ed. Cambridge University Press, New York (2009)
Hand, D.J., Daly, F., Lunn, A.D., McConway, K.J., Ostrowski, E.: A Handbook of Small Data Sets. Chapman & Hall, London (1994)
Hilbe, J.M.: Negative Binomial Regression. Cambridge University Press, New York (2008)
Hosmer, D.W., Lemeshow, S.: Applied Logistic Regression. Wiley, New York (1989)
Hosmer, D.W., Lemeshow, S.: Applied Survival Analysis. Wiley, New York (1999)
Iverson, C., Christiansen, S., Flanagin, A., et al.: American Medical Association Manual of Style: A Guide for Authors and Editors, 10th ed. Oxford University Press, New York (2007)
Kirkwood, B.R., Sterne, J.A.C.: Essential Medical Statistics. 2nd ed. Blackwell, Malden (2003)
Peat, J., Barton, B.: Medical Statistics: A Guide to Data Analysis and Critical Appraisal. Blackwell, Malden (2005)
Petrie, A., Sabin, C.: Medical Statistics at a Glance, 2nd ed. Blackwell, Malden (2005)
Riffenburgh, R.H.: Statistics in Medicine, 2nd ed. Elsevier Academic Press, Burlington (2006)
Rosner, B.: Fundamentals of Biostatistics, 6th ed. Thomson Brooks/Cole, Belmont (2006)

Chapter-Specific References[2]

1. Newsom-Davis, T., Poulter, D., Gray, R., et al.: Case report: malignant teratoma of the uterine corpus. BMC. Cancer. **9**, 195 (2009). doi:10.1186/147-12407-9-195

[1] In writing the book, we consulted several sources for reference material, data sets or both. They are listed under the heading "General References and Data Sources."

[2] The references listed under the heading "Chapter-Specific References" are cited in this chapter.

2. de Paleville, D.T., Topp, R.V., Swank, A.M.: Effects of aerobic training prior to and during chemotherapy in a breast cancer patient: a case study. J. Strength Cond. Res. **21**(2), 635–637 (2007)
3. Kim, J., Lim, S., Shin, A., et al.: Fatty fish and omega-3 acid intakes decrease the breast cancer risk: a case-control study. BMC Cancer. **9**, 216 (2009). doi:10.1186/1471-2407-9-216
4. Rajaraman, P., Simpson, J., Neta, G., et al.: Early life exposure to diagnostic radiation and ultrasound scans and risk of childhood cancer: case-control study. BMJ. **342**, d472 (2011). doi:10.1136/bmj.d472
5. Sakata, R., McGale, P., Grant, E.J., Ozasa, K., Peto, R., Darby, S.C.: Impact of smoking on mortality and life expectancy in Japanese smokers: a prospective cohort study. BMJ. **345**, e7093 (2012). doi:10.1136/bmj.e7093
6. Clemson, L., Fiatarone Singh, M.A., Bundy, A., et al.: Integration of balance and strength training into daily life activity to reduce rate of falls in older people (the LiFE study): randomised parallel trial. BMJ. **345**, e4547 (2012). doi: 10.1136/bmj.e4547
7. Noman, A., Ang, D.S.C., Ogston, S., Lang, C.C., Struthers, A.D.: Effect of high-dose allopurinol on exercise in patients with chronic stable angina: a randomised, placebo controlled crossover trial. Lancet. **375**, 2161–2167 (2010)
8. Schulze-Rath, R., Hammer, G.P., Blettner, M.: Are pre- or postnatal diagnostic X-rays a risk factor for childhood cancer? A systematic review. Radit. Environ. Biophys. **47**, 301–312 (2008)
9. Dosoretz, A.M., Chen, M., Salenius, S.A., et al.: Mortality in men with localized prostate cancer treated with brachytherapy with or without neoadjuvant hormone therapy. Cancer. **116**, 837–842 (2010)
10. Centers for Disease Control and Prevention.: About the behavioral risk factor surveillance system (BRFSS). http://www.cdc.gov/brfss/about/about_brfss.htm. Accessed 19 March 2013
11. IBM Corp. Released 2013. IBM SPSS Statistics for Windows, Version 22.0. Armonk, NY: IBM Corp
12. Bissonauth, V., Shatenstein, B., Fafard, E., et al.: Weight history, smoking, physical activity and breast cancer risk among French-Canadian women non-carriers of more frequent BRCA1/2 mutations. J. Cancer. Epidemiol. **2009**, 11 (2009). doi:10.1155/2009/748367
13. Franco, C., Yoo, W., Franco, D., Xu, Z.: Predictors of end stage renal disease in African Americans with lupus nephritis. Bull. NYU. Hosp. Jt. Dis. **68**(4), 251–256 (2010)
14. Srinivas-Shankar, U., Roberts, S.A., Connolly, M.J., et al.: Effects of testosterone on muscle strength, physical function, body composition, and quality of life in intermediate-frail and frail elderly men: A randomized, double-blind, placebo-controlled study. J. Clin. Endocrinol. Metab. **95**(2), 639–650 (2010)
15. Shaikh, A.S., Saleem, A.F., Mohsin, S.S., et al.: Anthracycline-induced cardiotoxicity: prospective cohort study from Pakistan. BMJ Open. **3**, e003663 (2013). doi:10.1136/bmjopen-2013-003663
16. Turakhia, M.P., Santangeli, P., Winkelmayer, W.C., et al.: Increased mortality associated with digoxin in contemporary patients with atrial fibrillation. J. Am. Coll. Cardiol. **65**, 660–668 (2014)

Chapter 2
Introduction to SPSS

Abstract This chapter introduces several basic SPSS procedures that are used in the analysis of a data set. The chapter explains the structure of SPSS data files, how to open an SPSS data file, and how to import into SPSS data contained in an Excel file. The chapter also explains how to select cases for an analysis, display variables listed in dialog boxes in alphabetical order, label and print output, paste output into a Microsoft Word document, and save data and output as SPSS or Excel files.

2.1 Overview

Throughout the book we take a hands-on approach to teaching statistics by asking you to carry out many of the statistical procedures yourself with SPSS. In this chapter, we show you how to open an SPSS data file and how to import data into an SPSS file from a Microsoft Excel spreadsheet. We show you how to modify and save a data file, how to display variables listed in dialog boxes in alphabetical order, how to label and print output, how to paste your output into a Microsoft Word document, and how to export your output into Excel.

Often it is necessary to limit an analysis of data to a subset of respondents. For example, you might want to include only women in your analysis or only respondents whose answers to a particular question were within a certain range. In this chapter, we show you one way by which you can select out a subset of cases for analysis.

The data that we will use are responses of residents of New York state in 2005 to telephone interview questions asked by the Centers for Disease Control and Prevention (CDC) Behavioral Risk Factor Surveillance System (BRFSS). BRFSS has been conducting annual cross-sectional studies of health conditions and risk behaviors in the USA since 1984. As we will soon see, the data set from 2005 consists of a large number of *categorical* and *quantitative* variables. Examples of categorical variables are the respondent's sex, marital status, and educational level. Examples of quantitative variables are the respondent's age, body mass index, and the number of days per week of exercise.

W. H. Holmes, W. C. Rinaman, *Statistical Literacy for Clinical Practitioners*,
DOI 10.1007/978-3-319-12550-3_2

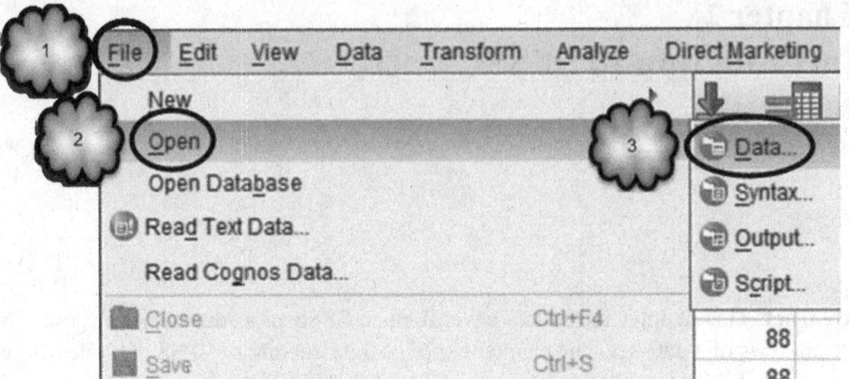

Fig. 2.1 Accessing the Open Data dialog

2.2 Opening SPSS Data Files

We will begin by opening an SPSS data file, **CDC BRFSS.sav** [1].

Double-Clicking The easiest way to open an SPSS data file is to navigate to it (e.g., with Window's *Explore* utility) and double-click it. In a few moments, SPSS will open and display the data file in its *Data Editor*.

From Within SPSS If SPSS is already running, you can open a data file within SPSS by following the sequence displayed in Figs. 2.1 and 2.2. Within SPSS, select its *File menu* at the top of the screen and then choose Open and Data. (To save some effort on our part, hereafter we will refer to a sequence of keystrokes such as this one as **File** > **Open** > **Data**.) An alternative method for opening the dialog box is to click the *Open data document* icon, located just beneath the *File menu* tab. SPSS will then display the *Open Data* dialog box. In the *Look in* window, navigate to the location of the data file, click the file so that it appears in the *File name* window, and then click **Open**.

Importing an Excel Spreadsheet It is often convenient to build a data set with Excel, and then analyze those data with SPSS. To import an Excel spreadsheet into SPSS, use the *Open Data* dialog box. There in the *Files of type* window, click on the downward pointing arrow and select *Excel*. Any Excel files at the location to which you have navigated will now appear. Click on the file you wish to open to move it to the *File name* window. Click **Open** and the *Opening Excel data source* dialog box will appear. If the first row of the Excel file contains the names of the variables (a good idea, by the way), then be sure that *Read variable names from the first row of data* is checked. Otherwise, uncheck this instruction. Click **OK**. This sequence of keystrokes is displayed in Figs. 2.3, 2.4, and 2.5. SPSS will now convert the Excel spreadsheet to an SPSS data file.

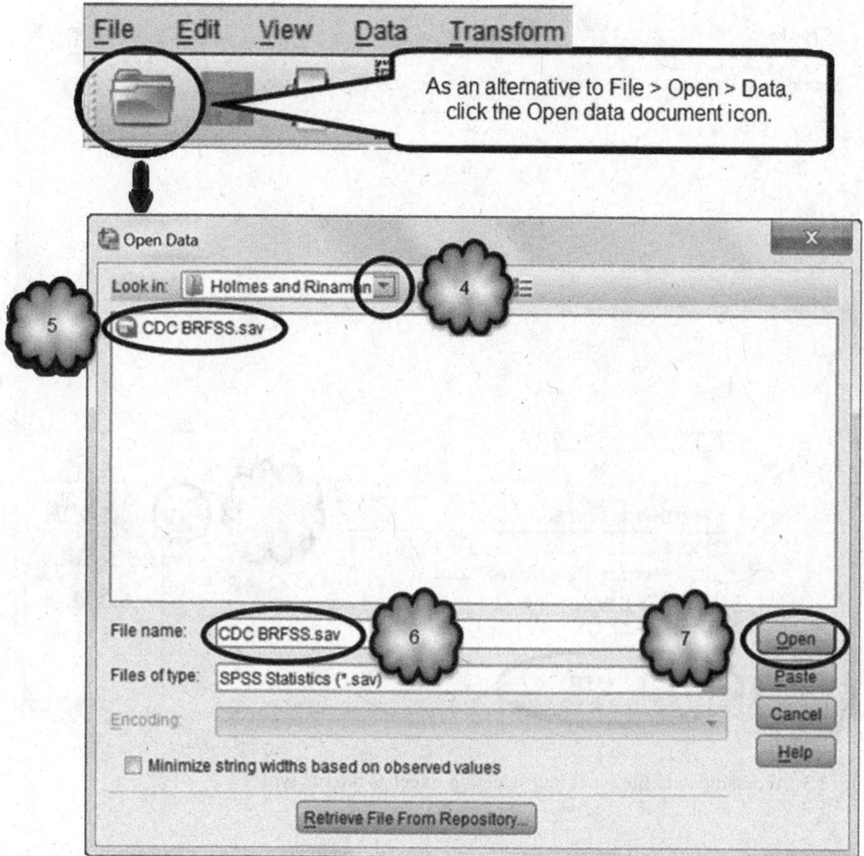

Fig. 2.2 Opening a data set with the Open Data dialog

2.3 Structure of SPSS Data Files: Data and Variable Views

Regardless of how you open a data file, once it is open you will see in the lower left-hand corner two tabs labeled *Data View* and *Variable View*, as shown in Fig. 2.6.

One of these two views will be active, and the tab for the active view will be highlighted. In Fig. 2.6, *Data View* is active. The view that is selected when a data file is opened depends on which view was active when the file was last saved.

Data View Click the *Data View* tab if it is not currently active. We will look at the *Variable View* window in a moment. A portion of the *Data View* page of the file is shown in Fig. 2.7. Note the layout of the data: Variables run across the top of the columns while respondents (SPSS refers to these as *cases*) run down the rows.

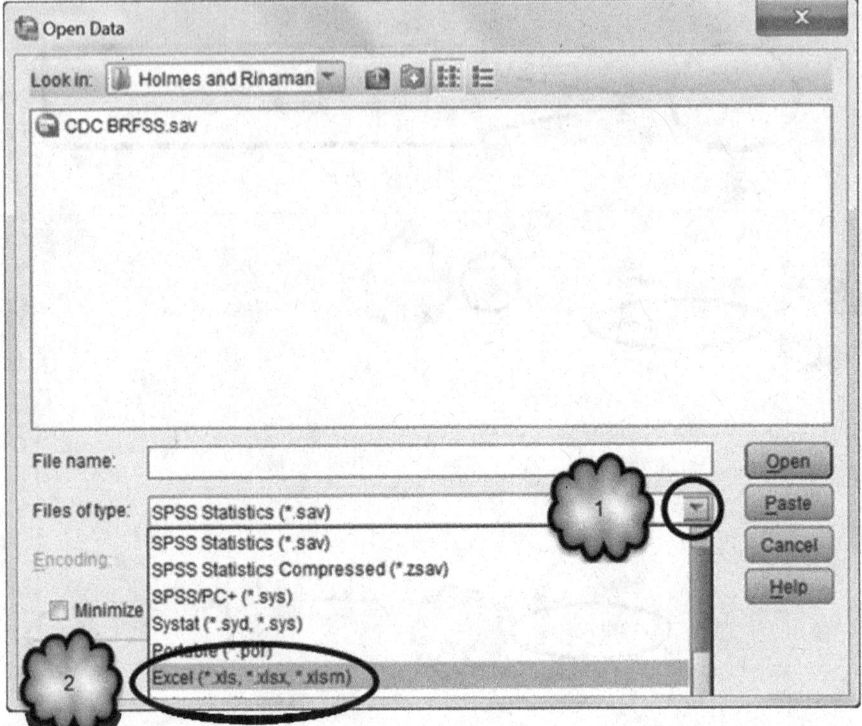

Fig. 2.3 Accessing data file types and selecting Excel as the file type

Variable View Click the *Variable View* tab in the lower left-hand corner and study the internal structure of the file. In Variable View, each row represents each of the variables and its associated properties. There are 11 properties altogether. The first five are displayed in Fig. 2.8. The 11 properties are as follows.

- **Name** This is the name that appears at the top of each column of the *Data View*. There are some limitations on names. Names must begin with a letter or one of the characters @, #, or $, and can contain no more than 64 characters. Only @ can be used in variable names that you define. The rest of the variable name can be a combination of letters, numbers, and underbars, but they cannot contain any blank spaces or other unusual symbols. Underscore, @, #, and $ are not considered unusual characters.
- **Type** There are different data types. The most common with this kind of data file are *String* and *Numeric*. String refers to variables that contain text. Numeric variables contain values that are numbers. To change the data type, click the *Type* cell. A button with an ellipsis will appear. Click the button to bring up the *Variable Type* dialog box, select the appropriate data type, and then click **OK**. These steps are displayed in Figs. 2.9 and 2.10.

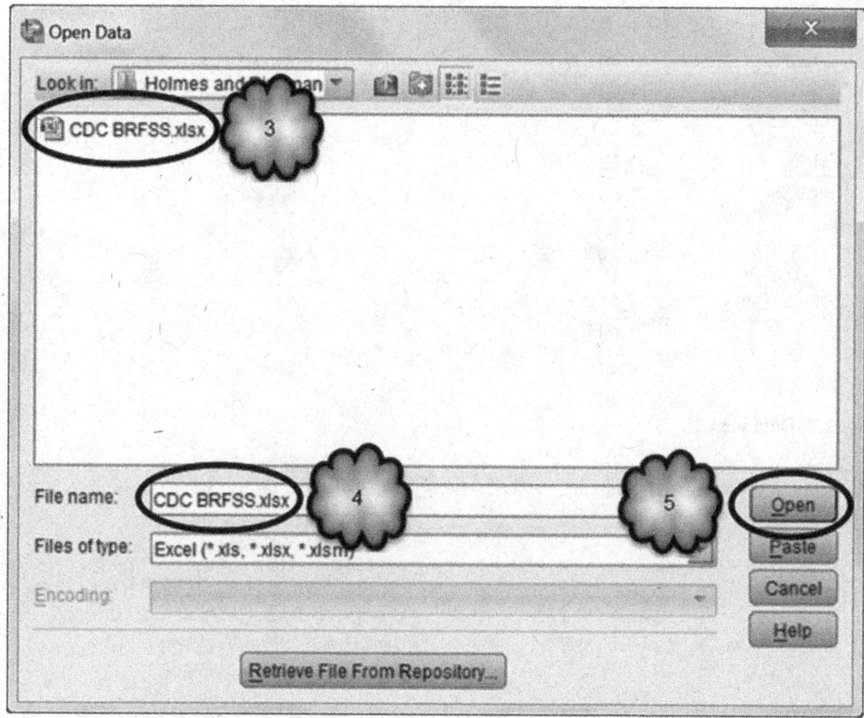

Fig. 2.4 Opening the Excel file

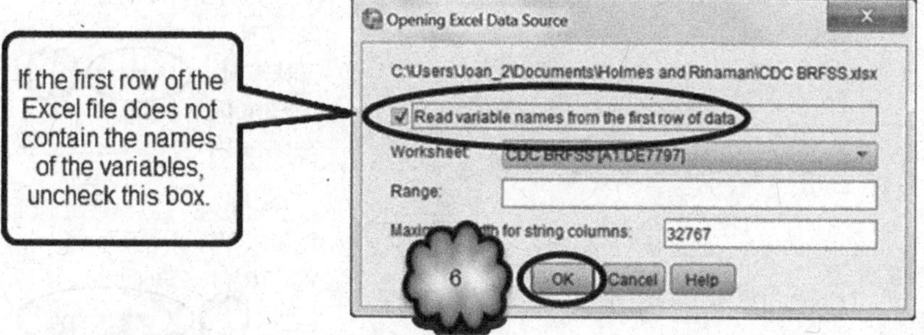

Fig. 2.5 Completing the import process

Fig. 2.6 Data view and variable view tabs

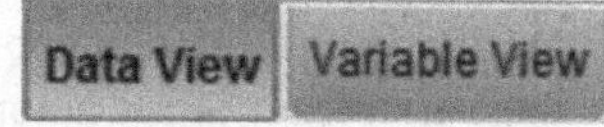

	@_GEOSTR	IMONTH	GENHLTH	PHYSHLTH	MENTHLTH	POORHLTH
1	1	07	2	88	88	.
2	1	12	3	88	88	.
3	1	02	2	88	88	.
4	1	02	2	88	2	1
5	1	04	1	88	88	.
6	1	06	2	88	1	88
7	1	03	3	88	6	7
8	1	07	2	88	28	10
9	1	06	1	88	88	.
10	1	12	2	88	15	88

Fig. 2.7 Data view

	Name	Type	Width	Decimals	Label
1	@_GEOSTR	Numeric	2	0	STRATUM CODE
2	IMONTH	String	6	0	MONTH OF INTERVIEW
3	GENHLTH	Numeric	1	0	GENERAL HEALTH
4	PHYSHLTH	Numeric	2	0	NUMBER OF DAYS PHYSICAL HEALTH NOT GOOD
5	MENTHLTH	Numeric	2	0	NUMBER OF DAYS MENTAL HEALTH NOT GOOD
6	POORHLTH	Numeric	2	0	DAYS HEALTH IMPAIRED LAST MO
7	HLTHPLAN	Numeric	1	0	HAVE HEALTH CARE COVERAGE

Fig. 2.8 Variable view

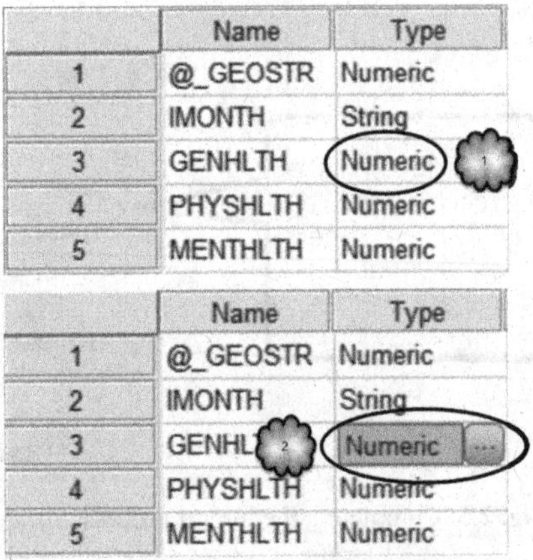

Fig. 2.9 Accessing the Variable Type dialog

	Name	Type
1	@_GEOSTR	Numeric
2	IMONTH	String
3	GENHLTH	Numeric
4	PHYSHLTH	Numeric
5	MENTHLTH	Numeric

	Name	Type
1	@_GEOSTR	Numeric
2	IMONTH	String
3	GENHLTH	Numeric ...
4	PHYSHLTH	Numeric
5	MENTHLTH	Numeric

- **Width** This is the number of characters that SPSS will allow to be entered for the variable. It is set automatically when you enter data. You change this by clicking the *Width* cell for that variable and then clicking the up or down arrow to get the desired width. Figure 2.11 displays an example for a variable named **GENHLTH**.

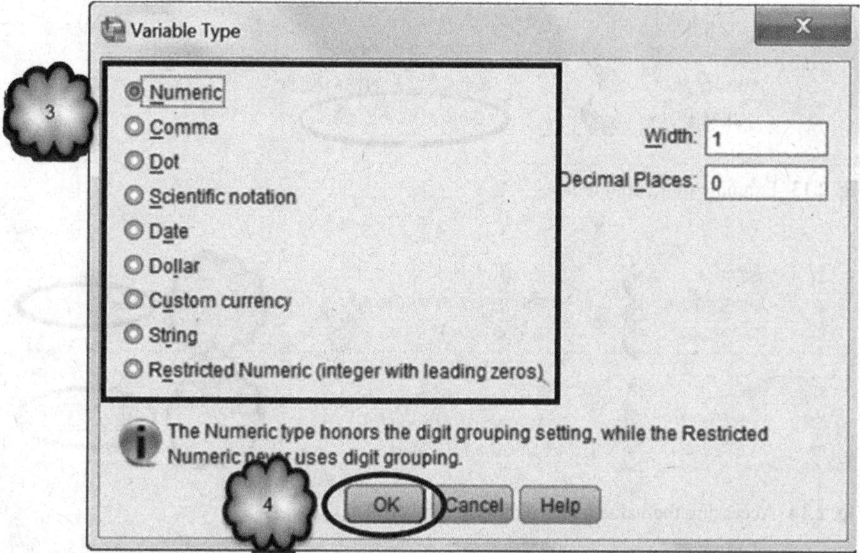

Fig. 2.10 Assigning a variable type

Fig. 2.11 Example of a numeric variable whose values consist of one character

	Name	Type	Width
1	@_GEOSTR	Numeric	2
2	IMONTH	String	6
3	GENHLTH	Numeric	1

Fig. 2.12 Changing the number of decimal places

	Name	Type	Width	Decimals
1	@_GEOSTR	Numeric	2	0
2	IMONTH	String	6	0
3	GENHLTH	Numeric	1	0

- **Decimals** This value is the number of decimal places that are displayed in the *Data View* for each value of that variable. It does not alter the values that are actually stored in the data set. As shown in Fig. 2.12, you change the number of decimal places by clicking on the *Decimals* cell and then clicking the up or down arrow to obtain the desired number of decimal places.
- **Label** This gives a more descriptive name for the variable. If this cell is not empty, the label will be displayed in any output. Figure 2.13 displays the variable label for **GENHLTH**.

It is highly recommended that every variable has a descriptive label. Because some variables names can be cryptic or uninformative, we will refer to variables by their labels rather than by their names. When we refer to a variable for the first time, we will also include the variable name in brackets and the variable number in parentheses. For example, **NUMBER OF DAYS PHYSICAL HEALTH**

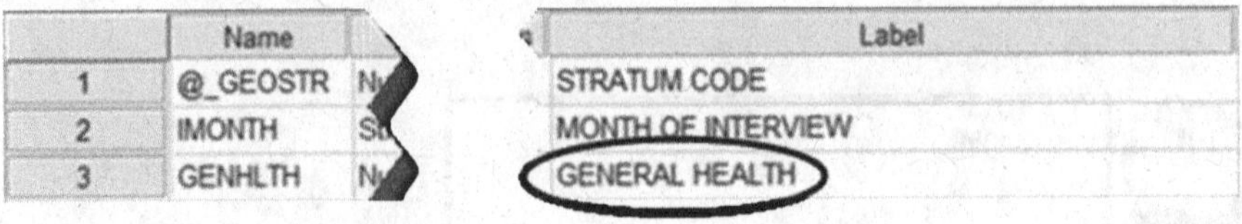

Fig. 2.13 Example of a variable label

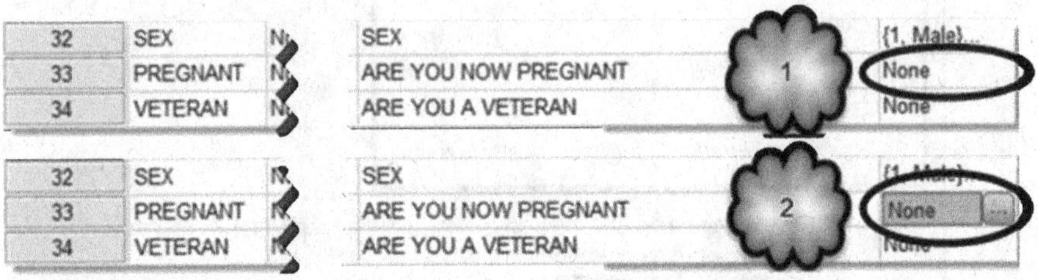

Fig. 2.14 Accessing the value labels dialog

NOT GOOD is the fourth variable in the data set, so on our first mention of it we would refer to it as **NUMBER OF DAYS PHYSICAL HEALTH NOT GOOD** [*PHYSHLTH*] (variable 4). Sometimes we will also include the value labels as well. For example, **SEX** [*SEX*] (variable 32; 1=Male; 2=Female).

- **Values** Categorical data are stored in the *Data View* with numerical values representing each category. The *Values* cell allows you to associate each numerical value with a plain language value. This should be done for all categorical variables. For example, female respondents were asked if they were pregnant. Their responses were entered into the variable, **ARE YOU NOW PREGNANT** [*PREGNANT*] (variable 33; 1=Yes, 2=No, 7=Do not know/Not Sure, 9=Refused). To enter the value labels, you would click the *Values* cell of this variable and then the button with the ellipsis to bring up the *Value Labels* dialog box. Next, you would enter each numerical value for the variable in the *Value* box, the plain language label in the *Label* box, and click the **Add** button. When you finish, you would click **OK**. Figures 2.14, 2.15, and 2.16, and 2.17 display these steps.

Practicing Entering Value Labels

Since understanding the results of data analysis is easier if value labels are used, practice entering a set of value labels for the categorical variable, **HAVE HEALTH CARE COVERAGE** [*HLTHPLAN*] (variable 7; 1=Yes; 2=No; 7=Do not know/Not sure; 9=Refused). This variable stores answers to the question, "Do you have any kind of health care coverage, including health insurance, prepaid plans such as HMOs, or government plans such as Medicare?"

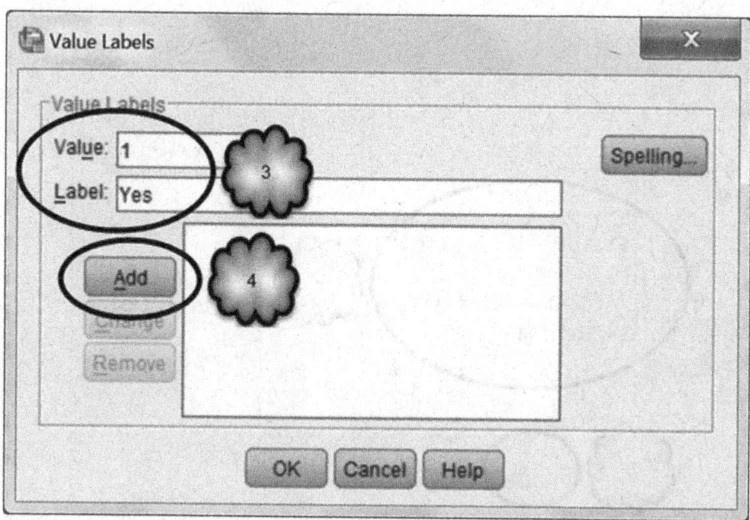

Fig. 2.15 Labeling a value

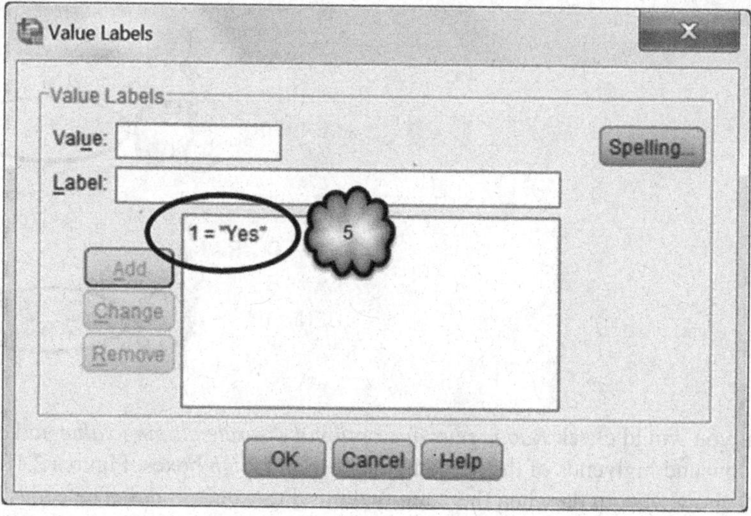

Fig. 2.16 Value Labels dialog showing one value labeled

- **Missing** Usually missing data appear in the *Data View* as periods. Sometimes special numerical values, such as 9999, are used to indicate missing data. You can set these by clicking the *Missing* cell for that variable and then the button with the ellipsis to bring up the *Missing Values* dialog box. If you have three or fewer missing value codes, you would check *Discrete missing values* and enter one code in each of the boxes. If there are more than three missing value codes, but they are within a range that does not contain any nonmissing value codes,

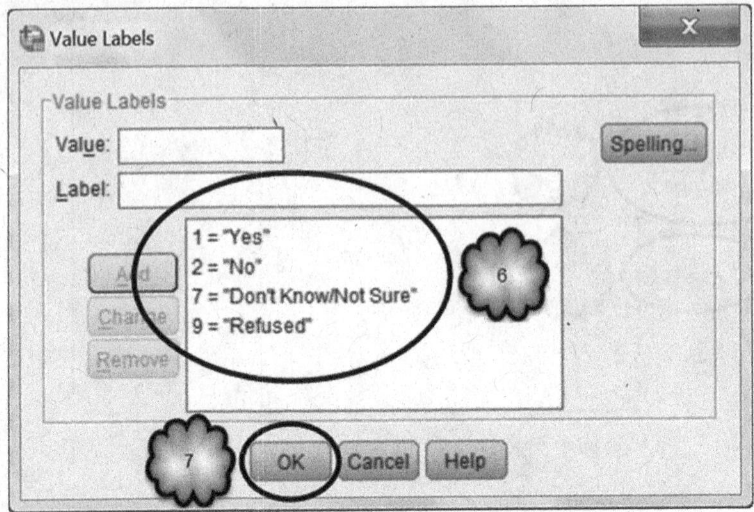

Fig. 2.17 Value Labels dialog showing all values labeled

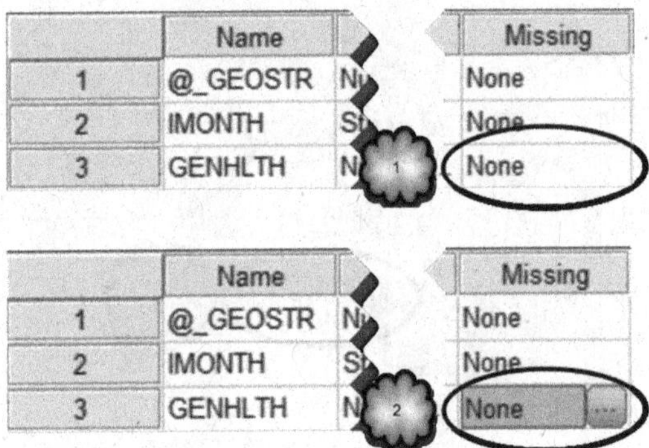

Fig. 2.18 Accessing the Missing Values dialog

then you would check *Range plus one optional discrete missing value* and enter the low and high ends of the range in the *Low* and *High* boxes. Figures 2.18 and 2.19 show what to do when there are two missing values codes. The codes happened to be 7 and 9.

The BRFSS data set contains examples of treating some responses as missing. This is because participants sometimes responded to interview questions by saying that they were not sure or by refusing to answer. We saw an example when we entered value labels for the variable, **ARE YOU NOW PREGNANT**. Most women replied either yes or no, but some said that they did not know or were not sure, and others would not give an answer. The CDC recorded all of the responses but considered not knowing, not being sure, and refusing to answer as missing data.

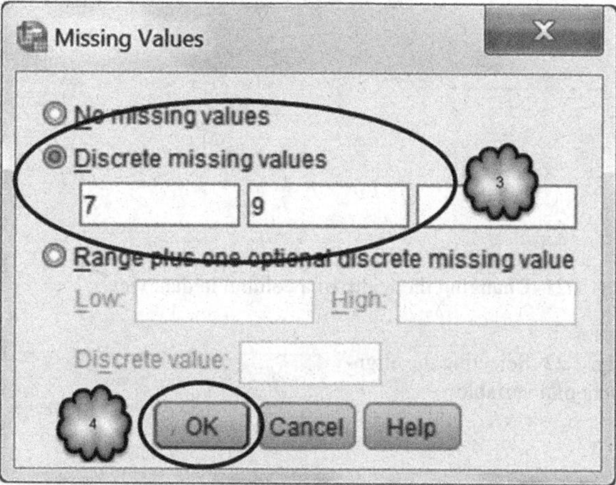

Fig. 2.19 Selecting the discrete missing values option and entering two missing values codes

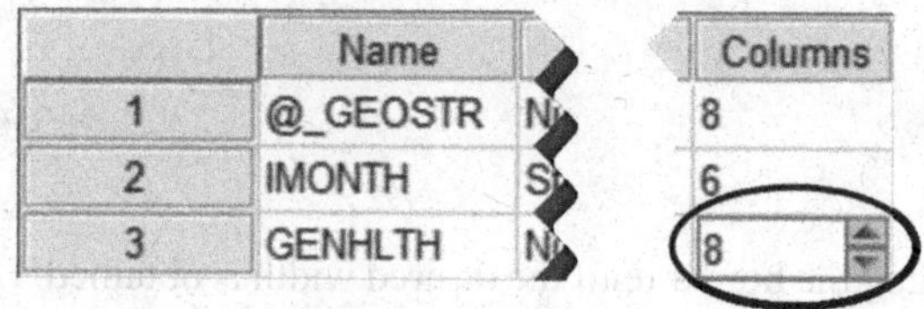

Fig. 2.20 Changing the width of a column in variable view

Practicing Declaring Missing Values

Treating certain responses as missing occurs often, so let us take a moment to practice declaring missing values on a variable in the BRFSS data set. We have already declared missing values for some of the variables. One is **GENERAL HEALTH** [*GENHLTH*] (variable 3). This variable contains the answer to the question, "Would you say that in general your health is excellent, very good, good, fair or poor?" The CDC used a value of 7 to indicate that the respondent did not know or was not sure, and a value of 9 to indicate that the respondent refused to answer. To declare these values as missing, we followed the sequence displayed in Figs. 2.18 and 2.19. Now it is your turn. Declare missing values for the variable, **HAVE HEALTH CARE COVERAGE** [*HLTHPLAN*] (variable 7; 1=Yes; 2=No; 7=Do not know/Not sure; 9=Refused).

- **Columns** This value gives the width, in number of characters, of the column that is displayed in the *Data View* for the variable. As shown in Fig. 2.20, you can change in *Variable View* the column width by clicking the *Columns* cell and then clicking the up or down arrows to get the desired width.

If you are in *Data View* you can do this by placing the cursor over the right-hand border of the desired variable. When the cursor becomes a double-headed arrow,

	@_GEOSTR	IMONTH	GENHLTH	PHYSHLTH
1	1	07	2	88
2	1	12	3	88
3	1	02	2	88

Fig. 2.21 Changing the width of a column in data view

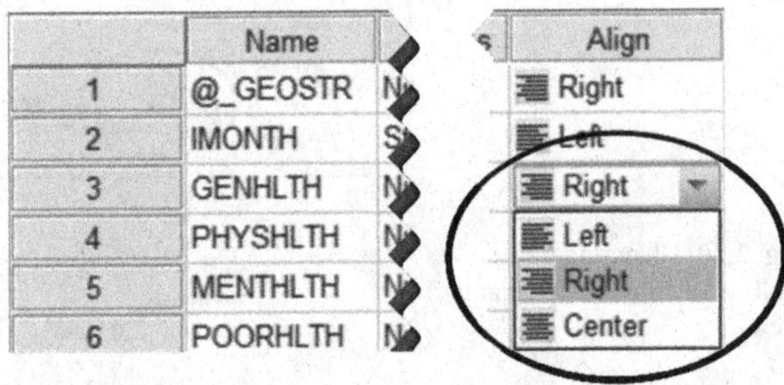

Fig. 2.22 Selecting the alignment of a variable

drag the border until the desired width is obtained. Figure 2.21 shows as an example **GENERAL HEALTH**.

- **Align** This shows whether the values for the variable will be aligned on the left, center, or right. Typically, string data are left aligned and numeric data are right aligned. As shown in Fig. 2.22, you can change the alignment by clicking the *Align* cell, clicking the arrow button, and then selecting the desired alignment.
- **Measure** SPSS recognizes three scales of measurement—scale, ordinal and nominal. Quantitative data (e.g., body mass index) are *scale* variables. Categorical data are *nominal* if there is no natural order to the categories (e.g., gender) or *ordinal* if there is a natural order to the categories (e.g., body mass index category—normal, overweight, or obese). Many statistical procedures require that data have the measure type appropriate to those procedures. SPSS cannot identify the type. It is up to the user to do that. To assign the type of measure of each variable, click its *Measure* cell, and then click a button with an arrow to display the three measure types. Select the desired measure type. Figure 2.23 displays the three measure types for the variable, GENHLTH.
- **Role** Variables in SPSS can play a variety of roles. For example, one variable might be used to predict the value of another. The predictor variable would be considered the *input* variable while the predicted variable would be considered the *target* variable. Some dialogs have the ability to preselect variables based on the variables' assigned roles. By default, all variables are assigned to the input role. As shown in Fig. 2.24, to change a variable's role, click its *Role* cell, click the arrow button to display the role options, and select the desired role.

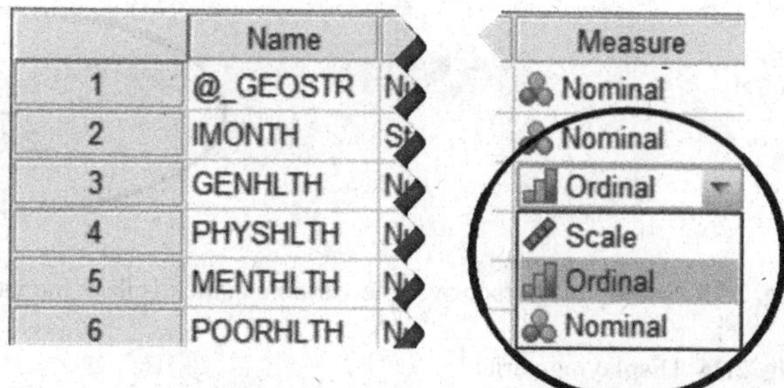

Fig. 2.23 Assigning a measure type

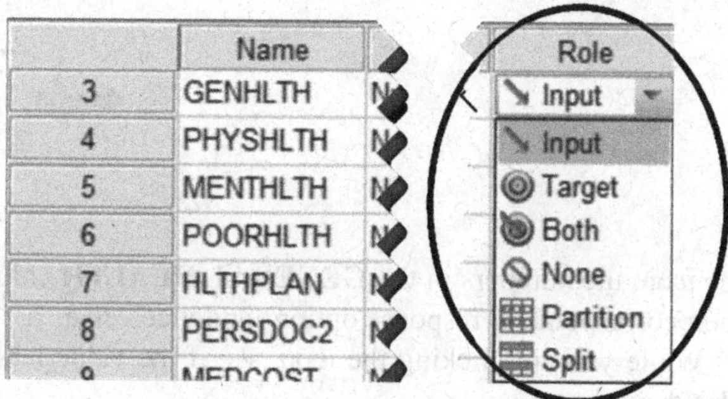

Fig. 2.24 Changing the role of a variable

Answer the following questions about the assigned properties of the variable, **GENERAL HEALTH.**

2.3.1 Is the variable string or numeric?
2.3.2 Is the variable nominal, ordinal, or scale?
2.3.3 What is the values label for a variable value of 3?

Back to Data View Click on the *Data View* tab and find the column with the variable name, **GENHLTH**. If the column is too narrow to show entirely either the name of the variable or the variable's data entries, widen the column as described earlier. You may widen other columns as you wish.

Place the cursor over the variable name. The variable's label, **GENERAL HEALTH,** will appear, as shown in Fig. 2.25. Slide the cursor over some of the other variable names and their labels will also appear.

Study the data that have been entered in the **GENERAL HEALTH** column. The entries may appear as either numbers or their value labels, depending on whether SPSS has been asked to display the numerical values or the value labels. Recall that each of the numerical entries represents the participant's response to the question about his or her general health. To see the numerical values and the responses that they represent, click the *Value Labels* icon. You will find it at the top of *Data View.* In SPSS 22, it looks like the middle icon displayed in Fig. 2.26. After each click of

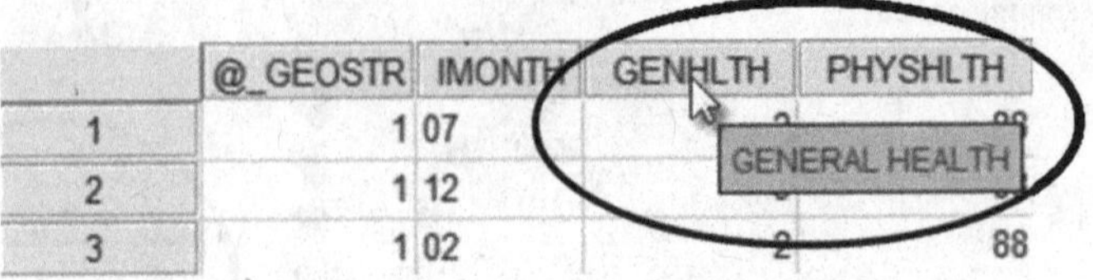

Fig. 2.25 Sliding the cursor over the variable name displays the variable label

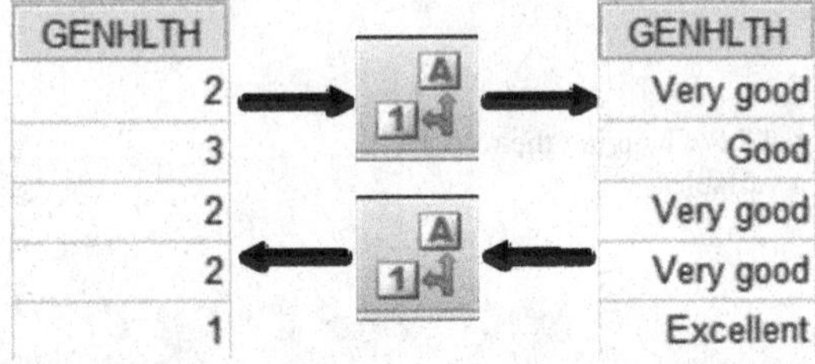

Fig. 2.26 Displaying variable values and their corresponding labels

the icon, the numbers in the **GENERAL HEALTH** column will be translated into their corresponding response options and vice versa.

While you are clicking the icon, see if the value labels you entered earlier are also displayed.

When the value labels listed in the **GENERAL HEALTH** column are displayed, the entries of most of the remaining variables remain numerical. There are two reasons for this: either the value labels for those variables have not been entered, or the variables are quantitative rather than categorical. For example, **BODY MASS INDEX** [*@_BMI4*] (variable 78) and **BODY MASS INDEX—THREE LEVELS CATEGORY** [*@_BMI4CAT*] (variable 79) are coded numerically. However, the numerical entries of **BODY MASS INDEX** reflect quantity, so this variable has no value labels. **BODY MASS INDEX—THREE LEVELS CATEGORY** has ordinal categories and so it has value labels.

2.4 Saving SPSS Data Files

We will be using this data set in other chapters. If you wish to keep the value labels you just entered, save your data file to your account. When we return to the data in future sessions, you can upload into SPSS the data file that you have saved rather than the file that you first opened in this session.

As an SPSS File To save the file, select **File > Save As** from the menu at the top of the screen. In the resulting *Save Data As* dialog box, locate the destination where you want to save the file, enter a name for the file, and click the **Save** button. The data file will be saved with the name that you assigned to it with a **.sav** extension. These steps are displayed in Figs. 2.27 and 2.28.

Fig. 2.27 Accessing the Save Data As dialog

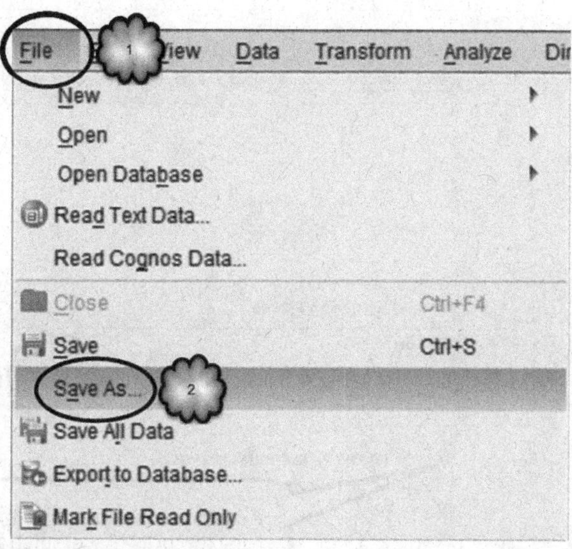

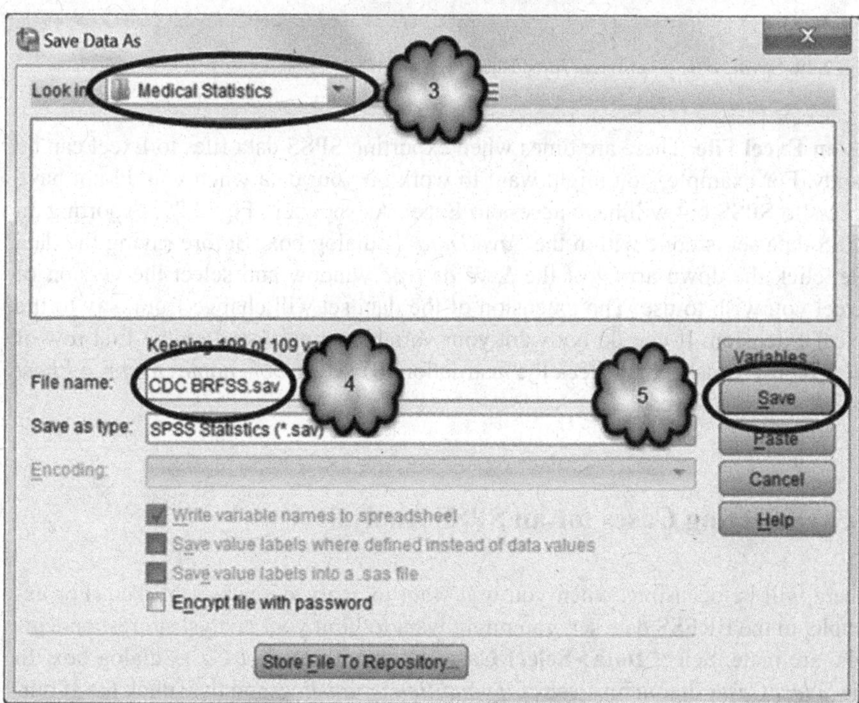

Fig. 2.28 Saving data as an SPSS data file

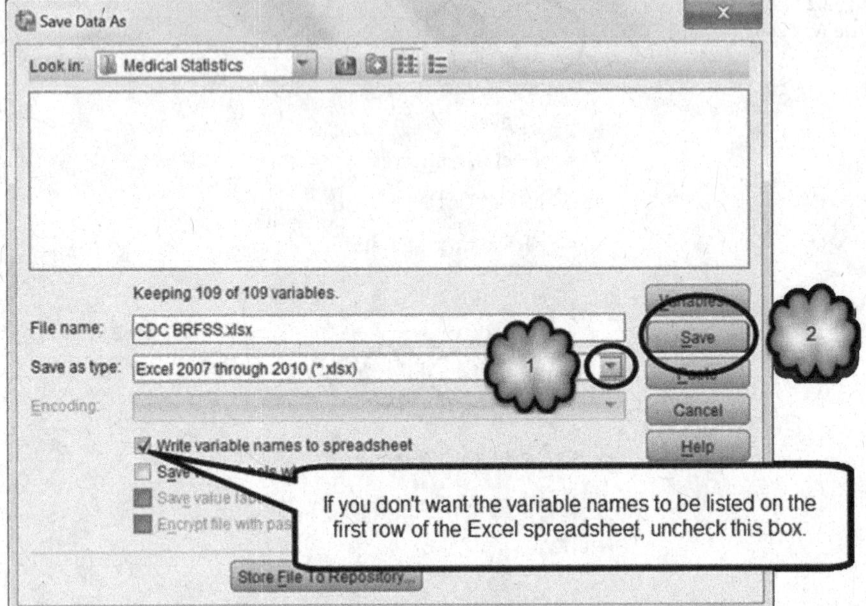

Fig. 2.29 Saving data as an Excel spreadsheet

As an Excel File There are times when exporting SPSS data files to Excel can be handy. For example, you might want to work on your data when you do not have access to SPSS but will have access to Excel. As shown in Fig. 2.29, exporting an SPSS data set is done within the *Save Data As* dialog box. Before saving the data file, click the down arrow of the *Save as type* window and select the version of Excel you wish to use. The extension of the data set will change from **.sav** to the Excel extension. If you do not want your variable names listed on the first row of the Excel spreadsheet, uncheck the instruction, *Write variable names to spreadsheet* before clicking **Save**.

2.5 Selecting Cases for an SPSS Analysis

There will be occasions when you will want to analyze a subset of data. For example, in the BRFSS data set, you might want to limit your analysis to respondents who are male. Select **Data>Select Cases** to open the *Select Cases* dialog box. In the *Select Cases* dialog box, select *If condition is satisfied,* and then click the **If** button to open the *Select Cases: If* dialog box. Highlight the variable **SEX** from the list of variables on the left and move it into the blank box to the right by clicking on the button that displays an arrow pointing to the right. Resist the temptation to type the variable name. It is too prone to typographical errors. Next, either type in an equals

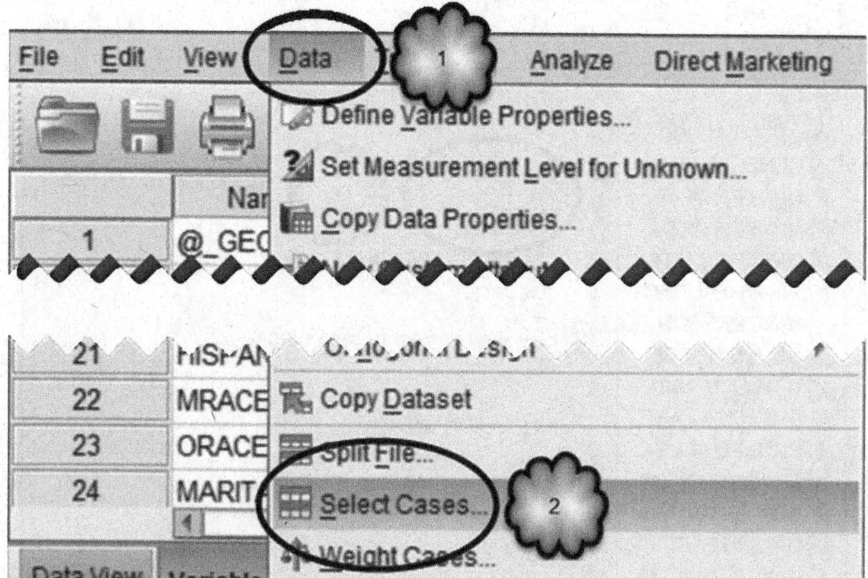

Fig. 2.30 Accessing the select cases dialog

sign or click the "=" button in the keypad area of the dialog box. Then either type in the number 1 or click the "1" button. Finally, click the **Continue** button. You will have now set up an *If condition* by which you are asking SPSS to select for analysis only those respondents whose sex has been entered as 1. Since a value of 1 represents males, you ask SPSS to select only male respondents. Back in the *Select Cases* dialog box, ask SPSS to execute your command by clicking **OK**. These steps are shown in Figs. 2.30, 2.31, 2.32, 2.33 and 2.34.

SPSS will execute the command and then automatically open its *Viewer* window. This window displays a *log* or record of the instructions SPSS just executed. The instructions are expressed in the language or *syntax* of SPSS, and tell us that SPSS has selected respondents for whom **SEX** had been coded as "1."

Return to the *Data Editor* by selecting **Window>CDC BRFSS.sav,** and select *Data View* if it is not active. Scroll over to the column that displays each respondent's sex and note that each row of data that belongs to a woman is now preceded by a diagonal line. These rows will not be included in any analysis that follows. In addition, if you scroll over to the last variable you will notice that a new variable, **filter_$,** has been created. It contains a zero for each case that is not included in subsequent analyses and a one for those cases that will be used in subsequent analyses. The zero is labeled *Not Selected* and the one is labeled *Selected.* Figure 2.35 displays the variables, **SEX and filter_$,** for ten cases.

Selecting Cases by Category To illustrate how analysis with selected cases works and to generate some output for later tasks, we will generate a frequency table for

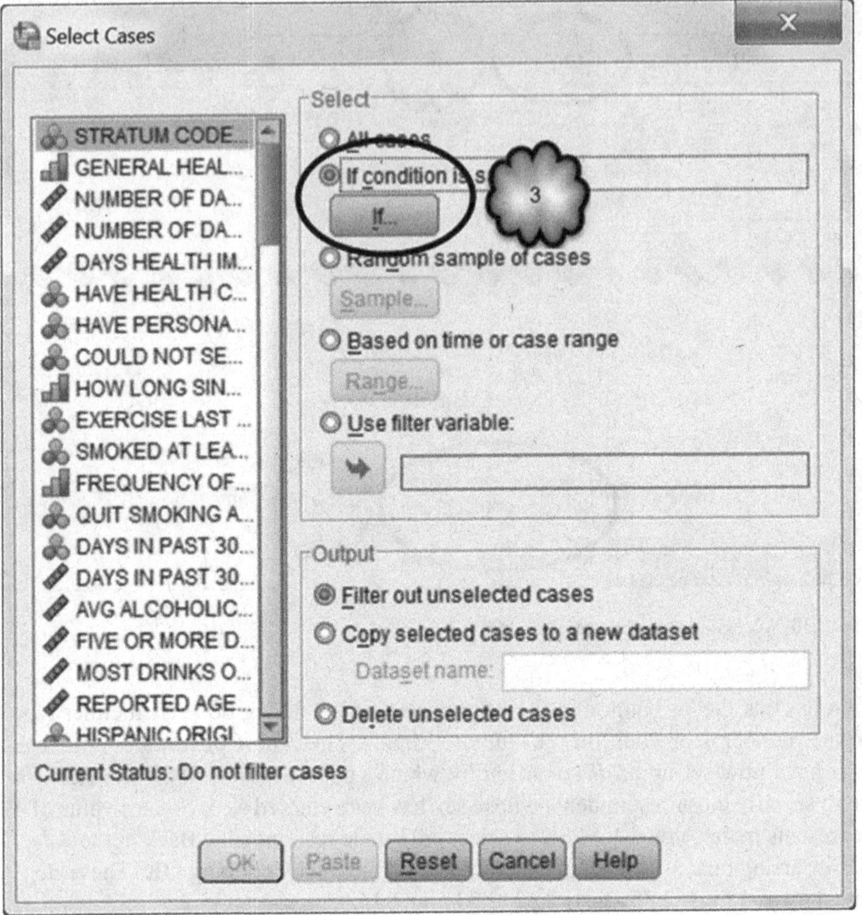

Fig. 2.31 Accessing the select cases: if dialog

the variable **GENERAL HEALTH**. An explanation of how to use a frequency table is a topic of Chap. 3. For now, do not concern yourself with that aspect of what we are doing. Select **Analyze > Descriptive Statistics > Frequencies** to open the *Frequencies* dialog box shown below. Move **GENERAL HEALTH** to the *Variables* box by highlighting it and clicking the right pointing arrow. Then click **OK**. Figures 2.36, 2.37, and 2.38 show you what to do.

SPSS will generate a frequency table and automatically display it in the *Viewer*. The output can also be found in Table 2.1. Note the number of cases included in the analysis. As a result of our including only men in the frequency analysis, the resulting total number of cases is far less than that of the entire sample.

We will generate a second frequency table but this time limit the analysis to female respondents. Return to **Data > Select Cases**. In the dialog box, make your way back to the *If condition,* "SEX = 1." Replace the "1" with a "2." One way to do this

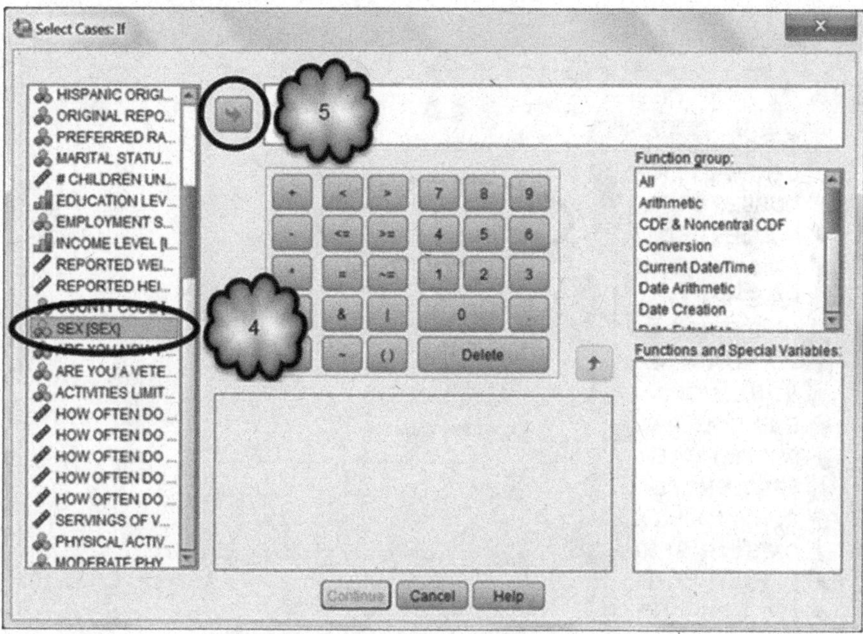

Fig. 2.32 Selecting a variable to be included in the if condition

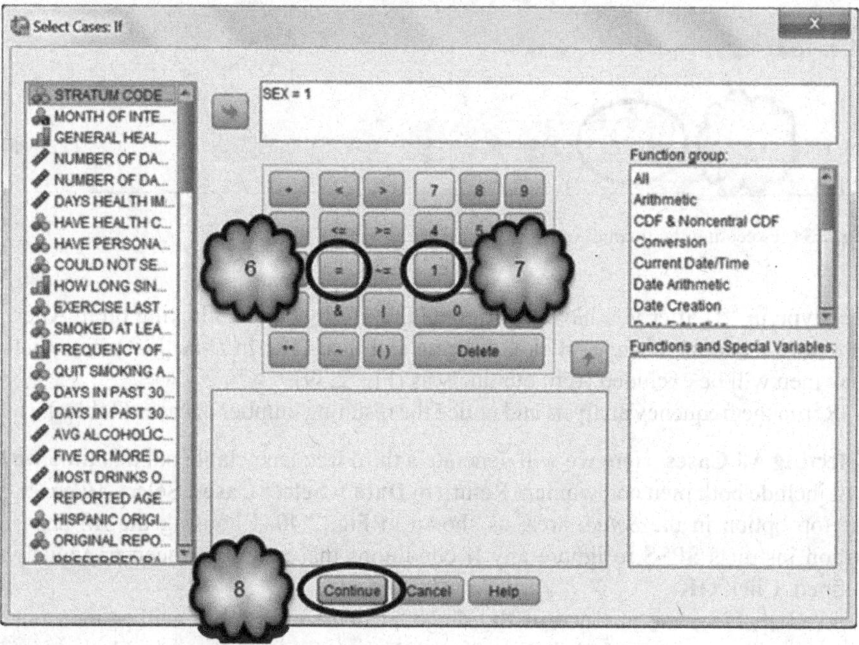

Fig. 2.33 Creating the if condition

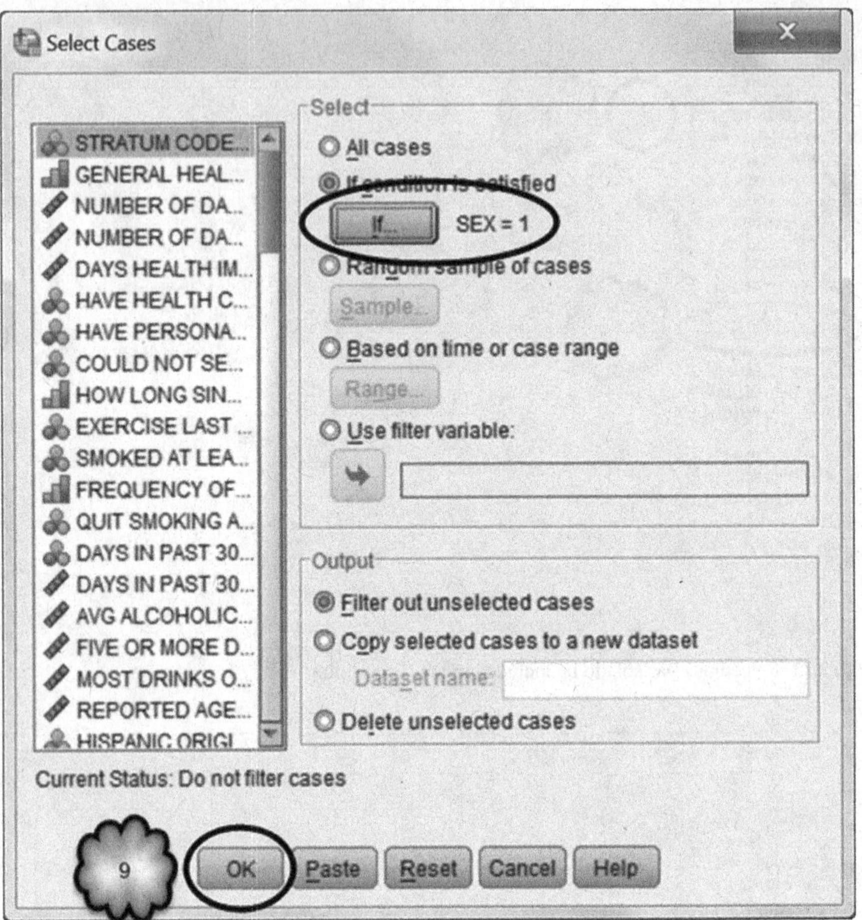

Fig. 2.34 Executing the if condition

is to type in "2" after you have highlighted the "1" by double-clicking on it. After you have made the change, click **Continue** and then **OK**. In *Data View,* note that now men will be excluded from our analysis (Fig. 2.39).

Rerun the frequency analysis and notice the resulting number of cases (Table 2.2).

Selecting All Cases Here we will generate a third frequency table but this time we will include both men and women. Return to **Data > Select Cases.** Select *All cases,* the top option in the *Select* area, as shown in Fig. 2.40. Choosing the *All cases* option instructs SPSS to ignore any If conditions that may have been previously defined. Click **OK.**

In *Data View,* the absence of the diagonal lines means that neither men nor women will now be excluded (Fig. 2.41). Notice that the filter variable has not changed—it is still set to exclude men. SPSS includes all cases by deactivating the filter variable.

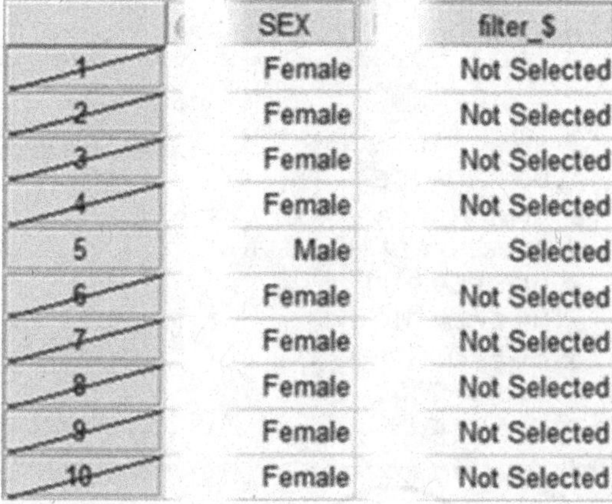

Fig. 2.35 Data view after selecting males

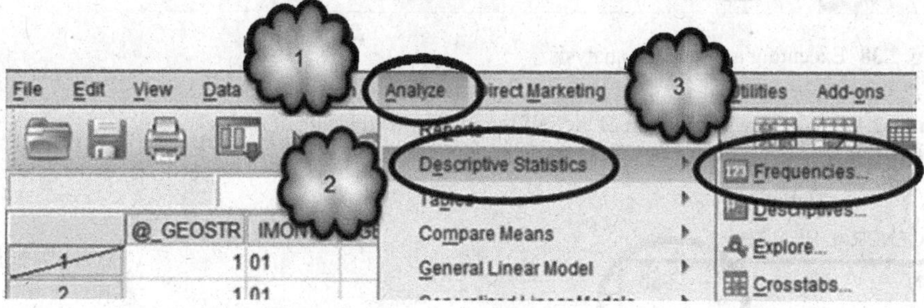

Fig. 2.36 Accessing the Frequencies dialog

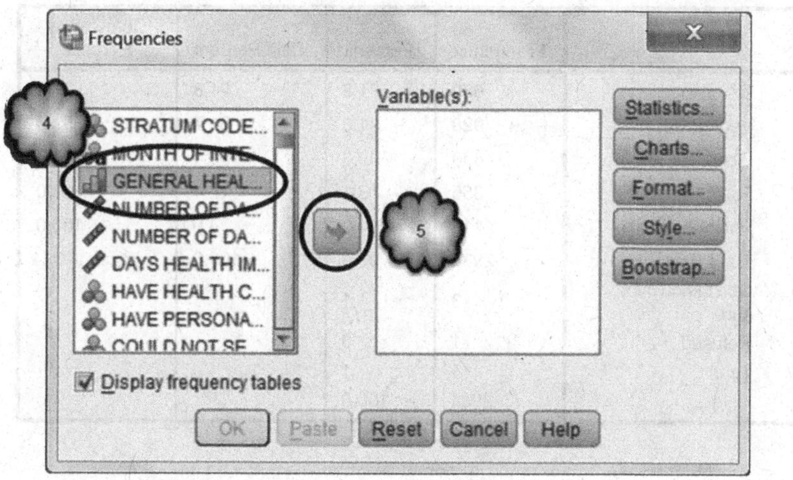

Fig. 2.37 Selecting a variable for a frequency analysis

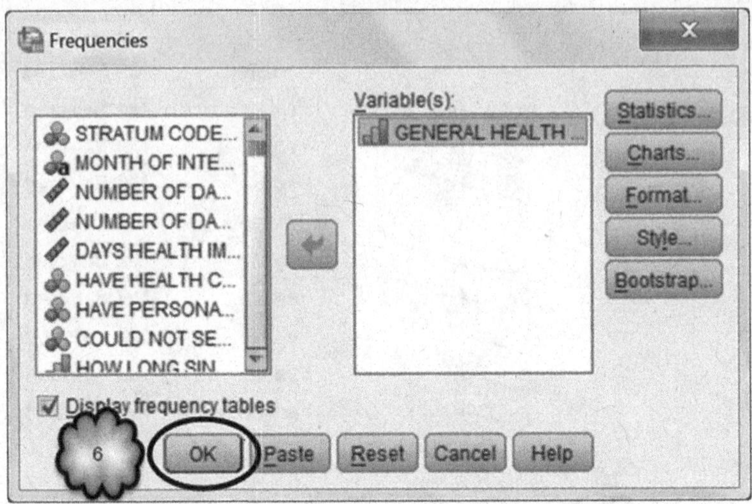

Fig. 2.38 Executing a frequency analysis

Table 2.1 Frequency distribution of the self-reported general health of males

Frequencies

Statistics

GENERAL HEALTH

N	Valid	2930
	Missing	4

GENERAL HEALTH

		Frequency	Percent	Valid Percent	Cumulative Percent
Valid	Excellent	639	21.8	21.8	21.8
	Very good	928	31.6	31.7	53.5
	Good	890	30.3	30.4	83.9
	Fair	355	12.1	12.1	96.0
	Poor	118	4.0	4.0	100.0
	Total	2930	99.9	100.0	
Missing	Don't know/Not sure	3	.1		
	Refused	1	.0		
	Total	4	.1		
Total		2934	100.0		

Fig. 2.39 Data view after selecting females

	SEX	filter_$
1	Female	Selected
2	Female	Selected
3	Female	Selected
4	Female	Selected
5	Male	Not Selected
6	Female	Selected
7	Female	Selected
8	Female	Selected
9	Female	Selected
10	Female	Selected

Table 2.2 Frequency distribution of the self-reported general health of females

Frequencies

Statistics

GENERAL HEALTH

N	Valid	4847
	Missing	15

GENERAL HEALTH

		Frequency	Percent	Valid Percent	Cumulative Percent
Valid	Excellent	1013	20.8	20.9	20.9
	Very good	1612	33.2	33.3	54.2
	Good	1393	28.7	28.7	82.9
	Fair	624	12.8	12.9	95.8
	Poor	205	4.2	4.2	100.0
	Total	4847	99.7	100.0	
Missing	Don't know/Not sure	13	.3		
	Refused	2	.0		
	Total	15	.3		
Total		4862	100.0		

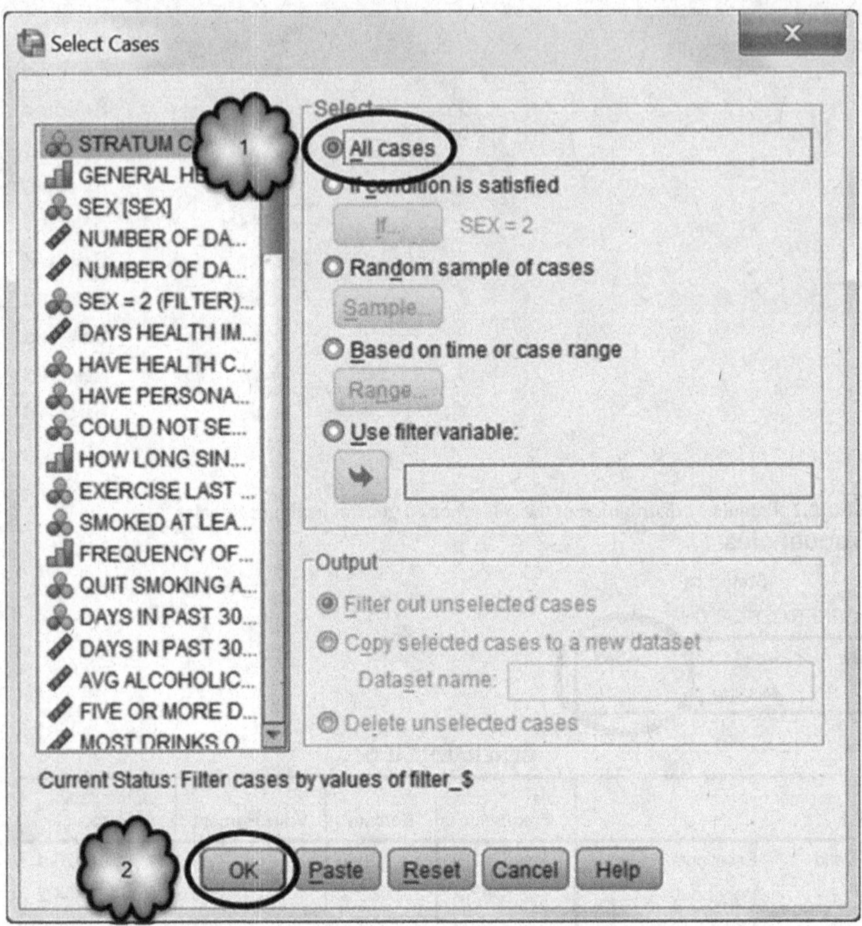

Fig. 2.40 Selecting all cases

Fig. 2.41 Data view after selecting both males and females

	SEX	filter_$
1	Female	Selected
2	Female	Selected
3	Female	Selected
4	Female	Selected
5	Male	Not Selected
6	Female	Selected
7	Female	Selected
8	Female	Selected
9	Female	Selected
10	Female	Selected

Table 2.3 Frequency distribution of the self-reported general health of the entire sample

Frequencies

Statistics

GENERAL HEALTH

N		
N	Valid	7777
	Missing	19

GENERAL HEALTH

		Frequency	Percent	Valid Percent	Cumulative Percent
Valid	Excellent	1652	21.2	21.2	21.2
	Very good	2540	32.6	32.7	53.9
	Good	2283	29.3	29.4	83.3
	Fair	979	12.6	12.6	95.8
	Poor	323	4.1	4.2	100.0
	Total	7777	99.8	100.0	
Missing	Don't know/Not sure	16	.2		
	Refused	3	.0		
	Total	19	.2		
Total		7796	100.0		

Rerun the frequency analysis. The output should be similar to that displayed in Table 2.3. Does the resulting number of cases seem right?

Selecting Cases by Range of Responses In this section, we focus only on those respondents whose answers to a question about their general health were coded within a 1 ("Excellent") to 5 ("Poor") range. That is, we will exclude those who gave no answer, said that they did not know, etc. As we have already seen, one way to do this is to declare values of 7 and 9 as missing (see Sect. 2.3). Another way to do this is to ask SPSS to limit our analysis to respondents whose answers to the **GENERAL HEALTH** question were coded 1, 2, 3, 4, or 5. One way to do this is to set the *If condition* in the *Select Cases* dialog box to "GENHLTH<6" (without the quotation marks). Set this condition (the "<" sign can either be typed in from the keyboard or "clicked in" from the dialog box keypad), and then generate the frequency table. Only the five response categories should be listed in the output (Table 2.4).

Selecting Cases by More Than One Condition Often it is necessary to select cases based on more than one condition. For example, in the CDC data set, we might want to limit an analysis to females who reported that they were in excellent general health. Let us see how cases can be selected based on more than one *If condition*.

Table 2.4 Frequency distribution of general health without missing values

Frequencies

Statistics

GENERAL HEALTH

N	Valid	7777
	Missing	0

GENERAL HEALTH

		Frequency	Percent	Valid Percent	Cumulative Percent
Valid	Excellent	1652	21.2	21.2	21.2
	Very good	2540	32.7	32.7	53.9
	Good	2283	29.4	29.4	83.3
	Fair	979	12.6	12.6	95.8
	Poor	323	4.2	4.2	100.0
	Total	7777	100.0	100.0	

	GENHLTH	SEX	filter_$
1	Excellent	Female	Selected
2	Good	Female	Not Selected
3	Fair	Female	Not Selected
4	Very good	Female	Not Selected
5	Good	Male	Not Selected
6	Good	Female	Not Selected
7	Excellent	Female	Selected
8	Very good	Female	Not Selected
9	Very good	Female	Not Selected
10	Very good	Female	Not Selected

Fig. 2.42 Data view after selecting females in excellent general health

If we wish to limit our analysis to women in excellent health, we can make use of the "and" logical operator (&). In the *Select Cases* dialog box, enter the following *If condition:* "SEX=2 & GENHLTH=1." The "&" symbol can be clicked in from the dialog keypad. As an alternative, the word "and" can be typed in from the keyboard instead. Click **Continue** and then **OK**. In *Data View,* notice that only women who reported to be in excellent health were selected (Fig. 2.42).

Imagine that we wanted to expand our selection to include women who reported that they were in either excellent or very good health. To select these cases, we would

Fig. 2.43 Data view after selecting females in either excellent or very good general health

	GENHLTH	SEX	filter_$
1	Excellent	Female	Selected
2	Good	Female	Not Selected
3	Fair	Female	Not Selected
4	Very good	Female	Selected
5	Good	Male	Not Selected
6	Good	Female	Not Selected
7	Excellent	Female	Selected
8	Very good	Female	Selected
9	Very good	Female	Selected
10	Very good	Female	Selected

use both the "and" (&) and the "or" (|) logical operators. In the *Select Cases* dialog box, enter the following condition: "SEX=2 & (GENHLTH=1 | GENHLTH=2)." The "|" symbol is the logical OR operator and can be clicked in from the dialog box keypad. As an alternative, the word "or" could be typed in from the keyboard instead. Click **Continue** and then **OK**. Inspection of *Data View* should reveal that we have selected only women who reported to be in either excellent or very good health (Fig. 2.43).

2.6 Sorting a Dialog Box Variables List

When a data file has a large number of variables, as is the case with the CDC data set, finding a particular variable from a dialog box listing can be frustrating. Fortunately, SPSS allows users to alphabetize the order by which the variables displayed in a dialog box are listed. To do so, right-click a variable in the list. From the resulting menu, choose whether to have the variables displayed by name or label, and then choose *Sort Alphabetically*. The variables will then be listed in the dialog box in alphabetical order. This procedure does not change the actual order of the variables within the data file. Figures 2.44, 2.45, and 2.46 show how to display variable labels alphabetically in the *Select Cases* dialog box.

2.7 Labeling SPSS Output

The output generated by the frequency procedure does not identify the subset of cases included in the analysis, and the log tells us only that the cases selected were those for whom **SEX** had been coded as a "1." It would be convenient if we could add commentary to the output indicating that the respondents were men. Here is one way.

In the *Viewer's* right-hand pane, double-click the heading *Frequencies*. This will either generate a text box that surrounds the heading, or produce an SPSS Output Text window. Figure 2.47 shows a text box.

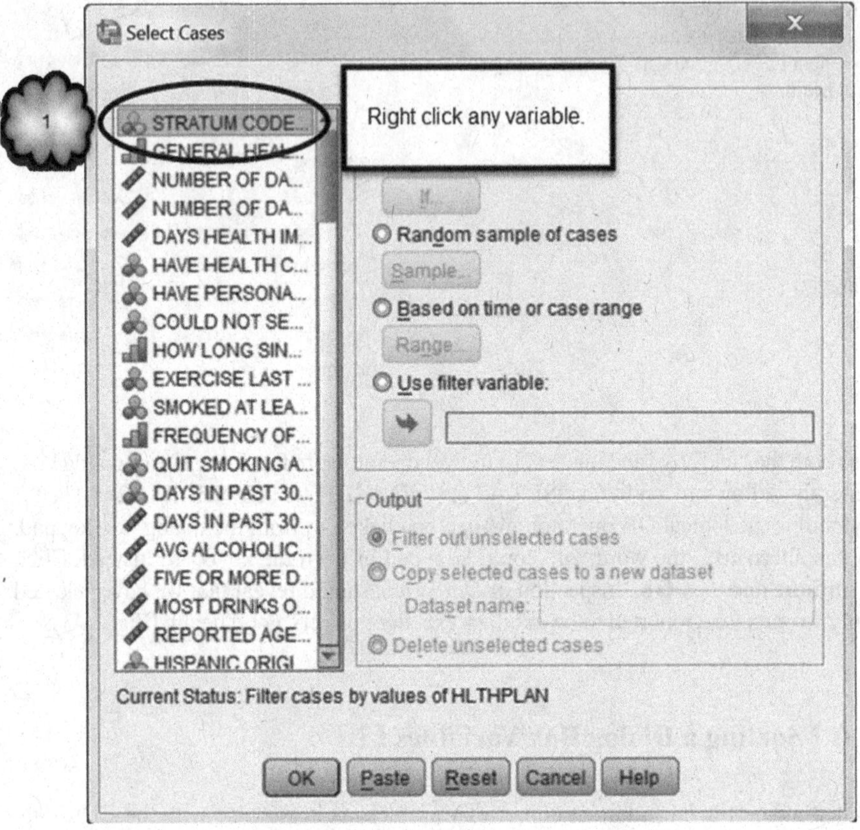

Fig. 2.44 Accessing the Sort Alphabetically option

Place the cursor to the right of the heading and type a description of the output that identifies the cases that were included in the analysis. For example, you might type, "Men only." Entering a colon or a space after "Frequencies" will make your output label easier to read, e.g., "Frequencies: Men only." To close the text box, double-click any white space outside of it. To close the Output Text window, click the **X** in the upper right hand corner. The end result will be output similar to that shown in Table 2.5.

2.8 Printing and Pasting SPSS Output

Sometimes you will want to print output or copy and paste output to a Word document.

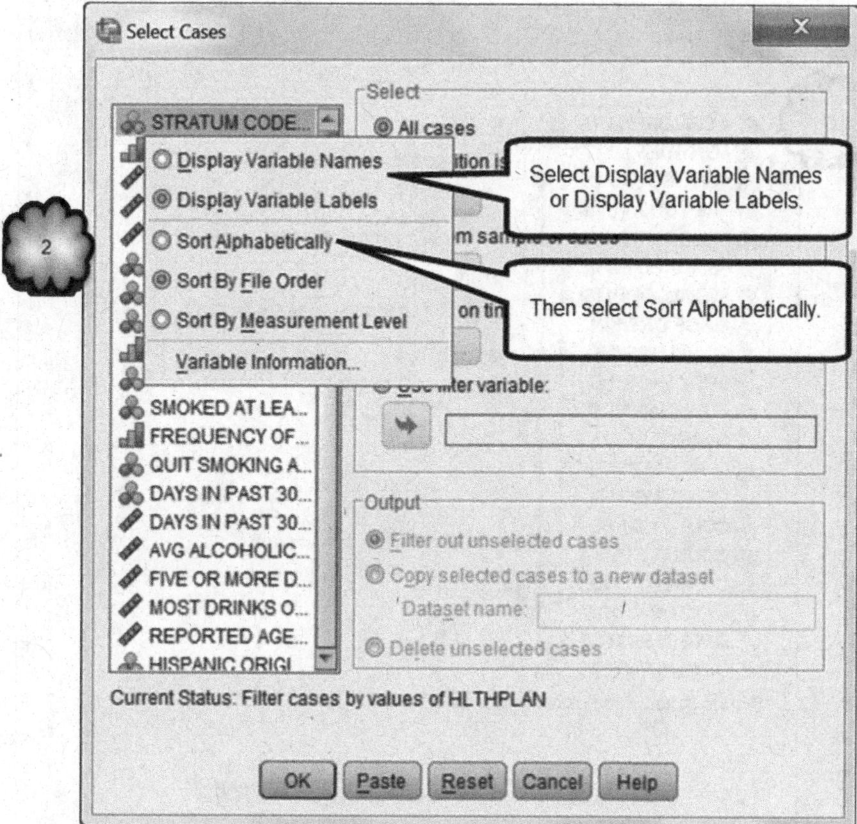

Fig. 2.45 Selecting the Sort Alphabetically option

Printing SPSS allows us to print either all of the output in the *Viewer*, or only selected portions. To print the entire output file, select **File > Print** or press the *Ctrl* and *P* keys simultaneously (i.e., press **Ctrl+P**) while the cursor is in the output window. Select the printer you wish to use and click **OK**.

To print selected portions of output, first select the output you wish to print by clicking it. You may use either the left or right output pane. To select more than one portion of output for printing, hold down the *Ctrl* key while you click the output that you wish to print. Then select **File > Print** to open the *Print* dialog box. Confirm that in the *Print Range* area, the option, *Selected output,* has been chosen, and click **OK**.

Pasting into a Word Document There may be times when you want to paste a portion of the output from SPSS into a Word document. One way to do this is to click the output that you wish to paste, and select **Edit>Copy** (or press **Ctrl+C**). Move to the location in your Word document where you want to place the output, and execute Word's paste command (e.g., **Edit>Paste** or **Ctrl+V**).

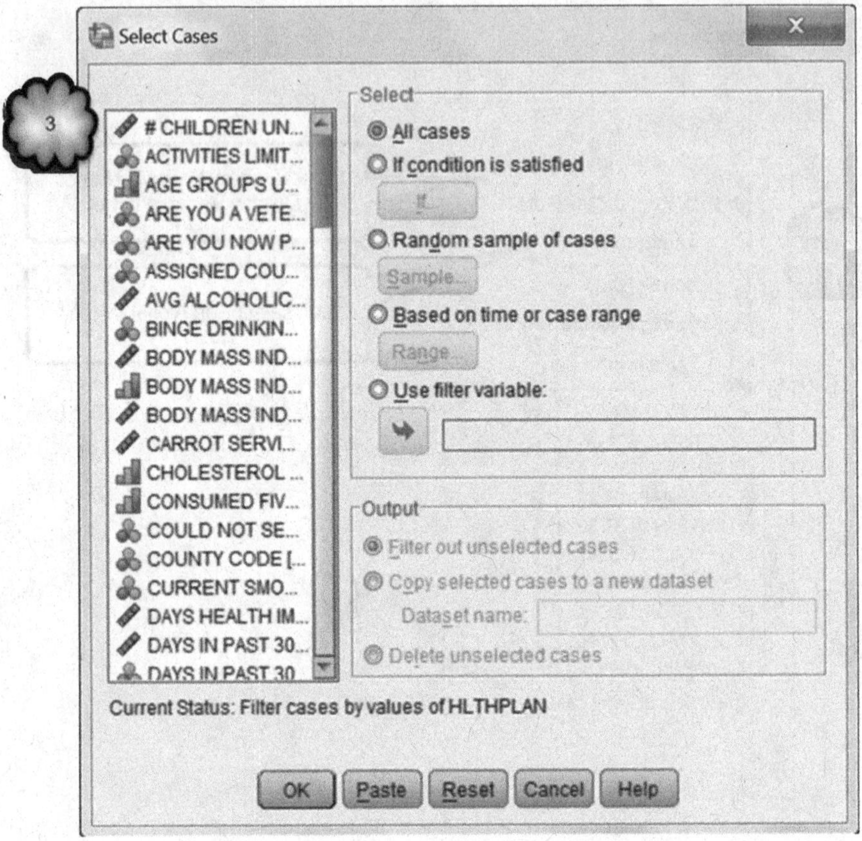

Select Cases

3

CHILDREN UN...
ACTIVITIES LIMIT...
AGE GROUPS U...
ARE YOU A VETE...
ARE YOU NOW P...
ASSIGNED COU...
AVG ALCOHOLIC...
BINGE DRINKIN...
BODY MASS IND...
BODY MASS IND...
BODY MASS IND...
CARROT SERVI...
CHOLESTEROL ...
CONSUMED FIV...
COULD NOT SE...
COUNTY CODE [...
CURRENT SMO...
DAYS HEALTH IM...
DAYS IN PAST 30...
DAYS IN PAST 30

Select
All cases
If condition is satisfied
If...
Random sample of cases
Sample...
Based on time or case range
Range...
Use filter variable:

Output
Filter out unselected cases
Copy selected cases to a new dataset
Dataset name:
Delete unselected cases

Current Status: Filter cases by values of HLTHPLAN

OK Paste Reset Cancel Help

Fig. 2.46 Select cases dialog displaying variables in alphabetical order by variable labels

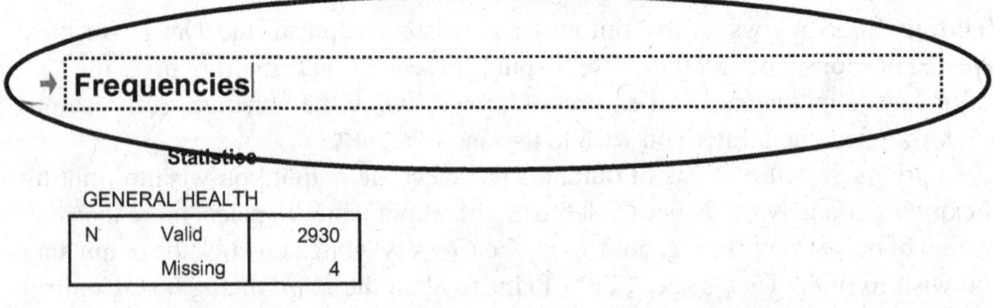
Frequencies

Statistics

GENERAL HEALTH

N	Valid	2930
	Missing	4

GENERAL HEALTH

		Frequency	Percent	Valid Percent	Cumulative Percent
Valid	Excellent	639	21.8	21.8	21.8
	Very good	928	31.6	31.7	53.5
	Good	890	30.3	30.4	83.9

Fig. 2.47 Text box for an output heading

Table 2.5 Output with an edited heading

Frequencies: Men Only.

Statistics

GENERAL HEALTH

N	Valid	2930
	Missing	4

GENERAL HEALTH

		Frequency	Percent	Valid Percent	Cumulative Percent
Valid	Excellent	639	21.8	21.8	21.8
	Very good	928	31.6	31.7	53.5
	Good	890	30.3	30.4	83.9
	Fair	355	12.1	12.1	96.0
	Poor	118	4.0	4.0	100.0
	Total	2930	99.9	100.0	
Missing	Don't know/Not sure	3	.1		
	Refused	1	.0		
	Total	4	.1		
Total		2934	100.0		

2.9 Saving and Exporting SPSS Output Files

SPSS output can be saved as an SPSS output file or exported to other formats, such as an Excel or a PDF file.

Saving the Output File Saving output as an SPSS file is straightforward. From *Viewer*, select **File>Save As**. In the resulting dialog box, select the location where the file is to be saved, enter a name for the file, and click **Save**. The output file will be saved with the name that you assigned to it with a **.spv** extension.

Exporting to an Excel or a PDF File If you want to save your output as either an Excel or PDF file, select **File>Export** from the output window. In the *Export Output* dialog box, indicate in the *Objects to Export* area how much of the output you want. Select *All* if you want to export the entire output file and you want to include additional information that SPSS collects behind the scenes such as data about processing times. This additional information does not appear on screen but can be included in the exported file. Select *All visible* if you want to export the entire file but do not want the data behind the scenes. Choose *Selected* if you have clicked a subset of results to export. In the *Type* box, click the down arrow and select either a version of *Excel* or *Portable Document Format*. Then click **Browse,** navigate to where you wish to save the file, name it, and click **OK**. These steps are displayed in Figs. 2.48 and 2.49.

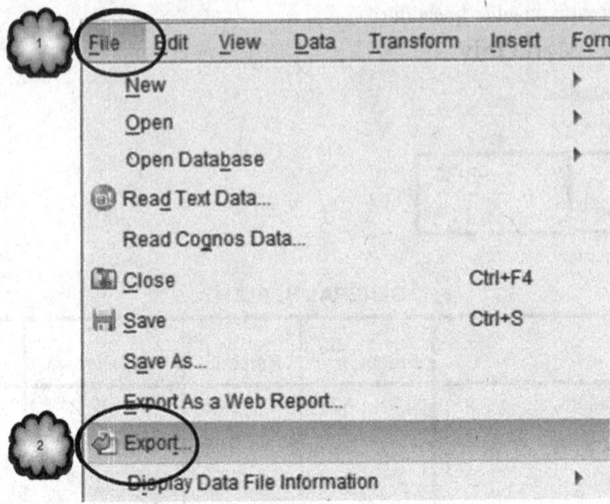

Fig. 2.48 Accessing the Export Dialog

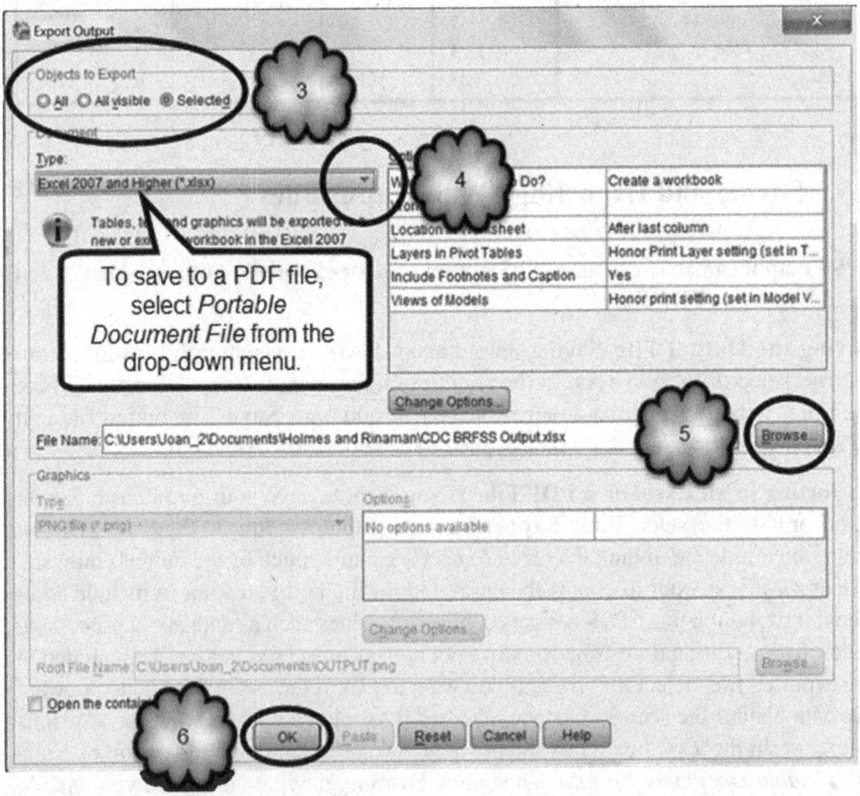

Fig. 2.49 Exporting SPSS output to Excel

2.10 Exercise Questions

The following questions refer to data found in **CDC BRFFS.sav**.

1. Participants interviewed by the CDC were asked: "Now thinking about your physical health, which includes physical illness and injury, for how many days during the past 30 days was your physical health not good?" Their answers are stored in the variable, **NUMBER OF DAYS PHYSICAL HEALTH NOT GOOD** [*PHYSHLTH*] (variable 4; 77=Do not know/Not sure; 99=Refused). Responses of "none" were coded by the CDC as 88.

   a. In the jargon of SPSS, what is the *name* of the variable?
   b. In the jargon of SPSS, what *type* of variable is it?
   c. How many decimal places do its entries show?
   d. Does this variable currently have any value labels? Should it? Why or why not?
   e. What values of this variable have been declared as missing data?
   f. In the jargon of SPSS, what is the type of *measure* that has been assigned? Is this measure type correct? Why or why not?
   g. What was the answer of the third case to this question? Was this case male or female?

2. The variable, **MARITAL STATUS** [*MARITAL*] (variable 24) is categorical, not quantitative, yet it is listed in *Variable View* as numeric. How can a categorical variable be numeric?
3. This chapter asked you to enter value labels and declare missing values for the variable, **HAVE HEALTH CARE COVERAGE** [*HLTHPLAN*] (variable 7; 1=Yes; 2=No; 7=Do not know/Not sure; 9=Refused).

   a. Conduct a frequency analysis of that variable. Be sure that the output displays the value labels.
   b. Repeat the analysis but this time limit it to women between the ages of 25 and 35. Age is stored in the variable, **REPORTED AGE IN YEARS** [*AGE*] (variable 20). Label the resulting output "Women between 25 and 35."

Data Set and Reference

1. CDC BRFSS.sav obtained from: Centers for Disease Control and Prevention (CDC). Behavioral Risk Factor Surveillance System Survey Data. US Department of Health and Human Services, Centers for Disease Control and Prevention, Atlanta (2005). Public domain. For more information about the BRFSS, visit http://www.cdc.gov/brfss/. Accessed 16 Nov 2014

Chapter 3
Describing the Distribution of a Categorical Variable

Abstract This chapter introduces graphical and numerical techniques for describing the distribution of a categorical variable. Frequency tables are described. Bar charts and pie charts are covered as graphical methods. The SPSS commands to create these are discussed. In addition, the procedure for transforming a variable in SPSS is discussed. Finally, the methods for copying SPSS charts into Microsoft Word are covered.

3.1 Overview

In Chap. 1, we said that clinical practice is continuously informed by the findings of clinical research, and that those findings are based on empirical evidence or data. But the well-known adage notwithstanding, data cannot speak for themselves, at least not literally. Researchers must make sense out of them. To interpret a set of data, researchers begin by using *descriptive statistics* and *graphical techniques* to describe or summarize its *distribution*. There are many of these statistical tools from which to choose, but they generally fall into two broad categories: those appropriate for *quantitative variables* and those for *categorical*. A quantitative variable has two important properties. It takes on values that reflect quantity, and equal intervals between the values correspond to equal differences in quantity. Weight measured in pounds is an example. Pounds reflect quantity of weight. For instance, a patient who weighs 125 pounds is heavier than one who weighs 100 pounds. Moreover, equal differences in pounds correspond to equal differences in weight. For instance, a difference of 25 pounds corresponds to the same difference in weight whether the difference is between a patient who weighs 100 pounds and a patient who weighs 125 pounds, or between a patient who weighs 125 pounds and one who weighs 150 pounds. A categorical variable lacks either the first or both of these properties.

As we saw in Chap. 2, there are two types of categorical variables. Values of a *nominal* variable do not reflect differences in quantity. Instead the values identify the group or category to which the patient is said to belong. Gender and ethnicity are examples. Values of an *ordinal* variable reflect differences in amount, but equal intervals between the values do not necessarily correspond to equal differences in quantity. Instead the values reflect a rank order. Educational level is an example.

W. H. Holmes, W. C. Rinaman, *Statistical Literacy for Clinical Practitioners*,
DOI 10.1007/978-3-319-12550-3_3

Patients who graduated from college have more education (we hope) than patients who graduated from high school, and high school graduates have more education than patients who did not attend high school. But the difference in education between a college graduate and a high school graduate cannot be assumed to be equal to the difference in education between a high school graduate and someone who never attended high school.

In this chapter, we will focus on some of the descriptive statistics and graphical techniques appropriate for categorical variables: *frequencies, percentages, frequency tables,* and *bar and pie charts*. In the next chapter, we will describe methods appropriate for quantitative variables. The Centers for Disease Control and Prevention (CDC) data set that we used in the previous chapter has a number of quantitative and categorical variables, so we will use that data set in both chapters.

Sometimes clinical researchers transform a quantitative variable into a categorical one. For example, body mass index (BMI) is a quantitative variable that is often converted into a categorical variable. In the CDC data set, respondents whose BMI was less than 25 were categorized as "Neither overweight nor obese," respondents whose BMI was 25 or over but less than 30 were categorized as "Overweight," and respondents whose BMI was 30 or over were categorized as "Obese." Sometimes researchers transform a categorical variable into one that has fewer but broader categories. For example, respondents to the CDC survey reported their general health in terms of the following categories: "Excellent," "Very good," "Good," "Fair" and "Poor." This produced a categorical variable, **GENERAL HEALTH** [*GENHLTH*] (variable 3), that has five values. This variable was transformed into a new one, **HEALTH STATUS** [*@_RFHLTH*] (variable 58), with two values, "Good or Better Health" and "Fair or Poor Health." To get a feel for how transformations work, we will transform some variables in this chapter.

3.2 Frequency Tables

Frequencies and Percentages When a variable is categorical, the number of times each of its values occurs in a set of data is counted. These counts are called *frequencies.* When a count or frequency is divided by the total count and multiplied by 100, the result is a *percentage* or *percent.* The frequencies or percentages of the values of a variable constitute its *distribution.* In this section, we will look at the distribution of various categories of BMI in the CDC BRFSS data set. Respondents were categorized as "Neither overweight nor Obese" if their BMI were less than 25, "Overweight" if their BMI were equal to or greater than 25 but less than 30, and "Obese" if their BMI were equal to or greater than 30. To determine the frequencies of these categories, we will create a frequency table.

Load the data file, **CDC BRFSS.sav** [1], into SPSS as you did in the previous chapter. Check that the value labels for the variable, **BODY MASS INDEX-THREE LEVELS CATEGORY** [*@_BMI4CAT*] (variable 79; 1 = Neither overweight nor obese, 2 = Overweight, 3 = Obese, 9 = Don't know/Refused/Missing) have been entered and that 9 has been declared as missing. Next, select **Analyze > Descriptive Statis-**

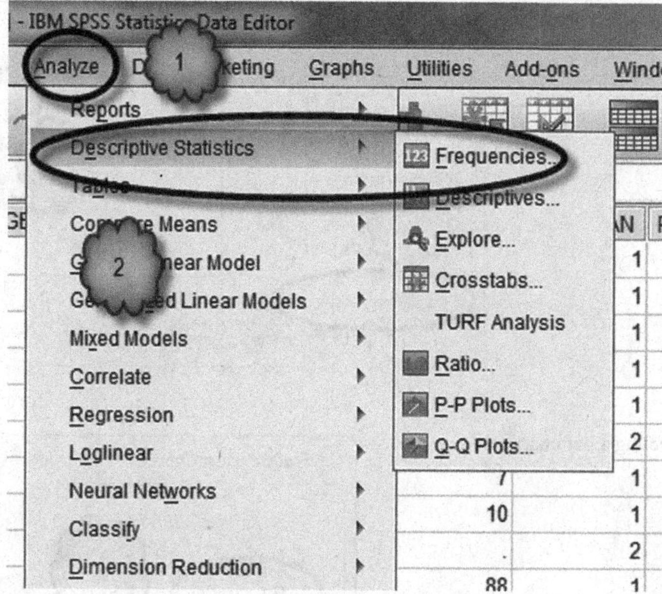

Fig. 3.1 Selecting the frequencies procedure

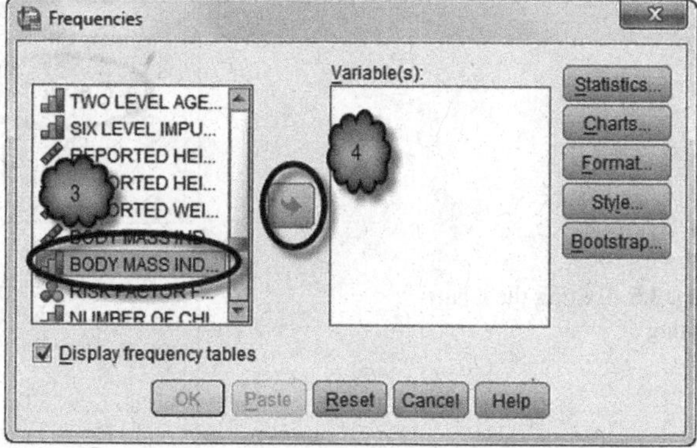

Fig. 3.2 Selecting the variable to be analyzed

tics>Frequencies to bring up the *Frequencies* dialog box. From the list of variables on the left of the dialog box, click the variable **BODY MASS INDEX-THREE LEVELS CATEGORY**. Move that variable to the *Variable(s)* area on the right by clicking on the arrow immediately to the left of the *Variable(s)* area. Check in the lower left corner of the dialog box that *Display frequency tables* has been checked. Next, click the **Charts** button to bring up the *Frequencies: Charts* dialog box. Select *Bar charts* and *Frequencies*. Click **Continue** and then **OK**. Figures 3.1, 3.2, 3.3, 3.4, 3.5, 3.6 show these steps.

SPSS will generate the output that you requested and display it in the *Viewer,* as shown in Fig. 3.7.

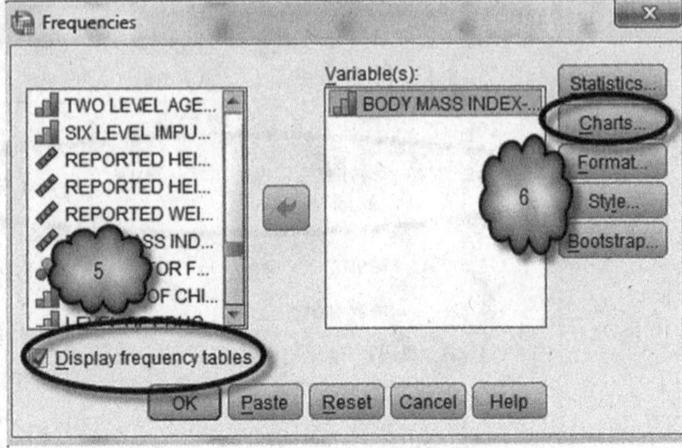

Fig. 3.3 Generating the frequency table and the Charts dialog

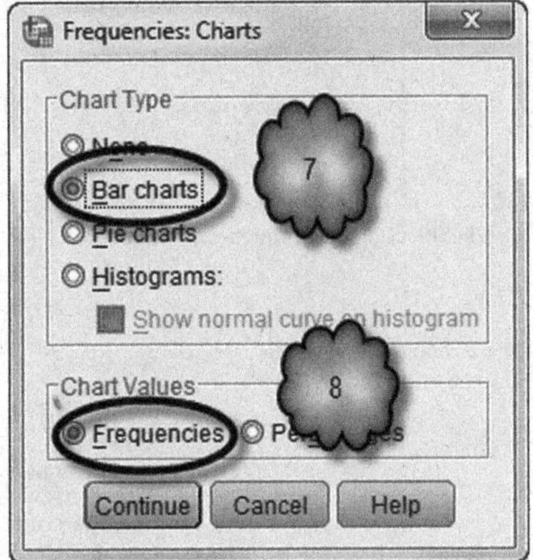

Fig. 3.4 Selecting a bar chart

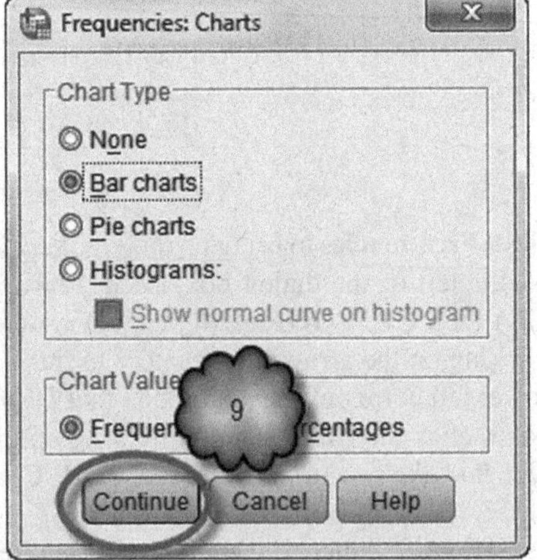

Fig. 3.5 Exiting the Charts dialog

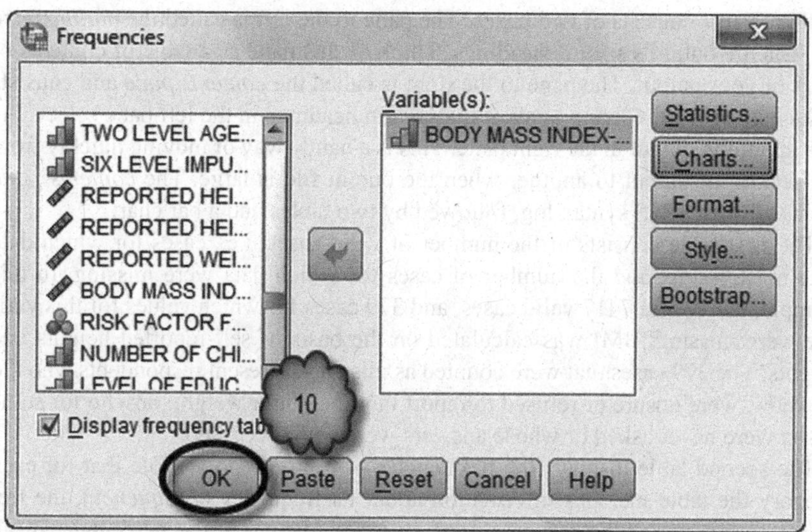

Fig. 3.6 Conducting the analysis

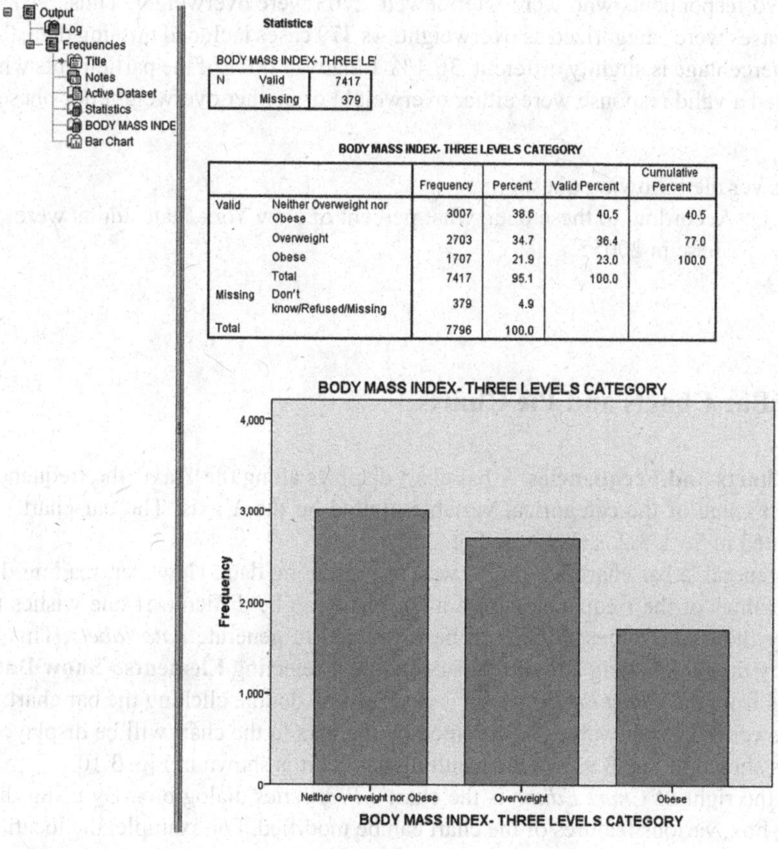

Output
Log
Frequencies
Title
Notes
Active Dataset
Statistics
BODY MASS INDE
Bar Chart

Statistics

BODY MASS INDEX- THREE LE

N	Valid	7417
	Missing	379

BODY MASS INDEX- THREE LEVELS CATEGORY

		Frequency	Percent	Valid Percent	Cumulative Percent
Valid	Neither Overweight nor Obese	3007	38.6	40.5	40.5
	Overweight	2703	34.7	36.4	77.0
	Obese	1707	21.9	23.0	100.0
	Total	7417	95.1	100.0	
Missing	Don't know/Refused/Missing	379	4.9		
Total		7796	100.0		

BODY MASS INDEX- THREE LEVELS CATEGORY
4,000
3,000
2,000
1,000
0
Frequency
Neither Overweight nor Obese
Overweight
Obese
BODY MASS INDEX- THREE LEVELS CATEGORY

Fig. 3.7 Output from the frequencies procedure

The *Viewer* consists of two panes. The pane to the left is called the *outline pane* and lists the output's section headings. Think of this pane as a table of contents or index of your output. The pane to the right is called the *contents pane* and consists of the output itself. Clicking any of the section headings in the left pane selects the corresponding output in the right pane. This is a handy way of moving quickly from one section of output to another when the output file is large. The *contents pane* begins with an SPSS syntax log, followed by two tables and a bar chart.

The first table consists of the number of valid cases, i.e., cases for which data were not missing, and the number of cases for which data were missing. In this example, there were 7417 valid cases, and 379 cases for which values for this variable were missing. BMI was calculated on the basis of self-reported heights and weights. The 379 cases that were counted as missing represent respondents who did not know, were unsure or refused to report their height or weight, or who for some reason were never asked or whose answers were never recorded.

The second table displays the frequencies of each category. Note that for each category the table includes information about its frequency (*Frequency*), the frequency expressed as the percentage of all cases (*Percent*), the percentage of all cases without missing values (*Valid Percent*), and the total percentage of valid cases in the category and the categories above it (*Cumulative Percent*). For example, of the 7796 respondents who were interviewed, 2703 were overweight. Thus, 34.7% of all cases were categorized as overweight. As 379 cases included missing data, the valid percentage is slightly different, 36.4%. Finally, 77.0% of the participants who provided a valid response were either overweight or neither overweight nor obese.

Answer the following question:

3.2.1 According to these data, what percent of New York State adults were obese in 2005?

3.3 Bar Charts and Pie Charts

Bar Charts and Frequencies A bar chart displays along the *Y*-axis the frequency of each value of the categorical variable plotted on the *X*-axis. The bar chart we generated in Sect. 3.2 is shown in Fig. 3.8.

In general, a bar chart is a useful way of presenting data. However, reading the exact values of the frequencies from a bar chart can be difficult. If one wishes to display the exact values, SPSS can be instructed to generate *data labels*. This is done by double clicking any of the bars and then selecting **Elements>Show Data Labels** from the *Chart Editor* which is accessed by double clicking the bar chart in the viewer. The exact values represented by the bars in the chart will be displayed. This is shown in Fig. 3.9, and the resulting bar chart is shown in Fig. 3.10.

To the right of *Chart Editor* is the chart's *Properties* dialog box. By using this dialog box, various features of the chart can be modified. For example, the location

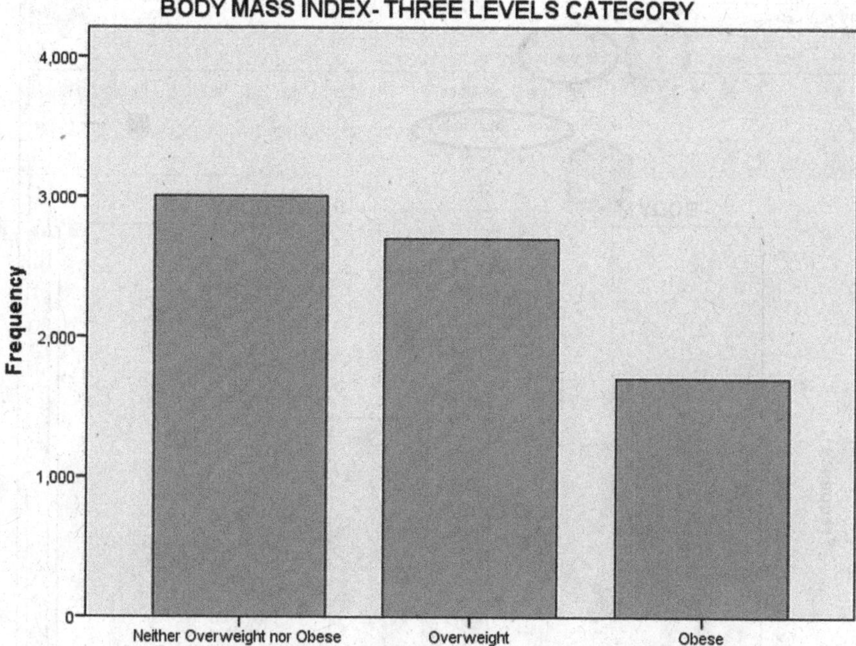

Fig. 3.8 A bar chart

of data labels can be changed by double clicking one of the data labels and then clicking the *Data Value Labels* tab, clicking the *Custom* option in the *Label Position* area, selecting one of the three location icons, and clicking **Apply**. This is shown in Fig. 3.11. To exit the *Chart Editor* and the *Properties* dialog box, click the **X** in the upper right-hand corner of the *Chart Editor*.

Many other aspects of an SPSS chart can be modified. For example:

- To modify the numerical entries along the *Y*-axis, click any number assigned to the *Y*-axis and enter changes in the Minimum, Maximum, Major Increment or Origin boxes under the *Properties Scale* tab. This is shown in Fig. 3.12.
- To add a title, select **Options > Title** in *Chart Editor* and enter a title in the title text box. To adjust the title's position or its overall look (e.g., its font or color), use the *Text Layout* and *Text Style* tabs of the *Properties* dialog box. Click anywhere outside the title text box when finished. This is shown in Fig. 3.13.
- To change the background color and remove the frame around the graph, click once within the body of the graph and use the *Properties Fill & Border* tab. This is shown in Fig. 3.14.
- To make changes to the label of the *X*- or *Y*-axis, click the label to select it, click again to edit the text, and use the *Properties Text Layout* and *Text Style* tabs as necessary. Click anywhere outside the text box when finished.
- To add text within the body of the graph, select **Options > Text Box** from *Chart Editor*, enter the information in the resulting text box, drag the box to its desired

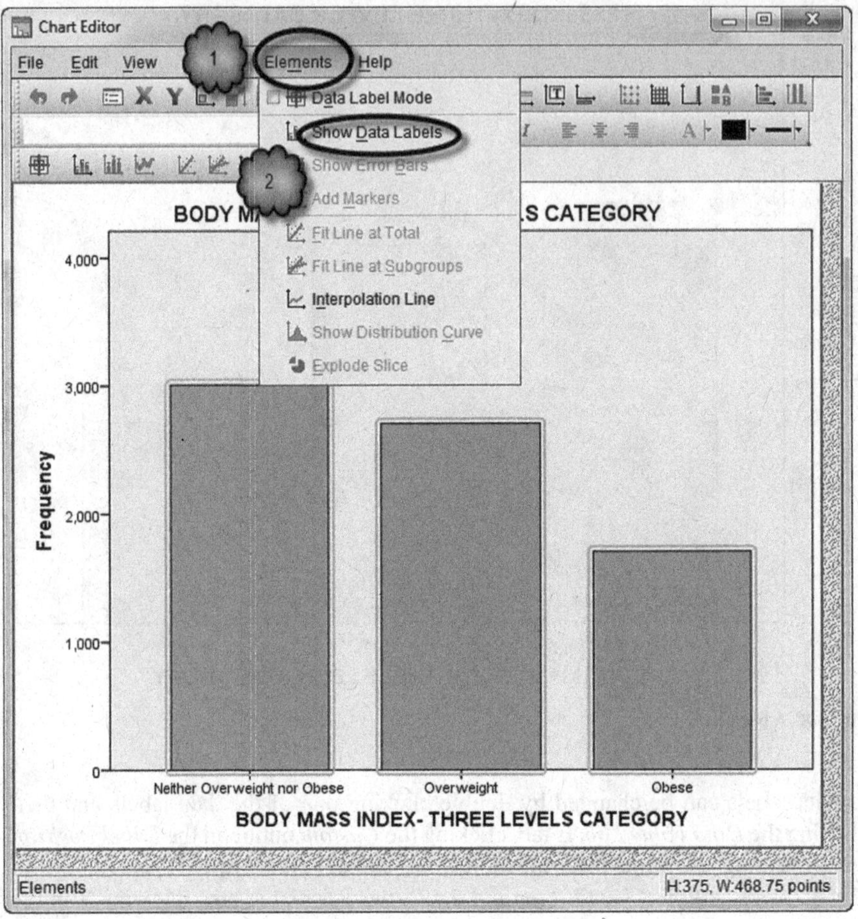

Fig. 3.9 Selecting show data labels

location and click anywhere outside the box when finished. To remove the text box, click it and press the delete key.

The chart in Fig. 3.15 shows how the bar chart might look with a few edits using many of the tools described above.

Bar Charts of Percentages Sometimes a bar chart of percentages is more useful than one showing the number of cases. To generate a chart showing percentages, select *Percentages* instead of *Frequencies* in the *Frequencies: Charts* dialog box. This was done to generate the graph that is shown in Fig. 3.16.

Charts with Transposed Axes Sometimes the two axes of a bar chart are transposed. An example is the chart that is shown in Fig. 3.17. This is the same chart as

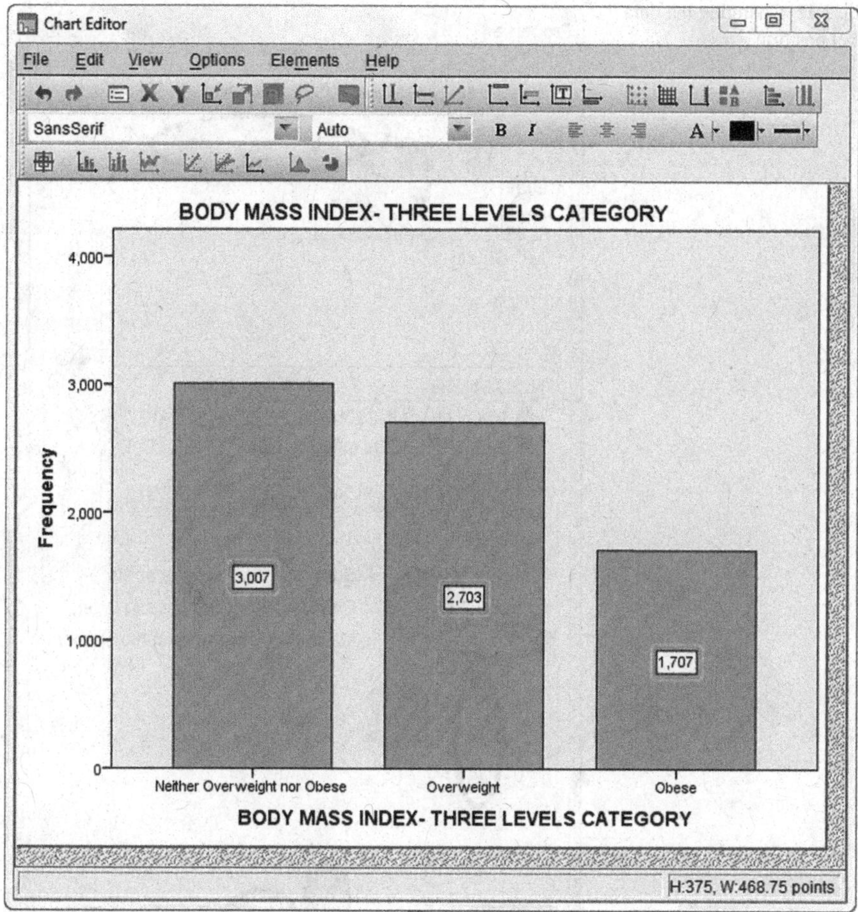

Fig. 3.10 Bar chart with data labels

the one shown in Fig. 3.16, except that several edits were made and the axes were transposed by selecting **Options > Transpose Chart** in *Chart Editor*.

Pie Charts An alternative to displaying percentages in terms of the heights of bars of a bar chart is in terms of the size of slices of a pie chart. The pie chart that is shown in Fig. 3.18 displays the distribution of the three categories of BMI. The pie chart was generated by conducting a frequency analysis in which the *Pie charts* option of the *Frequencies: Charts* dialog box was selected. Selecting **Elements > Explode slice** in the *Chart Editor* resulted in the pie chart shown in Fig. 3.19. In both pie charts, data labels were added in the manner explained above.

Chart Builder In SPSS, bar and pie charts can be generated without conducting a frequency analysis. This is done by selecting **Graphs > Chart Builder**. This will open two dialog boxes. The first informs us that before creating a chart, each of our

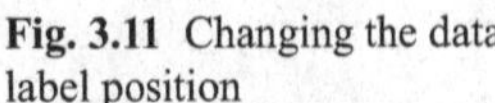

Fig. 3.11 Changing the data label position

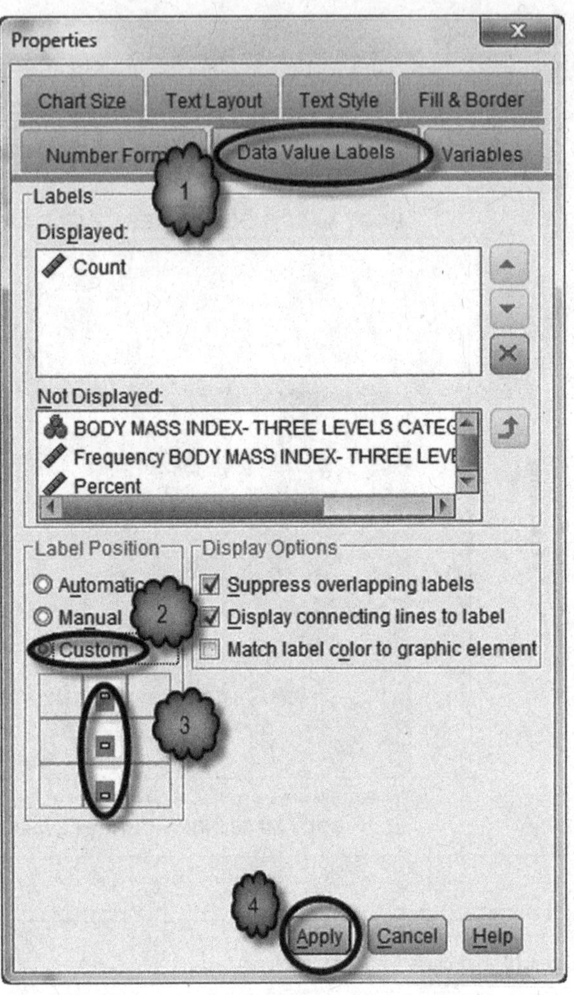

variables should have the appropriate measure type assigned to it, and if the variable is categorical, its value labels should be defined. We can click *Define Variable Properties* to change measure types or create value labels, or we can click **OK** to go directly to the *Chart Builder*. In this example, we can click **OK**. To create our bar chart in *Chart Builder*, select *Bar* from the *Gallery*. Drag the picture of the first bar chart (the one in the upper left hand corner) to the area just above it. This will open another dialog box, *Element Properties*, to the right of *Chart Builder.* In *Chart Builder*, drag **BODY MASS INDEX-THREE LEVELS CATEGORY** from the *Variables* area to the *X-Axis* box under the picture of the bar chart that you had just dragged. Clicking **OK** at this point will produce a bar chart. Figures 3.20, 3.21, 3.22, 3.23, 3.24 summarize these steps.

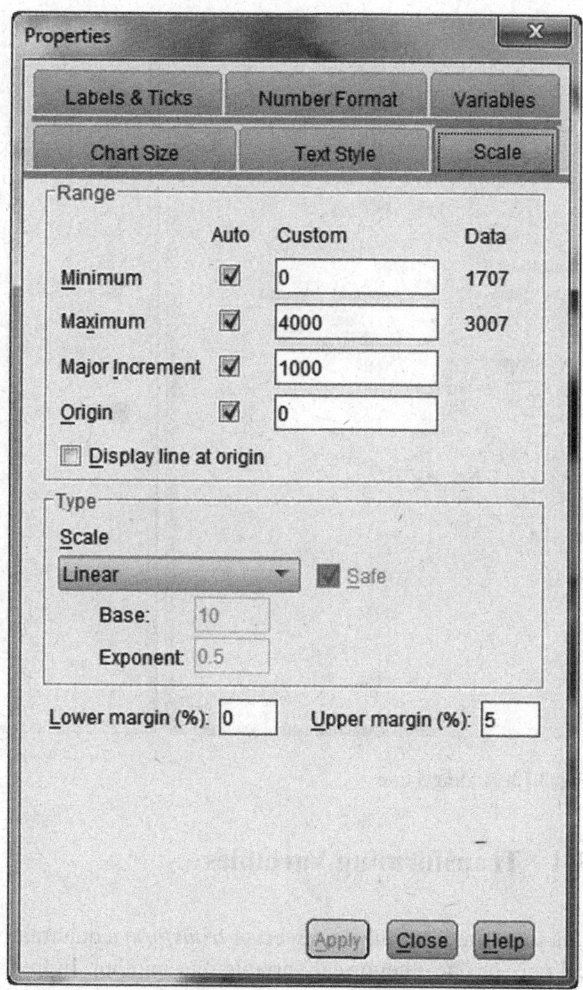

Fig. 3.12 Changing the Y-axis scale

To get a graph of percentages instead of number of cases, go to the *Element Properties* dialog box before clicking **OK.** There select *Percentage(?)* from the list of options in the *Statistic* drop-down menu and click **Apply**. Back in *Chart Builder*, click **OK** to generate the chart. These steps are shown in Figs. 3.25 and 3.26.

Data labels and the look of the graph can be controlled by using *Chart Editor* in the same way as explained earlier.

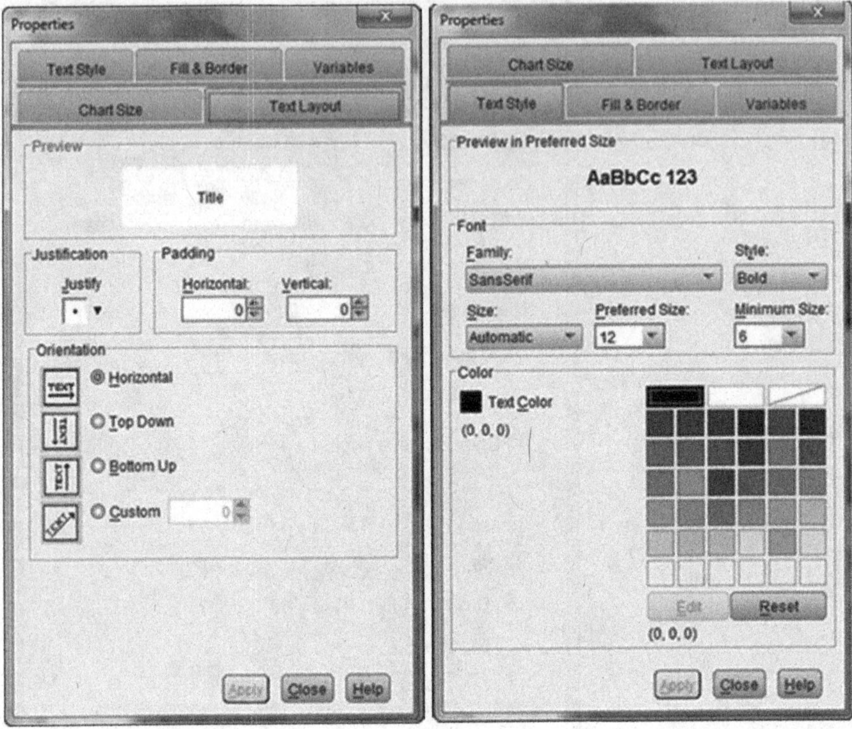

Fig. 3.13 Adding a title

3.4 Transforming Variables

It is sometimes useful to convert or *transform* a quantitative variable into a categorical one, or one categorical variable into another. In this section, we will look at an example of each of these transformations.

Recoding a Quantitative Variable As we saw earlier, the CDC data set includes a variable that represents three categories of BMI. Let us create a new categorical variable that adds a fourth group—people who are underweight (BMI < 18.50). One way to do this is depicted in Figs. 3.27, 3.28, 3.29, 3.30, 3.31, 3.32, 3.33, 3.34. That is, select **Transform > Recode into Different Variables**. In the *Recode into Different Variables* dialog box, click the third from the last variable of the data set, **BODY MASS INDEX** [*BMI*] (variable 107), and move it to the *Input Variable → Output Variable* box by clicking the right-pointing arrow. In the *Output Variable* area, type a variable name and a variable label for the new variable into the *Name* and *Label* boxes. In our example, we happened to name the new variable BMIFourCategories (variable names cannot contain spaces), and to label it, BMI Four Categories. Click

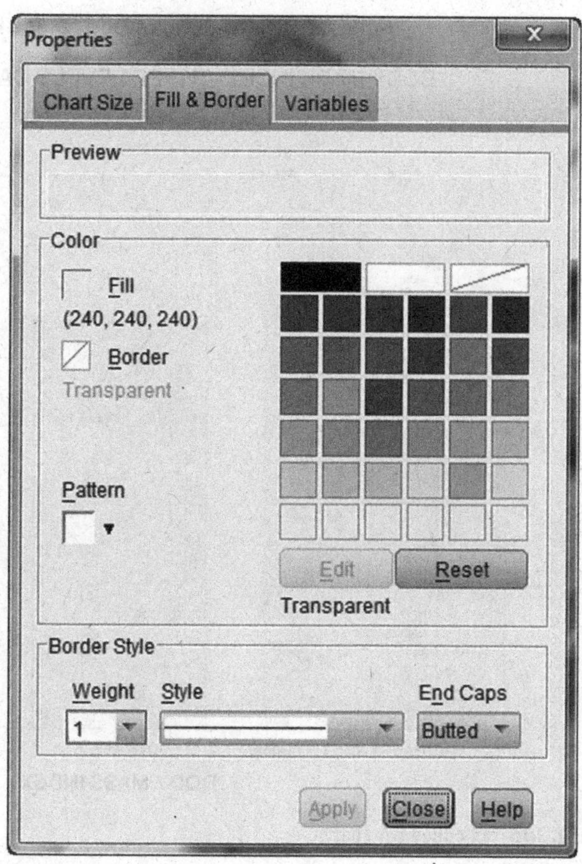

Fig. 3.14 Changing the fill and border

Change and then *Old and New Values*. In the *Old and New Values* dialog box, select *Range* in the *Old Value* area and enter the range of values for our first category, which will be the underweight group. To be sure that we included all qualifying cases, set the range to 0 through 18.49. In the *New Value* area, select *Value* and enter 1 in the box. Click **Add**. Repeat setting the ranges for the second, third and fourth categories (18.50 through 24.99, 25 through 29.99, and 30 through 80). These categories will be the normal, overweight and obese groups, respectively. Any missing values in the old variable should be copied into the new one, so select *All other values* in the *Old Value* area and *Copy old values* in the *New Value* area, and click **Add**. Now click **Continue** and execute the transformation by clicking **OK**.

SPSS will create the new variable and store it in the very last column of *Data View*, and print the following syntax in the output.

```
RECODE BMI (0 thru 18.49=1)  (18.5 thru 24.99=2)  (25 thru 29,99=3)
(30 thru 80=4)    (ELSE=Copy)  INTO BMIFourCategories.
VARIABLE LABLES BMIFourCategories 'BMI Four Catergories'.
EXECUTE.
```

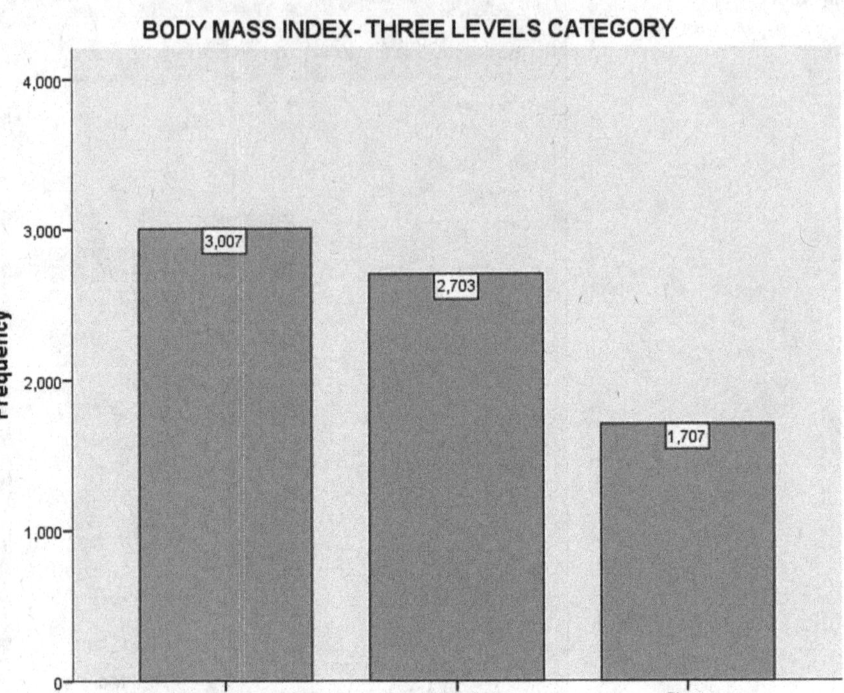

Fig. 3.15 An edited bar chart

After labeling the values of the new variable, we conducted a frequency analysis that generated the frequency table shown in Table 3.1.

> Answer the following question:
> 3.4.1 According to these data, what percent of New York state residents in 2005 was underweight?

Recoding a Categorical Variable The CDC asked respondents the following question: "In general, how satisfied are you with your life?" The response alternatives were "Very satisfied," "Satisfied," "Dissatisfied," and "Very dissatisfied." The respondents' answers are stored in the ordinal variable, **SATISFACTION W/ LIFE** [*LSATISFY*] (variable 50; 1 = Very satisfied; 2 = Satisfied, etc.). If we wished,

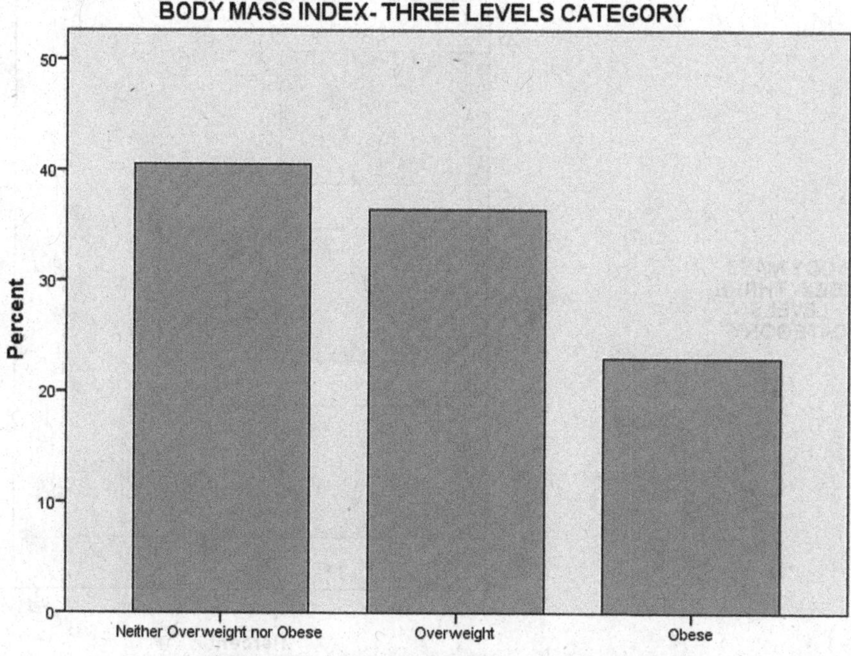

Fig. 3.16 A bar chart of percentages

we could recode this variable. For example, we could combine the first two groups into a category called "Satisfied or Very Satisfied" and the last two groups into a category called "Dissatisfied or Very Dissatisfied." To do this, we would follow the same general procedure that we used for recoding a quantitative variable. We leave this for you to do as an exercise question.

3.5 Copying SPSS Charts into MS Word Documents

In this section, we will review how to copy an SPSS chart into a Microsoft Word document. Right-click the chart you've created and choose *Copy* from the resulting menu. As an alternative, you can double click the graph to open *Chart Editor* and choose *Copy Chart* from the **Edit** menu. Next, place the cursor in the Word document where you wish to copy the chart, and execute Word's paste command (e.g., **Edit > Paste** or **Ctrl + V**). The chart should now appear. If the size of the chart needs to be adjusted, use Word's *Format Picture* dialog box to resize it.

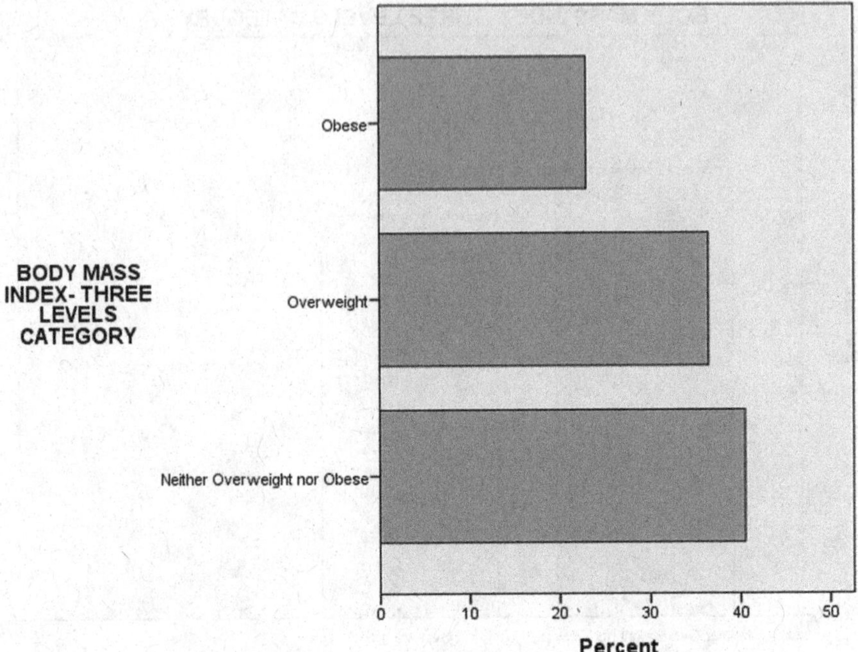

Fig. 3.17 A transposed bar chart

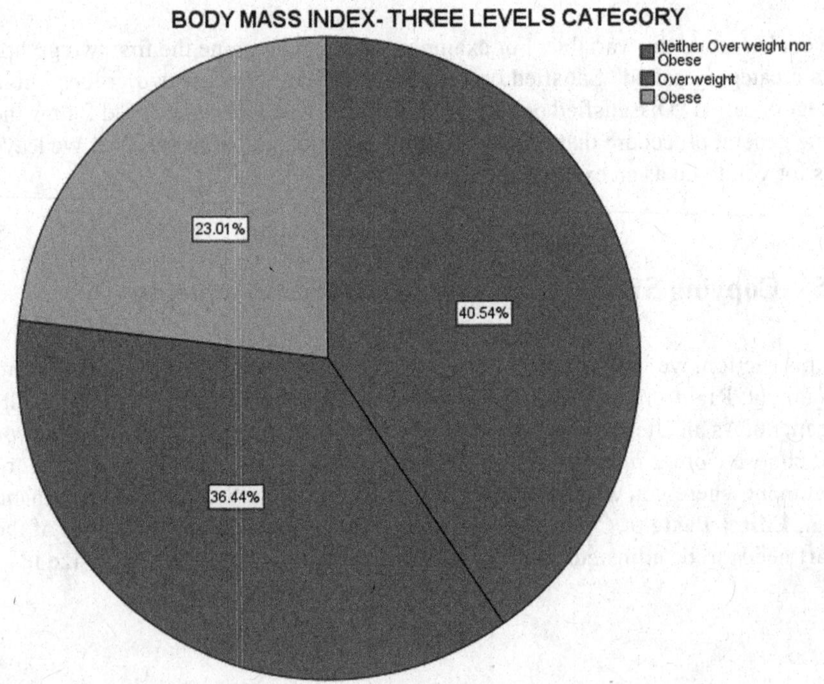

Fig. 3.18 A pie chart

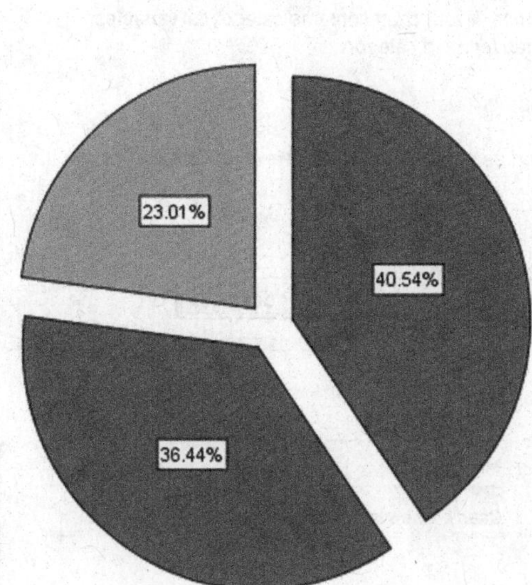

Fig. 3.19 An exploded pie chart

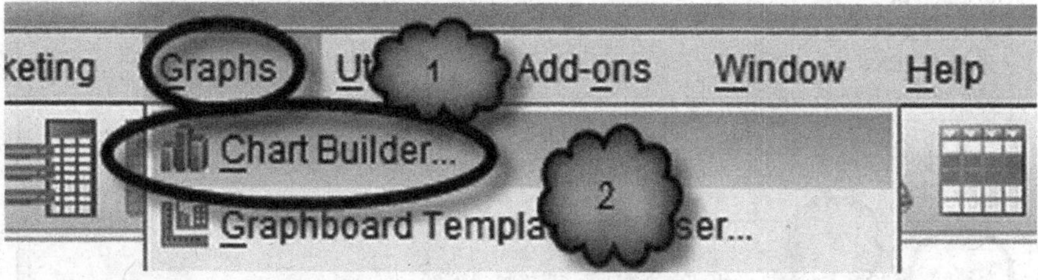

Fig. 3.20 Selecting the chart builder

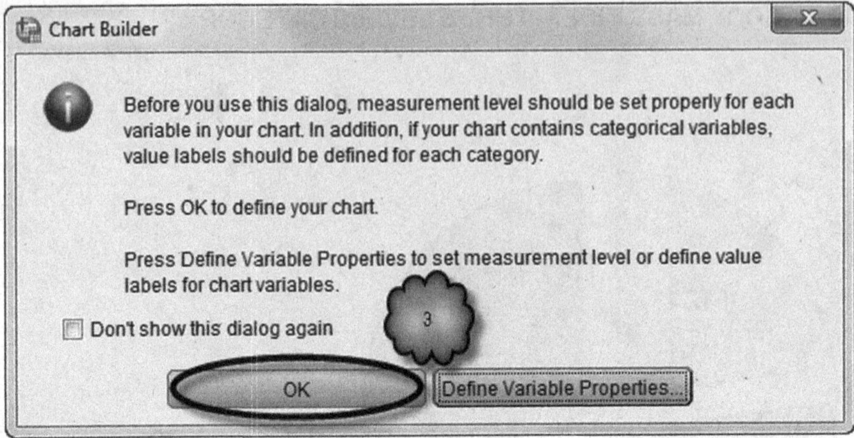

Fig. 3.21 Accepting existing variable properties

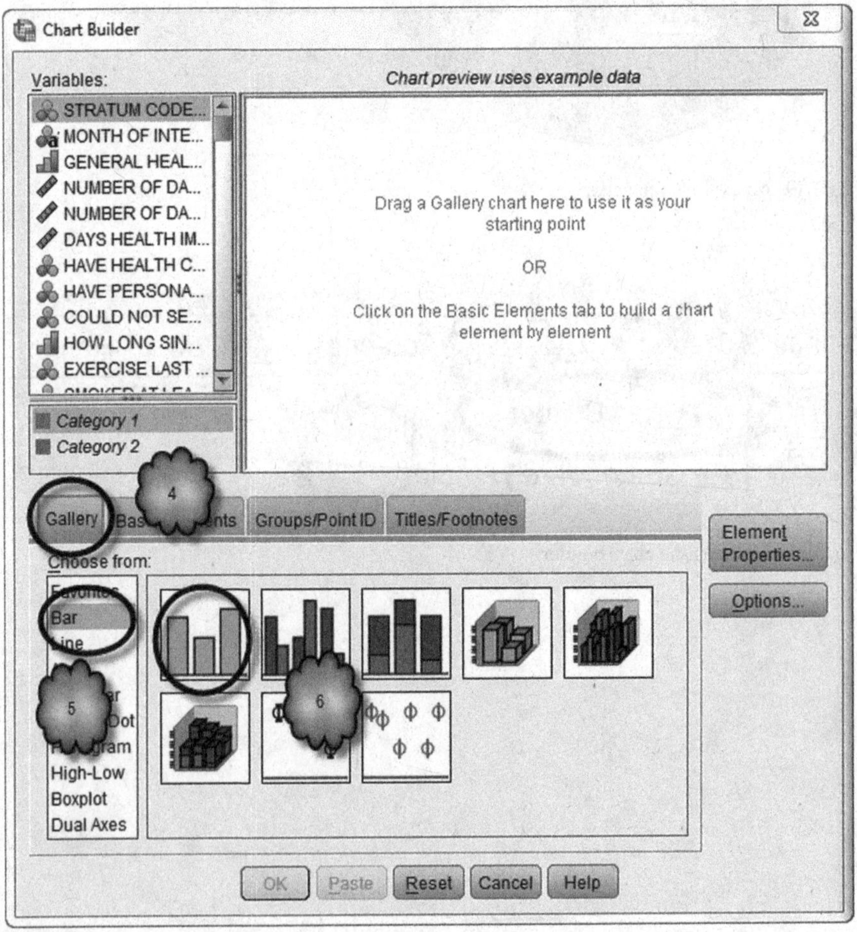

Fig. 3.22 Selecting a bar chart

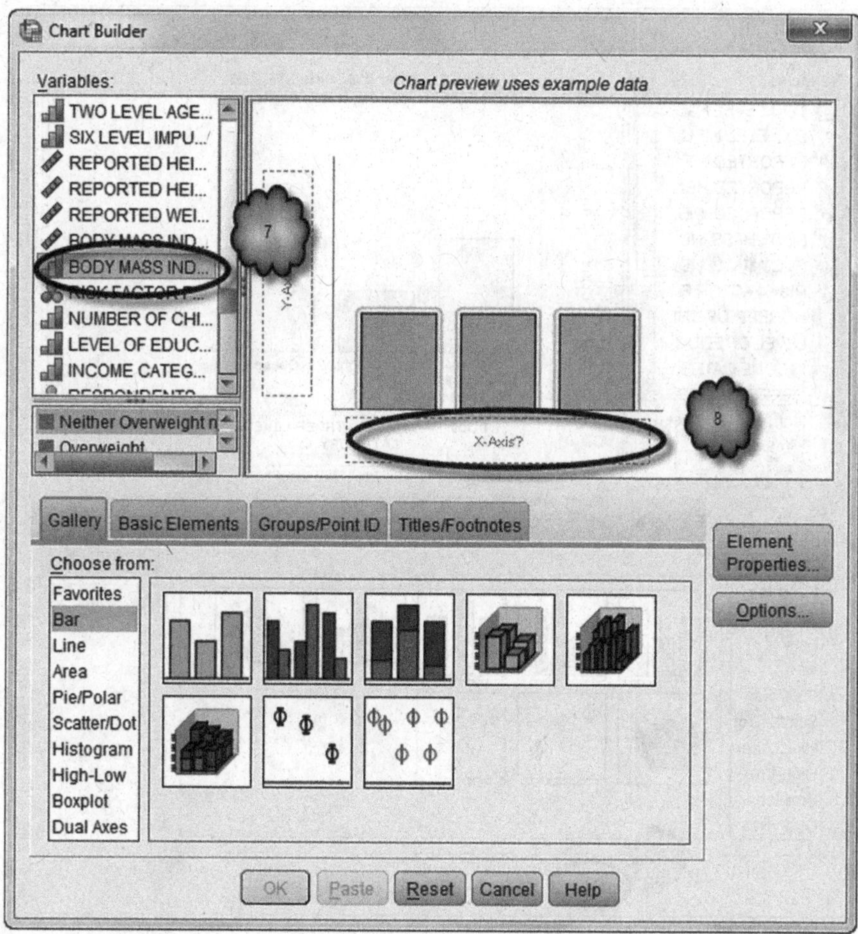

Fig. 3.23 Selecting the variable to plot

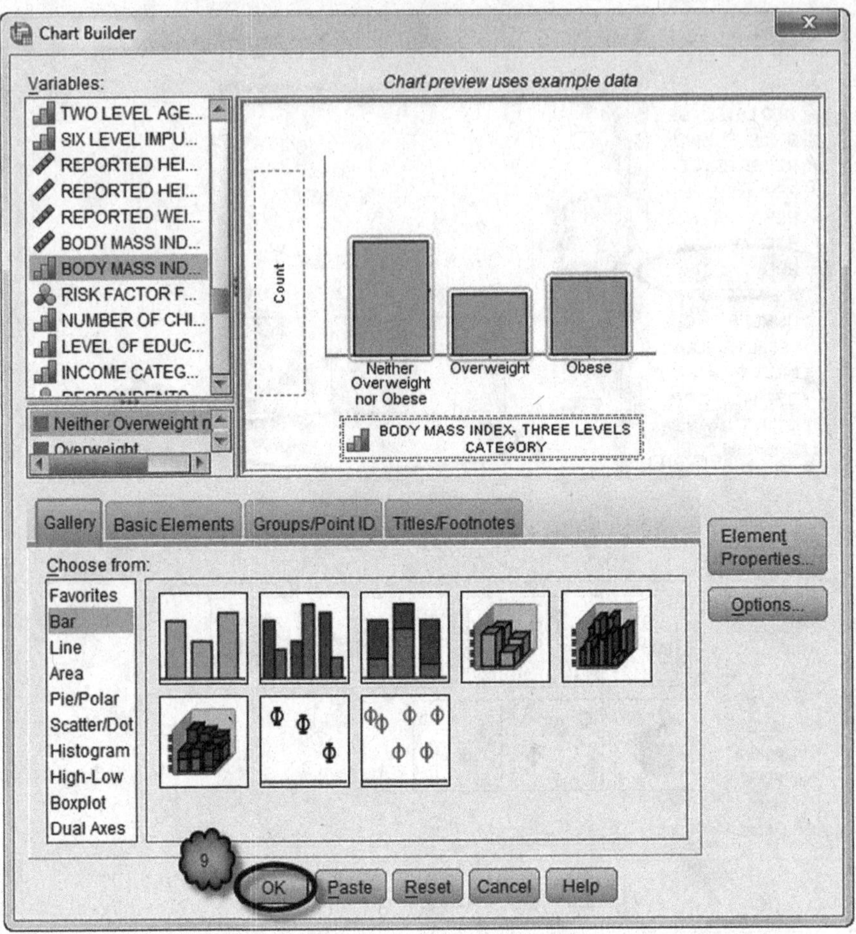

Fig. 3.24 Drawing the bar chart

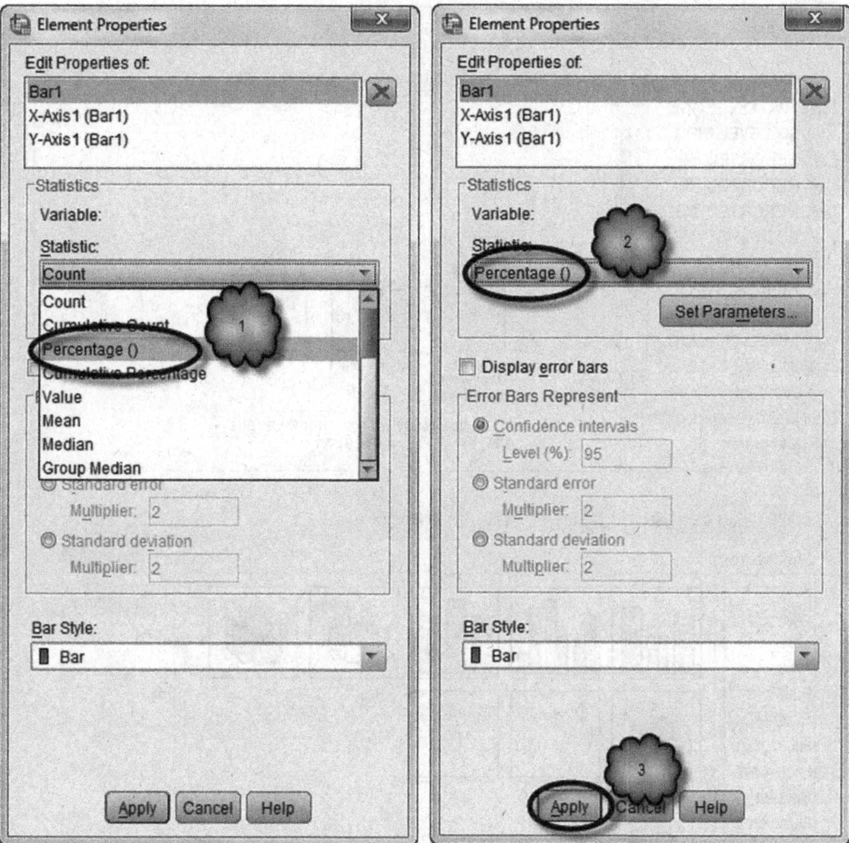

Fig. 3.25 Creating a bar chart of percentages

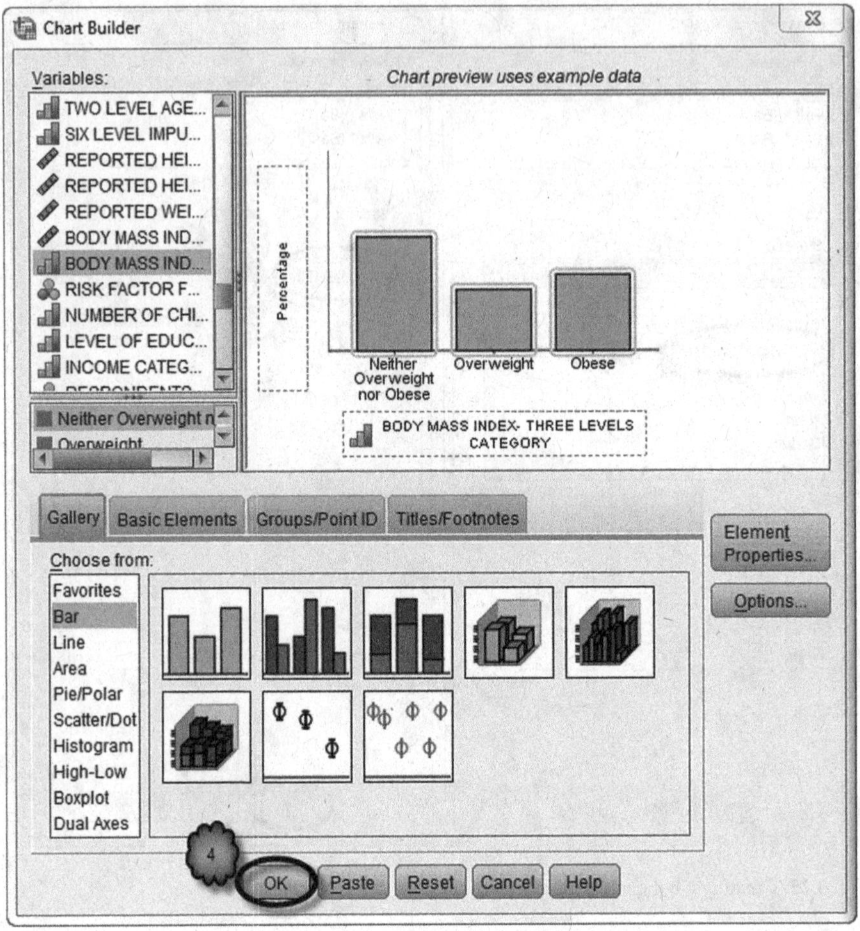

Fig. 3.26 Drawing the bar chart of percentages

Fig. 3.27 Selecting the recode procedure

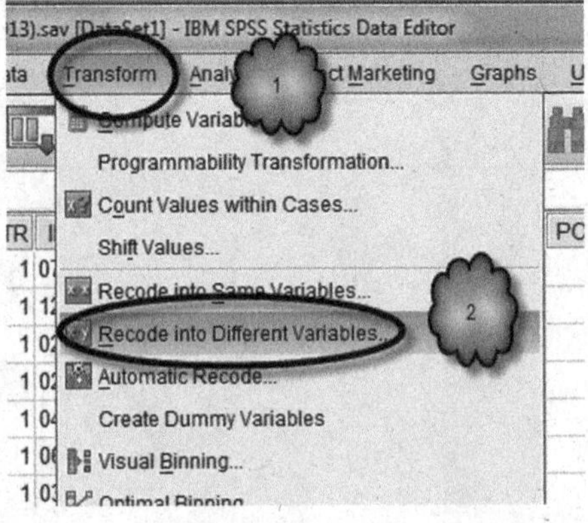

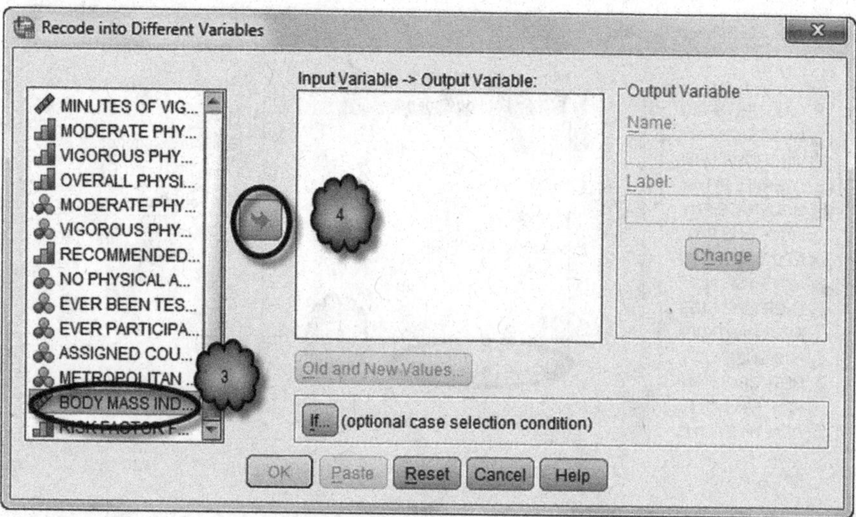

Fig. 3.28 Selecting the variable to recode

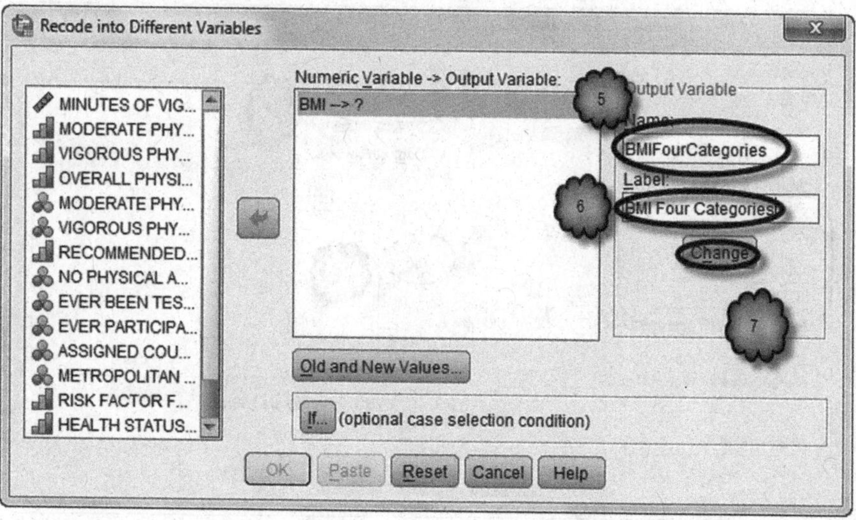

Fig. 3.29 Creating the new variable name and label

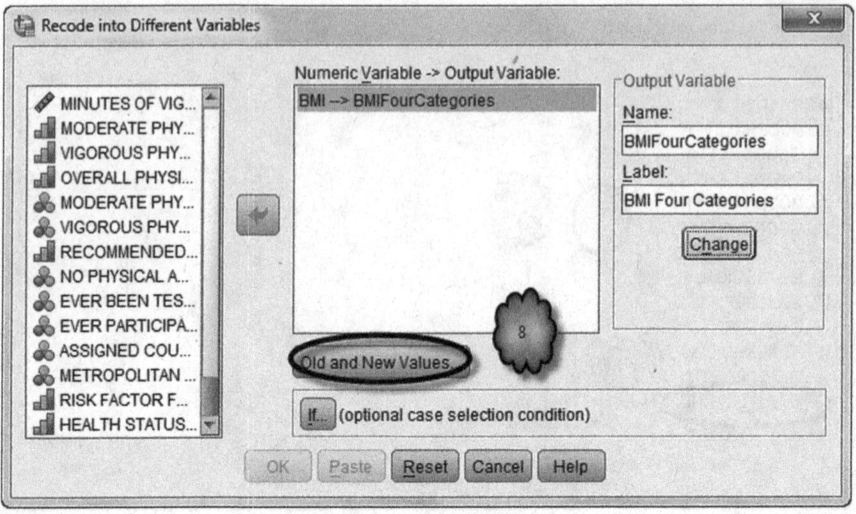

Fig. 3.30 Selecting the define old and new values dialog

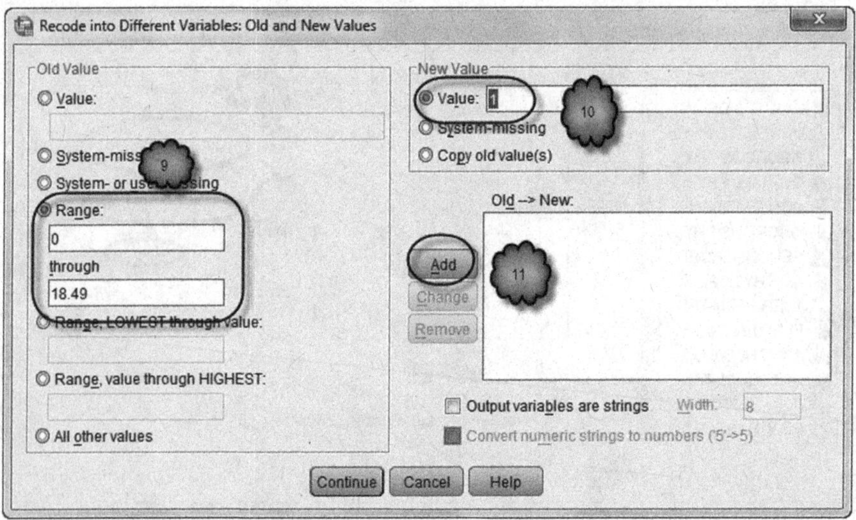

Fig. 3.31 Creating the underweight category

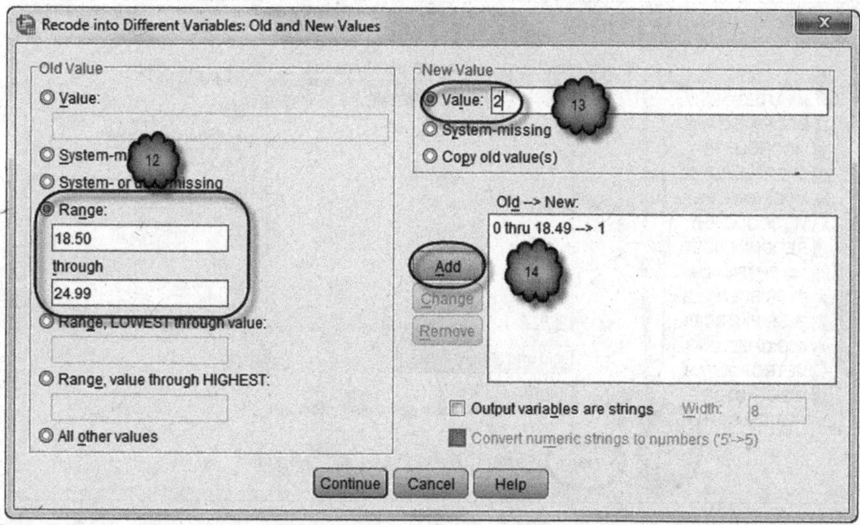

Fig. 3.32 Creating the normal category

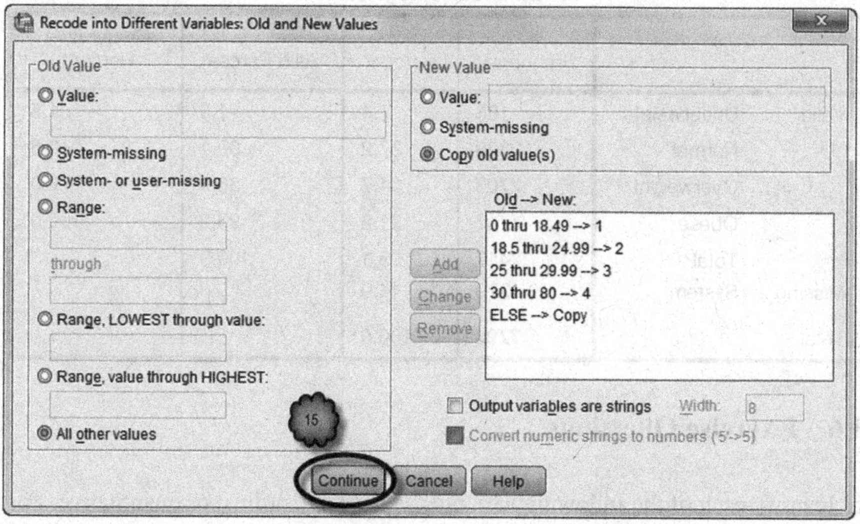

Fig. 3.33 Completing the new variable definition

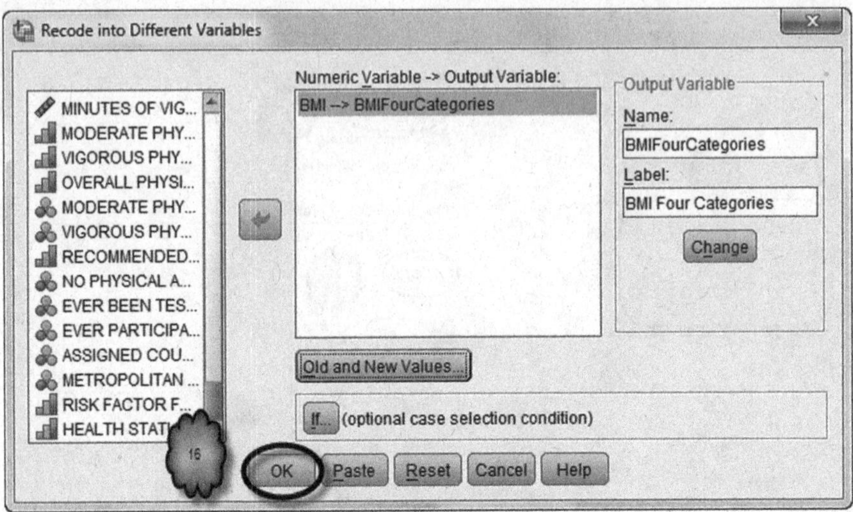

Fig. 3.34 Creating the new variable

Table 3.1 Analysis of recoded variable

BMI Four Categories

		Frequency	Percent	Valid Percent	Cumulative Percent
Valid	Underweight	108	1.4	1.5	1.5
	Normal	2899	37.2	39.1	40.5
	Overweight	2703	34.7	36.4	77.0
	Obese	1707	21.9	23.0	100.0
	Total	7417	95.1	100.0	
Missing	System	379	4.9		
Total		7796	100.0		

3.6 Exercise Questions

1. Identify each of the following variables as nominal, ordinal or quantitative. For each, explain your answer.

   a. Body temperature
   b. Blood type
   c. Blood pressure
   d. Cause of death
   e. Disease stage (e.g., mild, moderate or severe)

Table 3.2 Frequency table for life satisfaction

LIFE SATISFACTION

		Frequency	Percent	Valid Percent	Cumulative Percent
Valid	Satisfied or Very Satisfied	6840	87.7	93.9	93.9
	Dissatisfied or Very Dissatisfied	445	5.7	6.1	100.0
	Total	7285	93.4	100.0	
Missing	7	46	.6		
	9	19	.2		
	System	446	5.7		
	Total	511	6.6		
Total		7796	100.0		

2. Conduct a frequency analysis of the variable, **SATISFACTION W/LIFE** [*LSATISFY*] (variable 50; 1= Very satisfied; 2= Satisfied, 3= Dissatisfied, 4= Very dissatisfied; 7 and 9 are missing values).
3. Generate a bar chart of percentages for a new variable called **LIFE SATISFACTION**. The new variable will have two categories. The first category will be called "Satisfied or Very Satisfied." The second category will be called "Dissatisfied or Very Dissatisfied."
4. Table 3.2 displays the frequency table for the variable, **LIFE SATISFACTION**. Answer the following questions.
   a. What percentage of the sample gave valid responses?
   b. What is a "valid" response?
   c. What percentage of the sample is dissatisfied or very dissatisfied?
5. Figure 3.35 displays three pie charts of the distribution of **LIFE SATISFACTION**. One is for married people, one for those who are divorced, and one for those who are separated.
   a. According to these data, would you say that adult New York residents in 2005 were generally satisfied or dissatisfied with their lives? Explain.
   b. According to these data, does it appear that life satisfaction has something to do with marital status? Explain.

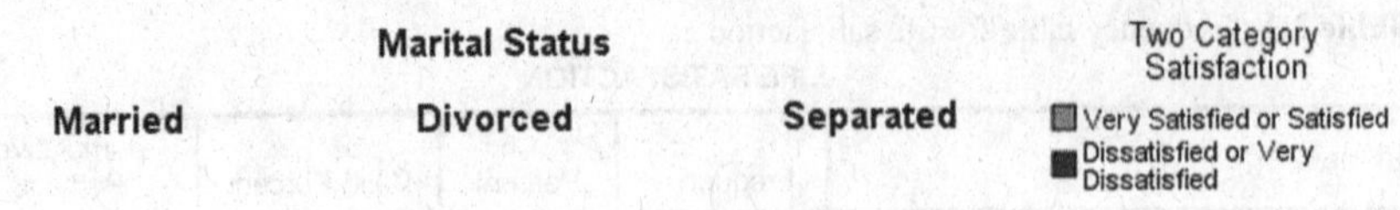

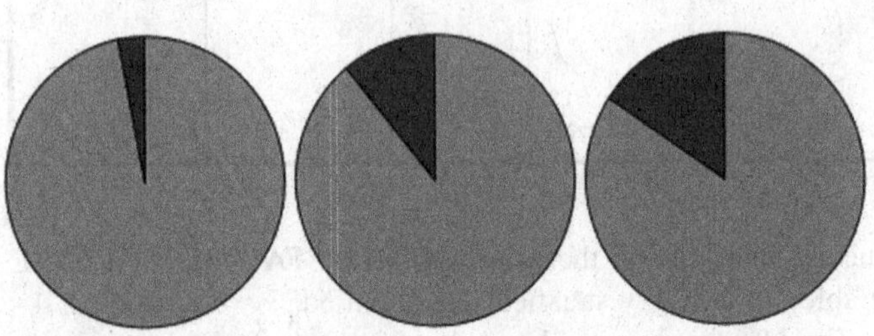

Fig. 3.35 Pie charts of the distribution of life satisfaction

Data Set and Reference

1. CDC BRFSS.sav obtained from: Centers for Disease Control and Prevention (CDC): Behavioral risk factor surveillance system survey data. US Department of Health and Human Services, Centers for Disease Control and Prevention, Atlanta, Georgia (2005). Public domain. For more information about the BRFSS, visit http://www.cdc.gov/brfss/. Accessed 16 Nov 2014

Chapter 4
Describing the Distribution of a Quantitative Variable

Abstract This chapter reviews measures of central tendency and spread, and graphical techniques that are commonly used to describe the distributions of quantitative data. Included are the arithmetic mean and median; interquartile range, variance and standard deviation; skewness, kurtosis, and outliers; and histograms, stem-and-leaf plots, box plots, and clustered bar charts. The standard error of the mean and the 95 % confidence interval are described briefly. The chapter concludes with a discussion of transformations and the geometric mean.

4.1 Overview

We pointed out in Chap. 3 that it is difficult to make sense of data without the use of descriptive statistics and graphs. In that chapter, we learned about frequency tables and bar and pie charts. However, the variables we studied were categorical. When describing the distribution of a quantitative variable, a different set of tools is required. In this chapter, we will review many of the descriptive statistics and graphical techniques for quantitative data.

Most of the descriptive statistics for a quantitative variable focus on data *within a single sample*. Some of these statistics focus on the overall shape of the distribution of the data within the sample. Others, called *measures of central tendency,* focus on the typical score within the sample. Still others, called *measures of spread,* attend to the variability of the sample scores. Other descriptive statistics focus on the variability of sample characteristics *across different samples* randomly drawn from the same population. Perhaps the most important of these are those that focus on the extent to which the mean of a set of scores varies from one sample to the next. In this chapter, we will study these various measures. We will also study some of the graphical methods for displaying the distribution of quantitative data: the *stem-and-leaf plot,* the *histogram,* and the *box plot*. Stem-and-leaf plots and histograms display the shape of the distribution of data. Box plots are useful for determining if the distribution of the data is skewed or symmetric and also whether there are any extreme observations, called *outliers*.

We will begin with data from residents of NY state in 2005 who were interviewed by the Centers for Disease Control and Prevention Behavioral Risk Factor

W. H. Holmes, W. C. Rinaman, *Statistical Literacy for Clinical Practitioners,*
DOI 10.1007/978-3-319-12550-3_4

Surveillance System (BRFSS). This is the same data set that we used in the previous chapter. This time we will focus on the respondents' body mass index (BMI). We will complete the chapter by turning to another data set. These data come from a study of the diagnostic value of prostate-specific antigen levels.

4.2 Describing the Distribution of a Sample

Load the data file, **CDC BRFSS.sav** [1], into. Select **SPSS Analyze > Descriptive Statistics > Explore** to bring up the *Explore* dialog box. Move **BODY MASS INDEX** [*BMI*] (variable 107) into the *Dependent List* box. In the *Display* area, check *Both* (in order to generate both statistics and graphs). Click the **Statistics** button to open the *Explore: Statistics* dialog box and check *Descriptives* and *Percentiles*. Click **Continue** to return to the main dialog box. Now click **Plots** to bring up the *Explore: Plots* dialog box. In the *Boxplots* area, select *Factor levels together*. In the *Descriptive* area, check *Stem-and-leaf* and *Histogram*. Return to the main dialog box by clicking **Continue**. Run the analysis by clicking **OK**. These steps are depicted in Figs. 4.1, 4.2, 4.3, 4.4, 4.5, 4.6 and 4.7.

Descriptive Statistics Study the resulting output. It contains a lot of information. We will begin with the descriptive statistics.

The *Case Processing Summary* (Table 4.1) tells the number of valid responses for the variable and the number of missing cases.

The *Descriptives* table (Table 4.2) gives the descriptive statistics. We will look at each one.

- **Mean** The mean is the arithmetic average of the data. It is a measure of central tendency, meaning that it is one way to describe where the data are centered. It should be used when the data are relatively symmetric and there are no outliers.

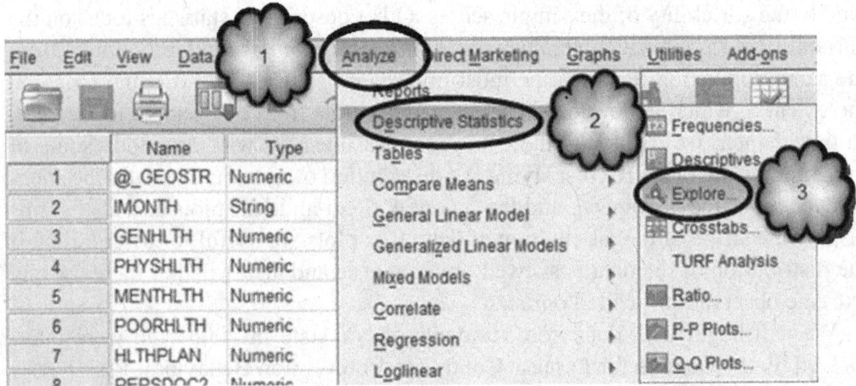

Fig. 4.1 Selecting Explore

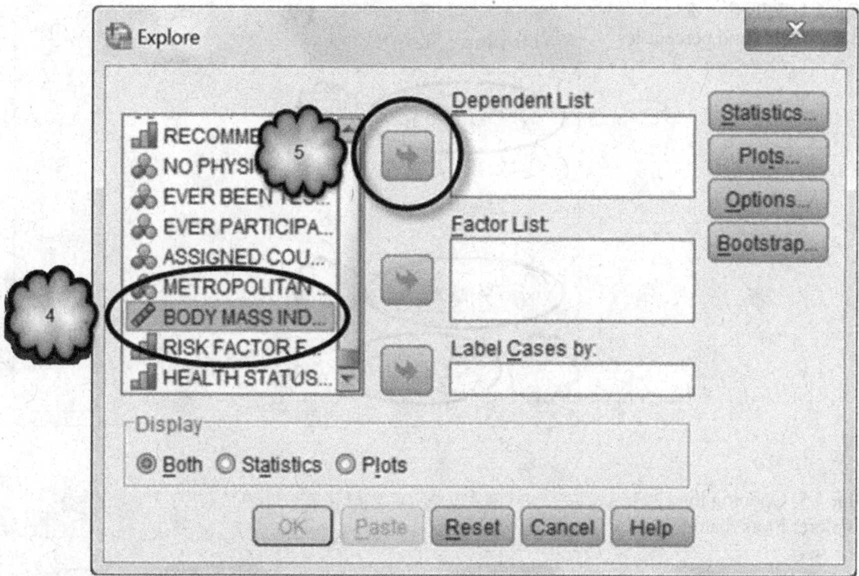

Fig. 4.2 Selecting the quantitative variable

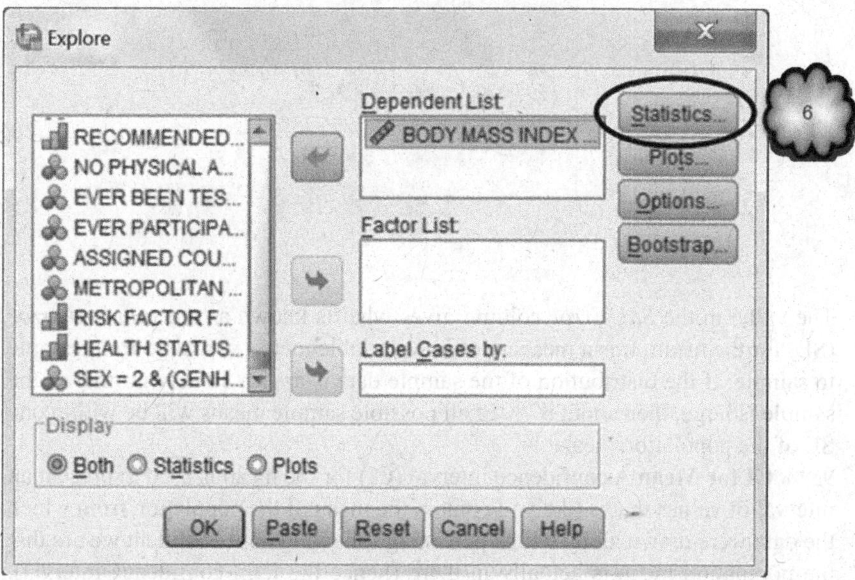

Fig. 4.3 Opening the Explore: Statistics dialog

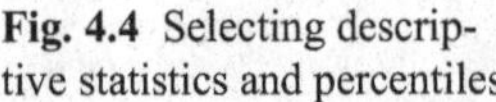
Fig. 4.4 Selecting descriptive statistics and percentiles

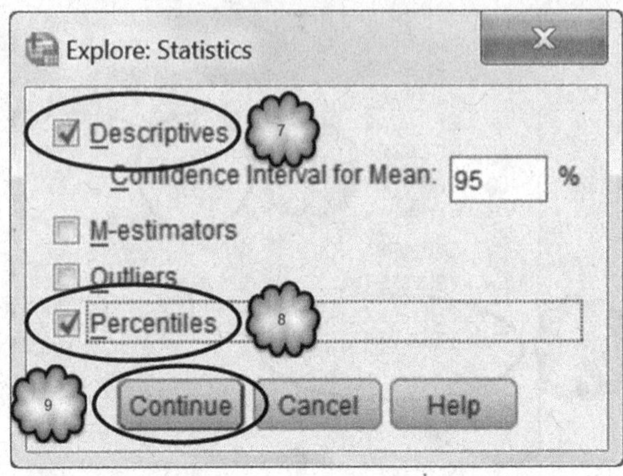

Fig. 4.5 Opening the Explore: Plots dialog

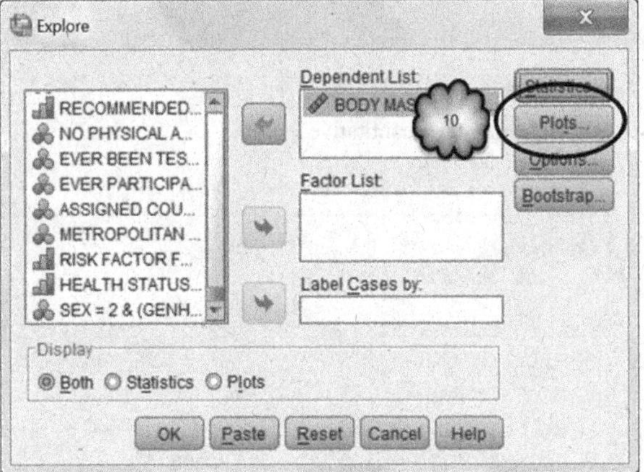

The value in the *Std. Error* column gives what is known as the *standard error* (SE) for the mean. It is a measure of how variable means would be from sample to sample. If the distribution of the sample data is approximately normal or the sample is large, then about 67 % of all possible sample means will be within one SE of the population mean.

- **95 % CI for Mean** A confidence interval (CI) for the mean is used to present an interval of values that is likely to contain the mean of the population from which the data were drawn along with a percentage showing how confident we are that the population mean is actually in there (hence the term confidence interval). The interpretation of the CI begins with the fact that there are a large number of samples than can be taken from the population. If we were to construct 95 % CIs for each one of these samples, then 95 % of these intervals would contain the population mean and 5 % would not. These will be discussed in more detail in the next chapter.

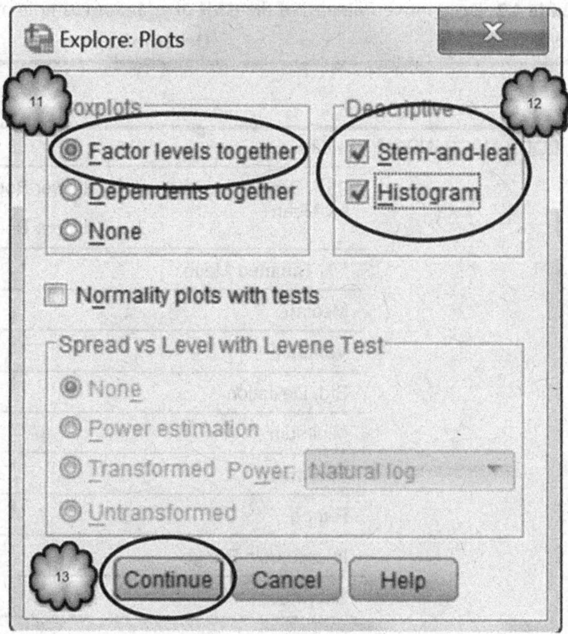

Fig. 4.6 Selecting a boxplot, a stem-and-leaf plot and a histogram

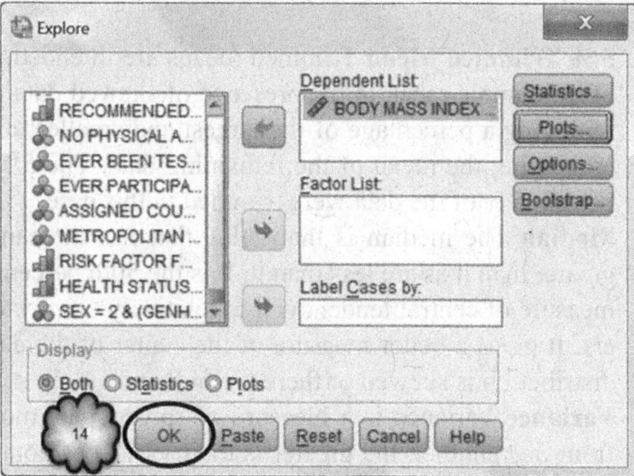

Fig. 4.7 Executing the explore procedure

Table 4.1 Number of valid and missing cases associated with the BMI of a random sample of NY state residents

Case Processing Summary

	Cases					
	Valid		Missing		Total	
	N	Percent	N	Percent	N	Percent
BODY MASS INDEX	7417	95.1%	379	4.9%	7796	100.0%

Table 4.2 Descriptive statistics of the BMI of a random sample of NY state residents

Descriptives

			Statistic	Std. Error
BODY MASS INDEX	Mean		26.8767	.06467
	95% Confidence Interval for Mean	Lower Bound	26.7499	
		Upper Bound	27.0034	
	5% Trimmed Mean		26.4811	
	Median		25.8800	
	Variance		31.024	
	Std. Deviation		5.56992	
	Minimum		9.63	
	Maximum		70.01	
	Range		60.38	
	Interquartile Range		6.42	
	Skewness		1.355	.028
	Kurtosis		3.584	.057

- **5 % Trimmed Mean** Trimmed means are intended to keep the good properties of the sample mean in the presence of skewed data or outliers. They do this by removing a percentage of the largest and smallest observations (trimming) and computing the mean of the remaining data. The 5 % indicates that the top and bottom 5 % of the data were trimmed in this case.
- **Median** The median is that value that has the same number of observations greater than it as are less than it. It is the 50th percentile of the data. It is another measure of central tendency. It is relatively unaffected by skewed data or outliers. It gives a better measure of the center of the data than the mean when the distribution is skewed or there are outliers.
- **Variance** Variance is a measure of spread. The more that sample scores vary from one another, the greater is their variance. Roughly speaking it is approximately the average squared distance between each observation and the mean.
- **Std. Deviation** The standard deviation is also a measure of spread. It is the square root of the variance. It is generally used more than the variance because it has the same units as the data. It should be used in those situations where you would use the mean to measure the center.
- **Minimum** The minimum, as its name implies, is the smallest observation in the data.
- **Maximum** The maximum, as its name implies, is the largest observation in the data.
- **Range** The range is a third measure of spread. It is the difference between the maximum and the minimum. Thus, it is the distance spanned by the data. It is easy to compute, but it is very sensitive to outliers.

- **Interquartile Range** The interquartile range is the difference between the 75th percentile and the 25th percentile of the data. The 25th, 50th, and 75th percentiles are known as the first, second, and third quartiles, respectively. So, the interquartile range is the distance between the first and third quartiles. That is, it is the distance spanned by the middle 50 % of the data. Like the median, it is relatively unaffected by outliers and should be used in those situations where you would use the median to measure the center of the data.
- **Skewness** Skewness is a measure of the shape of the distribution. It is a measure of asymmetry. The normal distribution is symmetric and has a skewness value of 0. A distribution that is positively skewed has a long right tail, while a distribution that is negatively skewed has a long left tail. According to SPSS, "a skewness value more than twice its standard error is taken to indicate a departure from symmetry." A positively skewed distribution will have a positive skewness, and a negatively skewed distribution will have a negative skewness.
- **Kurtosis** Kurtosis is a measure of the extent to which observations pile up around a central point. It is also called *peakedness.* Again, the standard of comparison is the normal distribution. Normal distributions have zero kurtosis. Distributions that have positive kurtosis cluster more and have longer tails than those in the normal distribution, while distributions that have negative kurtosis cluster less and have shorter tails.

The *Percentiles* table (Table 4.3) gives various percentiles for the data. The top row of the table gives the 5th, 10th, 25th, 50th, 75th, 90th, and 95th percentiles computed using a weighted average method. The percentiles computed using this method are the ones used to compute the interquartile range. The percentiles referred to as *Tukey's hinges* compute the 50th percentile in the same manner as the weighted average method. The 25th percentile, however, is obtained by finding the median of all the observations that fall below the median of the entire sample, and the 75th percentile is obtained by finding the median of all the observations that fall above the median of the entire sample.

Graphical Techniques Now let us look at the various graphs that are included in the output.

- **Histogram** Figure 4.8 displays a histogram. A histogram shows the shape of the distribution. The range of the data is broken up into a number of equal width subintervals called *bins*. The number of observations in each bin is determined, and a bar whose height is proportional to the number of observations in each bin is drawn over each bin. The mean, standard deviation, and sample size are displayed to the right of the plot.

Table 4.3 Percentiles of the BMI of a sample of NY state residents

Percentiles

		Percentiles						
		5	10	25	50	75	90	95
Weighted Average (Definition 1)	BODY MASS INDEX	19.7800	20.9220	23.0650	25.8800	29.4800	34.0400	37.2800
Tukey's Hinges	BODY MASS INDEX			23.0700	25.8800	29.4800		

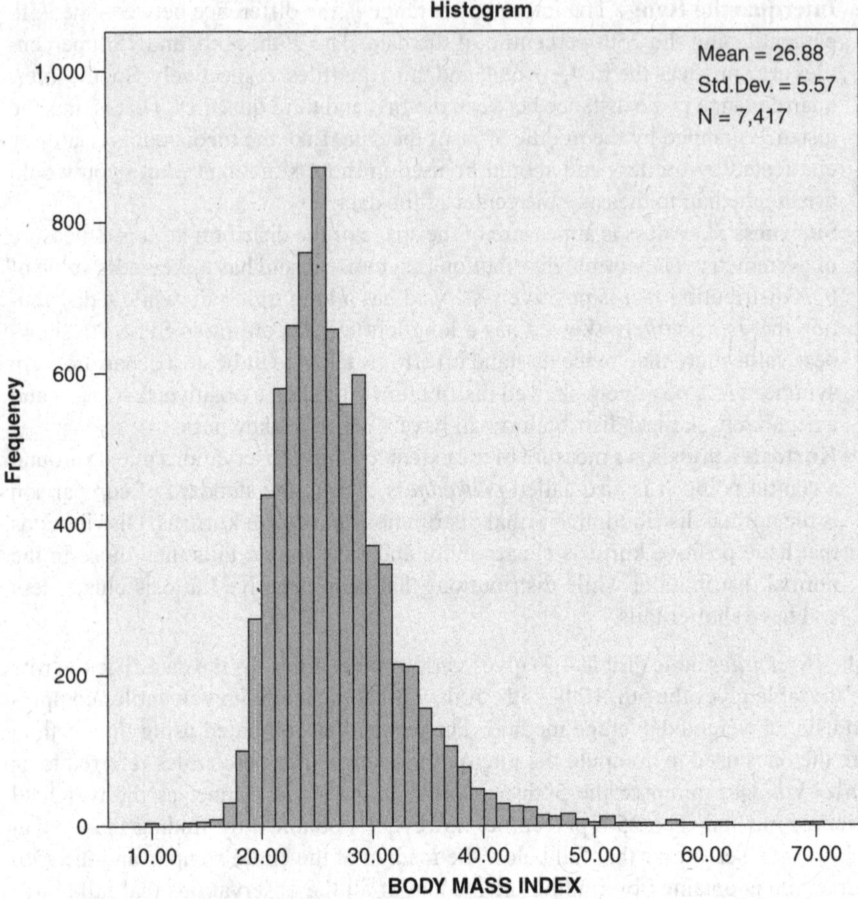

Fig. 4.8 Histogram of the BMI of a sample of NY state residents

- **Stem-and-leaf plot** Figure 4.9 displays a stem-and-leaf plot. It too shows the shape of the distribution of the data in a manner similar to a histogram, only rotated 90° clockwise. It has the additional feature that it orders the data. The values of the observations are subdivided into two parts—the stems and the leaves. For example, an observation of 78 might be divided so that the tens digit, 7, is the stem and the units digit, 8, is the leaf. The possible stems are listed on the left, and all of the leaves for each stem are listed to the right of the stem. The leaves are then ordered in ascending order from left to right. The numbers in the extreme left column are the number of observations in each stem. For example, there are 38 observations in the 17 stem.

- **Box plot** Figure 4.10 displays the final item in the output, a box plot of the data. It is useful for determining if the data are skewed or symmetric and for detecting

```
  2.00 Extremes    (=<13.4)
  3.00        14 .  &
  7.00        15 .  &
 17.00        16 .  6&
 38.00        17 .  67&&
115.00        18 .  0123355668899&
241.00        19 .  00112222344455556666777888 9
342.00        20 .  0011112222333444445556666777888888999
541.00        21 .  000000001111122333333334445555555566666666677788888899999 9
500.00        22 .  000001111222233333333344555555666666677777788888899999
603.00        23 .  0000000111111222222333333444444555566666666777777777888888889999
598.00        24 .  00000000001122222223333333344444444444444444555666677778888888899999
822.00        25 .  000000000000111111111111111111111112223344445555566666777777888888888888888888888888999999999
539.00        26 .  0011122233333344445555555555566666666666666666666666666678899
509.00        27 .  00011111112333333334444444444444455555555555556677788889999
460.00        28 .  00001111222223333333333344444444445556677777788899999
373.00        29 .  00001111222222233333333344566666777888 9999
338.00        30 .  00000011111112223444445667777778889999
254.00        31 .  00011122233333334556666778999
207.00        32 .  01111233333455666678 8999
165.00        33 .  0001233334555778 99&
137.00        34 .  002234445567889&
134.00        35 .  002233555557 9&
 79.00        36 .  01235666&
 86.00        37 .  012335668&
 51.00        38 .  014678&
  6.00        39 .  0
250.00 Extremes    (>=39.1)

Stem width:       1.00
Each leaf:        9 case(5)
```

Fig. 4.9 Stem-and-leaf plot of the BMI of a sample of NY state residents

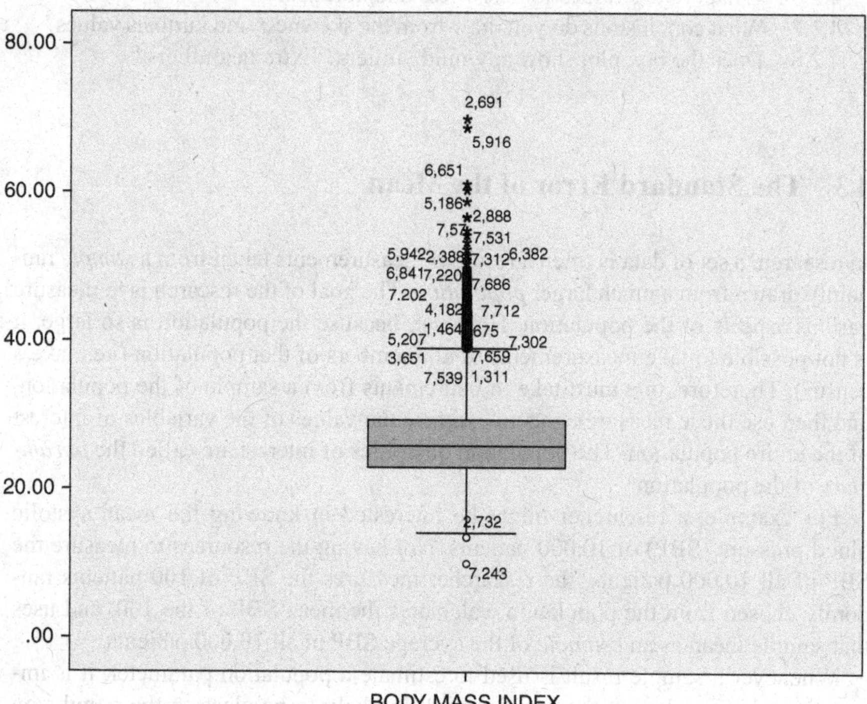

Fig. 4.10 Box plot of the BMI of a sample of NY state residents

outliers in the data. It consists of a box that uses the first quartile (the 25th percentile) as its lower boundary and the third quartile (the 75th percentile) as its upper boundary. A line is drawn in the box at the median (the 50th percentile). Next, lines called *whiskers* are drawn from each end of the box to a point determined by the width of the box. Finally, each observation that has a value more extreme than the whiskers is drawn with either a circle or an asterisk. These are outliers. Outliers with a circle are designated as *mild outliers,* and those with asterisks are designated as *extreme outliers.* The numbers are the case numbers in the data of the outliers.

Now that we have reviewed the output, see if you can answer the following questions:

4.2.1 How many respondents were included in the analysis?
4.2.2 What was the mean BMI? The median?
4.2.3 Do the values of the mean and median suggest that the distribution of BMI scores was skewed? If so, in the positive or negative direction?
4.2.4 Does your answer seem to be confirmed by the histogram or stem-and-leaf plot? How so?
4.2.5 What was the interquartile range? What BMI scores were its lower and upper boundaries?
4.2.6 What are the values for skewness and kurtosis?
4.2.7 What conclusions do you draw from the skewness and kurtosis values?
4.2.8 Does the box plot show any mild outliers? Extreme outliers?

4.3 The Standard Error of the Mean

In research, a set of data is often a result of measurements taken from a *sample* randomly drawn from a much larger *population.* The goal of the research is to measure various aspects of the population. However, because the population is so large, it is not possible to take measurements of all members of that population (i.e., take a census). Therefore, one must take measurements from a sample of the population, and then use those measurements to estimate the values of the variables of interest of the entire population. The population quantities of interest are called the *parameters* of the population.

For example, a researcher might be interested in knowing the mean systolic blood pressure (SBP) of 10,000 patients. Not having the resources to measure the SBP of all 10,000 patients, the researcher measures the SBP of 100 patients randomly chosen from the population, calculates the mean SBP of the 100, and uses that sample mean as an *estimate* of the average SBP of all 10,000 patients.

Whenever a sample result is used to estimate a population parameter, it is important to know whether the sample result is likely to be close to the population value. For example, if we try to estimate the mean SBP of 10,000 patients by using the mean SBP of 100 of those patients, we would want to know if the mean of 100 patients is approximately the same as the mean SBP of all 10,000. We will never know for sure because we will never measure the mean SBP of all 10,000 patients and compare that mean with the average of any given sample of 100 patients. However, we can get a sense of the goodness of the sample mean as an estimate of the population mean by noticing how much sample means vary from one sample to the next. In the output of *Explore* this is estimated by the *Std. Error* of the mean. The interpretation goes as follows. If the distribution is roughly normal or if the sample is large enough (a commonly used rule of thumb is 30 or more), then about 67 % of all sample means based on samples of the same size will be within one SE of the population mean. Furthermore, about 95 % will be within two SEs of the population mean, and about 99 % will be within three SEs of the population mean. So, if you consider the observed SE to be small, then the sample mean is likely to be relatively close to the population mean, but if you consider it to be large, then the sample would not be a very reliable estimate of the population mean.

The smaller the SE, the less the sample mean will vary across samples. Ideally, we want a sample mean that has a very low SE, for such a mean would tell us that its value is close to values of the means that we would obtain if we were to take many samples, and therefore close to the mean of the population from which we drew our sample. However, if the SE is large, we will not have much confidence that our sample mean gives us a good sense of the population mean. After all, how can we trust any particular sample mean as an estimate of the population mean if different samples give us very different results?

Our ability to trust that the average SBP of a sample of patients accurately reflects the average SBP of a population of 10,000 patients from which the sample was taken will be greater the larger our sample. This is because means based on larger samples tend to have smaller SEs. A sample of 200 patients will give us a more reliable estimate of the population SBP than would a sample of 100, for example. In addition, our trust in our sample result will be enhanced the more the SBP of the patients in the sample are similar to one another. This is because means based on samples from populations whose scores have small standard deviations tend to have small SEs. In addition, we should also try to lower the variability in SBP scores by following procedures for measuring blood pressure exactly the same each and every time SBP is measured. Large samples and standardization of measurement are key to reducing SEs and increasing our confidence in our sample means.

To see if you understand the concept of the standard error, tackle the following questions:

4.3.1 What is the standard error of the mean BMI?

4.3.2 If we were to repeat the CDC's interviews of NY state residents and found that the mean BMI was 28, would we be surprised? What about 25? Why?

4.4 Comparing Distributions Across Values of a Categorical Variable

So far we have looked at the distribution of a quantitative variable across an entire sample. However, distributions can vary across subsets of cases within a sample. For example, the distribution of BMI in the CDC sample might covary with the health status of the respondents or with the extent to which they engage in physical activity. In this section we will see if the distribution of BMI covaries with respondents' self-reports of their general health. We will leave the study of the relationship between BMI and physical activity to an exercise question. As before, we will use **Explore** to generate the descriptive statistics, but this time we will use **Chart Builder** to generate the graphs.

Descriptive Statistics Before we begin, be sure that 7 and 9 have been declared as missing values for the variable, **GENERAL HEALTH** [*GENHLTH*] (variable 3; 1=Excellent, …, 5=Poor). Then return to the **Analyze > Descriptive Statistics > Explore** dialog box and, as shown in Figs. 4.11 and 4.12, move **GENERAL HEALTH** into the *Factor List* box. We will be generating graphs with *Chart Builder,* so select *Statistics* in the *Display* area. Click **OK**.

Table 4.4 is an edited version of the resulting descriptives table.

Try answering the following questions:

4.4.1 Judging from the resulting table of descriptive statistics, does there appear to be a relationship between general health and average BMI?

4.4.2 How about between general health and the variability of BMI scores?

4.4.3 How would you describe those relationships?

Box Plots You should have noticed that the central tendency and spread of BMI increased as self-reported health decreased. A box plot can display these increases.

Select **Graphs > Chart Builder** and make your way to the *Chart Builder* dialog box. Then select *Boxplot* in the *Gallery* area. Drag the first box plot option into the window above it. Then drag **BODY MASS INDEX** [*BMI*] (variable 107) to the *Y*-axis and **GENERAL HEALTH** [*GENHLTH*] (variable 3) to the *X*-axis. Click **OK** to generate the box plot. These steps are displayed in Figs. 4.13, 4.14 and 4.15.

The box plot is reproduced in Fig. 4.16.

Answer the following questions:

4.4.4 How can we tell from the box plot that the median BMI increases as reported health varies from excellent to poor?

4.4.5 How can we tell from the box plot that the interquartile range increases as reported health varies from excellent to poor?

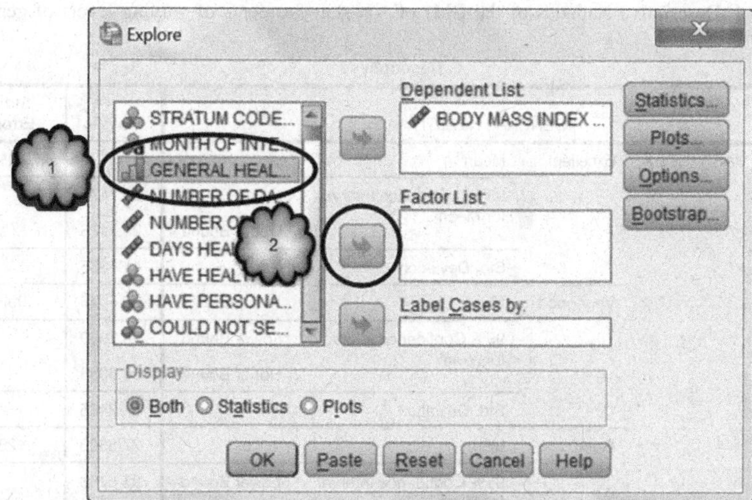

Fig. 4.11 Selecting a factor in Explore

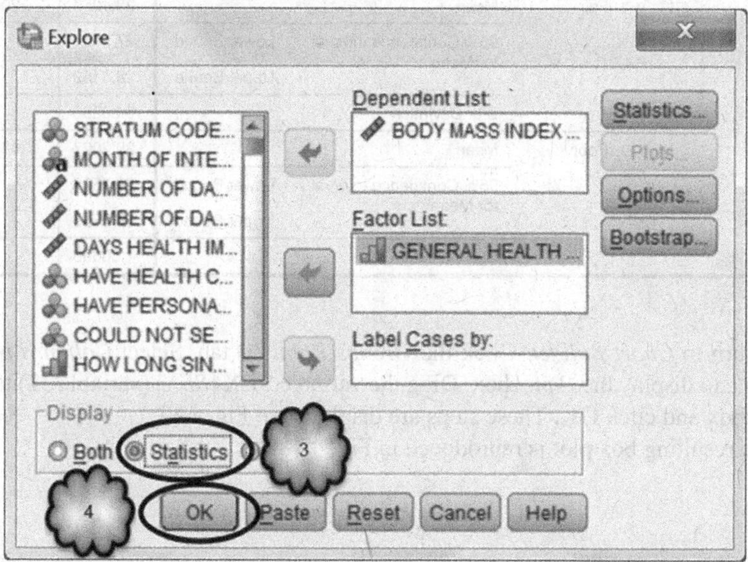

Fig. 4.12 Requesting output in Explore that displays statistics but not graphs

In the box plot of Fig. 4.16, the horizontal lines within the boxes and the heights of those boxes show the increases in the medians and interquartile ranges of BMI across the values of a single categorical variable. Box plots can also display distributions across levels of more than one categorical variable. For example, a box plot can display the relationship between BMI and general health for each gender.

Table 4.4 Descriptive statistics of the BMI of NY state residents of varying levels of general health

Descriptives

GENERAL HEALTH				Statistic	Std. Error
BODY MASS INDEX	Excellent	Mean		24.9477	.10198
		95% Confidence Interval for Mean	Lower Bound	24.7477	
			Upper Bound	25.1478	
		Std. Deviation		4.05865	
	Very good	Mean		26.4026	.09980
		95% Confidence Interval for Mean	Lower Bound	26.2069	
			Upper Bound	26.5983	
		Std. Deviation		4.92465	
	Good	Mean		27.8306	.12940
		95% Confidence Interval for Mean	Lower Bound	27.5768	
			Upper Bound	28.0843	
		Std. Deviation		6.01386	
	Fair	Mean		28.4057	.20867
		95% Confidence Interval for Mean	Lower Bound	27.9961	
			Upper Bound	28.8152	
		Std. Deviation		6.30856	
	Poor	Mean		29.2027	.43187
		95% Confidence Interval for Mean	Lower Bound	28.3529	
			Upper Bound	30.0525	
		Std. Deviation		7.56698	

Return to *Chart Builder.* Click the *Groups/Point ID* tab. Select *Columns panel variable* to display the *Panel* box. Drag the variable **SEX** [*SEX*] (variable 32) to the *Panel* box and click **OK.** These steps are displayed in Fig. 4.17.

The resulting box plot is reproduced in Fig. 4.18.

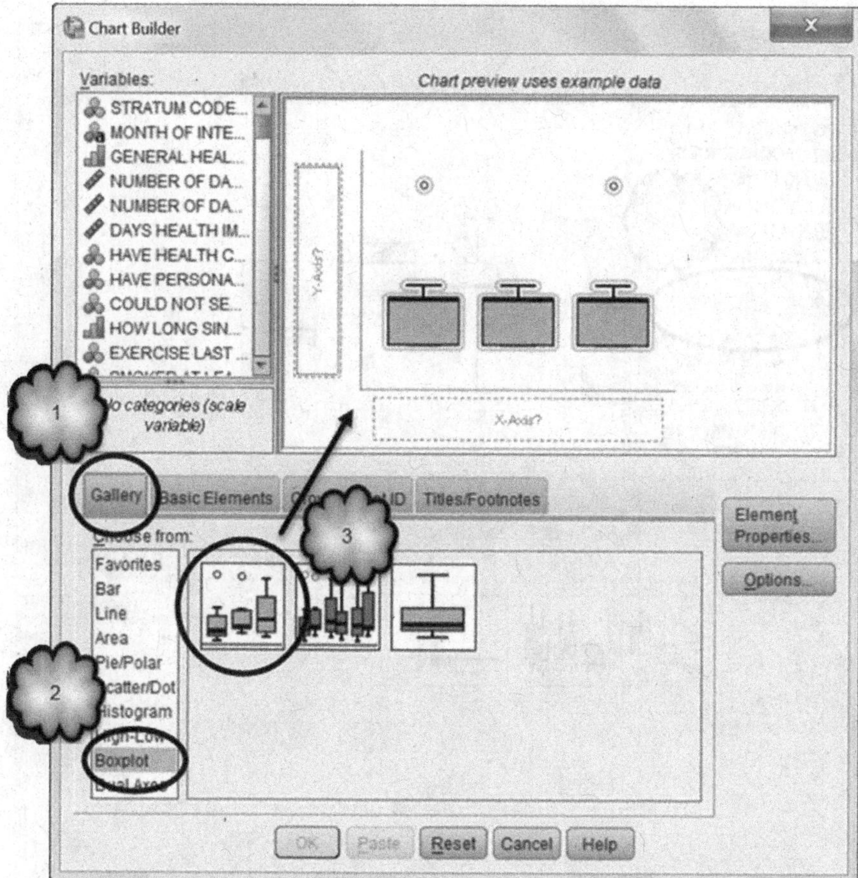

Fig. 4.13 Selecting a box plot in Chart Builder

> 4.4.6 Does the relationship between median BMI and general health seem to be similar for men and women?
> 4.4.7 Does the relationship between the interquartile range and general health seem to be similar for men and women?

Bar Charts Bar charts are frequently used to display various properties of a distribution across values of categorical variables. For example, the mean BMI of male and female respondents across levels of general health can be displayed in a *clustered bar chart*.

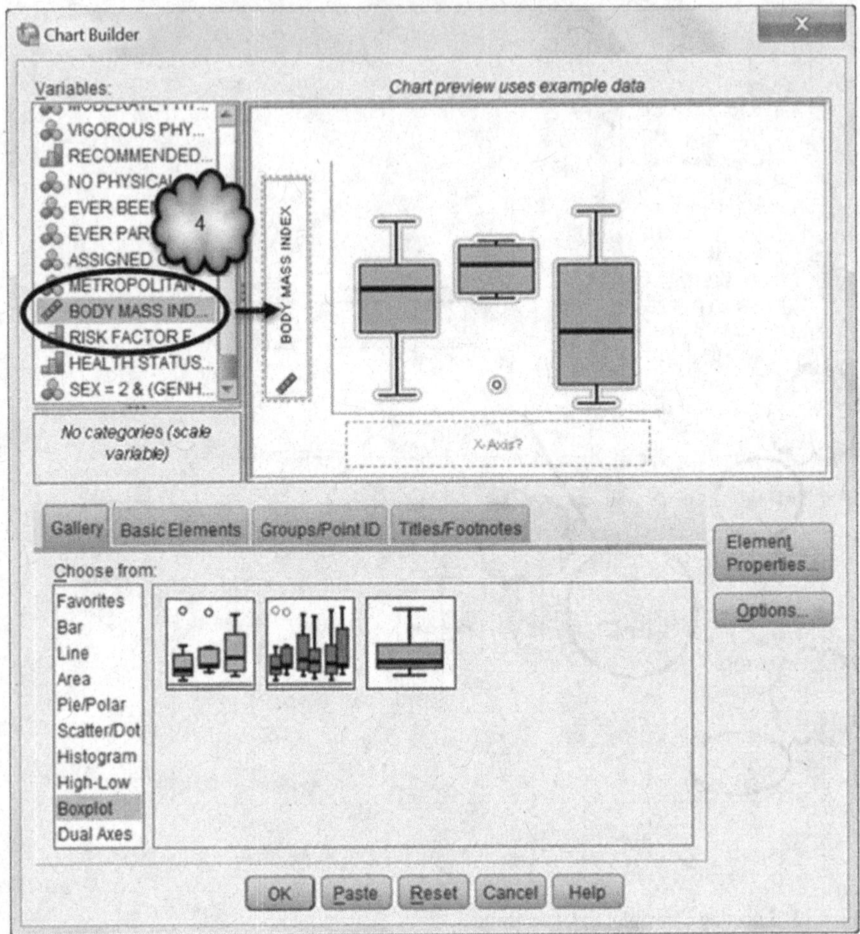

Fig. 4.14 Selecting a variable for the *Y*-axis

Return to *Chart Builder.* Select *Bar* from the *Gallery* and drag the picture of the second bar chart to the window immediately above it. Drag **GENERAL HEALTH** to the *X-Axis* box and drag **BODY MASS INDEX** to the *Y-Axis* box. In order to graph the relationship between BMI and general health separately for men and women, drag the variable, **SEX** into the *Cluster: set color* box. Click **OK** to generate the graph. These steps are displayed in Figs. 4.19, 4.20 and 4.21.

Figure 4.22 displays an edited version of the resulting clustered bar chart. (Because Fig. 4.22 is in grayscale rather than in color, we modified the formatting of the bars representing men and women).

Descriptive statistics other than the mean can also be displayed in a bar chart by making use of the *Element Properties* dialog box that can be found to the right of the *Chart Builder*. For example, in order to plot standard deviations instead of

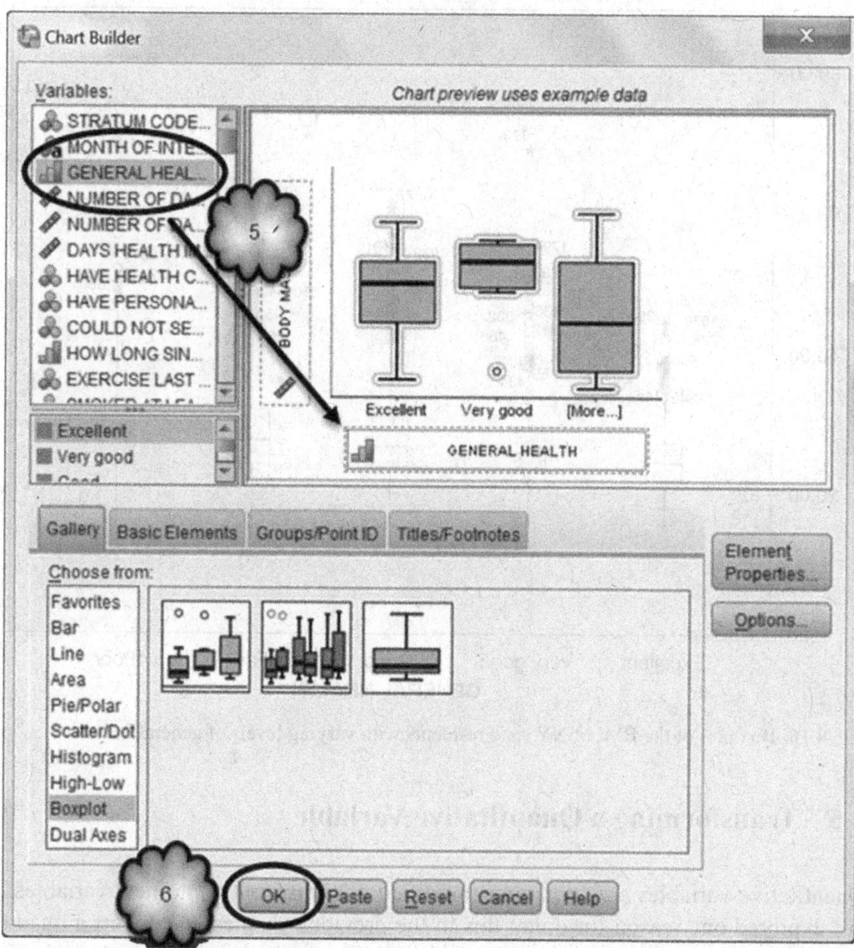

Fig. 4.15 Selecting a variable for the *X*-axis and generating the box plot

means, click *Mean* in the *Statistic* box of the *Element Properties* dialog box and select *Standard Deviation* from the drop down menu. Click **Apply** and notice that the *Y-Axis* box now reads *StdDev BODY MASS INDEX*. Click **OK** to generate a bar chart of standard deviations. These steps are displayed in Figs. 4.23, 4.24 and 4.25.

The clustered bar chart of the standard deviations is displayed in Fig. 4.26.

4.4.8 How would you describe the relationship between mean BMI and general health?

4.4.9 How about the relationship between the standard deviation and general health?

4.4.10 Do these relationships seem to be similar for men and women?

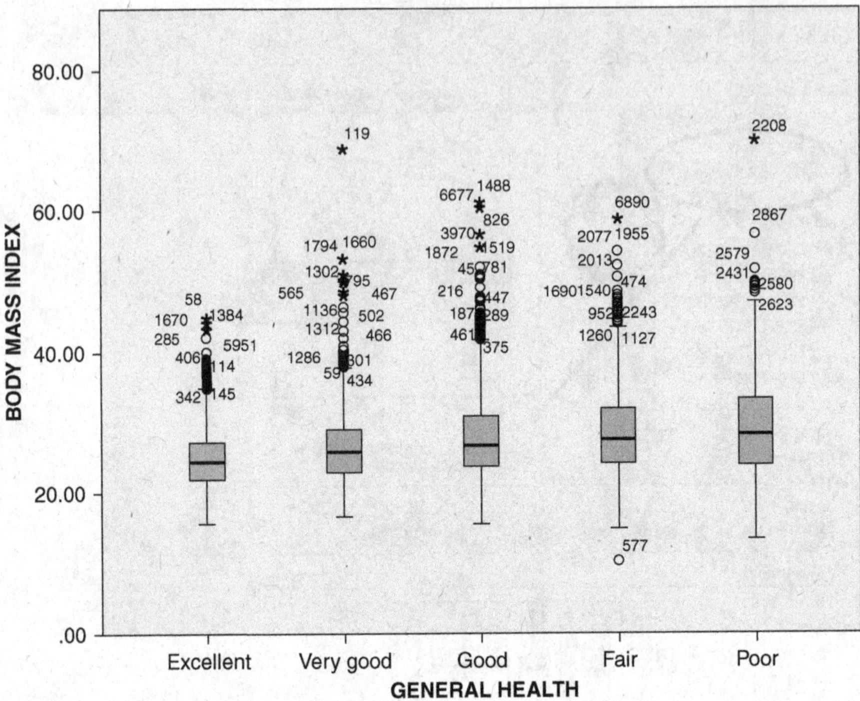

Fig. 4.16 Box plot of the BMI of NY state residents with varying levels of general health

4.5 Transforming a Quantitative Variable

Quantitative variables are sometimes modified or *transformed* into new variables. We explored one reason for doing this in the previous chapter: to convert a quantitative variable into a categorical variable. In this section, we will explore three additional reasons: to generate a new quantitative variable, to change the shape of a distribution, and to make the variability of data across two or more groups more nearly equal. To demonstrate, we will use data from a study of prostate cancer.

Generating a new quantitative variable Open **PSA.sav** [2]. This file consists of 301 men who reported to the urology department at the Naval Medical Center San Diego. Their prostate-specific antigen (PSA) levels (in ng/ml) are stored in the variable **Prostate-Specific Antigen Level (ng/ml)** [*psa*] (variable 5), and the volume (in ml) of their prostates is stored in Volume of Prostate (ml) [*vol*] (variable 6). From these two quantitative variables, a new quantitative variable was created, **Prostate-specific Antigen Density Level** [*psad*] (variable 7) in order to determine whether PSA density is superior to PSA levels in detecting the presence of prostate cancer. (In a later chapter, we will conduct an analysis to determine which one was better).

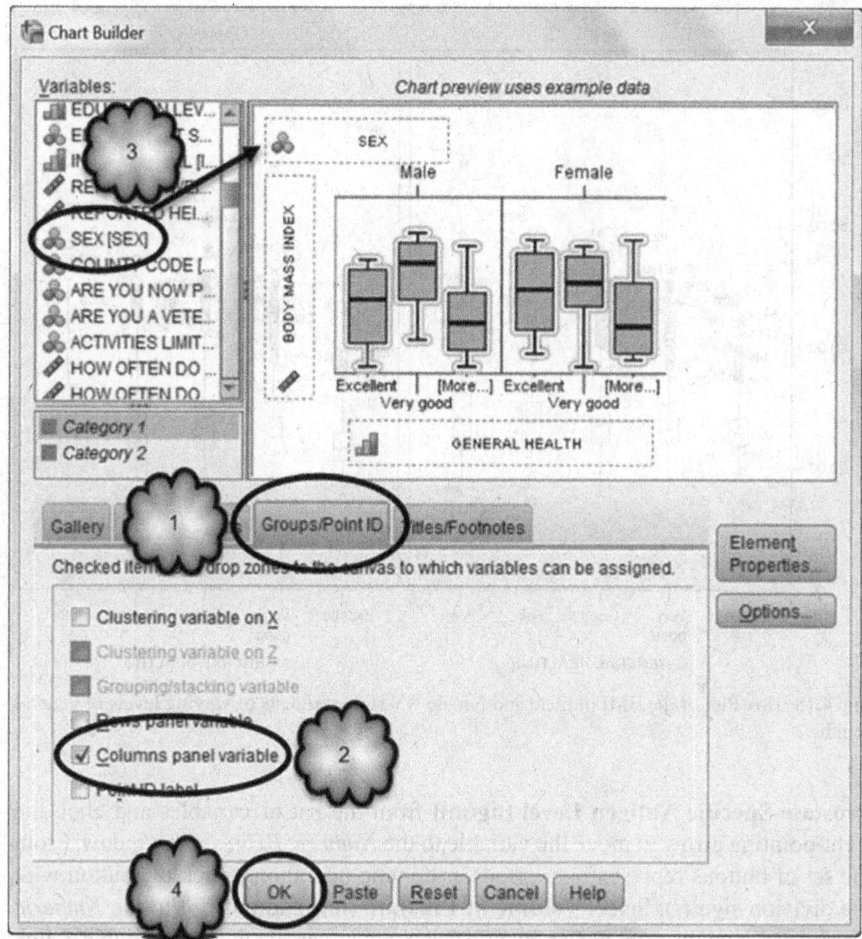

Fig. 4.17 Adding a columns panel variable to a box plot

To create the new variable, each patient's PSA level was divided by the volume of his prostate:

$$psad = psa/vol. \tag{4.1}$$

To conduct this transformation, choose **Transform > Compute Variable** to open the *Compute Variable* dialog box. In the *Target Variable* window, give the new variable a name, such as *PSADensity.* Remember from Chap. 2 that SPSS does not accept spaces in variable names. Next, give the new variable a variable label, such as **PSA Density**, by clicking **Type & Label** to open the *Type & Label* dialog box, entering the label into the *Label* window, and clicking **Continue.** Now select

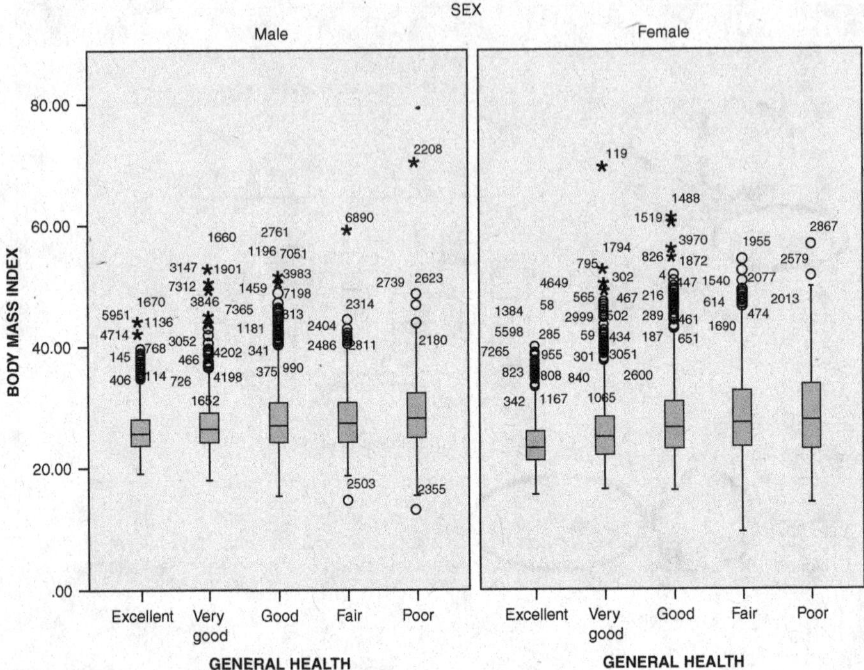

Fig. 4.18 Box Plot of the BMI of male and female NY state residents of varying levels of general health

Prostate-Specific Antigen Level (ng/ml) from the list of variables and click the right-pointing arrow to move the variable to the *Numeric Expression* window. From the set of buttons representing various arithmetic operations, click the button with the division sign (/). Select **Volume of Prostate (ml)** and move it to the *Numeric Expression* window. You have now told SPSS how to create the new variable. Click **OK** to execute the transformation. The steps for computing this new variable are displayed in Figs. 4.27, 4.28, 4.29, 4.30, 4.31 and 4.32.

The new variable will be stored in the last column of the data file. Go to *Data View* and scroll over to the last column to see the results of the transformation. Compare the values of the new variable with those of **Prostate-specific Antigen Density Level** [*psad*] (variable 7). The values of the two variables should be identical except for rounding error.

Changing the Shape of a Distribution Another purpose of a transformation is to change the shape of the distribution of a variable. For example, there are times when an analysis of a variable requires that the variable be normally distributed. If the variable is not normal, it might be possible to transform it into one that is, or at least into one that more closely approximates a normal distribution. The analysis would then be conducted on the transformed variable. One such transformation is a *log transformation*, which converts the values of a variable into their logarithmic

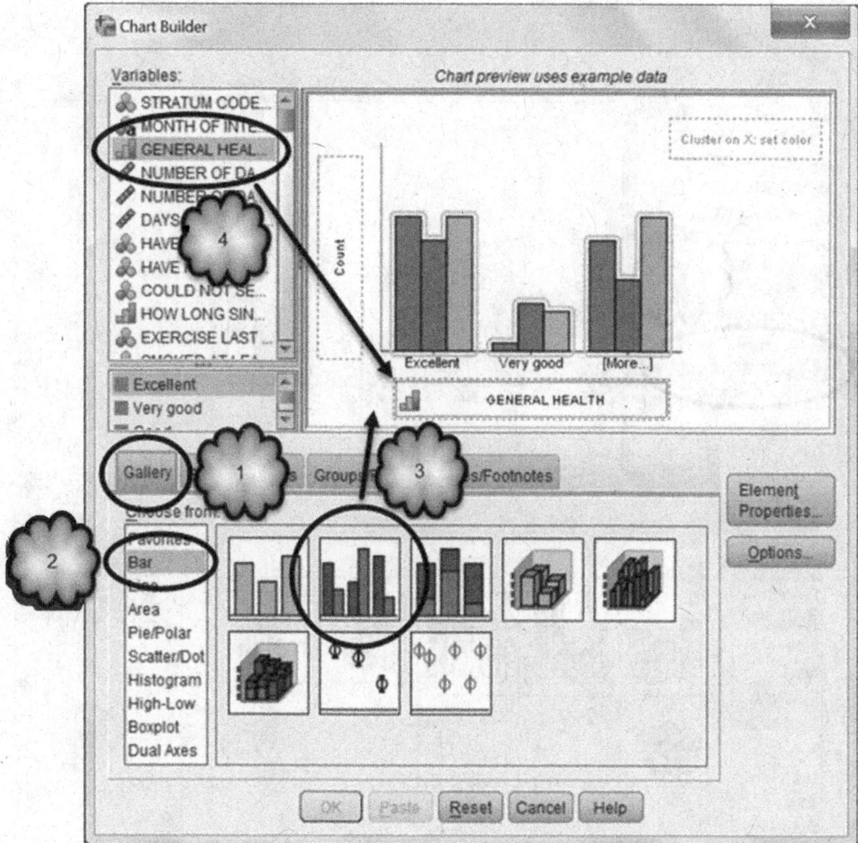

Fig. 4.19 Selecting clustered bar chart from the gallery and assigning a variable to the *X*-axis

equivalents. The statistical analysis is then conducted on the log values. A log transformation is used when the distribution of the original variable is positively skewed. As an example, let us look at the distribution of the variable, **prostate-specific antigen level (ng/ml)**, in the **PSA.sav** data set. Across the 301 patients, the PSA levels varied from 0.3 to 221.0.

To generate a histogram of the distribution, we could use *Explore*, but let us use instead *Chart Builder* which can also produce histograms. Return to *Chart Builder*. Select *Histogram* from the *Gallery* and drag the first histogram (called a *simple histogram*) in the row of histograms to the window above it. Drag **Prostate-Specific Antigen Level (ng/ml)** to the *X-Axis* box and click **OK.** These steps are displayed in Fig. 4.33.

The histogram is shown in Fig. 4.34. We can see that the data are not normally distributed. For example, most PSA levels are located to the extreme left, rather than in the middle of the distribution, and there are several extremely high values.

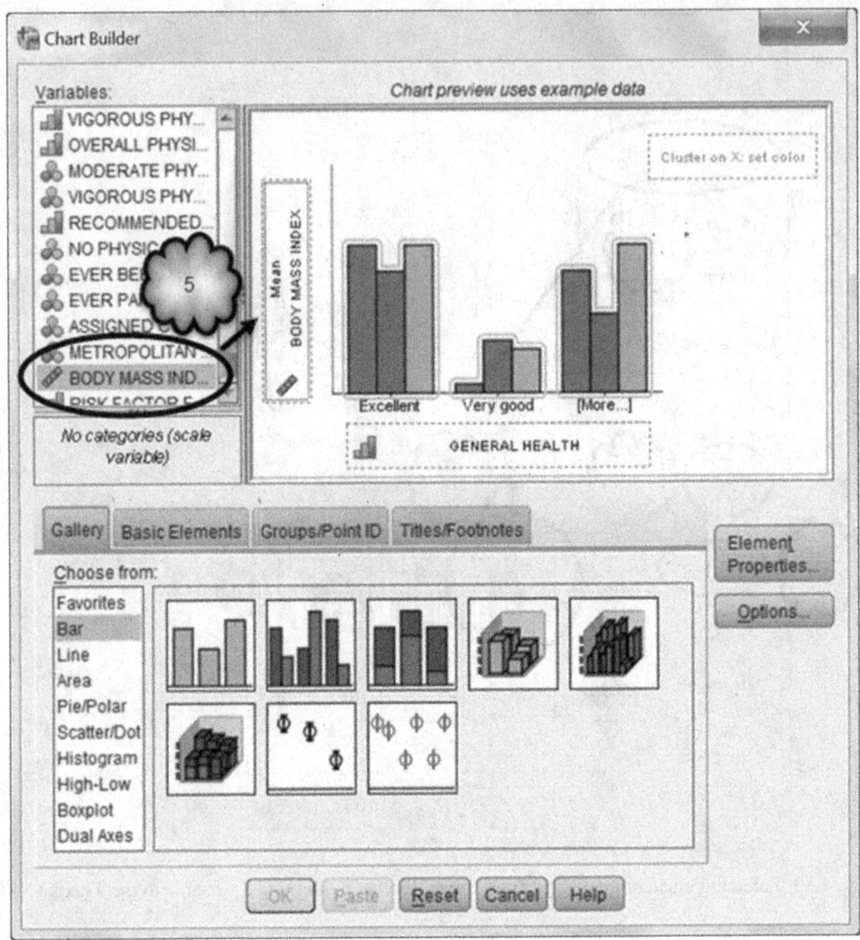

Fig. 4.20 Assigning a variable to the *Y*-axis of a clustered bar chart

Had we used *Explore* to generate the histogram, we would have seen that the skewness is 8.113 and its kurtosis is 87.725.

To make these positively skewed data more nearly normal, we can try a log transformation. Usually, this transformation involves taking either the log to the base 10 (log_{10}) or the natural logarithm (*ln*) of the variable. Here, we will do the former, although we could have just as easily taken the natural log. The $\log_{10}$ of a number is the value that when used as the exponent of 10 returns that number. For example, the $\log_{10}$ of 10 is 1 because 10^1 equals 10. The $\log_{10}$ of 100 is 2 because 10^2 equals 100. The $\log_{10}$ of 1 is zero because 10^0 equals 1. The $\log_{10}$ of values between 0 and 1 are negative. For example, the $\log_{10}$ of 0.5 is −0.301. Thus, the $\log_{10}$ of PSA levels of 0.5, 1, 10 and 100 would be −0.301, 0, 1 and 2. The $\log_{10}$ of our highest PSA level, 221, is 2.344.

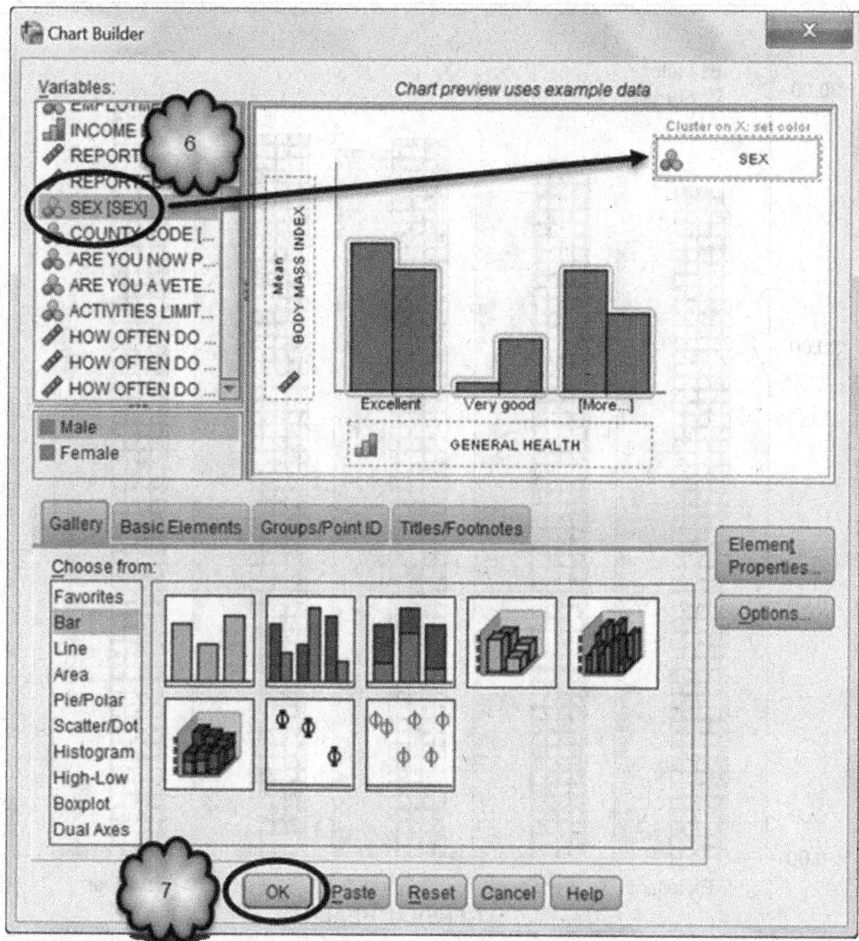

Fig. 4.21 Selecting a variable to be the cluster variable and generating the clustered bar chart

To conduct the log transformation, return to the *Compute Variable* dialog box. Click **Reset**. In the *Target Variable* window, enter a name for the new variable, such as *LogPSA*, and in the *Type & Label* dialog box, enter a variable label, such as **Log PSA**. To set up the numeric expression, select *Arithmetic* from the *Function group* window. In the *Function and Special Variables* window, select *Lg10* and click the up pointing arrow. Select **Prostate-Specific Antigen Level (ng/ml)** from the list of variables and click the right pointing arrow. These latter six steps are displayed in Figs. 4.35, 4.36 and 4.37.

The resulting histogram of the $\log_{10}$ of the PSA levels is displayed in Fig. 4.38.

We can see from the histogram that by taking the log of the PSA values, we have created a variable that still measures levels of PSA, but whose distribution more closely approximates a normal distribution than did the distribution of the

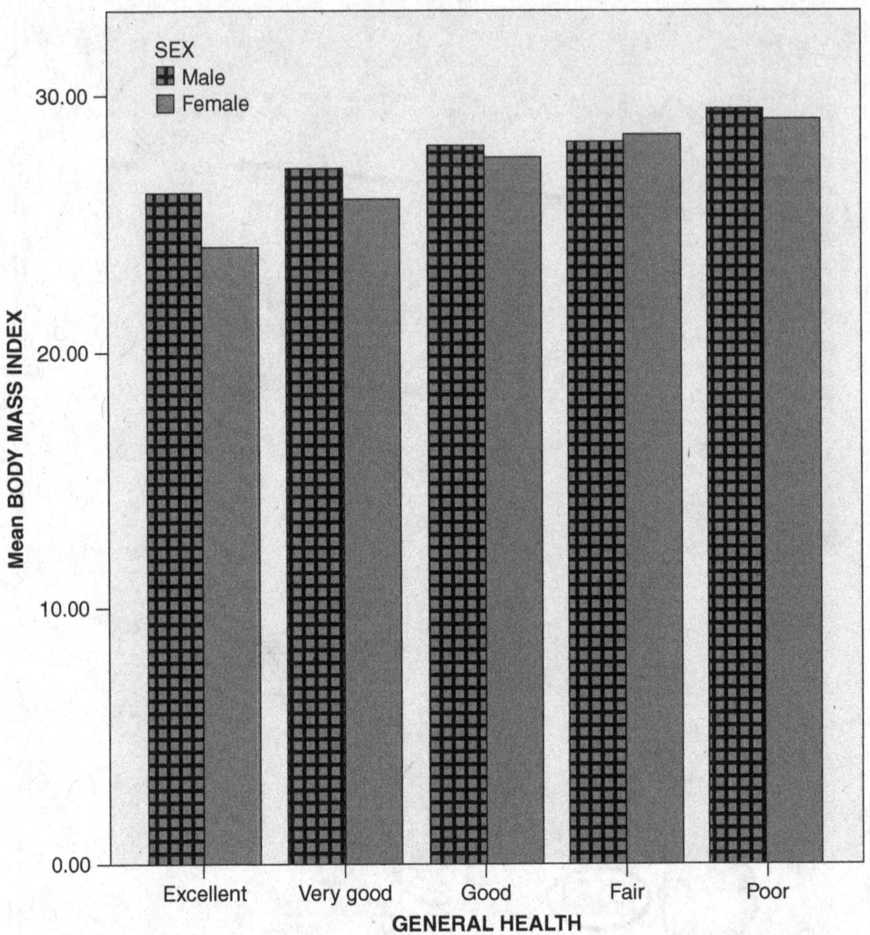

Fig. 4.22 Clustered bar chart displaying the mean BMI of male and female NY state residents of varying levels of general health

original values. If we had used *Explore* to generate the histogram of the log values, we would have seen that the skewness and kurtosis of the transformed variable are much closer to zero than they were for the original variable. The skewness of the transformed variable is −0.20, and its kurtosis is 0.832.

Medical researchers can use several other transformations to convert a nonnormal distribution into one that approximates a normal distribution. These include taking the reciprocal (dividing each value into one) or the square root of the variable if the distribution is positively skewed, and squaring the variable if the distribution is negatively skewed.

Equalizing Variability Across Groups There are times when a statistical comparison of the distribution of a variable across groups requires that the variability of

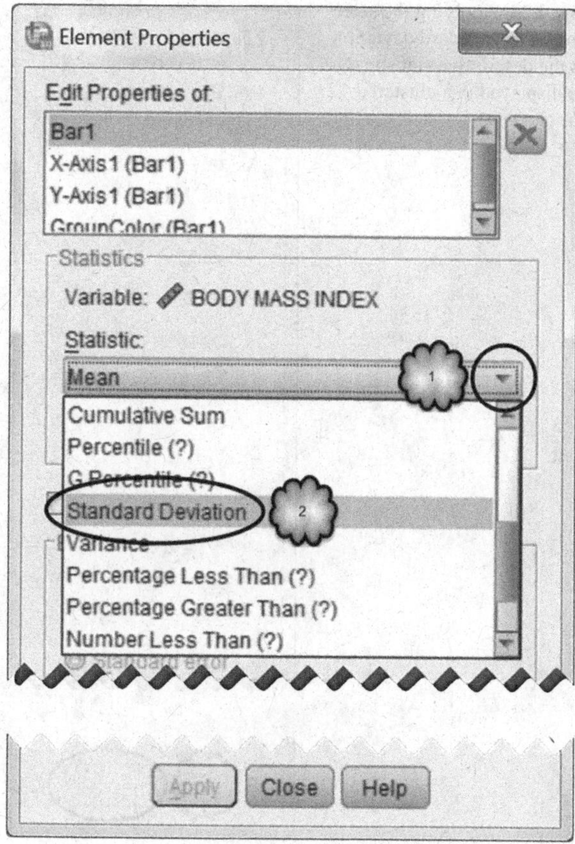

Fig. 4.23 Selecting the standard deviation as the descriptive statistic to be displayed in a clustered bar chart

the distribution be constant across those groups. If constancy is absent, then the data can sometimes be transformed to reduce the inequality of the variances. Several transformations can be tried, including taking the reciprocal or square root of the variable. A log transformation can also be effective. As an example of the latter, let us return to the **PSA.sav** data set. Table 4.5 displays some of the output generated by *Explore*. The data are the PSA levels and their $\log_{10}$ equivalents of two groups of patients: those who had prostate cancer and those who did not. Cancer was diagnosed by biopsy.

Answer the following questions:

4.5.1 What was the mean PSA level of patients with prostate cancer?

4.5.2 What was the mean PSA level of patients who were disease-free?

4.5.3 What were the standard deviations of the PSA levels of the two groups?

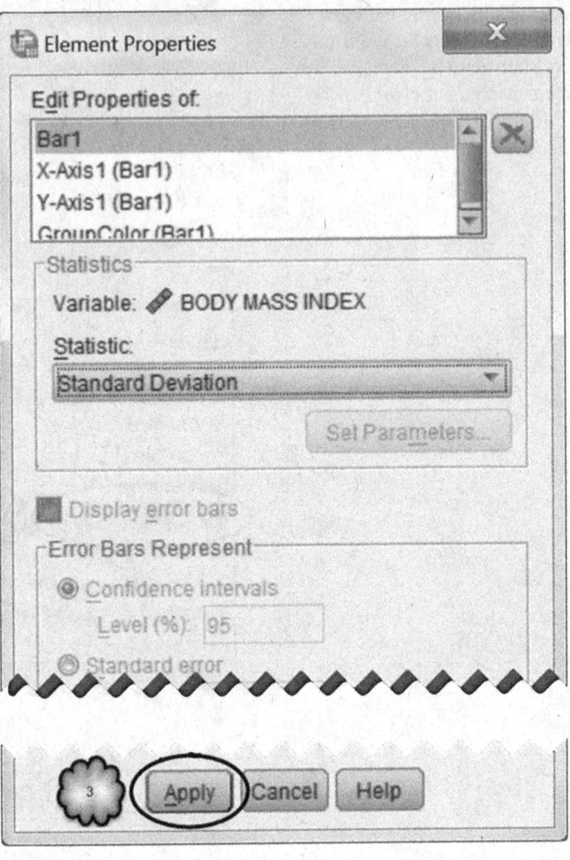

Fig. 4.24 Applying the selection of the standard deviation as the descriptive statistic to be displayed in a clustered bar chart

4.5.4 Were these two standard deviations similar?
4.5.5 What were the standard deviations of the $\log_{10}$ values of the two groups?
4.5.6 Were the standard deviations of the $\log_{10}$ values similar?

We can see from the output that the standard deviations of the PSA levels of the two groups of patients were very different while the standard deviations of the log values were similar. Consequently, if we wished to compare the average PSA levels of the two groups of patients with a measure of PSA that produces similar variability across the two groups, we could use log values of PSA. Our comparison though would be in terms of logarithms, not in terms of the original units of measurement. If after we had conducted our analysis, we wanted to express our findings in terms of the original PSA units, we would have to convert the results obtained with the transformed variable back into the original units of measurement. This is done by computing the *antilog* or *exponent* of the log. The exponent of a log is equal to the

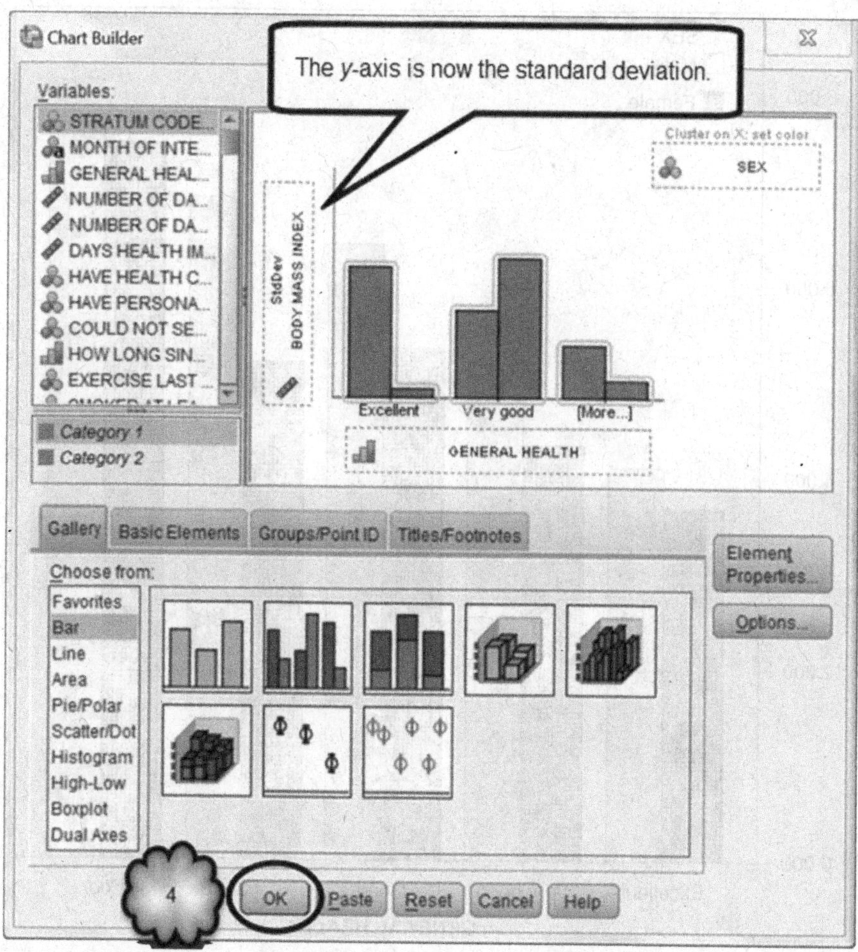

Fig. 4.25 Generating a clustered bar chart displaying the standard deviation of the BMI of men and women of varying levels of general health

base of the log raised to a power equal to the log. For example, according to the output above, the mean of the $\log_{10}$ PSA levels of patients with prostate cancer was 0.9105. If we raise 10 to the power of 0.9105 ($10^{0.9105}$), the result is 8.138. The exponent of 0.9105 is 8.138.

The mean of a variable is sometimes called the variable's *arithmetic mean.* In our example, the arithmetic mean of the PSA levels of patients with cancer was 15.548. The exponent of the mean of the log of the values of a variable is called the variable's *geometric mean.* In our example, the geometric mean of the PSA levels of the prostate cancer patients was 8.138. Geometric means are less sensitive to

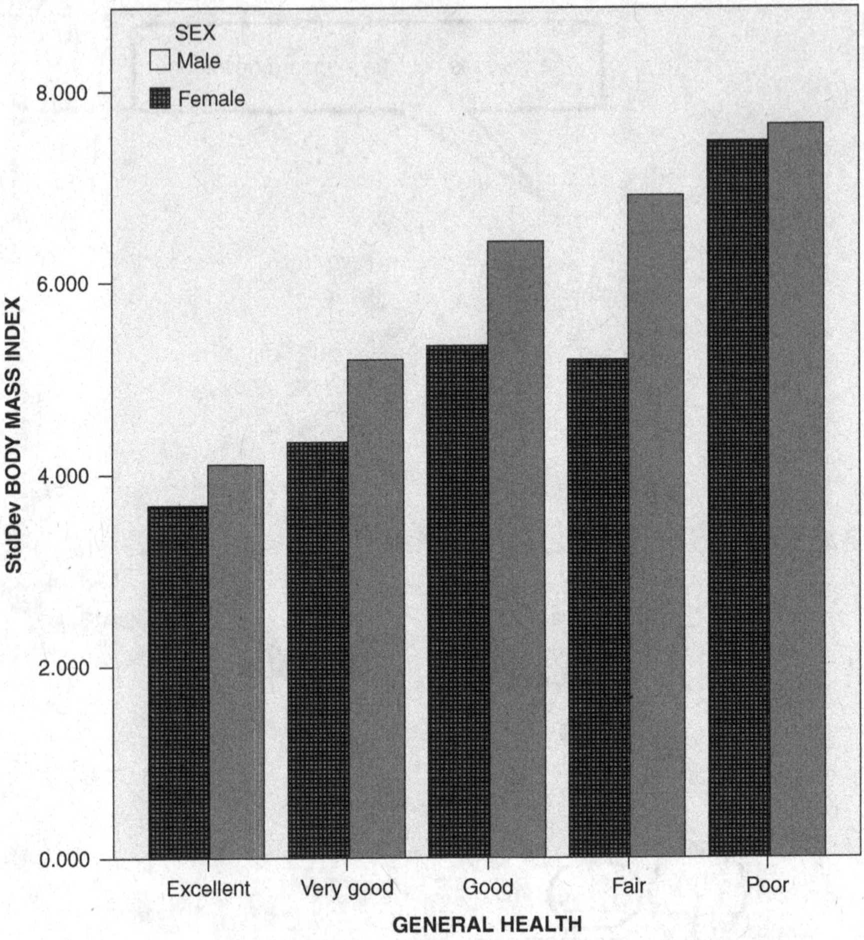

SEX
Male
Female
8.000
6.000
4.000
2.000
0.000
StdDev BODY MASS INDEX
Excellent
Very good
Good
Fair
Poor
GENERAL HEALTH

Fig. 4.26 Cluster bar chart of the standard deviations of the BMI of male and female NY state residents of varying levels of general health

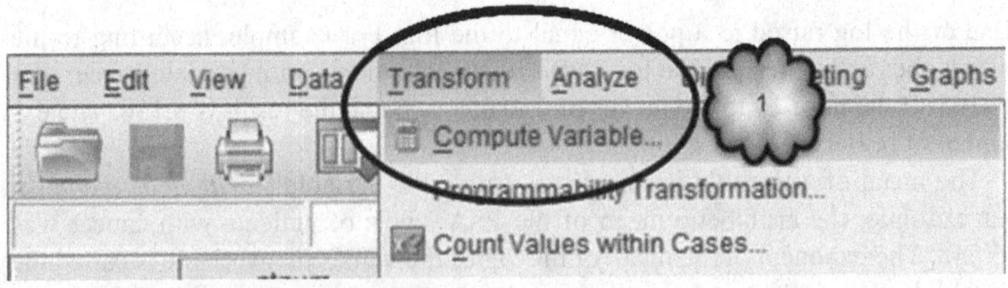

Fig. 4.27 Opening the Compute Variable dialog

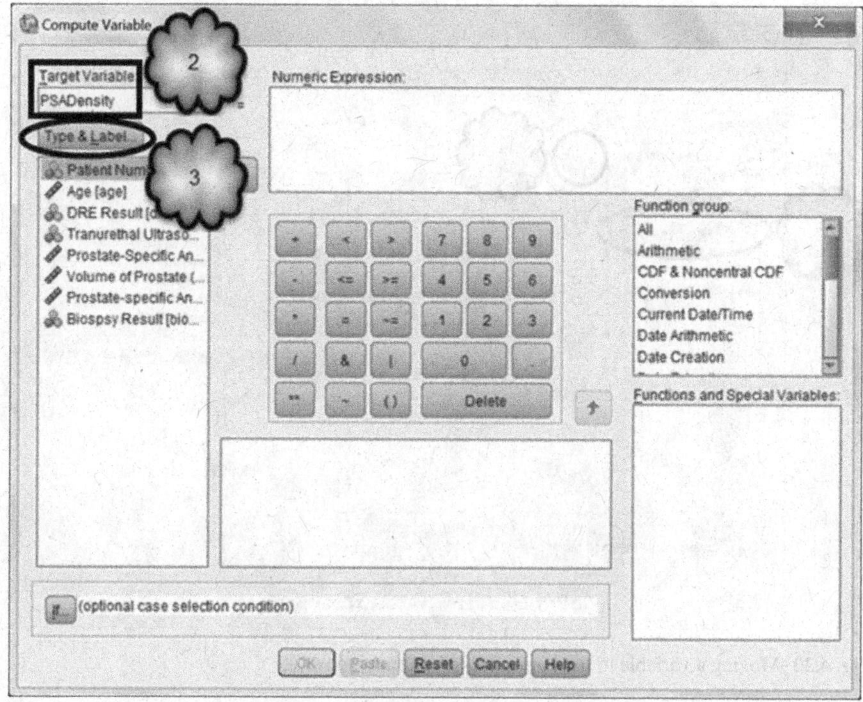

Fig. 4.28 Naming the new variable and opening the Type & Label dialog

Fig. 4.29 Labeling the variable

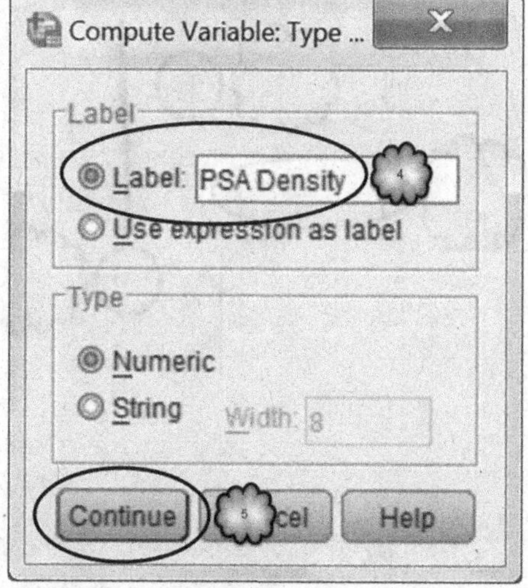

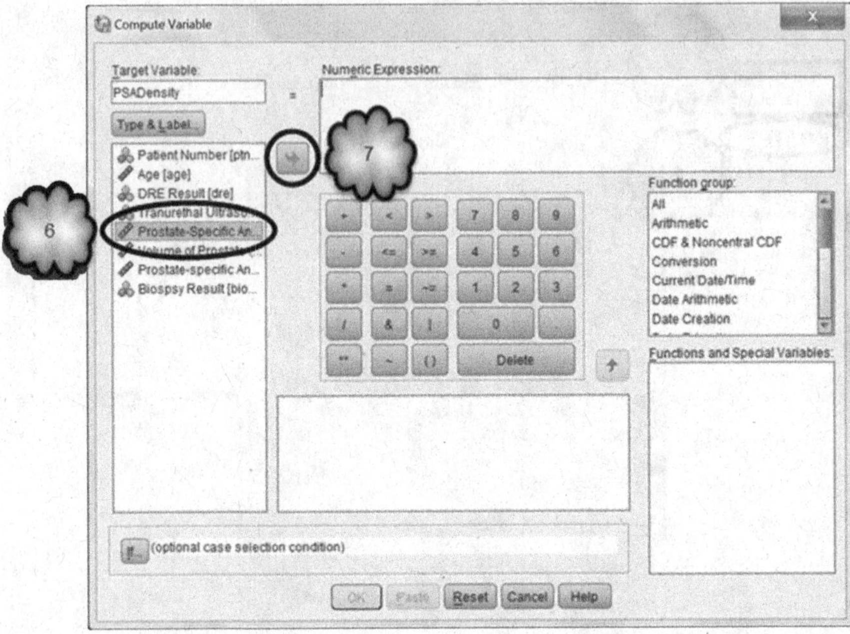

Fig. 4.30 Moving a variable to the numeric expression window

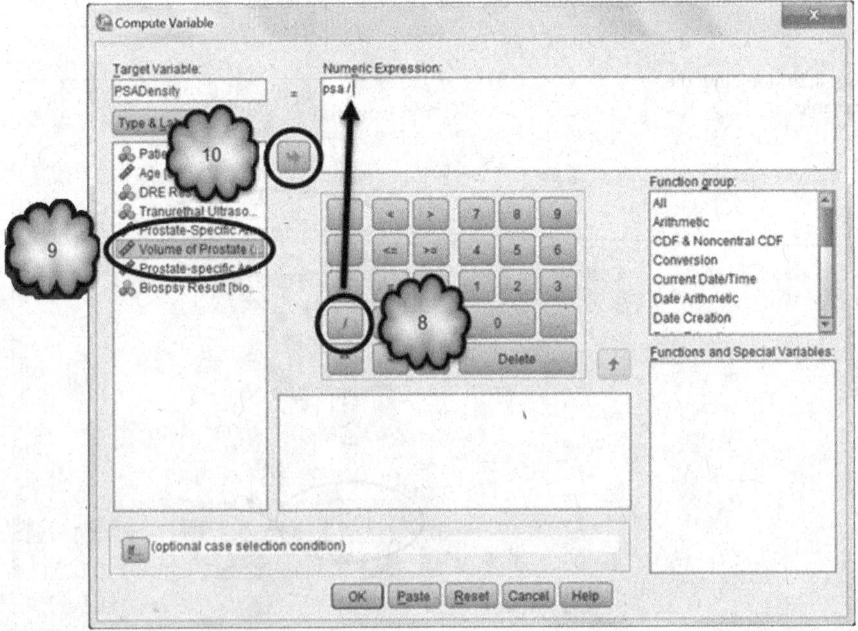

Fig. 4.31 Completing the numeric expression

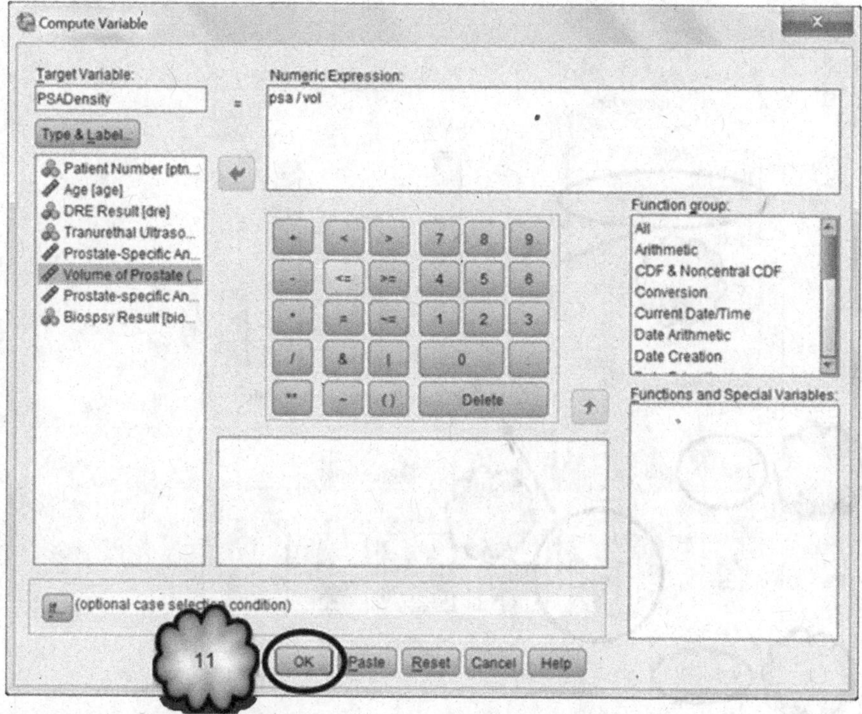

Fig. 4.32 Executing the transformation

extreme values than arithmetic means. As a result, when the distribution of a variable includes extreme values, the variable's geometric mean will be smaller than its arithmetic mean, as is the case in our example.

4.6 Exercise Questions

1. Return to the CDC data set. Respondents were asked whether they engage in moderate physical activity for at least 10 min at a time during a typical week. Respondents who answered in the affirmative were then asked the number of days per week they did so and the total time they spent per day engaged in that activity. The number of days per week is stored in the variable, **DAYS PER WEEK OF MOD. PHYS. ACT** [*MODPADAY*] (variable 44), and ranges from 1 to 7. Values of 77, 88 and 99 should be declared missing values. The number of minutes per day is stored in **MINUTES OF MODERATE PHYSICAL ACTIVITY** [@_*MODPAMN*] (variable 94), and ranges from 0 to 599. Using

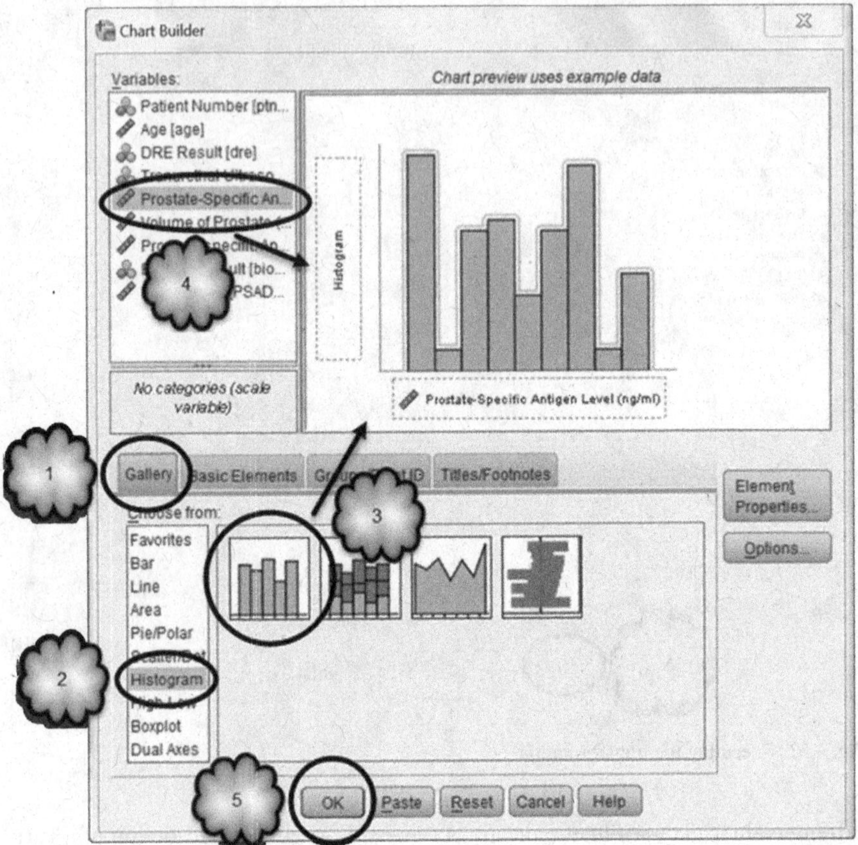

Fig. 4.33 Creating a histogram of a distribution of PSA levels

Explore, study the distribution of the number of minutes per day of moderate physical activity reported by respondents.

a. How many respondents were included in the analysis?
b. What was the mean number of minutes per day? The median?
c. Do the above values of the mean and median suggest that the distribution of minutes was skewed? If so, in the positive or negative direction?
d. What was the skewness of the distribution of minutes? Does this value indicate that the distribution was skewed? In which direction?
e. Did the distribution of minutes include outliers?
f. What was the interquartile range?
g. What was the range?

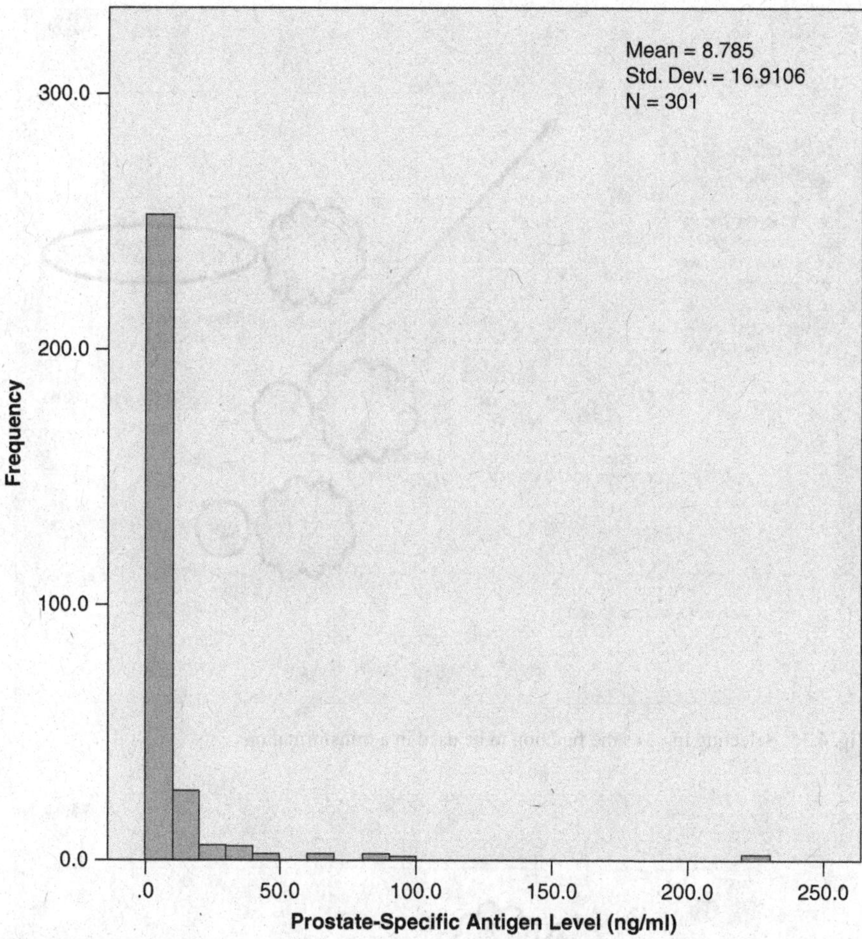

Fig. 4.34 Histogram of the distribution of the PSA levels of a sample of 301 men

h. We can be 95 % confident that on average, adult residents of NY state spend __________ to ___________ minutes per day engaged in moderate physical activity.

2. Using *Explore* once again, study the relationship between **BODY MASS INDEX-THREE LEVELS CATEGORY** [@*_BMI4CAT*] (variable 79) and **MINUTES OF MODERATE PHYSICAL ACTIVITY** [@*_MODPAMN*] (variable 94). Be sure that 9 has been declared a missing value for the BMI variable.

   a. For each category, report in Table 4.6 the mean number of minutes and the corresponding SE.

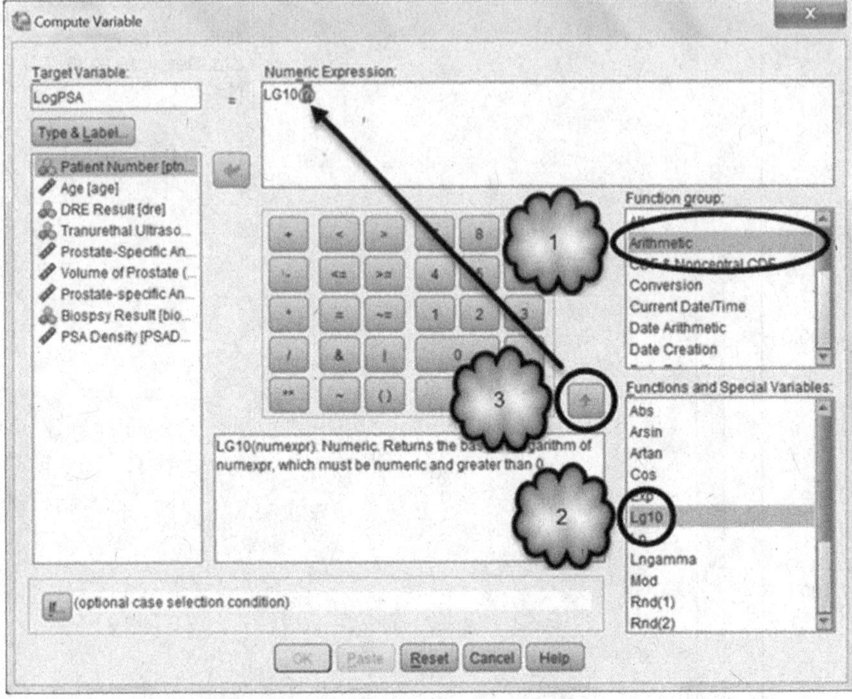

Fig. 4.35 Selecting $\log_{10}$ as the function to be used in a transformation

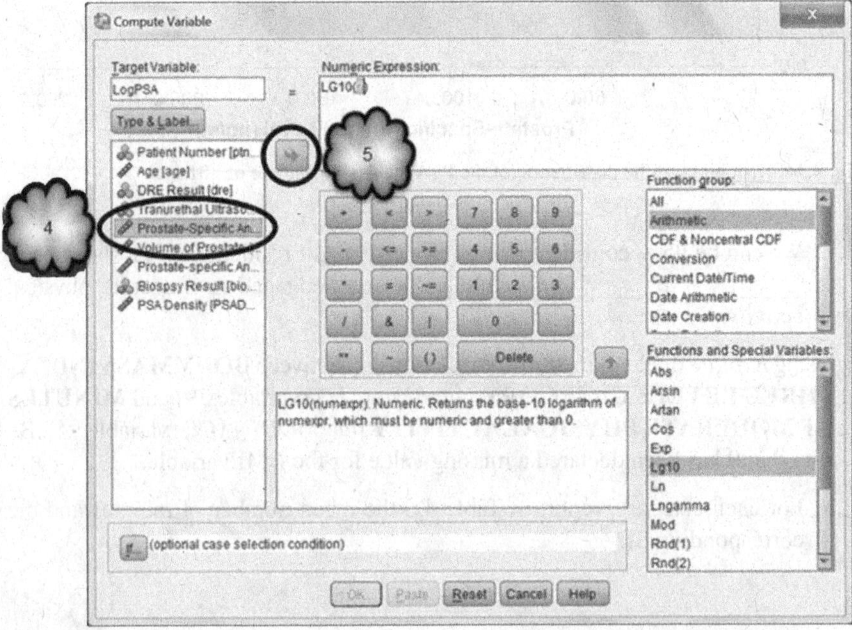

Fig. 4.36 Selecting a variable to be transformed into its logarithm equivalent

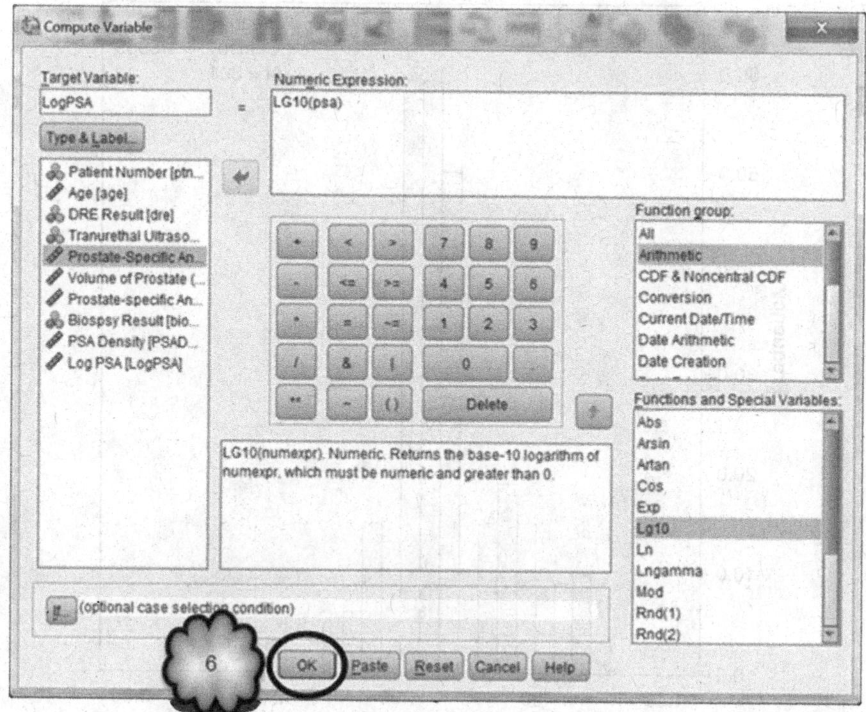

Fig. 4.37 Executing the logarithm transformation

b. Describe the relationship between BMI category and moderate physical activity.

3. Using *Chart Builder*, create a bar graph to determine if the relationship between BMI category and mean moderate physical activity that you described in 2b is the same across sex.

   a. Overall, which sex appears to engage in more minutes of moderate activity?
   b. Does the relationship between BMI and moderate activity appear to be the same for each sex?

4. In this question, focus on respondents who reported engaging in moderate physical activity for at least 10 min at a time. That is, use **Data > Select Cases** to limit the analysis to people for whom **MINUTES OF MODERATE PHYSICAL ACTIVITY** [*@_MODPAMN*] (variable 94) was greater than zero. Then, using *Transform*, create a variable, **MINUTES PER WEEK** [*MINUTES_WEEK*], that stores the number of minutes per week these respondents engaged in moderate physical activity: To create this variable, multiply **DAYS PER WEEK OF**

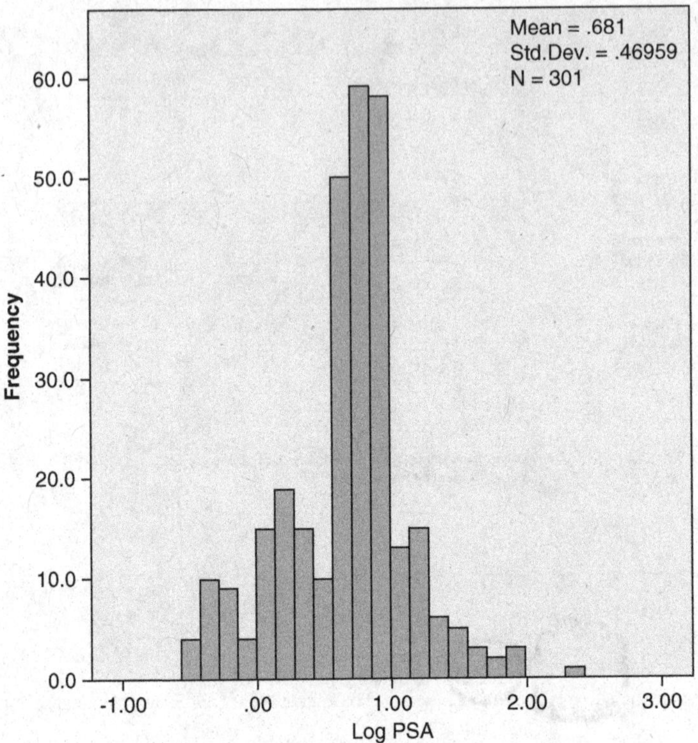

Fig. 4.38 Histogram of the distribution of the $\log_{10}$ PSA levels of a sample of 301 men

MOD. PHYS. ACT [*MODPADAY*] (variable 44) by **MINUTES OF MODERATE PHYSICAL ACTIVITY**:

$$MINUTES\_WEEK = \text{MODPADAY} * @\_\text{MODPAMN}. \quad (4.2)$$

Analyze the new variable with *Explore* and report in Table 4.7 the sample size, median and interquartile range for each sex.

5. Figure 4.39 is the distribution of minutes per week for men and women who engaged in moderate physical activity for at least 10 min at a time during a typical week. Figure 4.40 is the $\log_{10}$ transformation of those distributions. Table 4.8 displays the means and standard deviations of the four distributions.

   a. Does the log transformation appear to have normalized the distributions? Why or why not?
   b. Does the log transformation appear to have equalized the spread of the distributions? Why or why not?

Table 4.5 Descriptive statistics of the PSA Levels and their Log_{10} equivalents of patients with and without prostate cancer

Descriptives

Biopsy Result				Statistic	Std. Error
Prostate-Specific Antigen Level (ng/ml)	Cancer Present	Mean		15.548	2.8688
		95% Confidence Interval for Mean	Lower Bound	9.852	
			Upper Bound	21.244	
		Std. Deviation		27.9615	
	Cancer Absent	Mean		5.666	.3753
		95% Confidence Interval for Mean	Lower Bound	4.926	
			Upper Bound	6.406	
		Std. Deviation		5.3862	
Log PSA	Cancer Present	Mean		.9105	.04804
		95% Confidence Interval for Mean	Lower Bound	.8151	
			Upper Bound	1.0058	
		Std. Deviation		.46822	
	Cancer Absent	Mean		.5752	.03009
		95% Confidence Interval for Mean	Lower Bound	.5158	
			Upper Bound	.6345	
		Std. Deviation		.43189	

Table 4.6 BMI category and number of minutes per day engaged in moderate physical activity

BMI category	Mean	SE
Neither overweight nor obese		
Overweight		
Obese		

Table 4.7 Minutes per week of moderate physical activity of respondents engaging in such activity for at least 10 min at a time

Gender	Sample size	Median	Interquartile range
Male			
Female			

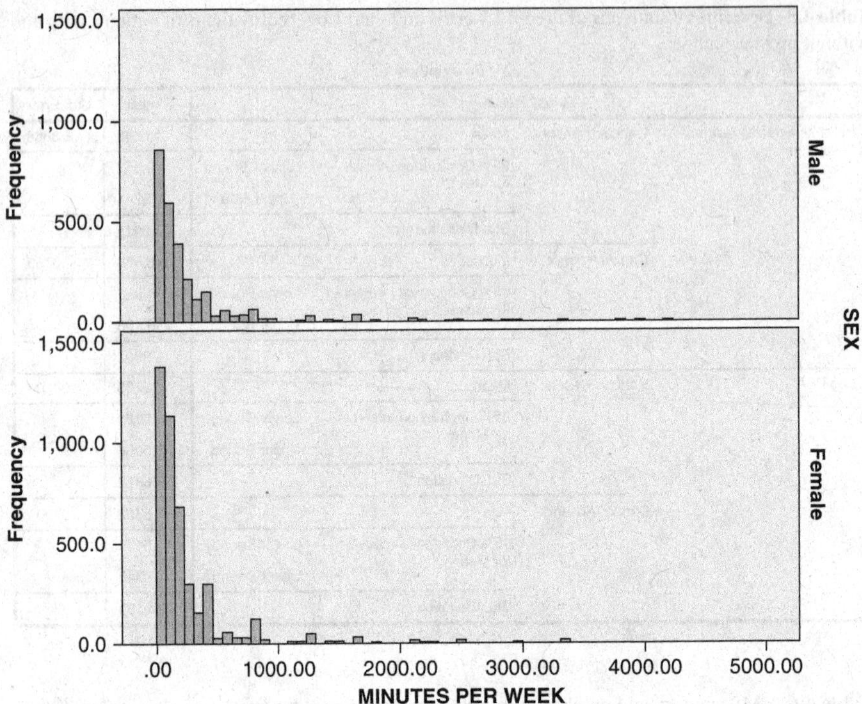

Fig. 4.39 Distribution of the number of minutes of exercise per week reported by a sample of male and female residents of NY state

c. The geometric mean (GM) for men was approximately 190.55. It was calculated with the following formula:

$$\mathrm{GM} = y^x. \tag{4.3}$$

What were the values of y and x that were used to calculate the geometric mean of men?

y=____________; x=____________.

d. Both the arithmetic and geometric means are measures of central tendency. Which provides the truer measure of the average number of minutes? Why?

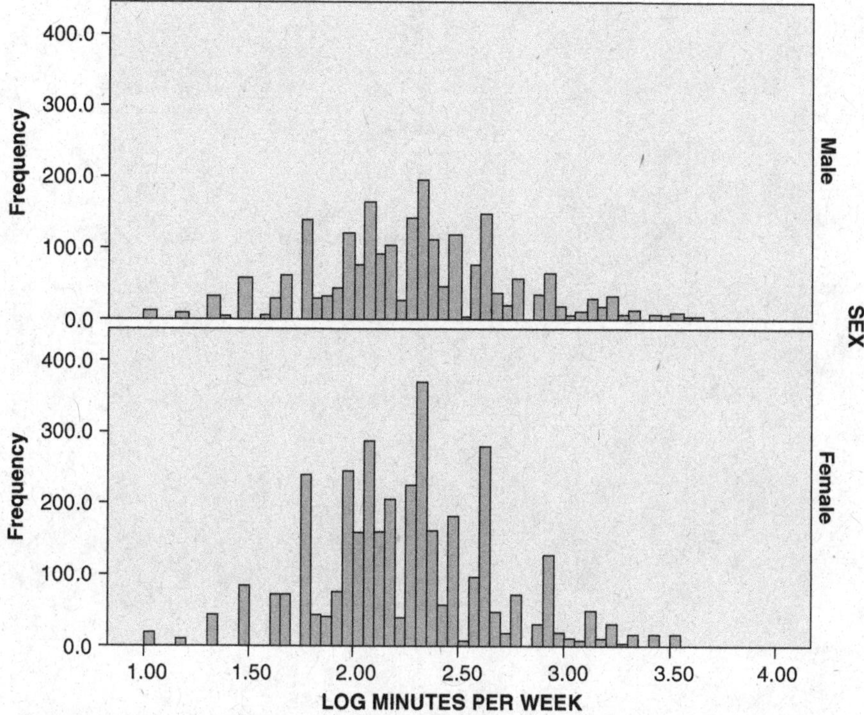

Fig. 4.40 Distribution of the $\log_{10}$ of the number of minutes of exercise per week reported by a sample of male and female residents of NY state

Table 4.8 Mean (SD) minutes and log minutes of exercise per week

Variable	Mean (SD)
Minutes per week	
Man	335.01 (465.65)
Woman	292.80 (400.88)
Log minutes per week	
Man	2.28 (0.45)
Woman	2.25 (0.42)

Data Sets and References

1. CDC BRFSS.sav obtained from: Centers for Disease Control and Prevention (CDC). Behavioral Risk Factor Surveillance System Survey Data. US Department of Health and Human Services, Centers for Disease Control and Prevention Public domain, Atlanta (2005). For more information about the BRFSS, visit http://www.cdc.gov/brfss/. Accessed 16 Nov 2014
2. PAS.sav obtained from: Riffenburgh, R.H.: Statistics in Medicine, 2nd edn. Elsevier, Burlington (2006). (With the kind permission of the Elsevier Books and Dr. Thomas K. Huisman)

Chapter 5
Introduction to Statistical Inference

Abstract This is an introduction to the two key tools for statistical inference. Confidence intervals on a population mean are introduced. This is followed by an introduction to the ideas behind hypothesis testing. They are applied to test a population mean. Since these procedures can depend, in the case of small samples, on the population distribution being normal, tests of this assumption are discussed. When the usual tests cannot be used, the Wilcoxon signed ranks test is introduced. This is followed by a discussion of statistical power and the difference between clinical significance and statistical significance.

5.1 Overview

In Chap. 2, we concentrated on becoming familiar with SPSS environment, seeing how to manipulate a data file to prepare it for analysis, how to save analysis, and how to transfer analysis from SPSS to a Word document. In Chap. 3, we learned how to describe the distribution of a categorical variable, while in Chap. 4, we learned how to describe the distribution of a quantitative variable by using measures of central tendency, measures of spread, skewness, and kurtosis. We also learned to describe the distribution of a quantitative variable graphically by constructing stem-and-leaf plots, histograms, and box plots. In all of the analyses, we have been interested in describing the distribution of our *sample* data. These types of analyses come under the general heading of *descriptive statistics*.

A logical, important question is whether or not the information gained from a sample is indicative of a similar pattern in the population from which the sample was drawn. For example, in a sample of quantitative data, we can compute the sample mean. This tells us something about the "center" of the data. What does this sample mean tell us about the "center" of the population (the population mean)? We are trying to use a sample result to *infer* a population quantity called a *population parameter*. This type of analysis is commonly referred to as *inferential statistics*. In this chapter, we focus on making inferences regarding the center of the population using a single sample from that population. Subsequent chapters will deal with other population parameters and research designs.

W. H. Holmes, W. C. Rinaman, *Statistical Literacy for Clinical Practitioners*,
DOI 10.1007/978-3-319-12550-3_5

In order to make valid inferences about population quantities, it is necessary that the data drawn from the population of interest are a random sample from the target population. This is the only way to ensure that the data are representative of the general population. For example, the data in the file **CDC BRFSS.sav** [1] consist of 7796 residents of New York State aged 18 or older who were interviewed in 2005 by the Centers for Disease Control and Prevention Behavioral Risk Factor Surveillance System (BRFSS). These were telephone interviews. The telephone numbers were obtained using a technique known as *random digit dialing*. It is exactly what it sounds like—telephone numbers from New York State were selected at random. To compensate for nonresponse and other factors, the results are then weighted to account for the possibility of systematic under- or overrepresentation of population subgroups. In this way, we can view these data as constituting a random sample of adults in New York State.

Not all statistical studies gather data in this manner. Suppose we are investigating the effect, if any, of a new drug on patients with hypertension, and we have a set of volunteers for the study. It is common practice to view these hypertensive patients as being representative of all persons with the condition, and to randomly assign patients to a treatment group and a control group. In this way, assuming that we have a random sample is reasonable.

In order to gain information regarding the value of a population parameter, we need to decide how to process the sample data. That is, we need to decide on what *statistic* to use. A statistic is a numerical value that is computed using sample data. For example, if we are interested in the population mean, we would typically use the sample mean as a basis for our analysis. Similarly, if we are considering the population standard deviation (SD), then the sample SD would be the statistic of choice. Since we are considering making inferences regarding the "center" of the population in this chapter, two of the three procedures we will investigate will start with the sample mean. The third procedure makes inferences about the population median and uses an entirely different approach.

Before we get into a detailed discussion of the procedures and how SPSS conducts them, it is necessary to review a little of the logic that underlies them. That is, we will discuss what *confidence intervals* (CIs) are and how to interpret them. We will also discuss what a *hypothesis test* is and how it works.

5.2 Confidence Intervals for a Population Mean

We introduced CIs in our discussion of the *Explore* procedure in the preceding chapter. CIs are methods that are intended to estimate the value of a population parameter. The value of the sample statistic that is associated with the parameter of interest can be used to get a good single number estimate for that parameter. However, since the value of the statistic will vary from sample to sample (a phenomenon known as *sampling variability*), you cannot assume that the value you get from a single sample will be equal to the value of the parameter. If the statistic is well chosen, you can be fairly confident that, on average, its value is pretty close to that of the parameter. However, given the nature of random sampling, you cannot always be certain.

The idea behind a CI is to derive a range (called the *confidence interval*) of possible values for the parameter that is reasonable given the value of the statistic and, along with that interval, provide a measure of how confident (called the *confidence level*) you are that the parameter is actually somewhere in that interval. Confidence levels are stated in percent. Since we would like to be very confident that the parameter is in your particular interval, confidence levels are usually chosen near 100 %. You cannot use 100 % because a 100 % CI would have to span all possible values for the parameter, and that would not serve to pin down the parameter's value. Common values are 90, 95, and 99 %, with 95 % being by far the one most frequently chosen.

The interpretation of the confidence level is as follows. Suppose, for the sake of example, we construct a 95 % CI for the population mean. This means that 95 % of all possible CIs will contain the true population mean, and 5 % will not. We do not know if the CI we just constructed is one of the good 95 % or one of the bad 5 %. However, since 95 % of all intervals will contain the population mean, we can say that we are 95 % "confident" that the population mean is in our interval.

The width of a CI depends on the confidence level chosen. Higher confidence levels result in wider CIs. Thus, a 99 % CI has a greater likelihood of containing the parameter of interest, but at the cost of being less precise. On the other hand, a 90 % CI is more precise, in the sense of being narrower, but at the expense of not containing the parameter of interest as often. A 95 % confidence level is a good compromise between 90 and 99 %. Other factors affect the width of a CI. If the underlying variability in the population is great, then CIs will be wider than for populations which are less variable everything else being constant. In addition, sample size affects the width of a CI. Larger sample sizes reduce the variability of the statistics on which CIs are based. The net effect is that CIs using larger sample sizes will be narrower than CIs based on smaller sample sizes, everything else being equal.

In this chapter, we use SPSS to construct CIs for the population mean. Although you will not need to construct CIs by hand, it is worthwhile that you be acquainted with how SPSS does it. When calculating a CI for a population mean, the statistic that serves as the basis for the interval is the sample mean. Generically, the symbol for the sample mean is $\overline{X}$. The variability in the population is measured using the sample SD, whose symbol is s. The sample size is denoted by n. The confidence level is accounted for by a multiplying factor called the *critical value*, denoted by t^*, obtained by using what is known as a t distribution. If the underlying population has a normal distribution, or if the sample size is large enough (a popular rule of thumb is $n \geq 30$), then using the t distribution is appropriate. The larger confidence levels result in higher values for t^*. The resulting formula for a CI for the population mean is

$$\overline{X} \pm t \times \frac{s}{\sqrt{n}} \tag{5.1}$$

We are presenting the formulas for the procedures in this chapter so that you know what SPSS uses. You will have no need to do these calculations by hand. Therefore, in succeeding chapters, we will not show the formulas. As you can see, the interval will be centered at the sample mean. Also, higher values of t^* (i.e., higher confi-

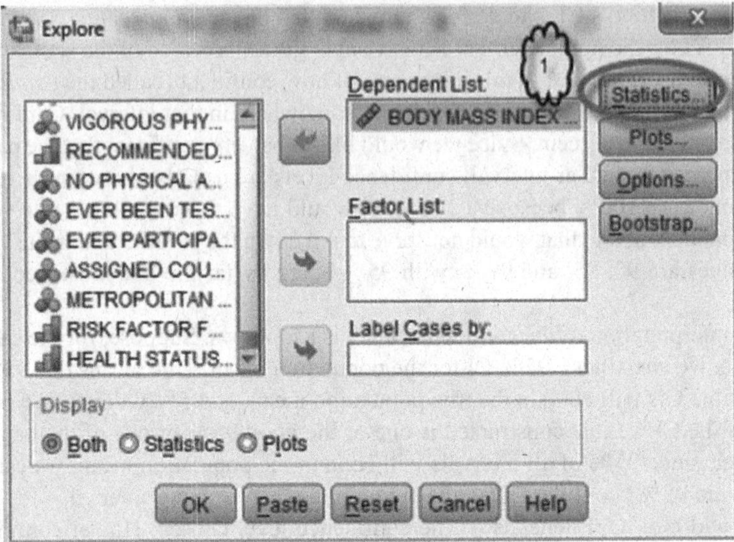

Fig. 5.1 Selecting the Explore: Statistics dialog

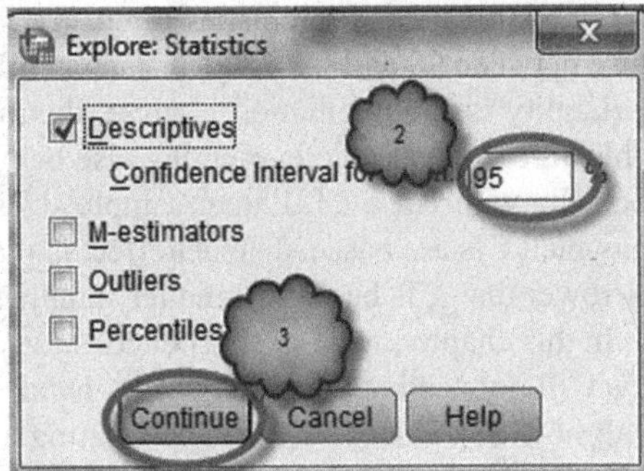

Fig. 5.2 Changing the confidence level

dence levels) and *s* contribute to wider intervals. In addition, higher values of *n* contribute to narrower intervals.

An example: the mean Body Mass Index (BMI) of New York state adults We wish to construct CIs for the variable, BODY MASS INDEX [*BMI*] (variable 107), found in the data file, **CDC BRFSS.sav**.

To generate the CIs with SPSS, load the data file. As we saw in Chap. 4, part of the standard output of the *Explore* procedure (**Analyze>Descriptive Statistics>Explore)** is a CI for the mean. The default interval has a confidence level of 95 %. This can be changed to any desired confidence level by clicking **Statistics** to open the *Explore: Statistics* dialog box shown in Figs. 5.1, 5.2, and 5.3. To change the confidence level, type the desired confidence level, in percent, in the *Confidence Interval for Mean* box and click **Continue**

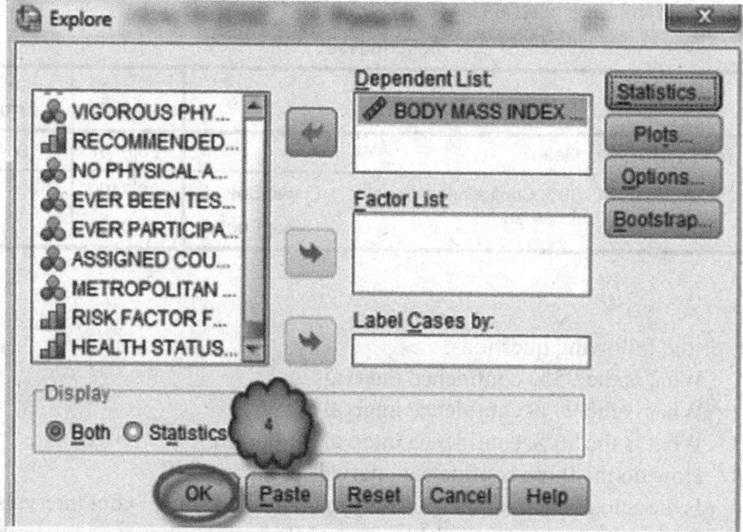

Fig. 5.3 Constructing the confidence interval

Table 5.1 95 % Confidence interval for body mass index

Descriptives

			Statistic	Std. Error
BODY MASS INDEX	Mean		26.8767	.06467
	95% Confidence Interval for Mean	Lower Bound	26.7499	
		Upper Bound	27.0034	

Table 5.2 90 % Confidence interval for body mass index

Descriptives

			Statistic	Std. Error
BODY MASS INDEX	Mean		26.8767	.06467
	90% Confidence Interval for Mean	Lower Bound	26.7703	
		Upper Bound	26.9830	

Use the *Explore* procedure to construct 95, 99, and 90 % CIs for the mean of **BODY MASS INDEX**. Study the resulting output.

The partial output displayed in Tables 5.1, 5.2 and 5.3 shows the 95, 90, and 99 % CIs for the mean of **BODY MASS INDEX,** respectively.

Table 5.3 99 % Confidence interval for body mass index

Descriptives

			Statistic	Std. Error
BODY MASS INDEX	Mean		26.8767	.06467
	99% Confidence Interval for Mean	Lower Bound	26.7100	
		Upper Bound	27.0433	

Answer the following questions:

5.2.1 What is the 95 % confidence interval?
5.2.2 What is the 99 % confidence interval?
5.2.3 What is the 90 % confidence interval?
5.2.4 How do the three confidence intervals compare?
5.2.5 Is the actual population mean body mass index in any of your intervals?
5.2.6 Which of your three confidence intervals is most likely to contain the true population body mass index?

5.3 Test of Hypotheses

The other statistical procedure that we will discuss is known as a *test of hypotheses*. While a CI is designed to provide a way to estimate the value of a population parameter, a statistical test is intended to decide between two statements about the value of a population parameter. Each statement about the value of the population parameter is a *hypothesis*.

Null and Alternative Hypotheses One hypothesis is referred to as the *null hypothesis*, and the other hypothesis is referred to as the *alternative hypothesis*. It is common practice for the null hypothesis to be the statement you feel should be false. The null hypothesis statement must always state that the parameter is equal to a specific value. The alternative hypothesis will state that the parameter is less than the value stated in the null hypothesis, greater than the value stated in the null hypothesis, or is not equal to the value stated in the null hypothesis. Which of these three versions of the alternative hypothesis should be used depends on the context of the problem.

There is some terminology that is commonly used in testing. When the alternative hypothesis is either greater than or less than, the alternative hypothesis is said to be *one-tailed* or *one-sided.* A test with a one-sided alternative hypothesis is referred to as a *one-tailed test* or a *one-sided* test. If the alternative hypothesis is not equal to, then the alternative is said to be *two-tailed* or *two-sided.* A test with a two-sided alternative hypothesis is referred to as a *two-tailed test* or a *two-sided test.*

As an example, suppose we wish to test hypotheses about the mean BMI of a population, and you believe that the mean BMI is <30 (not obese). One hypothesis would be that the mean BMI is <30. As a consequence, the other hypothesis would

Table 5.4 *P*-values for testing a population mean

Alternative Hypothesis	*p*-value
$\mu > \mu 0$	$\Pr(T \geq t)$
$\mu < \mu 0$	$\Pr(T \leq t)$
$\mu \neq \mu 0$	$2\Pr(T \geq \|t\|)$

be that the mean BMI is ≥30. Since the second statement contains equality, it becomes the null hypothesis. The statement that we believe is true becomes the alternative hypothesis. It is common practice to neglect the inequality part of the null hypothesis and simply restate it as that the mean BMI is equal to 30.

Test Statistics Once the null and alternative hypotheses have been formulated, we need a procedure for determining which hypothesis is better supported by the sample data. A typical starting point is the sample statistic that is associated with the parameter being tested. Since we will be discussing testing hypotheses about a population mean, the appropriate statistic will be $\overline{X}$, the sample mean. Using the sample statistic, we compute what is called the *test statistic*. The test statistic is computed assuming that the value of the parameter specified in the null hypothesis is true. This is why the null hypothesis must contain equality.

The formula for the test statistic for tests on a population mean is

$$T = \frac{\overline{X} - \mu_0}{s / \sqrt{n}}, \tag{5.2}$$

where T is the name of the test statistic, $\overline{X}$ is the sample mean, μ_0 is the value of the population mean specified in the null hypothesis, s is the sample standard deviation (SD), and n is the sample size. The use of μ_0 in the formula is how the test statistic assumes that the null hypothesis is true. The numerator in T is the distance that the sample mean is from the value of the population mean when the null hypothesis is true. The denominator in T is the *standard error of the mean* (*SEM*). Consequently, the test statistic for the population mean measures how many standard errors the sample mean is from the population mean when the null hypothesis is true. It is less likely that the null hypothesis is true when this distance, in standard error terms, is large.

Statistical Significance and *p*-Values In order to ascertain which hypothesis is better supported by the data we compute the probability of observing a value of our test statistic that is as extreme or more extreme than the value we compute when the null hypothesis is true. This probability is called the *p-value* of the test. The calculation of the *p*-value depends on the form of the alternative hypothesis. For tests on a population mean, the *p*-value calculations are as shown in Table 5.4. μ denotes the population mean, Pr denotes a probability, and t denotes the value of T calculated using sample data. The probability is calculated using a distribution known as the

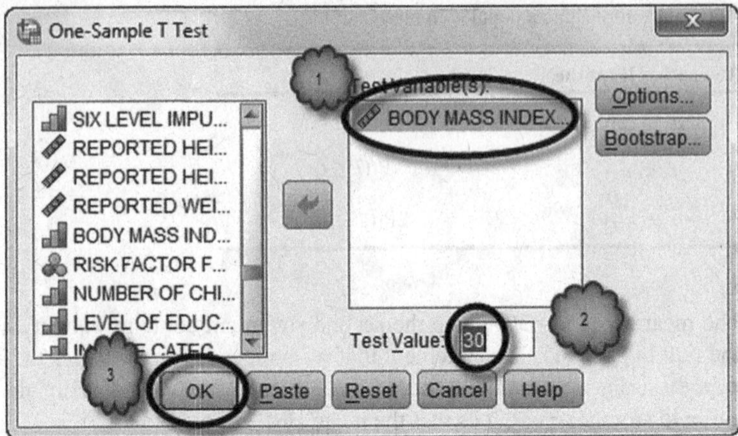

Fig. 5.4 Testing a population mean

t distribution. Using the t distribution is appropriate as long as we have a random sample, and either the population distribution is normal or the sample size is large enough (a typical rule of thumb is $n \geq 30$).

Small p-values are indicative of evidence against the null hypothesis. Typically, any p-value >0.1 is considered to be supportive of the null hypothesis. As p-values decrease below 0.1 we have increasingly stronger evidence that the null hypothesis is not true.

A term associated with p-values is *statistical significance.* A *significance level* is a value of the p-value. It is also known as an $\alpha-$ level (or alpha level). Common significance levels are 0.1, 0.05, and 0.01. Significance levels are often referred to in percentage terms by multiplying the significance level by 100. A test is termed to be *significant at level* α if the p-value is $\leq \alpha$. Thus, the statement "the test was significant at the 5 % level" indicates that the p-value was 0.05 or less. What this means is that, if we conduct repeated tests of our two hypotheses when the null hypothesis is true, we will find, in the long run, a significant result 5 % of the time.

An Example: The One Sample t-Test We want to test whether or not the mean BMI of the population of New York state adults is not in the obese range (i.e., <30). Therefore, we will use SPSS to test the null hypothesis that the mean BMI is 30 against the alternative hypothesis that the mean BMI is <30.

Select **Analyze>Compare Means>One-Sample T Test** to open the *One-Sample T Test* dialog box shown in Fig. 5.4. Select and move **BODY MASS INDEX** [*BMI*] (variable 107) to the *Test Variable(s)* box. Enter the value of the population mean specified by the null hypothesis (30) in the *Test Value* box.

Part of the standard output for this procedure is a CI for the difference from the value of the population mean specified by the null hypothesis. (This is an alternative method of constructing a CI for the population mean, if you enter a value of 0 in the *Test Value* box.) The default confidence level is 95 %. If you want to use another confidence level, click **Options** to open the *One-Sample T Test: Options* dialog box

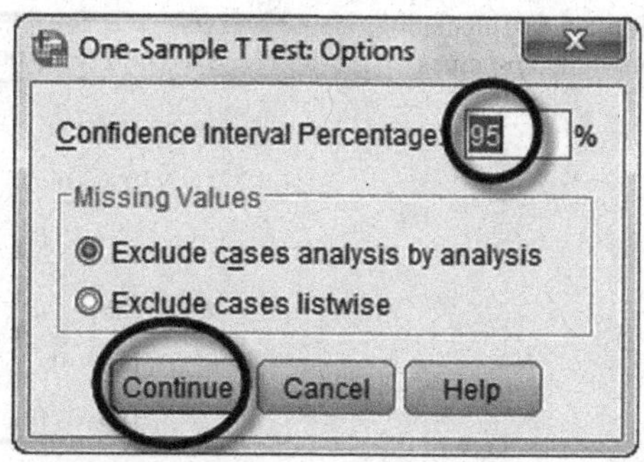

Fig. 5.5 Changing the confidence level

Table 5.5 Output for the *t*-test procedure

One-Sample Statistics

	N	Mean	Std. Deviation	Std. Error Mean
BODY MASS INDEX	7417	26.8767	5.56992	.06467

One-Sample Test

	Test Value = 30					
					95% Confidence Interval of the Difference	
	t	df	Sig. (2-tailed)	Mean Difference	Lower	Upper
BODY MASS INDEX	-48.293	7416	.000	-3.12335	-3.2501	-2.9966

shown in Fig. 5.5. Enter the desired confidence level, in percent, in the *Confidence Interval* box and click **Continue.**

Click **OK** to conduct the test. Study the resulting output.

The one-sample *t*-test generates two tables, reproduced in Table 5.5. The first table gives the sample size (*N*), the sample mean (*Mean*), the sample SD (*Std. Deviation*), and the SEM (*Std. Error Mean*). The SEM is the sample SD divided by the square root of the sample size. Recall that the SEM is the denominator in the test statistic, *T*.

The second table gives test results. At the top of the table is the value of the population mean used in the null hypothesis. The leftmost box of the bottom row of the table shows the variable that is being tested. The next box in the bottom row gives the value of the test statistic (*t*). The column headed *df* gives the *degrees of freedom* associated with the test. Degrees of freedom are a quantity that takes into account the size of our sample. Degrees of freedom for this *t* statistic are $n-1$. The value of *t* and the degrees of freedom are used to compute the *p*-value for the test. The next box headed *Sig. (2-tailed)* gives the *p*-value for the two-sided alternative.

If you want to conduct a one-tailed test, you can use this two-tailed *p*-value to obtain the one-sided *p*-value by using Table 5.6. Let *Sig* denote the two-tailed *p*-value.

The next box of the bottom row of the *One-Sample Test* table is headed *Mean Difference* and gives the value of $\overline{X} - \mu_0$. The next two boxes give the upper and lower limits of the CI (in our case a 95 % CI) for the mean difference.

Table 5.6 Calculating one-tailed *p*-values

Alternative Hypothesis	One-tailed *p*-value
$\mu > \mu_0$	
If $t > 0$:	*Sig/2*
If $t \leq 0$:	1 – *Sig/2*
$\mu < \mu_0$	
If $t < 0$:	*Sig/2*
If $t \geq 0$:	1 – *Sig/2*

Consult the output and answer the following questions.

5.3.1 What is the value of the sample mean?
5.3.2 What is the value of the sample standard deviation?
5.3.3 What is the sample size?
5.3.4 What is the value of *t*?
5.3.5 What are the degrees of freedom?
5.3.6 What is the *p*-value for testing that the population mean is equal to 30 against the alternative hypothesis that the population mean is 30?
5.3.7 Does your *p*-value give evidence that the null hypothesis is false?
5.3.8 Have the technical requirements that we have a random sample and either a normal population or a large sample size been satisfied?

5.4 Test of Normality

In those cases when the sample size is not large (i.e., <30) it is necessary to determine whether it is reasonable to assume that the underlying population has a normal distribution. The normal distribution is the familiar bell-shaped curve. We saw in the previous chapter that it is possible to look at a stem-and-leaf plot or a histogram to see if the general shape of the distribution follows a bell curve. But there are more definitive means available.

Open the file, **Bodymass.sav** [2]. It contains data on the BMI of 20 anorexic patients. It has the BMI at the beginning of a treatment program, the BMI at discharge, and the patient's preferred BMI based on the patient's stated preferred weight at admission. Suppose we wish to test the null hypothesis that the mean BMI at the beginning of the treatment program is 18.5 (not underweight) against the alternative hypothesis that the mean BMI at the beginning of the program is <18.5 (underweight). Since the sample size is only 20, we need to verify that it is reasonable to assume that the population distribution is normal.

Select **Analyze > Descriptive Statistics > Explore**. As shown below, place **Body mass at admittance** [*Admit*] (variable 2) in the *Dependent List* box. Click **Plots**

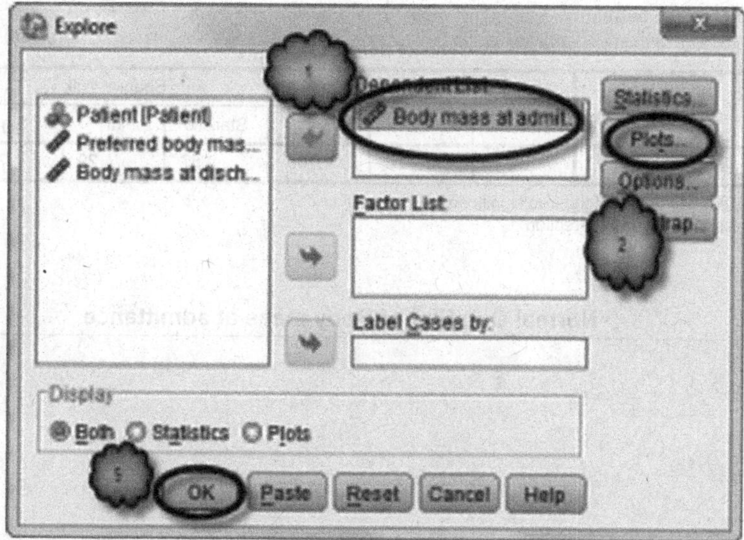

Fig. 5.6 Selecting plots in Explore

Fig. 5.7 Choosing normality plots with tests

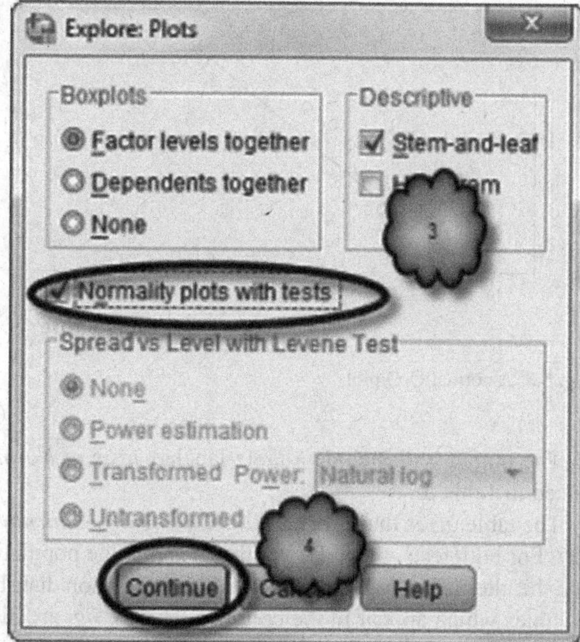

to open the *Explore: Plots* dialog box, and check *Normality plots with tests.* Click **Continue** followed by **OK**. These steps are shown in Figs. 5.6 and 5.7.

Table 5.7 Tests of normality

Tests of Normality

	Kolmogorov-Smirnov[a]			Shapiro-Wilk		
	Statistic	df	Sig.	Statistic	df	Sig.
Body mass at admittance	.097	20	.200*	.967	20	.700

*. This is a lower bound of the true significance.
a. Lilliefors Significance Correction

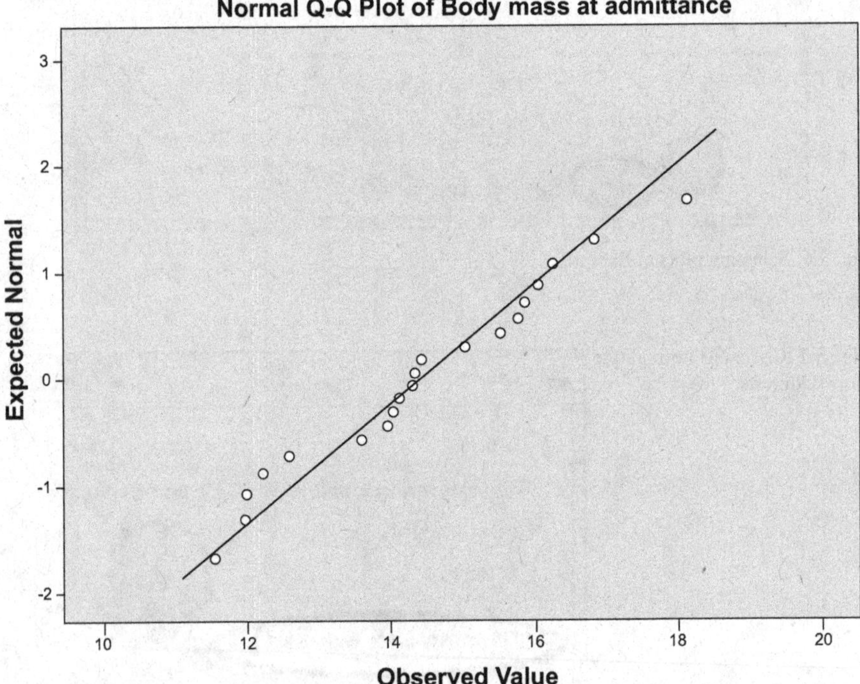

Fig. 5.8 A normal Q-Q plot

The output will include a table-labeled *Tests of Normality*. This table is reproduced in Table 5.7.

The table gives the results of the *Kolmogorov-Smirnov test* and the *Shapiro-Wilk test*. For both tests, the null hypothesis is that the population distribution is normal, and the alternative hypothesis is that the population distribution is not normal. If the *p*-values which appear in the columns labeled *Sig.* are higher than 0.1 it is reasonable to accept the null hypothesis that the population distribution is normal.

In addition to the test results, what is known as a *normal quantile-quantile plot* (or simply a *normal Q-Q plot*) appears following the stem-and-leaf plot. This plot is shown in Fig. 5.8. The term quantile is synonymous with percentile. If the sample

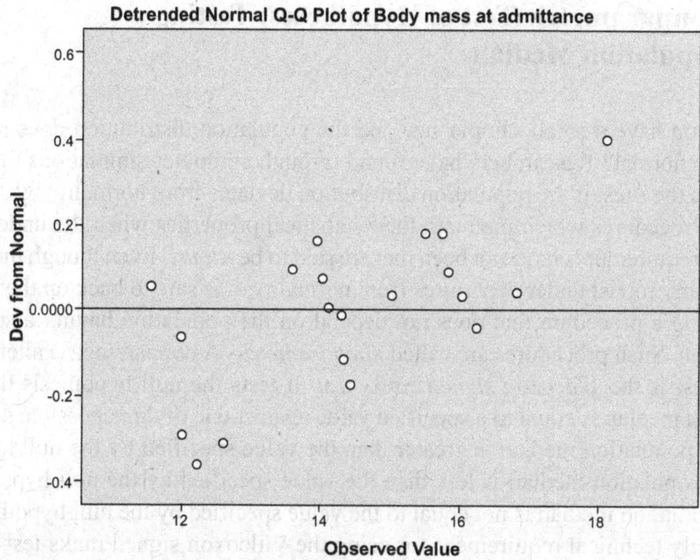

Fig. 5.9 A detrended normal Q-Q plot

results are consistent with a normal population distribution, the points on the plot should generally follow the straight line that is drawn. The points should be a random scattering about the line. Following the Q-Q plot is a *detrended normal Q-Q plot.* It is like the Q-Q plot except that the line is horizontal. The detrended plot is shown in Fig. 5.9.

Study the output and answer the following questions.

5.4.1 What is the p-value for the Kolmogorov-Smirnov test? What does it signify?

5.4.2 What is the p-value for the Shapiro-Wilk test? What does it signify?

5.4.3 Does the normal Q-Q plot indicate that a normal distribution is appropriate?

5.4.4 Should we use the t-test to determine whether or not the mean body mass index for anorexic patients entering treatment is <18.5?

5.4.5 If the answer to the previous question is "yes," have SPSS conduct the t-test of the null hypothesis that the mean body mass index for anorexic patients entering treatment is equal to 18.5 against the alternative hypothesis that the mean body mass index for anorexic patients entering treatment is < 18.5. Interpret your results.

5.5 Nonparametric Test of Hypotheses: Testing a Population Median

What if you have a small sample size and the population distribution does not appear to be normal? Researchers have found through computer simulations that it is safe to use the *t*-test if the population distribution deviates from normality by a slight amount. Procedures which maintain their statistical properties when the underlying technical requirements have not been met are said to be *robust*. Even though the *t*-test is reasonably robust under departures from normality, it is safe to back up the analysis by using a procedure that does not depend on the population having a specific distribution. Such procedures are called *nonparametric*. A nonparametric alternative to the *t*-test is the *Wilcoxon signed ranks test*. It tests the null hypothesis that the population median is equal to a specified value against one of three possible alternatives: the population median is greater than the value specified by the null hypothesis, the population median is less than the value specified by the null hypothesis, or the population median is not equal to the value specified by the null hypothesis.

The only technical requirement for using the Wilcoxon signed ranks test is that we must have a random sample. Even though the *t*-test is appropriate we will test the median BMI of the anorexic patients on admittance to treatment. We will test the null hypothesis that the median BMI is equal to 18.5 against the alternative that the median BMI is <18.5.

SPSS only conducts the Wilcoxon signed ranks test for an experimental situation known as *matched pairs*. We will discuss matched pairs in detail in Chap. 11. This procedure can, however, be adapted to conduct a single sample Wilcoxon signed ranks test by creating a new variable containing the value of the median specified by the null hypothesis. Select **Transform>Compute Variable**. As shown in Fig. 5.10, enter *nullmedian* in the *Target Variable* box and enter *18.5* in the *Numeric Expression*. Click **OK** to create the new variable.

To conduct the Wilcoxon test, select **Analyze>Nonparametric Tests>Legacy Dialogs>2-Related Samples** to open the *Two-Related-Samples Tests* dialog box shown below. Select **Body mass at admittance** and **nullmedian,** and move them as a pair to the *Test Pair(s) List* box by clicking the right pointing arrow. Make sure that *Wilcoxon* is checked in the *Test Type* area. Click **OK** to conduct the test. These steps are shown in Fig. 5.11. Study the output.

The output will include a *Test Statistics* box, shown in Table 5.8.

Z is the value of the test statistic, and *Asymp. Sig. (2-tailed)* gives the *p*-value for the two-sided alternative.

The *p*-value can be converted to a one-tailed *p*-value by using Table 5.9. For notation let $\tilde{\mu}$ denote the population median, $\tilde{\mu}_0$ denote the value of the population median specified by the null hypothesis, and *Sig* denote the two-sided *p*-value.

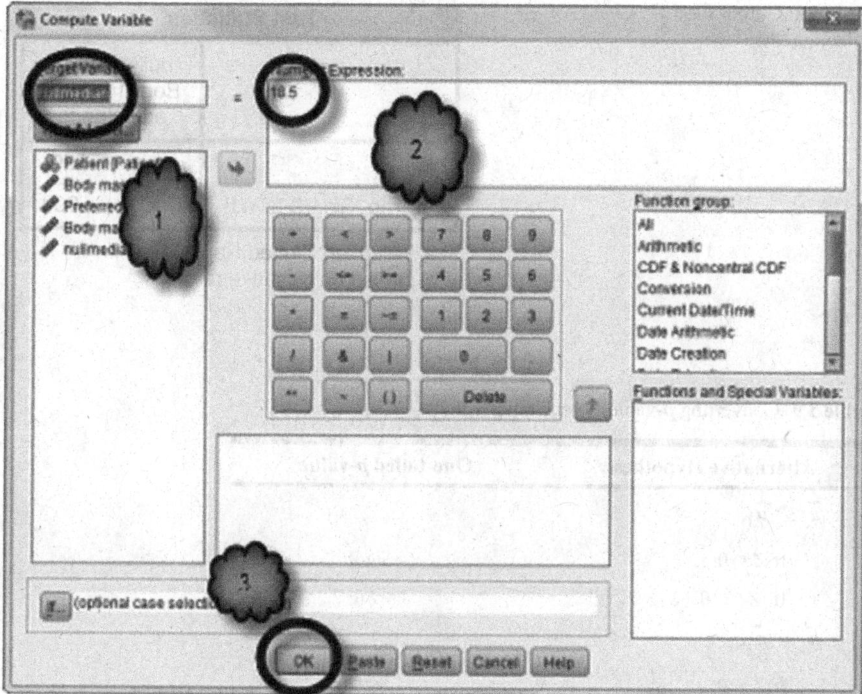

Fig. 5.10 Creating a new variable

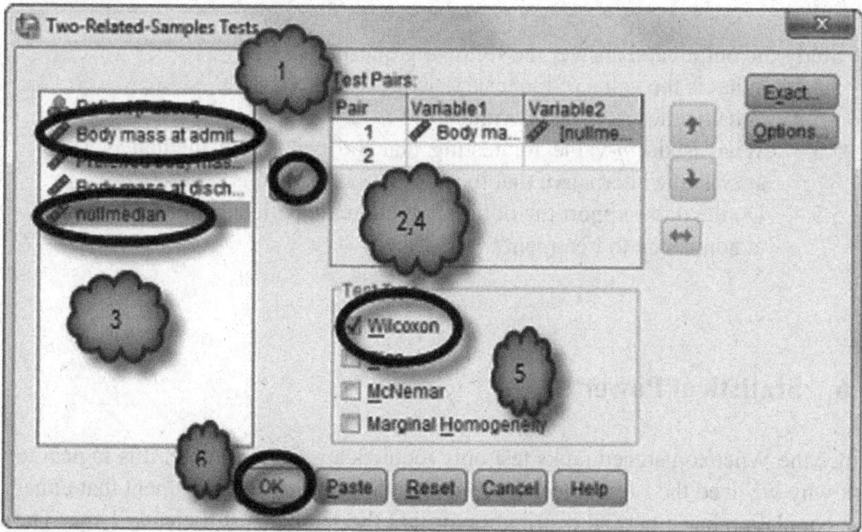

Fig. 5.11 Conducting the Wilcoxon test

Table 5.8 Output for the Wilcoxon test

Test Statistics[a]

	nullmedian - Body mass at admittance
Z	-3.920[b]
Asymp. Sig. (2-tailed)	.000

a. Wilcoxon Signed Ranks Test
b. Based on negative ranks.

Table 5.9 Converting p-values to one tail p-values

Alternative Hypothesis	One-tailed p-value
$\tilde{\mu} > \tilde{\mu}_0$	
If $Z < 0$:	$Sig/2$
If $Z \geq 0$:	$1 - Sig/2$
$\tilde{\mu} < \tilde{\mu}_0$	
If $Z < 0$:	$Sig/2$
If $Z \geq 0$:	$1 - Sig/2$

Study the output and answer the following questions.

5.5.1 What is the value of the test statistic?
5.5.2 What is the two-sided p-value?
5.5.3 What is the p-value for testing that the population median is 18.5 against the alternative that the population median is <18.5?
5.5.4 Do the data support the notion that anorexic patients are underweight at admission to treatment?

5.6 Statistical Power

Since the Wilcoxon signed ranks test only requires a random sample, it is logical to ask why we need the t-test, a test that imposes the additional requirement that either the population has a normal distribution or that the sample is sufficiently large. The answer lies in the *power* of the test. A statistical test that correctly finds evidence

Table 5.10 Output for *t* test

One-Sample Statistics

	N	Mean	Std. Deviation	Std. Error Mean
REPORTED HEIGHT IN INCHES	2916	69.76	3.011	.056

One-Sample Test

	Test Value = 70					
					95% Confidence Interval of the Difference	
	t	df	Sig. (2-tailed)	Mean Difference	Lower	Upper
REPORTED HEIGHT IN INCHES	-4.360	2915	.000	-.243	-.35	-.13

against the null hypothesis is said to be *more powerful* than a test that correctly finds evidence against the null hypothesis less often. It is a general rule that a test that places more restrictions on the population distribution is more powerful than one that does not. Therefore, when the requirements for using the *t*-test are met, it is used instead of the Wilcoxon signed ranks test. The *t*-test is more powerful than the Wilcoxon.

5.7 Clinical Versus Statistical Significance

Let's return to the data file, **CDC BRFSS.sav,** to test whether or not the mean reported height for males is 70 in. This will be a two-sided test of the null hypothesis that the mean height is 70 in. against the alternative hypothesis that the mean height is not equal to 70 in.

Begin by declaring the value of 999 as missing for the variable, **REPORTED HEIGHT IN INCHES** [*HTIN3*] (variable 75). Select those cases where **SEX** [*SEX*] (variable 32) is 1 (male). Now use **Analyze>Compare Means>One-Sample T Test** with **REPORTED HEIGHT IN INCHES** in the *Test Variable(s)* box and 70 in the *Test Value* box. Study the output shown in Table 5.10.

The output reports that the value for *t* is − 4.360, the degrees of freedom are 2915, and the resulting two-sided *p*-value is 0.000. (The reported *p*-value is rounded to the third decimal place. To see the exact value, double-click the output table and then double-click again the cell that displays the *p*-value.) The results of the *t*-test provide very strong evidence that the mean height for males is not 70 in. However, notice that the value of the sample mean is 69.76 in. In terms of the actual values, the sample mean is not *meaningfully* different from 70 in. When dealing with large sample sizes, small differences can be statistically significant. Although a difference may be statistically highly significant, that difference in practical or clinical terms may not be significant at all.

5.8 Exercise Questions

1. Do men who are 25 years old engage in moderate exercise on more than 4 days a week? Load SPSS data file, **CDC BRFSS.sav**. The variable of interest is **DAYS PER WEEK OF MOD. PHYS. ACT** [*MODPADAY*] (variable 44). Be sure that the values of 77, 88, and 99 have been declared as missing. Test the null hypothesis that the mean number of days for 25-year-old men who engage in moderate physical activity is 4 against the alternative hypothesis that the mean number of days is >4. In addition, construct a 99 % CI for the mean number of days that respondents engage in moderate physical activity.

    a. What is your sample size?
    b. What is the sample mean?
    c. What is the value of the test statistic, t?
    d. What are the degrees of freedom?
    e. What is the p-value for the test? Remember that we are running a one-sided test.
    f. What is your 99 % confidence interval?
    g. According to the results of the t-test, can we reject the null hypothesis? Why or why not?
    h. What are the technical requirements for using the t-test? Have they been satisfied? Explain.

2. Imagine that you are in charge of a treatment program for anorexia, and you want to know if your patients have a BMI > 18.5 at the time of discharge from the program. To find out, you analyze the data in SPSS data file, **Bodymass.sav**. The variable you are interested in is **Bodymass at discharge** [*Disch*] (variable 4). Note that the sample size is 20.

    a. Do the data indicate that a normal distribution is appropriate for the population?
    b. If so, conduct a t-test of the null hypothesis that the mean BMI is 18.5 against the alternative hypothesis that the mean BMI is > 18.5. If not, conduct a Wilcoxon signed ranks test that the median BMI is 18.5 against the alternative hypothesis that the median BMI is > 18.5.
    c. What is the value of your test statistic?
    d. What is the p-value for your test? Remember that we are running a one-sided test.
    e. Can you confidently conclude from these results that the average patient leaves your program with a BMI > 18.5? Why or why not?

3. Do patients with advanced colon cancer who are treated with ascorbate have an average survival time of 500 days? Use SPSS data file, **Patient.sav** [3], which contains data from patients with various types of cancer. Focusing on patients with colon cancer (use **Data > Select Cases**), analyze the variable, **Survival Days** [*Days*] (variable 2). Note that the sample size is 17.

Table 5.11 Normality test for PSA

Tests of Normality

	Kolmogorov-Smirnov[a]			Shapiro-Wilk		
	Statistic	df	Sig.	Statistic	df	Sig.
Prostate-Specific Antigen Level (ng/ml)	.314	301	.000	.358	301	.000

a. Lilliefors Significance Correction

a. Do the data indicate that a normal distribution is appropriate for the population of colon cancer patients?
b. If so, conduct a *t*-test of the null hypothesis that the mean survival time is 500 days against the alternative hypothesis that the mean survival time is not equal to 500 days. If not, conduct a Wilcoxon signed ranks test that the median survival time is 500 days against the alternative hypothesis that the median survival time is not equal to 500 days.
c. What is the value of your test statistic?
d. What is the *p*-value for your test?
e. Can you confidently conclude that the average survival time is not equal to 500 days? Why or why not?

4. The PSA levels and prostate volumes of 301 men were measured [4].
   a. According to the results of the tests of normality displayed in Table 5.11, are the PSA levels of men within the population from which the sample was taken normally distributed? Defend your answer.
   b. According to the normal Q-Q plot shown in Fig. 5.12, are the prostate volumes of men within the population from which the sample was taken normally distributed? Defend your answer.
5. How many hours per night do college seniors sleep during the week day? To find out, undergraduates were polled [5]. Sixteen were seniors. Because the sample size was small and the population distribution was not normal, a one sample *t*-test and a Wilcoxon signed ranks test were conducted. The *t*-test tested the null hypothesis that the mean number of hours of sleep per night obtained within the population of college seniors is equal to six against the alternative hypothesis that the mean number of hours of sleep per night obtained within the population of college seniors is >6. The Wilcoxon test tested the null hypothesis that the median number of hours of sleep per night is equal to 6 against the alternative hypothesis that the median number of hours of sleep is >6. The results of a two-tailed test for each analysis are reported below:
   - Sample mean: 6.56.
   - Sample median: 6.75.
   - One-sample *t*-test: $t_{15}=2.377$, $P=0.031$.
   - Wilcoxon signed ranks test: $Z=-2.087$, $P=0.037$.

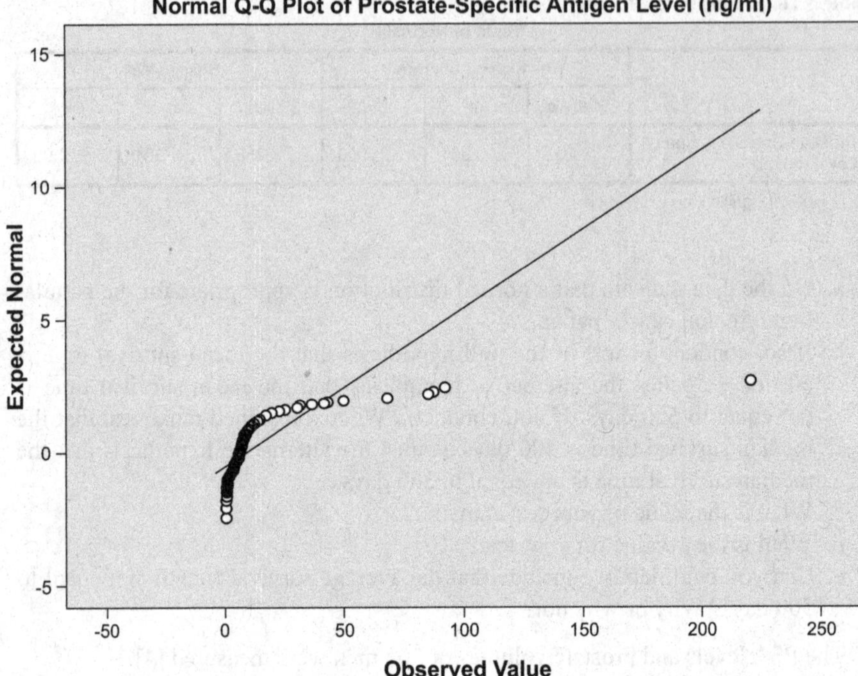

Fig. 5.12 Q-Q plot for PSA

a. The results of the two inferential tests are reported in the editorial style of the American Medical Association. For the value of *t*, the number "15" appears as a subscript. To what does the "15" refer?
b. According to the results of the one-sample *t*-test, what is the one-tailed *p*-value?
c. According to the results of the one-sample *t*-test, should we reject the null hypothesis that the population mean is equal to 6 hours of sleep in favor of the alternative hypothesis that the population mean is >6 h of sleep? Why or why not?
d. Do the results of the nonparametric test support or contradict the results of the *t*-test? Briefly defend your answer.
e. The sample mean (6.56 h) is about 0.5 h greater than the value stated in the null hypothesis (6 h). Is this finding statistically significant? Why or why not? In your opinion, is this finding clinically significant? Why or why not?

Data Sets and References

1. CDC BRFSS.sav obtained from: Centers for Disease Control and Prevention (CDC): Behavioral Risk Factor Surveillance System Survey Data. Atlanta, Georgia: US Department of Health and Human Services, Centers for Disease Control and Prevention (2005). Public domain. For more information about the BRFSS, visit http://www.cdc.gov/brfss/. Accessed 16 Nov 2014
2. Bodymass.sav obtained from: Hand, D.J., Daly, F., Lunn, A.D., McConway, K.J., Ostrowski, E.: A Handbook of Small Data Sets. Chapman & Hall, London (1994). (With the kind permission of the Routledge Taylor and Francis Group, and Professor Shelley L Channon)
3. Patient.sav obtained from: Hand, D.J., Daly, F., Lunn, A.D., McConway, K.J., Ostrowski, E.: A Handbook of Small Data Sets. Chapman & Hall, London (1994). With the kind permission of the Routledge Taylor and Francis Group, Dr. Linus Pauling, Jr. For context, see Cameron, E., Pauling, L.: Supplemental ascorbate in the supportve treatment of cancer: re-evaluation of prolongation of survival times in terminal human cancer. Proc. Natl. Acad. Sci. U S A **75**, 4538–4542 (1978)
4. PAS.sav obtained from: Riffenburgh, R.H.: Statistics in Medicine, 2nd ed. Elsevier Academic Press, Burlington (2006). (With the kind permissson of the Elsevier Books and Dr. Thomas K. Huisman)
5. From: Bacchus, H.F., Boeltz, B.R., Rybinski, J.G., Brown, R.G., Holmes, W.H.: Sleep duration, body mass index, self-reported health and the academic performance of college students. Unpublished data, Le Moyne College, Syracuse (2009)

Data Sets and References

1. [illegible]
2. [illegible]
3. [illegible]
4. [illegible]
5. [illegible]
6. [illegible]

Chapter 6
Inference for Proportions

Abstract An important goal in clinical research is estimating the proportion of a population who has a particular disease or who will acquire the disease over a given period of time, and identifying factors that are associated with the occurrence of the disease. This chapter reviews how confidence intervals and tests of hypotheses are used to estimate prevalence and incidence from sample data, and how various measures of association based on sample proportions—the difference between two proportions, relative risk and the odds ratio—are used to identify risk factors.

6.1 Overview

Researchers are often interested in the frequency with which a patient characteristic, medical condition or disease is encountered within a population. With regard to disease, researchers often document *prevalence* and *incidence*. Prevalence refers to the proportion of a population who has the disease at a given point in time. For example, an investigator might be interested in knowing the proportion of residents of NY state who had hypertension *at the end of* the year 2005. Incidence refers to the proportion of a population who acquire a disease over a given period of time. For example, a researcher might be interested in knowing the proportion of NY state residents who *became* hypertensive *during* the year 2005. In some instances, researchers wish to know whether the proportion of a population with a given characteristic, condition, or illness is equal to, greater than, or less than some particular value. For example, an investigator might wish to know whether the proportion of a population who needed to see a doctor but could not because of the cost associated with an office visit is no more than some value, say, 10 %.

Since researchers cannot examine the entire population, they need to estimate a population proportion using sample data. This means that they need to construct a confidence interval (CI) for the population value and to test hypotheses regarding the population proportion. SPSS does not have a built-in capability to construct CIs or test hypotheses regarding population proportions. SPSS does, however, provide the capability of writing external procedures to produce analysis that is not part of SPSS program. They are known as SPSS *scripts*. We shall see how to use previously written scripts to analyze population proportions.

W. H. Holmes, W. C. Rinaman, *Statistical Literacy for Clinical Practitioners*,
DOI 10.1007/978-3-319-12550-3_6

In addition, there are times when researchers want to compare the proportions of two independent populations. For example, they might wish to determine if a disease is more prevalent among men or women in order to determine whether the occurrence of the disease is related to the patient's sex. In these instances, researchers construct CIs for the difference between two population proportions and conduct tests of hypotheses regarding the difference between two population proportions. As is the case with a single proportion, SPSS does not have a built-in capability for performing these procedures but can make use of previously written scripts.

Estimating or testing the difference between two proportions can reveal whether the likelihood of developing a particular medical condition or disease is greater for people who share a certain characteristic or experience. Such characteristics or experiences are called *risk factors*. Risk factors can also be identified by using two proportions to compare the *probability* or *odds* of acquiring a disease for a person exposed to the factor to the probability or odds for a person not exposed. Often the comparison is made in terms of the ratio of the two probabilities or the two odds. When the ratio consists of two probabilities, the result is known as *relative risk*. When the ratio consists of two odds, the result is known as an *odds ratio*. Later in the chapter, we will explore these two statistics and learn how to instruct SPSS to compute them.

6.2 CIs for Population Proportions

Suppose that we are interested in determining the proportion of people in a population that has a certain condition. The population parameter of interest here is the population proportion. The mathematical symbol for it is p. (Do not confuse this symbol for p-value.) Looking back at our discussion of CIs for the population mean, we note a couple of things. First, the basic form for the CI was

$$\textit{Statistic} \pm (\textit{Critical value})\,(\textit{Standard error}) \tag{6.1}$$

Second, the statistic was the sample statistic corresponding to the population parameter. That is, the sample mean is the statistic associated with the population mean. The same holds true for a CI for a population proportion. Before getting to the details we need to define some terms. An observation that has the condition of interest is said to be a *success*. An observation that does not have the condition of interest is said to be a *failure*. The statistic associated with the population proportion is the *sample proportion*. Its symbol is $\hat{p}$ and is called *p hat*. If we let X denote the number of successes in our sample and let N denote the sample size, then *p hat* is computed by dividing the number of successes by the sample size. That is,

$$\hat{p} = X / N. \tag{6.2}$$

We need these terms in order to understand how to complete the dialog box for constructing the CIs and conducting the tests that we will be discussing in this chapter.

CIs for a proportion have the same interpretation as those for the population mean. That is, 95 % confidence means that 95 % of all possible CIs based on samples of the same size from the same population will contain the population proportion and 5 % will not.

An Example As an example, let us construct a 95 % CI for the proportion of adults living in NY state in 2005 who were obese. Load the data file, **CDC BRFSS.sav** [1], into SPSS. Be sure that 9 has been declared as a missing value for **BODY MASS INDEX-THREE LEVELS CATEGORY** [*@_BMI4CAT*] (variable 79) Select **Analyze > Descriptive Statistics > Frequencies** and enter **BODY MASS INDEX-THREE LEVELS CATEGORY** in the *Variable(s)* box and click **OK**. This will generate the frequency table in Table 6.1. The value in the *Frequency* column for the category labeled *Obese* will be the number of successes in the sample (X), and the value in the *Frequency* column for the category labeled *Total* will be the sample size (N). You will need these to construct the CI. Note that the valid percent divided by 100 is the sample proportion.

As we mentioned in the overview, SPSS does not have a built-in capability to construct CIs for a population proportion. SPSS does have a capability to write external programs called *scripts* that can perform procedures that are not part of SPSS. A script has been written to construct CIs for a single population proportion. It is called **ciprop.sbs**. Your instructor will tell you where to find it. The procedure used by the script is appropriate as long as there are at least 10 successes and 10 failures in the sample.

To run the script select **Utilities > Run Script**. This will open the *Run Script* dialog box shown in Fig. 6.1. In the *Look in* window, make your way to the script. Run the script by either double-clicking the script or by clicking the script followed by **Run**. This will open the *Confidence Interval for a Proportion* dialog box shown in Fig. 6.2.

Table 6.1 Frequency table for three categories of body mass index

BODY MASS INDEX- THREE LEVELS CATEGORY

		Frequency	Percent	Valid Percent	Cumulative Percent
Valid	Neither Overweight nor Obese	3007	38.6	40.5	40.5
	Overweight	2703	34.7	36.4	77.0
	Obese	1707	21.9	23.0	100.0
	Total	7417	95.1	100.0	
Missing	Don't know/Refused/Missing	379	4.9		
Total		7796	100.0		

The number of cases = X, while the total number of valid cases = N.

The valid percent divided by 100 = X/N, the sample proportion of obesity.

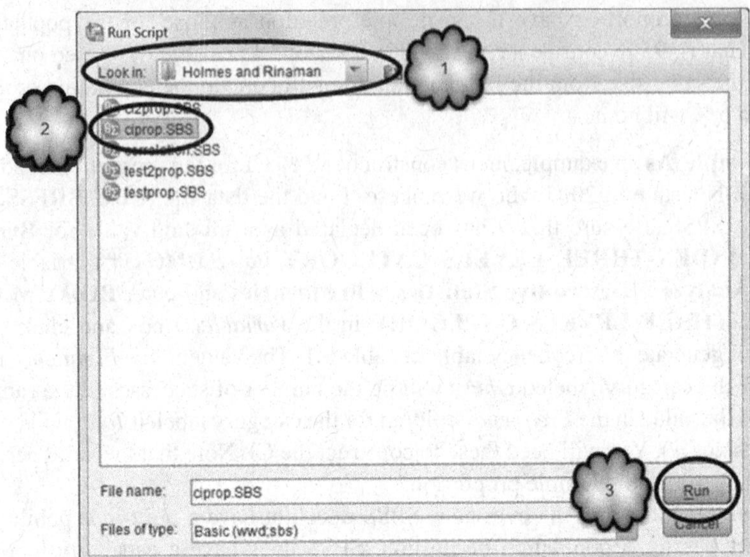

Fig. 6.1 Selecting the script, Confidence Interval for a Single Population Proportion

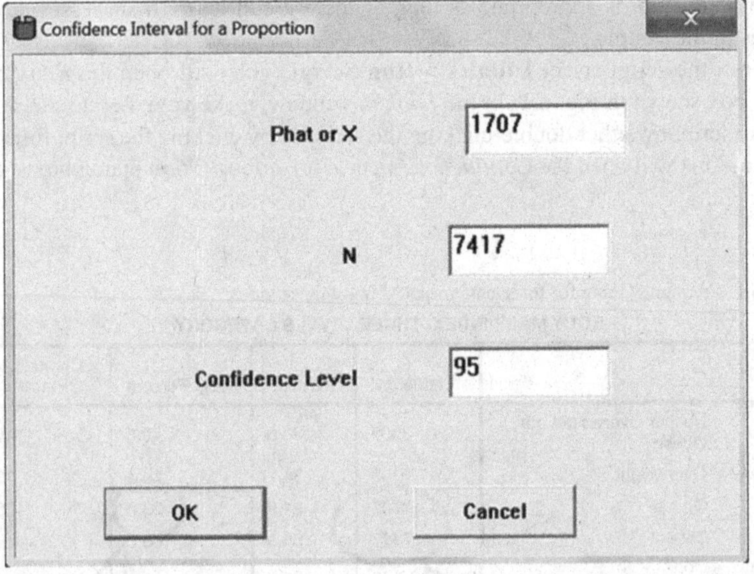

Fig. 6.2 Generating a 95% confidence interval for a single population proportion

If you have the value for *p hat,* enter it in the *Phat or X* box. If you have the number of successes (*X*), enter it in the *Phat or X* box. Enter the sample size (*N*) in the *N* box. Enter the desired confidence level in percent in the *Confidence Level* box. The resulting dialog box should look like the one in Fig. 6.2.

Click **OK** to construct the CI. The output is reproduced in Table 6.2.

Table 6.2 95 % Confidence interval for the proportion of obese NY state residence

95% Confidence Interval for P

	N	X	Phat	Lower	Upper
	7417	1707	0.230147	0.2205675	0.2397264

Answer the following questions:

6.2.1 What is the value of *N*?

6.2.2 What is the value of *p hat*?

6.2.3 What are the confidence limits for the proportion of the population that is obese?

6.2.4 Does your CI contain the true proportion?

6.3 Testing a Single Proportion

There are situations where one wants to test whether or not the proportion of the population that has a certain condition is equal to a specified value. This is the null hypothesis. The possible alternative hypotheses are that the population proportion is less than the value specified by the null hypothesis, the population proportion is greater than the value specified by the null hypothesis, or the population proportion is not equal to the value specified by the null hypothesis. The appropriate alternative hypothesis will be dictated by the context of the investigation. Similar to the case for testing population means, the test statistic is based on a sample statistic—in this case, the sample proportion, *p hat*—and it computes a *p*-value. The *p*-value is interpreted in the same way that *p*-values for testing the population mean are interpreted.

An Example We wish to test whether or not less than 10 % of the population needed to see a doctor within the last 12 months but could not because of the cost of an office visit. The relevant variable in the Centers for Disease Control and Prevention (CDC) data file is **COULD NOT SEE DR. BECAUSE OF COST** [*MEDCOST*]. (variable 9; 1 = Yes, 2 = No, 7 = Don't know/Not sure, 9 = Refused).

Declare values of 7 and 9 as missing and assign the value labels. Select **Analyze > Descriptive Statistics > Frequencies**. Enter **COULD NOT SEE DR. BECAUSE OF COST** in the *Variable(s)* box and click **OK**. Study the output which should include the frequency table displayed in Table 6.3.

The value in the *Frequencies* column for *Yes* will be the number of successes (*X*), and the value in the *Frequencies* column for *Total* will be the sample size (*N*).

As was the case for CIs, SPSS does not have a built-in capability to conduct tests on a single population proportion, so we have provided a script, **testprop.sbs**, for you. The procedure that it implements is appropriate if the sample size times the

Table 6.3 Frequency of NY state residents unable to see a doctor because of cost

COULD NOT SEE DR. BECAUSE OF COST

		Frequency	Percent	Valid Percent	Cumulative Percent
Valid	Yes	742	9.5	9.5	9.5
	No	7034	90.2	90.5	100.0
	Total	7776	99.7	100.0	
Missing	Don't know/Not Sure	15	.2		
	Refused	5	.1		
	Total	20	.3		
Total		7796	100.0		

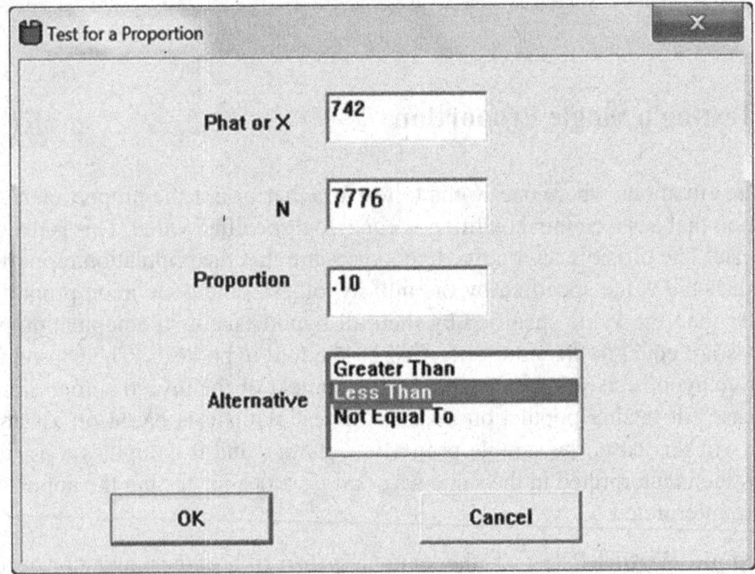

Fig. 6.3 Generating a test of proportion against a one-tailed alternative hypothesis

proportion specified by the null hypothesis is at least 10 and the sample size times 1 minus the proportion specified by the null hypothesis is at least 10.

To run the script, select **Utilities** > **Run Script**. Run the **testprop.sbs** script to open the *Test for a Proportion* dialog box. As was the case with the CI script, enter either the value of *p hat* or the number of successes (*X*) in the *Phat or X* box, and the sample size (*N*) in the *N* box. Enter the proportion specified by the null hypothesis in the *Proportion* box. Select the appropriate alternative hypothesis by clicking on it in the *Alternative* box. The resulting dialog box should look like the one in Fig. 6.3.

Click **OK** to conduct the test. The output is reproduced in Table 6.4.

Table 6.4 Results of a one-tailed test of a population proportion

Test of P = .10 vs. P Less Than.10

	N	X	Phat	Z	P-value
	7776	742	9.542181E-02	-1.345707	8.919852E-02

Answer the following questions:

6.3.1 What is the sample size?

6.3.2 What is the value of *p hat*?

6.3.3 What is the value of *Z*?

6.3.4 What is the *p*-value for the test?

6.3.5. What does the test lead you to conclude regarding whether or not less than 10 % could not visit a doctor because of the cost?

6.4 CIs for the Difference Between Two Population Proportions

There are situations where researchers will want to compare two population proportions. For example, an investigator might be interested in comparing the proportion of men who are obese to the proportion of women who are obese to determine whether sex is a risk factor for obesity. One way to compare two population proportions is to construct a CI for the difference between the two proportions. As was the case with inferences regarding a single population proportion, SPSS does not have a built-in capability for comparing two proportions. SPSS scripts are provided to address this need. It is appropriate to use the script if you have at least five successes and five failures in each sample.

An Example We wish to construct a 95 % CI for the difference between the proportion of men who are obese and the proportion of women who are obese. We will be using the variable **BODY MASS INDEX-THREE LEVELS CATEGORY**[*@_BMI4CAT*] (variable 79).

Before running **Analyze > Descriptive Statistics > Frequencies** to get the summary statistics needed for the script, we need to split the file according to gender so that we can obtain summary statistics separately for men and women. Select **Data > Split File** to open the *Split File* dialog box. Check *Organize output by groups* and enter **SEX** [*SEX*] (variable 32; 1 = Male, 2 = Female) in the *Groups Based on* box. Click **OK**. Splitting the file will result in a separate analysis for each distinct value of the grouping variable, **SEX**. Figures 6.4, 6.5 and 6.6 review these steps.

Run **Analyze > Descriptive Statistics > Frequencies** on **BODY MASS INDEX-THREE LEVELS CATEGORY.** Study the output.

The frequency table for each sex is reproduced in Tables 6.5 and 6.6. Now that we have obtained the numbers of obese respondents and the sample sizes of each

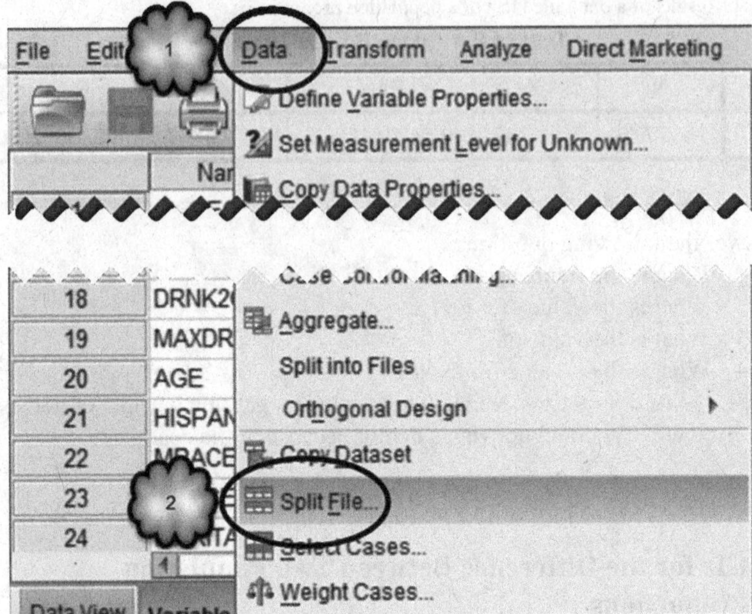

Fig. 6.4 Opening the Split File dialog

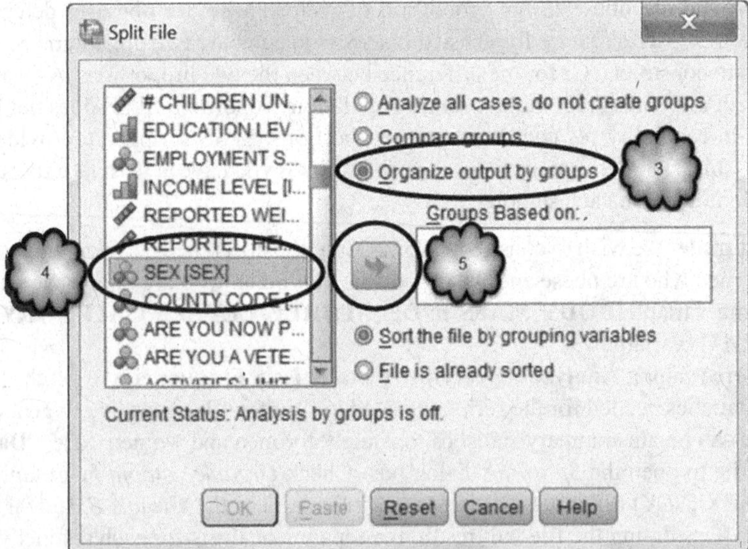

Fig. 6.5 Organizing the output by sex

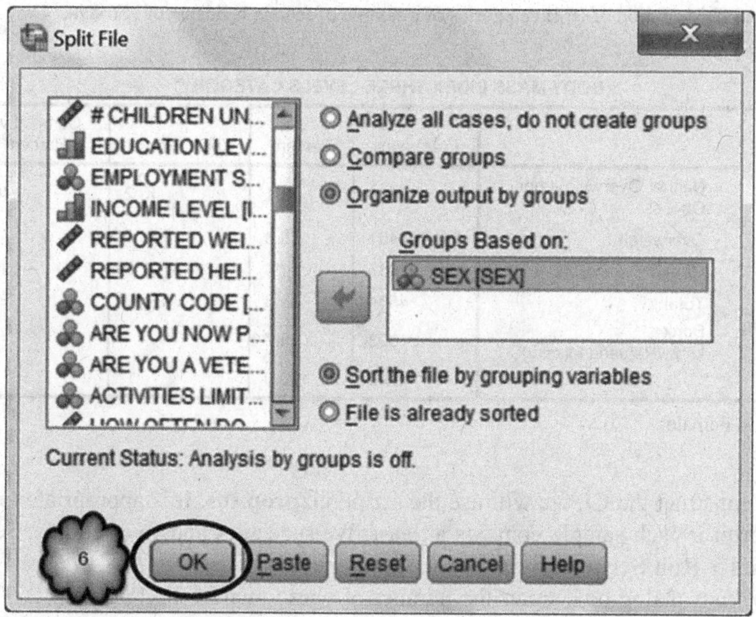

Fig. 6.6 Splitting the data file by sex

Table 6.5 Distribution of BMI categories of a sample of male residents of NY state

SEX = Male

BODY MASS INDEX-THREE LEVELS CATEGORY[a]

		Frequency	Percent	Valid Percent	Cumulative Percent
Valid	Neither Overweight nor Obese	911	31.0	31.6	31.6
	Overweight	1302	44.4	45.2	76.8
	Obese	670	22.8	23.2	100.0
	Total	2883	98.3	100.0	
Missing	Don't know/Refused/Missing	51	1.7		
Total		2934	100.0		

a. SEX = Male

sex, we can construct the CI for the difference between the proportions of men and women who are obese.

We will construct the CI for the difference between the two proportions by subtracting the women from the men. The group that is being subtracted from is called generically *population 1*, and the group that is being subtracted is called generically *population 2*. That is, the difference is *population 1 minus population 2*. So, in this case *population 1* will be the men and *population 2* will be the women.

Table 6.6 Distribution of BMI categories of a sample of female residents of NY state

SEX = Female

BODY MASS INDEX-THREE LEVELS CATEGORY[a]

		Frequency	Percent	Valid Percent	Cumulative Percent
Valid	Neither Overweight nor Obese	2096	43.1	46.2	46.2
	Overweight	1401	28.8	30.9	77.1
	Obese	1037	21.3	22.9	100.0
	Total	4534	93.3	100.0	
Missing	Don't know/Refused/Missing	328	6.7		
Total		4862	100.0		

a. SEX = Female

To construct the CI, we will use the script, **ci2prop.sbs**. It is appropriate to use this script if each sample contains at least five successes and five failures. Select **Utilities > Run Script** and run the script to open the *Conf. Int. Diff. between Two Proportions* dialog box. Enter the number of obese men in the *Phat 1 or X1* box, the sample size for the men in the *N1* box, the number of obese women in the *Phat 2 or X2* box, and the sample size for the women in the *N2* box. Enter the desired confidence level in the *Confidence Level* box. The resulting dialog box should look like the one shown in Fig. 6.7.

Click **OK** to construct the CI. Table 6.7 displays the resulting output.

Answer the following questions:

6.4.1 What were the sample sizes for the men and the women?

6.4.2 What were the values of *p hat* for the men and for the women?

6.4.3 What are the confidence limits for the difference between the proportion of men who are obese and the proportion of women who are obese?

6.4.4 Is this interval consistent with there being no difference in the population between men and women with regard to obesity?

6.5 Testing Two Proportions

When comparing two proportions, a test of whether or not two proportions are equal can be conducted. The null hypothesis is that the two proportions are equal. The possible alternative hypotheses are that one proportion is greater than the other, one proportion is less than the other, or the two proportions are not equal to each other. Again, the context of the investigation indicates which alternative hypothesis is appropriate.

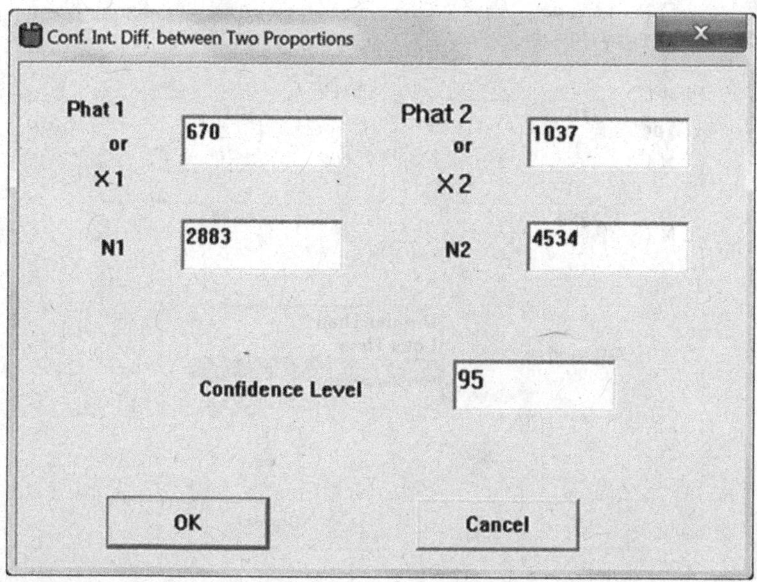

Fig. 6.7 Generating a 95% confidence interval for the difference between two population proportions

Table 6.7 95% confidence interval for the difference between two population proportions

95% Confidence Interval for P1 - P2

	N	X	Phat	Lower	Upper
One	2883	670	0.2323968	-1.599581E-02	2.335672E-02
Two	4534	1037	0.2287164		

An Example We wish to test whether or not the proportion of men who are obese is equal to the proportion women who are obese. The null hypothesis will be that the two proportions are equal, and the alternative hypothesis will be that the two proportions are not equal. As we did when we constructed the **CI**, *population 1* will be the men and *population 2* will be the women.

The condition that must be satisfied in order to use the script that is appropriate for this situation is a little complicated. First, unsplit the file by selecting **Data > Split File,** checking *Analyze all cases, do not create groups*, and clicking **OK.** Now run **Analyze > Descriptive Statistics > Frequencies** on **BODY MASS INDEX-THREE LEVELS CATEGORY** to compute the proportion of respondents who are obese. You may recall from Sect. 6.2 that the proportion of the entire sample that is obese is 0.23. If each sample size times this proportion is at least 5, and if each sample size times 1 minus this proportion is at least 5, then the procedure implemented by the script is appropriate.

To conduct the test, select **Utilities > Run Script** and run the script **test2prop.sbs** to open the *Test for Equality of Two Proportions* dialog box. Enter the number

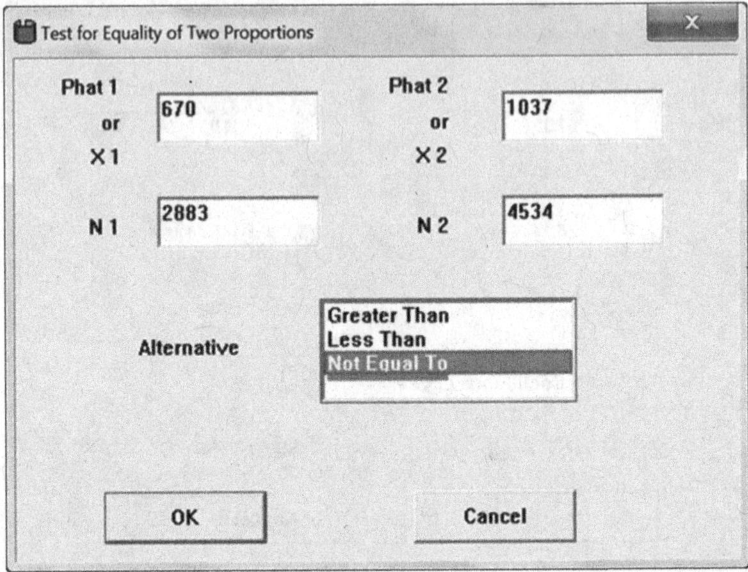

Fig. 6.8 Generating a two-tailed test of the difference between two proportions

Table 6.8 Results of a two-tailed test of the difference between two proportions

Test of P1 = P2 vs. P1 Not Equal To P2

	N	X	Phat	Z	P-value
One	2883	670	0.2323968	0.3670656	0.7135701
Two	4534	1037	0.2287164		

of obese men in the *Phat 1 or X1* box, the sample size for the men in the *N1* box, the number of obese women in the *Phat 2 or X2* box and the sample size for the women in the *N2* box. Select the appropriate alternative hypothesis (*Not Equal To*) by clicking it in the *Alternative* box. The resulting dialog box should look like the one shown in Fig. 6.8.

Click **OK** to conduct the test. Table 6.8 displays the resulting output.

Answer the following questions:

6.5.1 What are the sample sizes for the men and women?

6.5.2 What are the sample proportions (p *hat*) for the men and women?

6.5.3 What is the value of Z?

6.5.4 What is the p-value for the test?

6.5.5 Does the test indicate that the proportion of men who are obese is different from the proportion of women who are obese?

6.5.6 Have the necessary conditions for using this procedure been met?

6.6 Relative Risk and Odds Ratios

Risk factors are associated with but have not been shown to *cause* the conditions or diseases of interest. As we pointed out in Chap. 1, to establish that a factor causes a particular outcome, it would be necessary to show that the factor preceded the outcome in time (causes come before their effects) and that the outcome was not due to the presence of some other variable or confounder that may have accompanied the factor. To establish these two conditions convincingly, an experiment would have to be conducted in which patients are at random either exposed or not exposed to the factor in question. The proportion of those exposed to the factor (the experimental group) who subsequently develop the outcome under investigation would then be compared to the proportion of those in the group not exposed (the control group).

For ethical reasons, suspected causal factors cannot be studied experimentally on humans. For example, it would be unethical to expose people to a suspected carcinogen to see if it really causes cancer. However, researchers can still establish that exposure to a factor is followed by an increase in the probability of disease or illness by conducting a *cohort study*. As with an experiment, this study tracks the incidence of an outcome in two groups, one which shares the risk factor and one which does not. The ratio of these two proportions yields a statistic called *relative risk*, the extent to which the probability of disease for those exposed to the risk factor is greater than that of those not exposed. If the relative risk is statistically significantly greater than 1, the researcher would have evidence that the variable under study is a risk factor.

By measuring how often new instances of the outcome occur after the two groups have been selected, the cohort study attempts to establish the appropriate time sequence regarding the risk factor and its outcome. However, because the two groups were not formed via random assignment, it is always possible that any observed difference in risk between the two groups was due to factors associated with the risk factor rather than to the risk factor itself. Therefore, relative risk in a cohort study is evidence regarding whether the factor under study is a risk factor but is not conclusive evidence that the factor is a cause of disease.

We saw in Chap. 1 that as useful as cohort studies are in identifying risk factors, they can be difficult and expensive to conduct. For example, cohort studies can take a long time to complete, patients can be difficult to track, and many patients may be lost to the study over time. Consequently, researchers may choose alternative designs to establish that exposure to a factor is associated with a higher likelihood of disease or illness. Although these designs have their weaknesses, they are often relatively easy, quick and inexpensive to conduct. Two such designs are the *case-control study* and the *cross-sectional study*. Chapter 1 provides details about these two designs, so here we will give a quick overview.

In a case-control study, the researcher works backward from the disease to the suspected risk factor. First, two groups of people are identified. One, called cases, already has the condition or illness. The second, called controls, does not. The researcher then counts the number of cases and controls that had been exposed to the risk factor and determines whether the proportion of cases that had been exposed to the factor is greater than the proportion of controls. In a cross-sectional study, the researcher collects data from a sample of people without first selecting them on the basis of either the risk factor (as would be the case in a cohort study) or disease (as would be the case in a case-control study). The researcher then divides the sample into those who it turns out had been exposed to the risk factor and those who had not, and determines if the prevalence of disease in the first group is greater than in the second.

Risk is defined as the probability of developing a negative health outcome over a given period of time. Consequently, it is impossible for either the case-control or cross-sectional study to assess risk as neither design identifies people who have yet to experience the outcome and then follows them forward in time to determine the proportion who during a specified time interval experience the outcome. Unable to measure risk, researchers using case-control or cross-sectional studies cannot calculate relative risk. But researchers can calculate the *odds ratio,* a statistic that determines the extent to which the odds of experiencing the outcome in question is greater for the group of people who had been exposed to the risk factor than for the group who had not been exposed.

Unless the outcome is rare, an odds ratio will not equal the relative risk, so it usually can not be used to make conclusions about how much more at risk people become when they are exposed to a risk factor. But odds ratios can always be used to determine if a risk factor and an outcome are related to one another. If the odds ratio is statistically significantly greater than 1, the researcher has evidence that the factor under study is a risk factor.

Relative Risk Let us analyze the CDC data to determine if being overweight is a risk factor for poorer health. At this point, you may have recognized the CDC survey as an example of a cross-sectional study. If so, you realize that in order to use the CDC data to estimate risk, we would have to assume that the variable we are calling a potential risk factor (being overweight) preceded in time the variable we are calling an outcome (poorer health). This is a tenuous assumption, but making it will allow us to use these data as an example.

Reverse coding the risk factor and the outcome variable. When using SPSS to calculate relative risk or odds ratios, cases that were exposed to the risk factor should be identified with a numerical code that is lower than the code used for cases that were not exposed to the risk factor. Unfortunately, in the CDC data set, the opposite is true: In the variable, **RISK FACTOR FOR OVERWEIGHT OR OBESE** [@_*RFBMI4*] (variable 80), respondents who were exposed to the risk factor (i.e., people who were either overweight or obese) are coded with a 2, while respondents who were not exposed (people who were neither overweight nor obese) are coded with a 1. So before we begin, we will have to reverse this coding.

Similarly, when using SPSS to calculate relative risk or odds ratios, cases that *experienced* the negative outcome should be identified with a numerical code that is *lower* than the code used for cases that did not experience the outcome. Unfortunately, in the CDC data set, the opposite is true: In the variable, **HEALTH**

STATUS [*@_RFHLTH*] (variable 58), respondents who experienced the outcome (i.e., people who were in fair or poor health) are coded with a 2, while respondents who did not experience the outcome (people who were in good or better health) are coded with a 1. So we will have to reverse this coding as well.

To reverse the coding of the two variables, we will use **Transform > Recode into Different Variables**. As this procedure was reviewed in earlier chapters, here we will just outline the steps needed to reverse the coding of our risk factor and outcome variable.

Select **Transform > Recode Into Different Variables** to bring up the *Recode into Different Variables* dialog box. Move **RISK FACTOR FOR OVERWEIGHT OR OBESE** to the *Input Variable → Output Variable* window. In the *Name* window, enter as a name for the new variable, **RISK_FACTOR_FOR_OVERWEIGHT_OR_OBESE_RECODED.** Then type a label for this new variable in the *Label* window, **RISK FACTOR FOR OVERWEIGHT OR OBESE RECODED**. Click **Change.** The dialog box should look similar to the one shown in Fig. 6.9.

Now click **Old and New Values** to bring up the *Recode into Different Variables: Old and New Values* dialog box. Into the *Value* window of the *Old Value* area, type a "1" (without the quotation marks). Into the *Value* window of the *New Value* area, type a "2." Click **Add.** Return to the *Value* window of the *Old Value* area and type in a "2," and then enter a "1" into the *Value* window of the *New Value* area. Again click **Add.** Finally, select *All other values* in the *Old Value* area and *Copy old value(s)* in the *New Value* area. Click **Add.** The dialog box should now look like the one shown in Fig. 6.10.

You will now have instructed SPSS to recode the old variable, **RISK FACTOR FOR OVERWEIGHT OR OBESE,** into a new variable, **RISK FACTOR FOR OVERWEIGHT OR OBESE RECODED,** such that cases that had been coded as

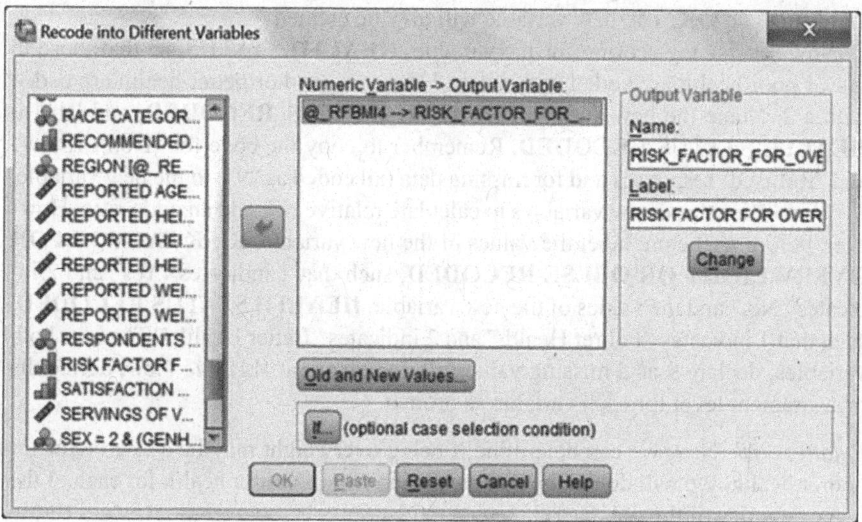

Fig. 6.9 Naming the output variable

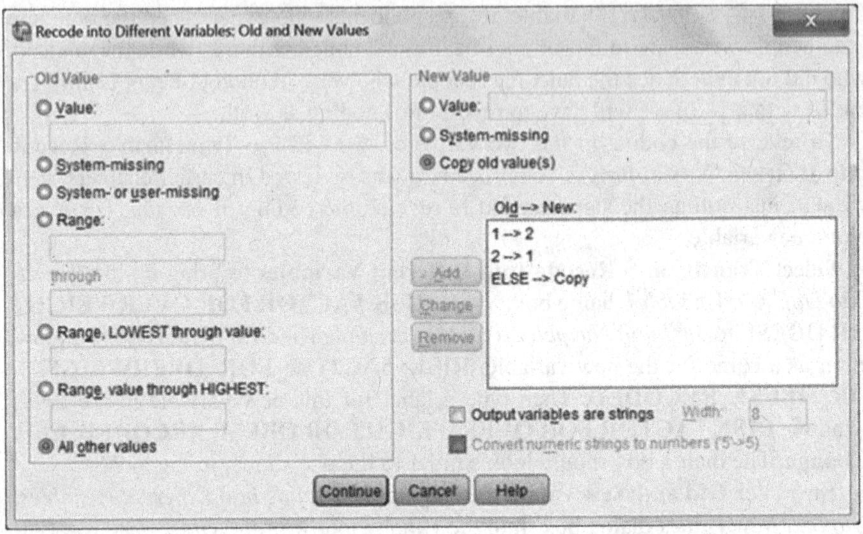

Fig. 6.10 Defining new values

1 in the old variable will now be coded as 2 in the new variable, and cases that had been coded as 2 in the old variable will now be coded as 1 in the new variable. By reversing the scoring that was used in the old variable, the new variable will identify respondents who are overweight or obese with a 1 instead of a 2, and those who are not overweight or obese with a 2 instead of a 1. You have also told SPSS to retain all remaining codes in the original variable. As a result, the code "9," which was used with the old variable for cases involving either responses of "Don't Know" or "Refused," or for missing values, will be copied over to the new variable. Now click **Continue** and **OK.** The new variable will now be created.

Now reverse the scoring for the variable, **HEALTH STATUS**, so that those in fair or poor health are coded with a 1 and those in good or better health are coded with a 2. Name the new variable, **HEALTH_STATUS_RECODED**, and label it **HEALTH STATUS RECODED.** Remember to copy the code for "Don't Know" and "Refused" responses and for missing data (all coded as "9") to the new variable.

We will use these new variables to calculate relative risk and an odds ratio. However, before we begin, label the values of the new variable, **RISK FACTOR FOR OVERWEIGHT OR OBESE RECODED**, such that 1 indicates "Yes" and 2 indicates "No," and the values of the new variable, **HEALTH STATUS RECODED**, such that 1 indicates "Poorer Health" and 2 indicates "Better Health." Then for both variables, declare 9 as a missing value. While you are at *Variable View*, define the measurement level for each variable as ordinal.

Relative Risk Now we can determine if being overweight may be a risk factor for poorer health. We will do this by comparing the risk of poorer health for each of the two categories of the risk factor.

Select **Analyze > Descriptive Statistics > Crosstabs** to bring up the *Crosstabs* dialog box. One purpose of the *Crosstabs* procedure is to generate a table displaying the distribution of cases across the combinations of the values of two categorical variables. In this instance, we want SPSS to display a table that shows the distribution of cases across the combinations of the two values of our risk factor, **RISK FACTOR FOR OVERWEIGHT OR OBESE RECODED**, and the two values of our outcome variable, **HEALTH STATUS RECODED**. SPSS requires that the risk factor defines the rows of the table and the outcome variable the columns. So move **RISK FACTOR FOR OVERWEIGHT OR OBESE RECODED** to the *Rows* window and **HEALTH STATUS RECODED** to the *Columns* window. To help us to understand the table that will be generated, click **Cells** to bring up the *Crosstabs: Cell Display* dialog box. Select *Row* in the *Percentages* area and then **Continue.** To instruct SPSS to calculate the relative risk and odds ratio statistics, click **Statistics** in the *Crosstabs* dialog box to bring up the *Crosstabs: Statistics* dialog box and select *Risk.* Click **Continue** and then **OK.** These steps are displayed in Figs. 6.11, 6.12, 6.13, 6.14, 6.15 and 6.16.

The output generated by this analysis is displayed in Tables 6.9, 6.10 and 6.11. Table 6.9 is a *Case Processing Summary* that tells us that we had 7400 valid cases, and 396 cases with missing values.

Table 6.10 is a *Crosstabulation* that displays the distribution of the valid cases across the combinations of the values of the two variables. Note that the first two rows of the table are defined by our risk factor and that the first two columns by our outcome variable. The bottom row is the total of the rows above it while the last column is the total of columns to the left of it.

The distribution of cases is represented both as counts and percentages. We see from the last column of the first row that there were a total of 4397 cases who were either overweight or obese. Of these 4397 cases, 837 or 19 % were in poorer health and 3560 or 81 % were in better health. We see from the last column of the second row that there were a total of 3003 cases who were neither overweight nor obese, of whom 384 or 12.8 % were in poorer health and 2619 or 87.2 % were in better health.

We can see from these data that for both weight groups, it was unlikely that respondents would be in poorer health. However, were those who were overweight

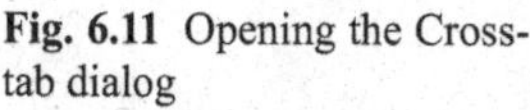

Fig. 6.11 Opening the Crosstab dialog

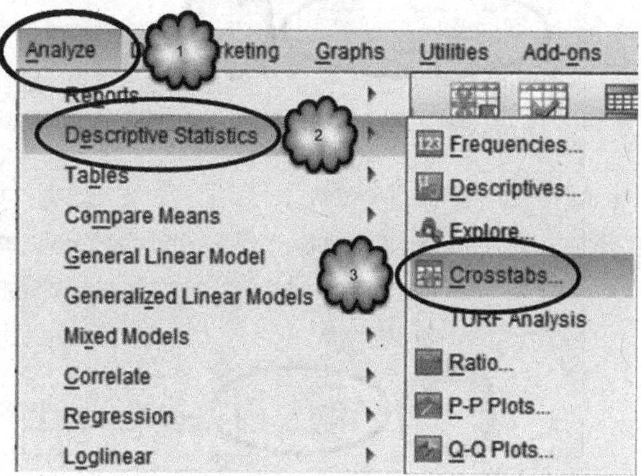

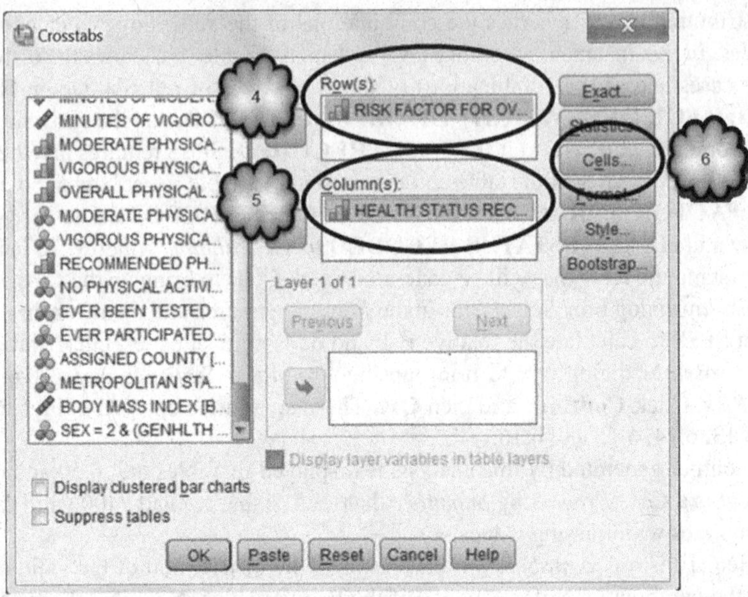

Fig. 6.12 Assigning the row and columns variables and opening the Cell Display dialog

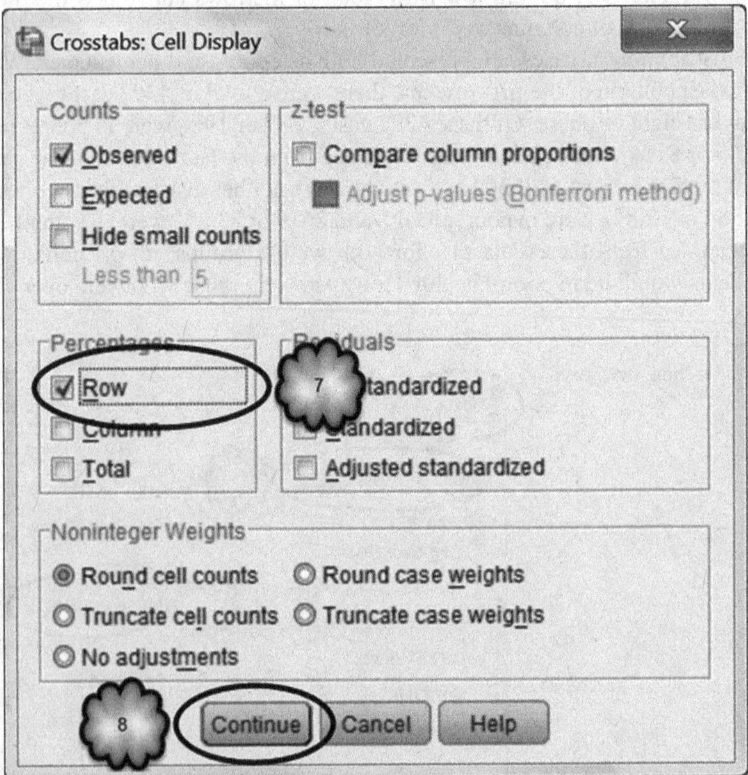

Fig. 6.13 Selecting row percentages

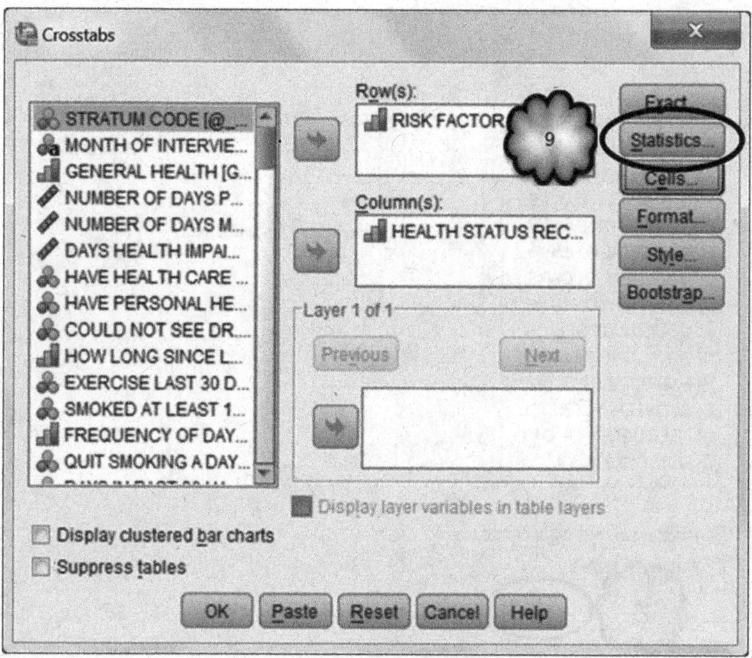

Fig. 6.14 Opening the Statistics dialog

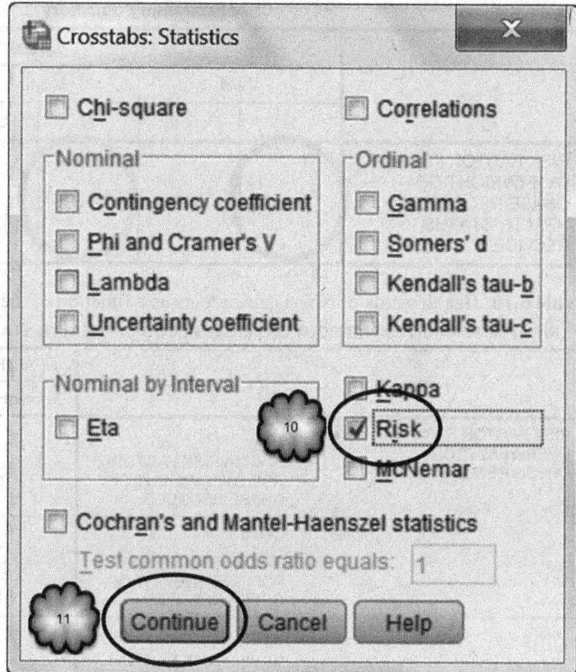

Fig. 6.15 Selecting risk estimates

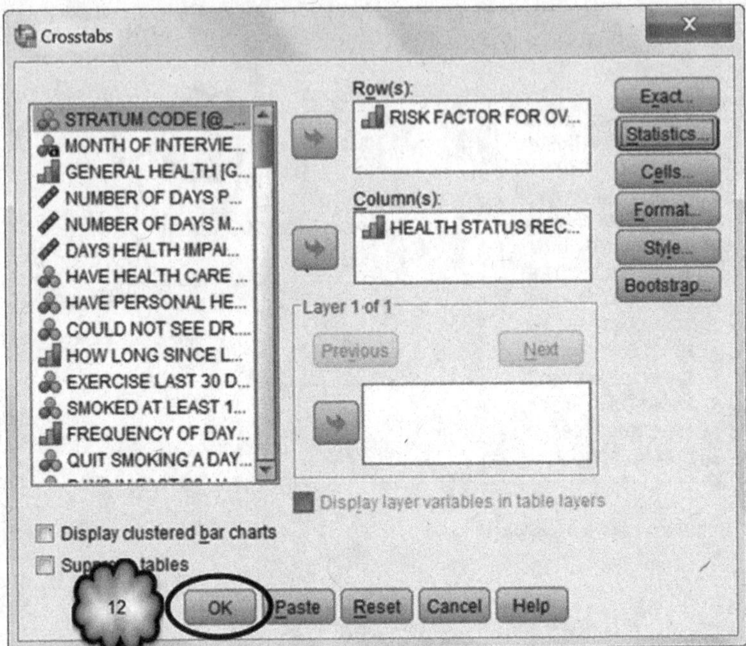

Fig. 6.16 Generating a cross-tabulation and risk estimates

Table 6.9 Number of valid and missing cases in the crosstabulation

Case Processing Summary

	Cases					
	Valid		Missing		Total	
	N	Percent	N	Percent	N	Percent
RISK FACTOR FOR OVERWEIGHT OR OBESE RECODED * HEALTH STATUS RECODED	7400	94.9%	396	5.1%	7796	100.0%

Table 6.10 Health status of NY state residents as a function of their BMI category

RISK FACTOR FOR OVERWEIGHT OR OBESE RECODED * HEALTH STATUS RECODED Crosstabulation

			HEALTH STATUS RECODED		
			Poorer Health	Better Health	Total
RISK FACTOR FOR OVERWEIGHT OR OBESE RECODED	Yes	Count	837	3560	4397
		% within RISK FACTOR FOR OVERWEIGHT OR OBESE RECODED	19.0%	81.0%	100.0%
	No	Count	384	2619	3003
		% within RISK FACTOR FOR OVERWEIGHT OR OBESE RECODED	12.8%	87.2%	100.0%
Total		Count	1221	6179	7400
		% within RISK FACTOR FOR OVERWEIGHT OR OBESE RECODED	16.5%	83.5%	100.0%

Table 6.11 Estimates of risk of poorer health

Risk Estimate

	Value	95% Confidence Interval	
		Lower	Upper
	Odds ratio and 95% Confidence Interval		
Odds Ratio for RISK FACTOR FOR OVERWEIGHT OR OBESE RECODED (Yes / No)	1.604	1.407	1.828
	Relative Risk and 95% Confidence Interval		
For cohort HEALTH STATUS RECODED = Poorer Health	1.489	1.332	1.664
For cohort HEALTH STATUS RECODED = Better Health	.928	.910	.947
N of Valid Cases	7400		

or obese *more likely* to be in poorer health than those who were neither overweight nor obese? To find out, we compare the proportion of poorer health for each group. As we saw in the preceding paragraph, 19 % of those who were overweight or obese were in poorer health while only 12.8 % of those who were neither overweight nor obese were in poorer health. Consequently, the relative risk is 19% to 12.8 % or 1.48. Respondents who were overweight or obese were almost 1.5 times as likely to be in poorer health compared to their thinner counterparts.

If the proportion of poorer health were equal in both weight groups, relative risk would equal 1. For example, if 12.8 % of both weight groups were in poorer health, the risk to both groups would be the same and relative risk would equal 1. However, in these data, relative risk was greater than 1. It appears that being overweight is a risk factor for poorer health.

We say "appears" because it is always possible that the value of relative risk that we obtain from our sample is due entirely to sampling variability. In this study, for example, it is possible that the value of relative risk is in fact 1 in the population from which the 7400 cases were drawn. Consequently, we need to determine how certain we can be that the population value is not equal to 1. One way to do this is by calculating a 95 % CI around the sample value. If the CI does not contain the value of 1, then we can be 95 % confident that the population value is not equal to 1. SPSS generates these CIs for us.

SPSS also generates relative risk values and displays them, along with the CIs, in the *Risk Estimate* table of the output, shown in Table 6.11.

To find the relative risk of being in poorer health if respondents are overweight or obese, inspect the row labeled, *For cohort HEALTH STATUS RECODED = Poorer Health*. In the column labeled *Value* you will find the sample value of relative risk, 1.489. (Since SPSS carries its calculations out to several decimal points, its values of relative risk are often a bit different from those we calculate by hand.) You will also find to the right of the value the lower and upper limits of the 95 % CI. As the interval does not include the value of 1, we can conclude with 95 % confidence that for residents of NY state, being overweight or obese is a risk factor for poorer health.

You may have noticed that in the *Risk Estimate* table, there is a row labeled, *For cohort HEALTH STATUS RECODED = Better Health*. This row refers to the relative chances of being in better health for respondents who are overweight or obese. This value is calculated in the same way that we calculated relative risk. (In fact, it could be referred to as a relative risk estimate but since we do not usually think of being in good health as a negative outcome, the term "risk" seems out of place in this context.) As you can see, the value is 0.928. What does this value mean? To find out, look at the column of the *Crosstabulation* table labeled, *Better Health*. What proportion of those who were overweight or obese enjoyed better health? What proportion of those who were neither overweight nor obese enjoyed better health? Which proportion is smaller? How much smaller? At this point you should see that the chances of being in better health for respondents who were obese were about 93 % of those of their thinner counterparts. Note that SPSS includes the 95 % CI for this value as well.

Odds Ratio Another statistic for determining whether a factor places people at risk is the odds ratio. As we explained above, using the odds ratio is more appropriate than using relative risk in our example as the CDC data come from a cross-sectional study. Similar to relative risk, an odds ratio reflects the relative likelihood of the occurrence of a negative outcome. However, while relative risk is expressed in terms of probabilities, an odds ratio is expressed in terms of odds.

Refer back to the *Crosstabulation* table. For those who were overweight or obese, 837 were in poorer health while 3560 were in better health. Thus for overweight or obese respondents, the odds of being in poorer health were 837 to 3560 or 0.235 to 1. What were the odds for those who were neither overweight nor obese? A check of the table reveals 384 to 2619, or 0.147 to 1.

We can see from these data that for both weight groups, the odds were against any respondent being in poorer health. However, were those who were overweight or obese more likely to be in poorer health than those who were neither overweight nor obese? To find out, we compare the two sets of odds and see that the odds of being in poorer health for those who were overweight or obese (0.235) are about 1.6 times as large as the corresponding odds for those who were neither overweight nor obese (0.147).-If being overweight or obese was not a risk factor for poorer health, then the odds for each of the weight groups would be equal and the odds ratio would equal 1. However, in these data, the odds ratio is greater than 1 and so it appears that being overweight is a risk factor for poorer health.

We say "appears" because, as with a relative risk estimate, it is always possible that the sample value of an odds ratio is due entirely to sampling variability. Consequently, we need to know the upper and lower limits of the 95 % CI constructed around the sample value to see if we can be 95 % confident that the population value is not equal to 1. SPSS generates the CIs for us and displays it along with the odds ratio in the first row of the *Risk Estimate* table. As you can see from that row, the odds ratio equals 1.604 and the 95 % CI does not contain the value of 1. Once again, we come to the confident conclusion that being overweight or obese is a risk factor for poorer health.

We might mention that there are two additional ways to calculate odds ratios. One involves the following three steps. First, multiply the two frequency counts in the upper left and lower right cells of the *Crosstabulation* table (837 and 2619 in this case). Then multiply the remaining two frequency counts (3560 and 384). Finally, divide the first product by the second. The second alternative method is to divide the relative risk of the negative outcome (in this case, 1.489) by the relative chances of the positive outcome (0.928).

Deriving an Odds Ratio from a Case-Control Study In the preceding example, we treated being overweight or obese as a risk factor and interpreted the relative risk and odds ratio to mean that people who are overweight or obese are more likely to develop poorer health. We cannot be sure, however, that being overweight was *followed* by a decline in health. For example, perhaps people who were in poorer health became less physically active and therefore gained weight. To overcome the problem of determining which variable came first in time, researchers can conduct a case-control study. In case-control studies, the degree of association, if any, between a suspected risk factor and an outcome is measured in terms of an odds ratio.

As an example of a case-control study, consider an investigation of whether age at first pregnancy is a risk factor for cervical cancer. A total of 366 women who had been pregnant at least once and were at the time of the study between the ages of 50 and 59 were selected. The cases were 49 women who had been diagnosed as having cervical cancer. The controls were 317 women who did not have the disease. For each group, the researchers counted the number of women who at their first pregnancy either were 25 years old or younger or were older than 25. Notice that in this study, the risk factor clearly preceded the outcome.

The data from this study can be found in **Cervical.sav** [2]. This file is constructed differently from others that we have seen so far. Instead of having 366 rows of data, one for each woman, we have only four, one row for each combination of the values of **Age at First Pregnancy** (25 or younger and Older than 25) and **Disease Status** (Cervical Cancer and Controls). Each row contains the number of women in each of the four combinations. For example, we have 42 women whose first pregnancy occurred when they were 25 or younger and who had been diagnosed with cervical cancer. Figure 6.17 displays the data file. We show you this type of data file to make the point that it is sometimes possible to conduct statistical analyses with SPSS from summary data.

	Count	Age	Status
1	42	25 or Younger	Cervical Cancer
2	203	25 or Younger	Controls
3	7	Older than 25	Cervical Cancer
4	114	Older than 25	Controls

Fig. 6.17 Cervical.sav data file

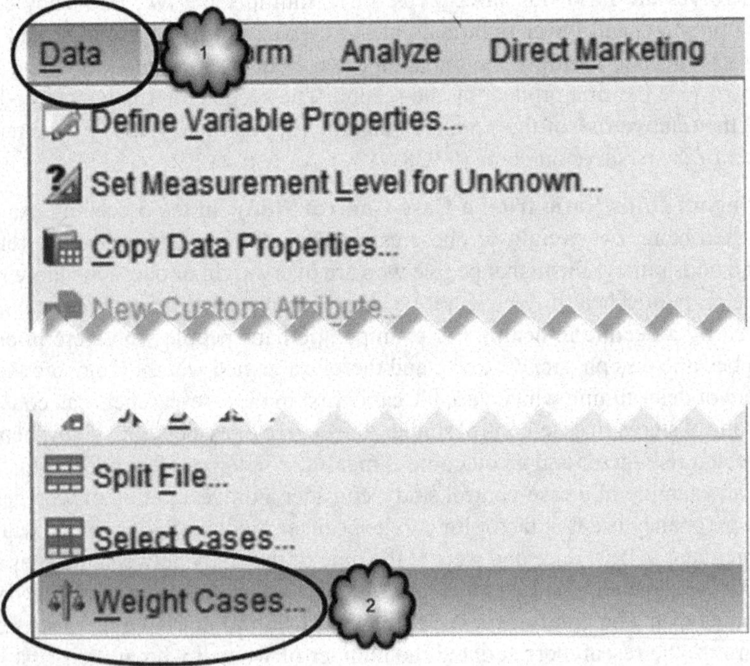

Fig. 6.18 Opening the Weight Cases dialog

Before we can calculate an odds ratio, we must convert our summary data into the original data set. Open the file and select **Data** > **Weight Cases** to bring up the following *Weight Cases* dialog box. Select *Weight cases by* and move **Number of Cases** to the *Frequency Variable* window. Click **OK.** These steps are displayed in Figs. 6.18 and 6.19.

Now you are ready to compute the odds ratio. Using the **Crosstab** procedure, ask SPSS to create a table with the risk factor (**Age at First Pregnancy)** as the row variable and the outcome (**Disease Status)** as the column variable, and to generate row percentages and risk statistics. Run the analysis. The output should be similar to the output shown in Tables 6.12 and 6.13.

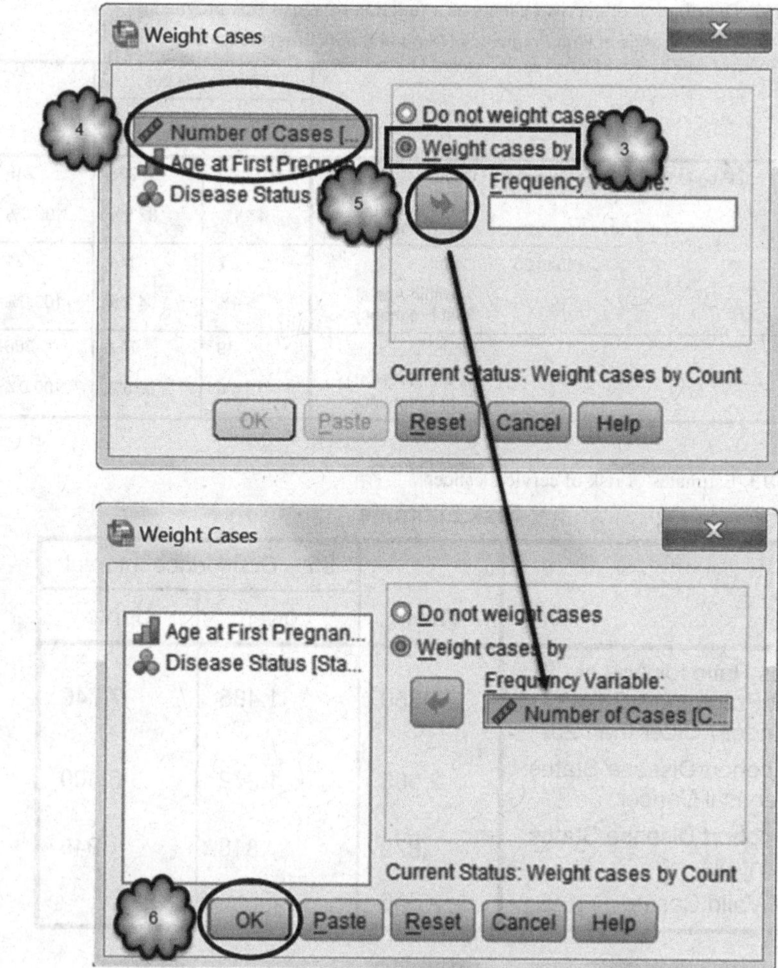

Fig. 6.19 Assigning the weight cases by variable and executing the weight cases procedure

Study the output and answer the following questions:

6.6.1 What are the odds that women who were 25-years old or younger at first pregnancy were diagnosed with cervical cancer?

6.6.2 What are the odds for women who were older than 25 at first pregnancy?

6.6.3 Are women who were 25-years old or younger at first pregnancy more or less likely to be diagnosed with cervical cancer?

6.6.4 How much more (or less)?

6.6.5 Does age at first pregnancy appear to be a risk factor for cervical cancer?

6.6.6 Can we be 95 % confident that age at first pregnancy is a risk factor?

Table 6.12 Distribution of cervical cancer as a function of age at first pregnancy

Age at First Pregnancy * Disease Status Crosstabulation

			Disease Status		
			Cervical Cancer	Controls	Total
Age at First Pregnancy	25 or Younger	Count	42	203	245
		% within Age at First Pregnancy	17.1%	82.9%	100.0%
	Older than 25	Count	7	114	121
		% within Age at First Pregnancy	5.8%	94.2%	100.0%
Total		Count	49	317	366
		% within Age at First Pregnancy	13.4%	86.6%	100.0%

Table 6.13 Estimates of risk of cervical cancer

Risk Estimate

		95% Confidence Interval	
	Value	Lower	Upper
Odds Ratio for Age at First Pregnancy (25 or Younger / Older than 25)	3.369	1.466	7.746
For cohort Disease Status = Cervical Cancer	2.963	1.372	6.400
For cohort Disease Status = Controls	.879	.818	.945
N of Valid Cases	366		

6.7 Exercise Questions

1. To answer the following questions, you will use the variable **INCOME CATEGORIES** [@_*INCOMG*] (variable 83; 1 ≤ US$ 15,000, 2 = US$ 15,000 to less than US$ 25,000, 3 = US$ 25,000 to less than US$ 35,000, 4 = US$ 35,000 to less than US$ 50,000, 5 = US$ 50,000 or more, 9 = Don't know/Not sure/Missing) in the **CDC BRFSS** data set. Be sure to declare the missing value before proceeding.

   a. What is the 90 % CI for the proportion of the population whose annual household income is less than $ 15,000?
   b. What is the 95 % CI for the proportion of the population whose annual household income is less than US$ 15,000?
   c. What is the 99 % CI for the proportion of the population whose annual household income is less than $ 15,000?

d. How do the widths of the three CIs you just reported differ from one another? Why are they different?

2. Using the variable **GENERAL HEALTH** [*GENHLTH*] (variable 3; 1=Excellent, 2=Very good, 3=Good, 4=Fair, 5=Poor, 7=Don't know/Not Sure, 9=Refused) in the **CDC BRFSS** data set, determine whether more than half of the adult population of NY state considers their general health to very good to excellent. Be sure that any missing values have been declared before you begin.
   a. How many people in the sample reported that they were in either very good or excellent health?
   b. What proportion of the people in the sample reported that they were in either very good or excellent health?
   c. What is the null hypothesis? What is the alternative hypothesis?
   d. Can we confidently conclude that more than half of the adult population of NY state consider themselves to be in very good to excellent health? Why or why not?
3. In Question 1, you conducted analyses on **INCOME CATEGORIES.** Recode this variable into a new variable so that people who earned less than US$ 15,000 are still coded as a 1 but all other non-missing values are coded as a 2. That is, a value of 1 will be those whose annual household income is less than US$ 15,000, and a value of 2 will be those whose annual household income is US$ 15,000 or more. Name the new variable something like, **INCOME CATEGORIES 2 GROUPS**. Now split the file (**Data > Split File)** according to this new variable and conduct analyses that will answer the following questions:
   a. How many people who earned less than US$ 15,000 reported that their general health was either very good or excellent?
   b. What proportion of people who earned less than US$ 15,000 reported that their general health was either very good or excellent?
   c. How many people who earned US$ 15,000 or more reported that their general health was either very good or excellent?
   d. What proportion of people who earned US$ 15,000 or more reported that their general health was either very good or excellent?
   e. What is the 95 % CI for the difference between these two proportions?
   f. Judging from the CI for the difference between the two proportions, can we be confident that the two population proportions are different? Why or why not?
   g. Check on your answer to f. above by testing whether the proportion of the population whose annual income is less than US$ 15,000 who report that their general health is either very good or excellent is different from the proportion of the population whose annual household income is US$ 15,000 or more who report that their general health is either very good or excellent. Were the two proportions significantly different?
   h. Were the requirements necessary for using the script in g. above satisfied? Why or why not?

Table 6.14 Distribution of lung cancer

Respondents kept birds	Respondents had lung cancer	
	Yes	No
Yes	98	101
No	141	328

Table 6.15 Distribution of injured collegiate athletes of varying physical flexibility

Flexibility at Beginning of Sports Season * Injured During the Sports Season Crosstabulation

			Injured During the Sports Season		
			Yes	No	Total
Flexibility at Beginning of Sports Season	Low	Count	12	21	33
		% within Flexibility at Beginning of Sports Season	36.4%	63.6%	100.0%
	High	Count	12	60	72
		% within Flexibility at Beginning of Sports Season	16.7%	83.3%	100.0%
Total		Count	24	81	105
		% within Flexibility at Beginning of Sports Season	22.9%	77.1%	100.0%

4. Researchers wanted to know whether owners of pet birds are at risk for contracting lung cancer. To find out, they asked 239 people who had lung cancer and 429 who did not whether they had kept birds as pets. The data are in **Petbirds.sav** [3]. The results of the study are shown in Table 6.14.

   a. Is this investigation an experiment, a cohort study, a case-control study or a cross-sectional study?
   b. To determine whether keeping pet birds is a risk factor, should we calculate relative risk or an odds ratio? Why?
   c. By hand calculate and report whichever statistic you think is appropriate.
   d. According to your calculations, does keeping pet birds seem to be a risk factor for contracting lung cancer? Why or why not?
   e. Open the data set, **Petbirds.sav**, and double check your calculations by instructing SPSS to conduct the relevant cross-tabulation.
   f. Does the 95 % CI include the value of 1?
   g. According to the 95 % CI, can we conclude that keeping pet birds is a risk factor for lung cancer? Why or why not?
   h. According to the 95 % CI, can we conclude that keeping pet birds is a cause of lung cancer? Why or why not?

5. A team of physician assistant students measured the physical flexibility of collegiate athletes at the beginning of a sports season to determine if lack of flexibility is a risk factor for being injured during the season [4]. The results of their analysis are displayed in Tables 6.15 and 6.16.

Table 6.16 Estimates of risk of injury

Risk Estimate

	Value	95% Confidence Interval	
		Lower	Upper
Odds Ratio for Flexibility at Beginning of Sports Season (Low / High)	2.857	1.114	7.328
For cohort Injured During the Sports Season = Yes	2.182	1.099	4.332
For cohort Injured During the Sports Season = No	.764	.578	1.008
N of Valid Cases	105		

a. Was this study an experiment, a cohort study, a case-control study or a cross-sectional study? Explain.
b. What was the risk of injury for athletes who were high in flexibility? Low in flexibility?
c. What was the relative risk of injury?
d. Was the relative risk of injury statistically significantly different from 1? How do you know?
e. What were the odds of injury for athletes low in flexibility?
f. What is the odds ratio? Does it indicate that low flexibility is a risk factor for injury?
g. Does the design of this study justify the use of relative risk or should the researchers use the odds ratio instead? Explain.

Data Sets and References

1. CDC BRFSS.sav obtained from: Centers for Disease Control and Prevention (CDC). Behavioral Risk Factor Surveillance System Survey Data. US Department of Health and Human Services, Centers for Disease Control and Prevention, Atlanta (2005). Public domain. For more information about the BRFSS, visit http://www.cdc.gov/brfss/. Accessed 16 Nov 2014
2. Cervical.sav obtained from: Graham, S., Shotz, W.: Epidemiology of cancer of the cervix in Buffalo, New York. J. Natl. Cancer Inst. **63**(1), 23–27 (1979). (Public domain)
3. Petbirds.sav obtained from: Kohlmeier, L., Arminger, G., Bartolomeycik, S., Bellach, B., Rehm, J., Thamm, M.: Pet birds as a independent risk factor for lung cancer: case-control study. Br. Med. J. **305**, 986–989 (1992). (With the kind permission of the BMJ Publishing Group Ltd.)
4. From: Barker, S., Jerome, J., Woods, D., Zaika, C., Brown, R.G., Holmes, W.H.: The Sit and Reach Test as a measure of flexibility for predicting lower extremity injury in Division III athletes. Unpublished data, Le Moyne College, Syracuse (2010)

Chapter 7
Relationships in Categorical Data

Abstract This chapter investigates relationships in categorical data. It begins with a discussion of contingency tables and clustered bar charts as descriptive measures. The chi-square test for contingency tables is discussed. If the two categorical variables are found to be related, then the strength of that relationship is measured using Cramér's *V* for nominal variables and Gamma for ordinal variables.

7.1 Overview

An important goal of science is to determine if one variable causes another. As we saw in Chap. 1, a first step toward establishing causal connections is to determine if the two variables in question are related. Once a relationship has been established, additional research can be conducted to determine if the relationship between the two variables is causal and if so, the direction of the causality. In this chapter, we look at several statistics that are used to determine whether two categorical variables are related. In Chap. 9, we will look at statistics that are used to determine whether two quantitative variables are related.

To better understand the association between two variables, it is helpful to generate a visual display of the relationship between those variables. When the variables are categorical, the relationship is depicted in the form of a two-way table called a *contingency table* or in the form of a graph called a *clustered bar chart*. When the variables are quantitative, the relationship between them is usually depicted in the form of a graph known as a *scatter plot*. In this chapter, we focus on how to interpret a contingency table. In Chap. 9, we will focus on how to interpret a scatter plot.

We pointed out in Chap. 5 that sample data are always subject to sampling variability. Random measurement errors and random differences across respondents guarantee that sample results will be affected by chance factors. We also pointed out that we can never know for sure the characteristics of a population. To overcome this, we will need to conduct a test of hypotheses.

In addition to determining whether two variables are related, measures of association can be used to quantify the strength of the relationship. Many do so along a scale ranging from 0 to −1 for negative relationships, and 0 to +1 for positive relationships. For data where it does not make sense for a relationship to have a

W. H. Holmes, W. C. Rinaman, *Statistical Literacy for Clinical Practitioners*,
DOI 10.1007/978-3-319-12550-3_7

direction (e.g., with some categorical data), these measures typically range from 0 to 1. The measures of association that we will study are *Cramér's V, gamma, Pearson correlation,* and *Spearman's Rho*. The last two are intended to be used when the data are quantitative, and they are the subject of Chap. 9. The first two are to be used when the two variables are categorical, and they are the subject of this chapter.

7.2 Contingency Tables

Using the CDC data set, we will construct what statisticians call a *contingency table* to see if there appears to be a relationship between the self-reported health of respondents and their sex. Since we are interested in whether self-reported health varies according to the sex of the respondent, it is common practice to refer to sex as the *explanatory variable,* and to refer to self-reported health as the *response variable.* When constructing a contingency table with two variables, the usual procedure is to have the explanatory variable be the column variable and the response variable be the row variable. We will create a contingency table with sex as the column variable and self-reported health as the row variable. The intersection of each column and row within the body of the table will display a count of the respondents of a particular sex who gave a particular response (e.g., the number of men who said that they were in excellent health), and the percentage of those of a particular sex who gave a particular response (e.g,, the percentage of all men in our sample who said that they were in excellent health).

Load the data file, **CDC BRFSS.sav [1],** into SPSS. Before proceeding be sure that 7 and 9 have been declared missing values for the variable, **GENERAL HEALTH** [*GENHLTH*] (variable 3). Begin by selecting **Analyze>Descriptive Statistics>Crosstabs**. This will open the *Crosstabs* dialog box. Move the variable **GENERAL HEALTH** into the *Row(s)* area, and the variable **SEX** [*SEX*] (variable 32) into the *Column(s)* area. We want to know for each sex the percent that gave each response. Of the men, what percent said they were in excellent health, were in very good health, and so on? Of the women, what percent said they were in excellent health, very good health, and so on? Since we decided to make **SEX** a column variable, each of these percentages is equal to the number of respondents in a given column-row combination divided by the total number of respondents in that column. To instruct SPSS to generate these percentages, click the **Cells** button to open the *Crosstabs: Cell Display* dialog box. As we want percentages calculated within each sex, and since **SEX** is our column variable, check *Column* in the *Percentages* area. Click **Continue** and then click **OK**. The steps for generating this analysis are displayed in Figs. 7.1, 7.2, and 7.3.

Interpreting a contingency table displaying column percentages SPSS will now generate a contingency table that shows the number of cases of men and women who chose each of the **GENERAL HEALTH** response categories. The table is reproduced in Table 7.1.

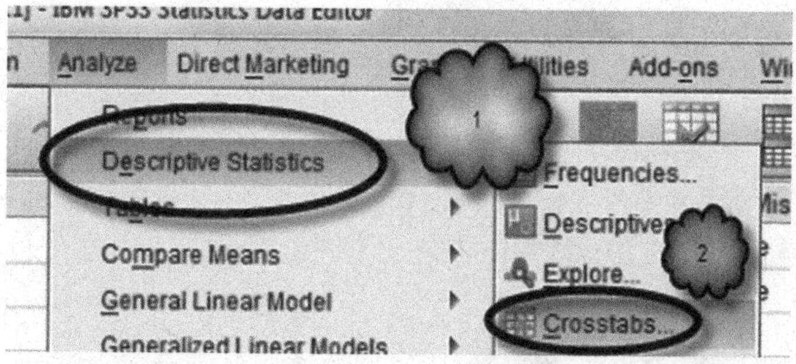

Fig. 7.1 Selecting crosstabs

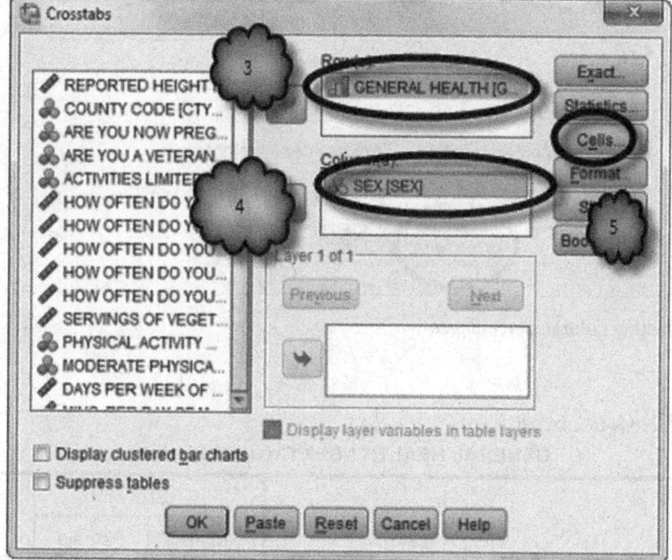

Fig. 7.2 Selecting the row and column variables and selecting the Cell Display dialog

The purpose of a contingency table is to reveal whether the distribution of respondents across the values of one variable depends or is contingent upon the values of the other variable. Study the contingency table and see if the distribution of respondents across the variable **GENERAL HEALTH** seems to depend on the respondents' sex.

The bottom row of the table provides the total for each sex and for all participants combined. According to the output, the sample consisted of 2930 men and 4847 women, for a total of 7777 respondents with valid responses. Note that each of these three numbers comes from one of the columns, and that the percentages reading down that column total to 100 %.

Each of the rows above the bottom row provides information about the number of men and women who gave the corresponding response. For example, 639 men or

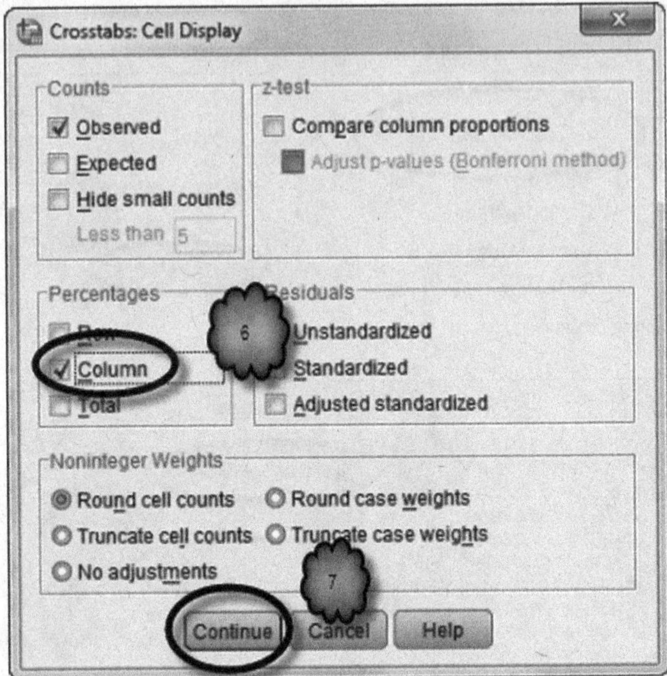

Fig. 7.3 Selecting column percentages

Table 7.1 A cross-tabulation

GENERAL HEALTH * SEX Crosstabulation

			SEX		Total
			Male	Female	
GENERAL HEALTH	Excellent	Count	639	1013	1652
		% within SEX	21.8%	20.9%	21.2%
	Very good	Count	928	1612	2540
		% within SEX	31.7%	33.3%	32.7%
	Good	Count	890	1393	2283
		% within SEX	30.4%	28.7%	29.4%
	Fair	Count	355	624	979
		% within SEX	12.1%	12.9%	12.6%
	Poor	Count	118	205	323
		% within SEX	4.0%	4.2%	4.2%
Total		Count	2930	4847	7777
		% within SEX	100.0%	100.0%	100.0%

21.8 % of the 2930 men said their health was excellent and 1013 women or 20.8 % of the 4847 women said they were in excellent health. Again note that we are reading the data within a given column and that the percentages within a column add up to 100 %.

Inspection of the table should tell us whether sex and reported general health are related. However, when interpreting a cross-tabulation, pay close attention to the percentages, especially when considering data where the number of respondents in each group differs greatly. In this sample, for example, there are many more women than men. Yet we see that the column percentages are very close for each gender. The similarity of the column percentages indicates that perceptions of overall health do not vary with a respondent's gender. The terminology here is to say that **SEX** and **GENERAL HEALTH** are *independent*.

In order to conclude that health varied with sex, we would have to see percentages within the columns that are different from column to column. For example, in the CDC data that we are analyzing, if 40 % of women said they were in excellent health contrasted with 25 % of men saying they were in excellent health, we might have reason to believe that women tend to be healthier than men.

We say that we *might* have reason to believe that women tend to be healthier than men because we are dealing with sample data. It is possible that a difference of this size (40 % of women versus 25 % of men) may not be inconsistent with what one might expect to see due to sampling variability. As we saw in Chap. 5, to know whether or not the trends we think we are seeing in our data are not just a fluke or the result of random factors is an important function of statistical analysis. We will return to this topic later in this chapter.

Interpreting a contingency table displaying row percentages The contingency table above displayed column percentages. When studying whether or not two variables are related, it is often useful to generate two contingency tables, one in which percentages are calculated within columns, another within rows. Let us look at the contingency table when it displays row percentages.

Return to the *Crosstabs: Cell Display* dialog box. Replace column percentages with row percentages and rerun the analysis.

The contingency table displaying the row percentages is shown in Table 7.2.

The frequencies within each cell of the cross-tabulation are exactly the same as before, but the percentages are different. This is because the percentages are read by reading across a given row. For example, recall that there were 639 men who reported that they were in excellent health. In the first analysis, 639 was 21.8 % of the 2930 men in the sample. In this analysis, 639 represents 38.7 % of the 1652 men and women in the sample who said that they were in excellent health.

In the first analysis, we could see that there was no relationship between sex and reported health because the column percentages in each row were quite close to each other. In this analysis, we can see that no relationship existed between sex and health by noting that the percentages of men and women in each row are essentially the same as the overall percentages of men and women in the sample.

Table 7.2 A contingency table with row percentages

GENERAL HEALTH * SEX Crosstabulation

			SEX		
			Male	Female	Total
GENERAL HEALTH	Excellent	Count	639	1013	1652
		% within GENERAL HEALTH	38.7%	61.3%	100.0%
	Very good	Count	928	1612	2540
		% within GENERAL HEALTH	36.5%	63.5%	100.0%
	Good	Count	890	1393	2283
		% within GENERAL HEALTH	39.0%	61.0%	100.0%
	Fair	Count	355	624	979
		% within GENERAL HEALTH	36.3%	63.7%	100.0%
	Poor	Count	118	205	323
		% within GENERAL HEALTH	36.5%	63.5%	100.0%
Total		Count	2930	4847	7777
		% within GENERAL HEALTH	37.7%	62.3%	100.0%

7.3 Clustered Bar Charts

Sometimes displaying a cross-tabulation as a bar chart is useful. In this section, we study a *clustered bar chart* of the cross-tabulation of **GENERAL HEALTH** and **SEX**.

As we did in Chap. 3, select **Graphs>Chart Builder** to open the *Chart Builder* dialog box. In the *Gallery,* select *Bar.* Now drag the clustered bar chart picture (the second chart from the left in the top row) to the empty window above it. Drag **GENERAL HEALTH** to the *X-Axis* box, and drag **SEX** to the *Cluster on X: set color* box. In the *Element Properties* dialog box, select *Percentage(?)* in the *Statistic* box. Click **Set Parameters** and select *Total for Each Legend Variable Category (same fill color).* Now click **Continue,** and then **Apply** followed by **OK** to produce the graph. These steps are displayed in Figs. 7.4, 7.5, 7.6, 7.7 and 7.8).

The resulting graph is reproduced in Fig. 7.9. Which of the two cross-tabulations in Sect. 7.2 does this graph seem to represent?

The graph in Fig. 7.9 shows the column percentages. To show the row percentages, we would return to *Chart Builder* and reverse the positions of the two variables by assigning **SEX** as the *X-Axis* variable and **GENERAL HEALTH** as the *Cluster on X: set color* variable. This would produce the graph shown in Fig. 7.10. Looking at this graph, would you say that men and women differed in their self-reported health? Remember, about 38 % of the sample was male.

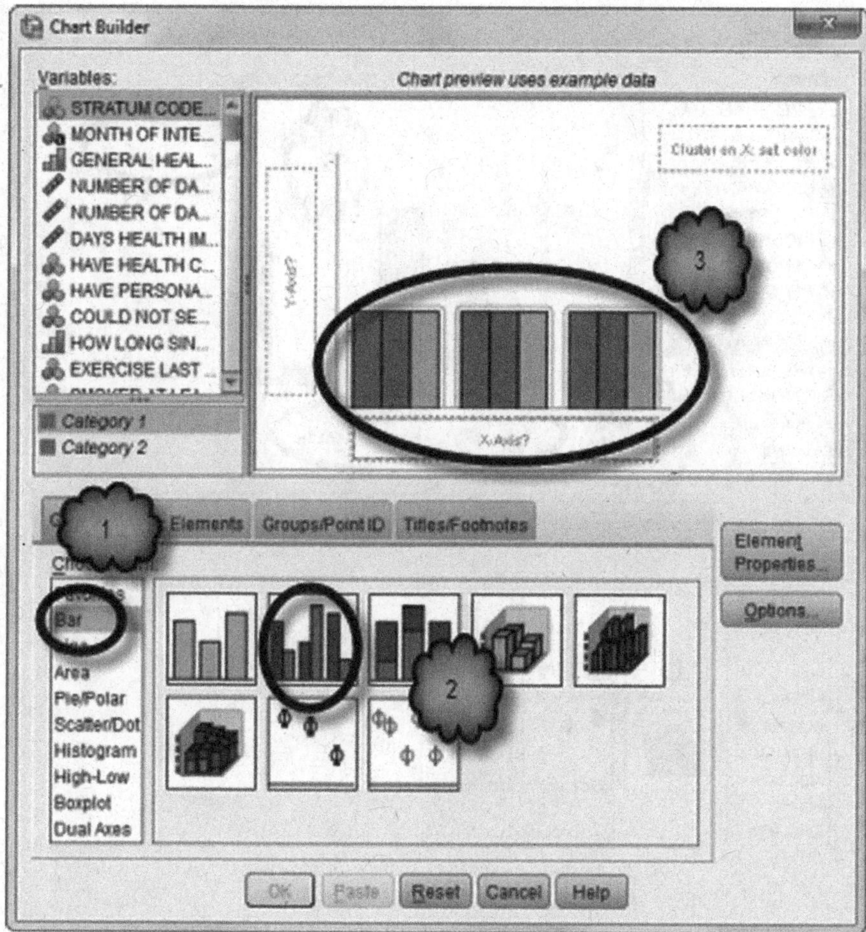

Fig. 7.4 Selecting the clustered bar chart

7.4 Testing Hypotheses About Whether Two Categorical Variables are Related

Imagine that we were to interview another random sample of 7000 or so New Yorkers. We would be very surprised if the data provided by the new sample turned out to be exactly the same as those of the present sample. In fact, we should be very suspicious of the sampling methodology if they were the same. Since sample data are subject to random fluctuation, it is always possible that any relationship we observe between two variables in a sample was due *only* to chance, a fluke that should not be taken to mean that the relationship we observed in the sample actually exists in the population from which the sample was taken.

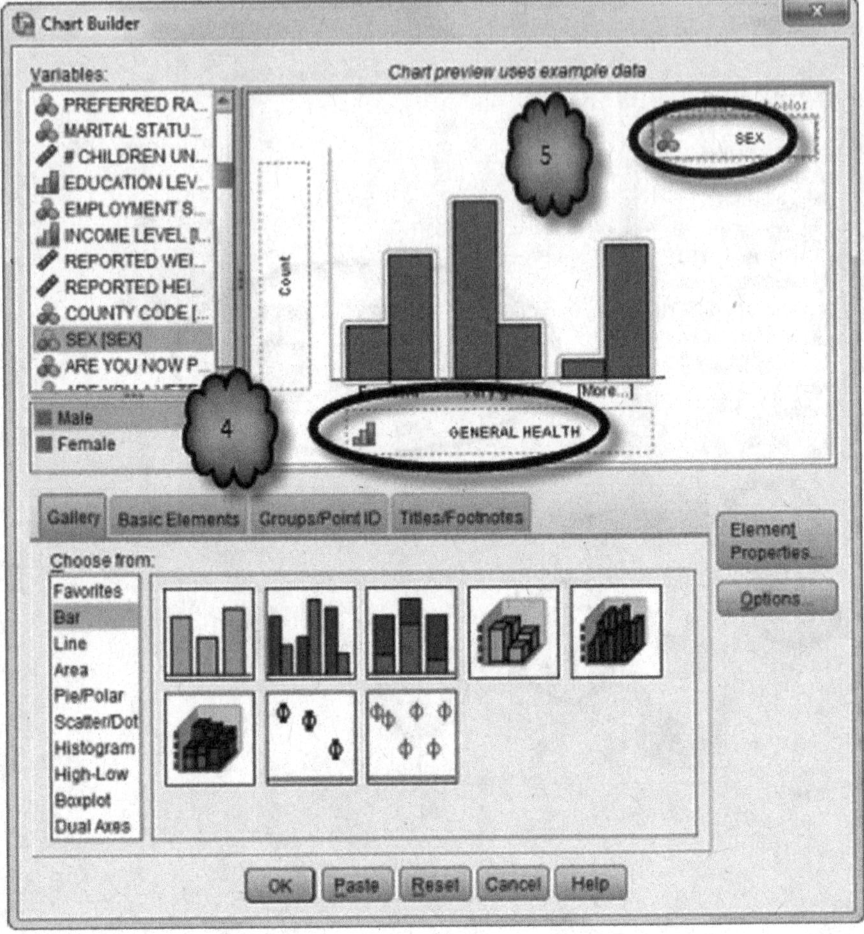

Fig. 7.5 Setting the X-axis and clustering variables

Instead of assuming that what is true of the sample is necessarily true of the population, we apply logic similar to that explained in Chap. 5 and conduct a test of hypotheses to decide between two claims about the population. One claim, the null hypotheses, states that in the population from which we took our sample, there is no relationship between the two variables of interest. The second claim, the alternative hypothesis, states that there is a relationship. Using the sample data, we test the null hypothesis by calculating the probability that the relationship between two variables observed in our sample would occur if the null hypothesis is in fact true. If that probability, which you will recognize as the *p*-value of the test, is small, we can then confidently conclude that the relationship we found in the sample is a true reflection of the relationship that exists in the population.

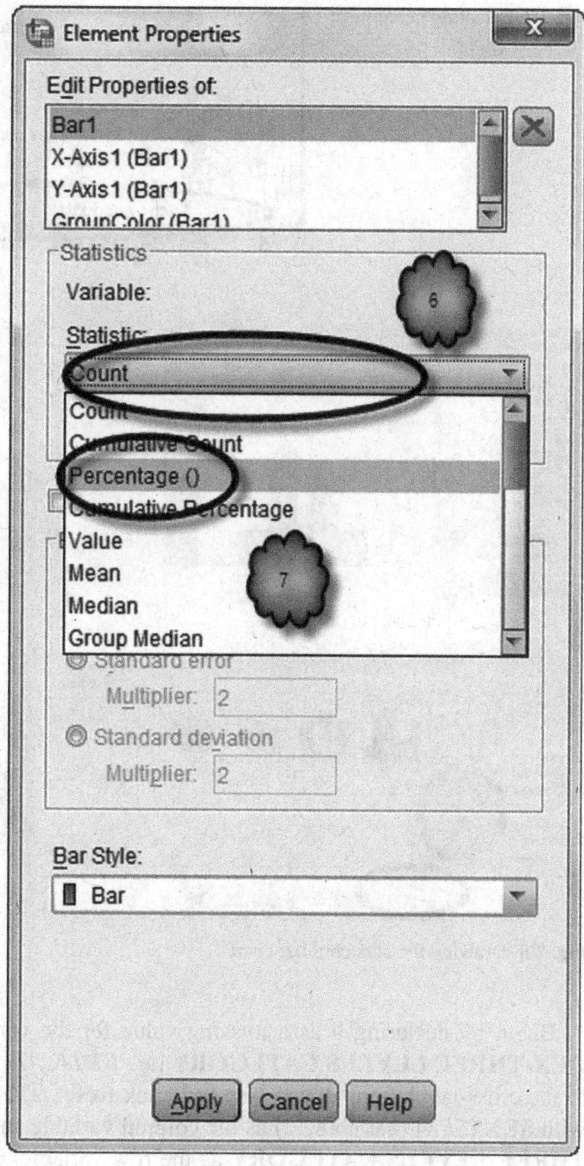

Fig. 7.6 Selecting a bar chart of percentages

Chi-square test When we are interested in whether or not two categorical variables are related in the population, the test of hypotheses we can conduct is known as a *chi-square test*. The test tries to decide between the null hypothesis that there is no relationship and the alternative hypothesis that there is. In this section, we use chi-square to explore the relationship between the nominal variable, sex (male versus female), and an ordinal measure of obesity (neither overweight nor obese, overweight, or obese).

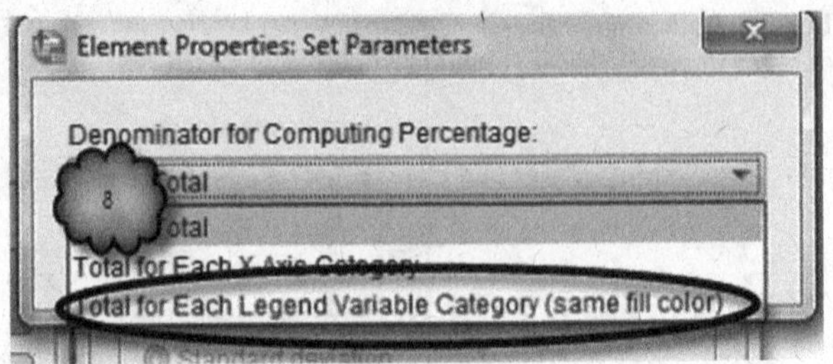

Fig. 7.7 Selecting percentage within each sex

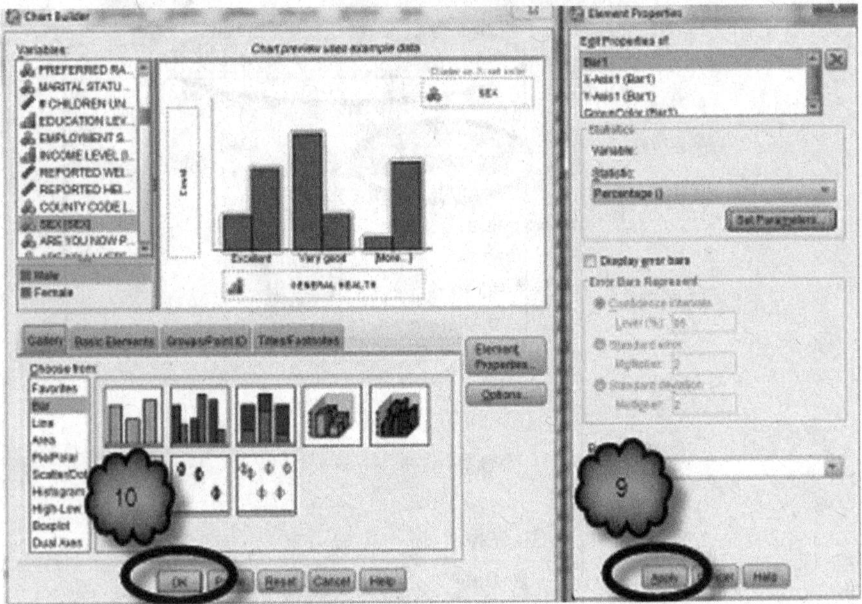

Fig. 7.8 Drawing the clustered bar chart

Begin by declaring 9 as a missing value for the variable, **BODY MASS INDEX-THREE LEVELS CATEGORY** [*@_BMI4CAT*] (variable 79). Next, return to the cross-tabulations dialog box and click **Reset**. Then set up a cross-tabulation with **SEX** [*SEX*] (variable 32) as the column variable and **BODY MASS INDEX-THREE LEVELS CATEGORY** as the row variable. Click **Statistics** and check *Chi-square.* Click **Continue** followed by **Cells**. Check column percentages and click **Continue**. Finally, to demonstrate another way to generate a graph of our results, check **Display clustered bar charts** in the main cross-tabulation dialog box. Click **OK.** These steps are displayed in Figs. 7.11, 7.12 and 7.13.

Study the output. The chi-square statistic that is of interest to us is labeled *Pearson Chi-square.* The *p*-value for the test appears in the *Asymp. Sig. (2-sided)* column.

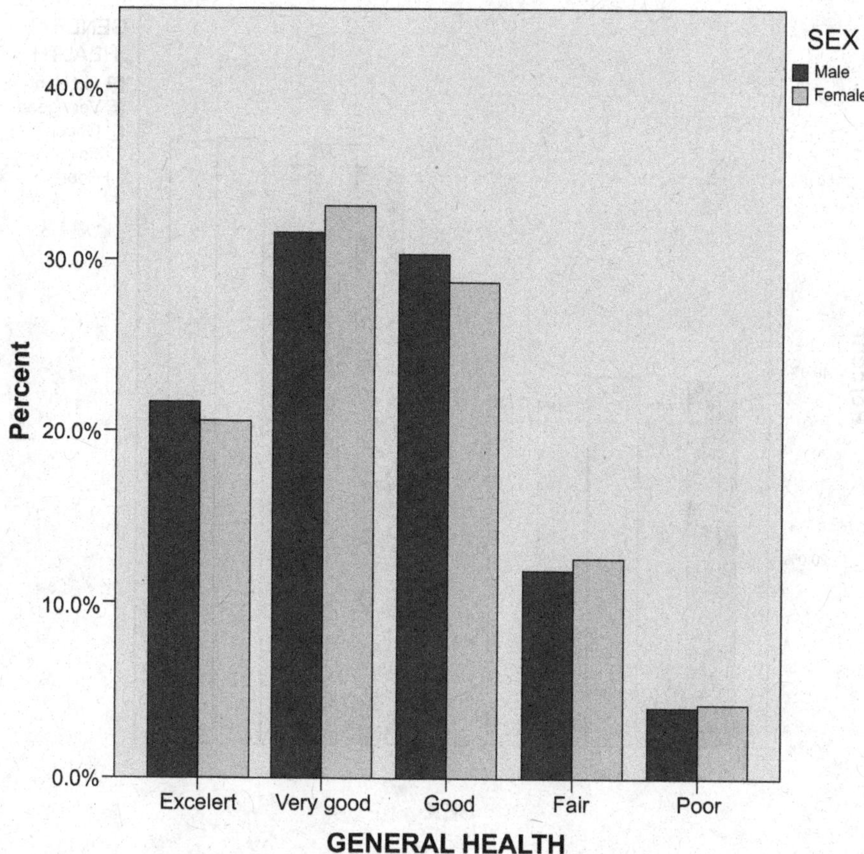

Fig. 7.9 A clustered bar chart

Statistical significance and the Type I Error Recall from Chap. 5 that scientists feel that we can rule out chance as the sole cause of a sample result whenever the p-value is ≤ 0.05. Whenever a p-value is ≤ 0.05, we know that if we took repeated samples and conducted the same test we would see a value of chi-square equal to or more extreme than what we found in only 5 % or fewer of those tests if the null hypothesis is true. When the p-value is this small, we say that the observed relationship between the two variables was *statistically significant at the 0.05 level*.

Another way of looking at this goes as follows. If we use 0.05 as our cutoff for saying that the observed relationship is statistically significant, 5 % of the time we will mistakenly conclude that a relationship we found between the two variables in our sample also exists in the population. In statistics, this mistake is known as a *Type I Error*. We never know when we have committed a Type I Error. However, we do know that if the null hypothesis is true we will make this mistake 5 % of the time. Scientists feel that a 5 % error rate is acceptable. In addition, it is common practice

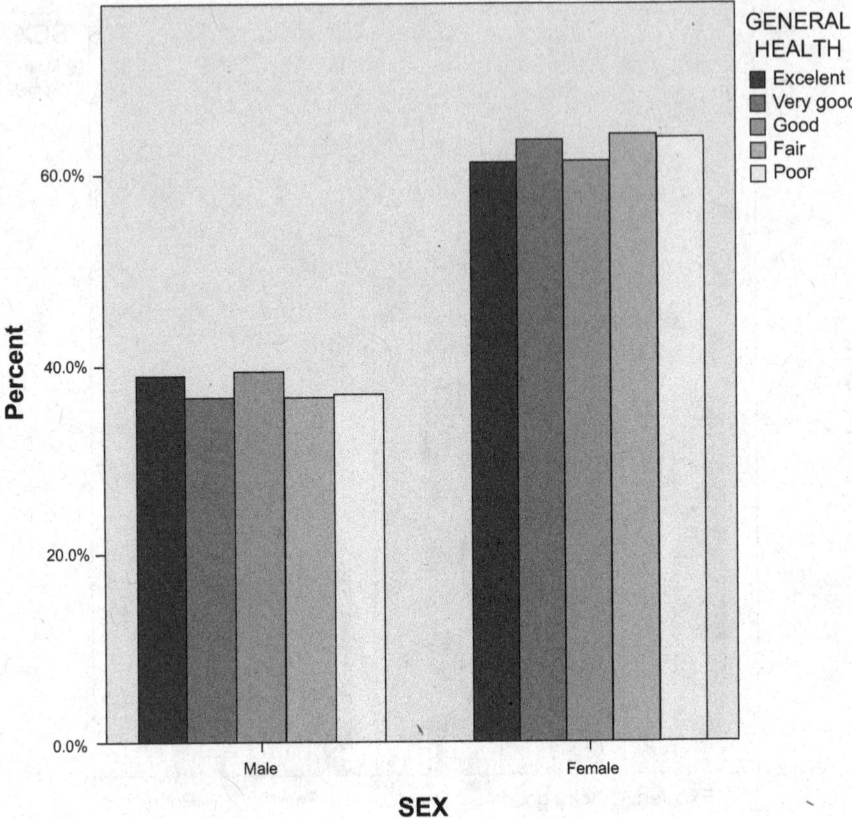

Fig. 7.10 A second clustered bar chart

for scientists to try to replicate each others' results. If the outcomes can be repeated, then the conclusion drawn is more likely to be valid.

Sometimes, an error rate of 5 % seems too high. This might be true if the implications of one's research are very important. In these cases, scientists will demand an even lower error rate. In such a situation, scientists might opt for a significance level of .01.

Any sample result associated with a *p*-value equal to or less than 0.05, 0.01, or 0.001 could be said to be statistically significant. Therefore, it is incumbent upon researchers to explain which *p*-value was used to determine whether results were to be labeled "significant." In addition, researchers are encouraged to report the exact *p*-value associated with each of their findings, e.g., $p=0.02$.

SPSS computes the *p*-value associated with many of its sample statistics. In some cases, it can calculate the exact *p*-value. In other cases, it calculates an approximate value.

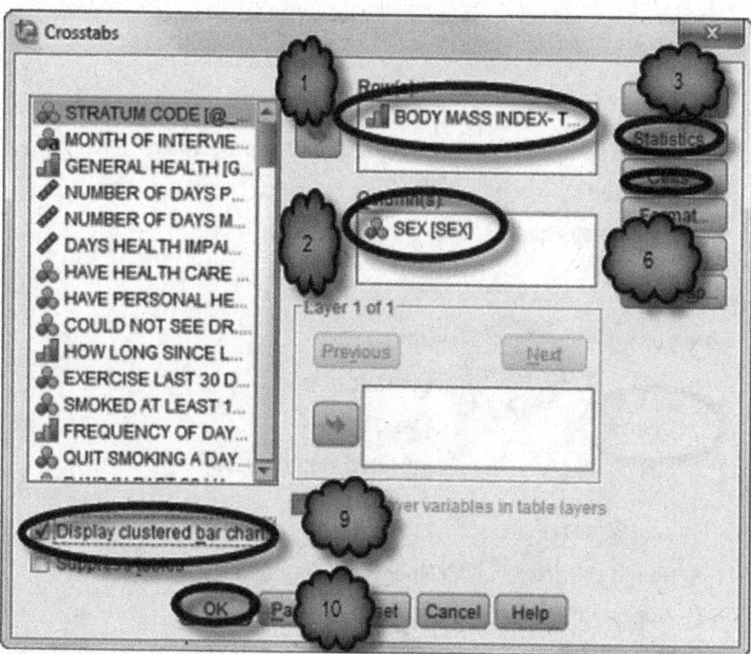

Fig. 7.11 Cross-tabulation dialog

Fig. 7.12 Requesting a chi-square test

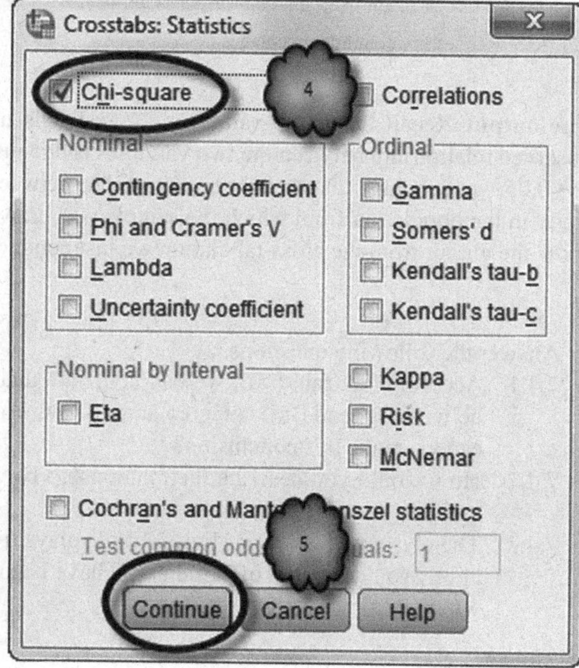

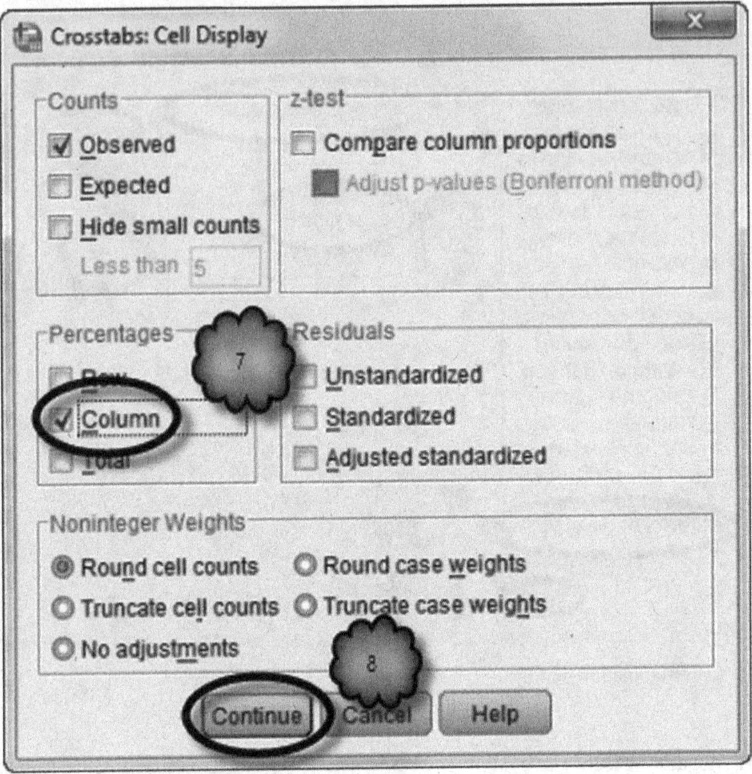

Fig. 7.13 Requesting column percentages

The output Recall that the *p*-value for the test tells us the probability that the observed relationship between the two variables is due just to chance. If the *p*-value is ≤0.05, we conclude that there is a relationship between the two variables under study in the population from which the sample was drawn. Table 7.3 and Fig. 7.14 show the output from the cross-tabulation we just conducted.

Answer the following questions.

7.4.1 According to Table 7.3, we can conclude that there is a relationship between sex and BMI category among New York State residents. Why can we make this conclusion?

7.4.2 How would you describe the relationship between sex and BMI category?

7.4.3 The clustered bar graph (Fig. 7.14) displays frequencies, not percentages. Would a graph of percentages have been more helpful? Why or why not?

Table 7.3 Crosstabs output

BODY MASS INDEX-THREE LEVELS CATEGORY * SEX Crosstabulation

			SEX		Total
			Male	Female	
BODY MASS INDEX-THREE LEVELS CATEGORY	Neither Overweight nor Obese	Count	911	2096	3007
		% within SEX	31.6%	46.2%	40.5%
	Overweight	Count	1302	1401	2703
		% within SEX	45.2%	30.9%	36.4%
	Obese	Count	670	1037	1707
		% within SEX	23.2%	22.9%	23.0%
Total		Count	2883	4534	7417
		% within SEX	100.0%	100.0%	100.0%

Chi-Square Tests

	Value	df	Asymp. Sig. (2-sided)
Pearson Chi-Square	191.497[a]	2	.000
Likelihood Ratio	192.439	2	.000
Linear-by-Linear Association	65.529	1	.000
N of Valid Cases	7417		

a. 0 cells (.0%) have expected count less than 5. The minimum expected count is 663.51.

7.5 Measuring the Strength of the Relationship: Cramér's *V*

The fact that a relationship observed in a sample is statistically significant means that it is very likely that the relationship also exists in the population. However, a significant relationship does not imply that the relationship is a strong one. For example, a weak relationship between two variables can still be significant if the size of the sample is sufficiently large. Consequently, when a relationship between two variables is found to be significant, often the next step is to determine how closely or strongly the two variables are associated with one another.

When both variables under study are categorical, a large number of *measures of association* are available. For the rest of the chapter, we focus on two of them, *Cramér's V* and *gamma*. First, Cramér's *V*. If either of the variables is nominal, Cramér's *V* is an appropriate measure of the degree to which the two variables are related. To demonstrate we will use the CDC data set to determine if sex (male or female) and access to health care (yes or no) are related.

To make interpretation of the output easier, begin by labeling the values of **HAVE HEALTH CARE COVERAGE** [*HLTHPLAN*] (variable 7; 1=Yes; 2=No) and declaring values of 7 and 9 for **HAVE HEALTH CARE COVERAGE** as missing. Open the *Crosstabs* dialog box and click **Reset.** Then using **SEX** [*SEX*] (variable 32) as the column variable and **HAVE HEALTH CARE COVERAGE** as the row

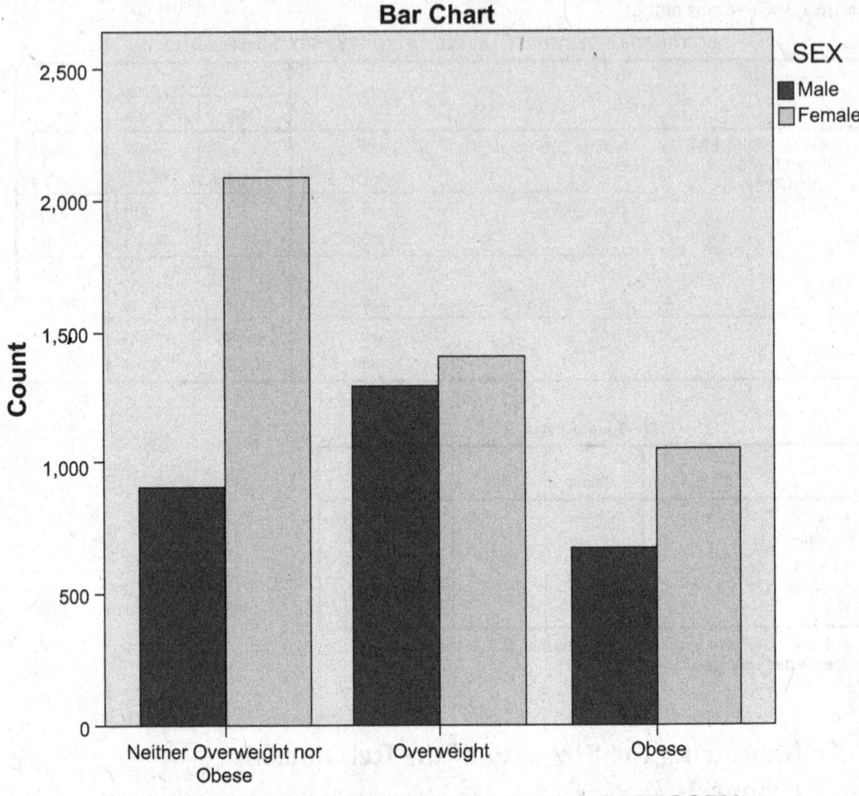

Fig. 7.14 Clustered bar graph

variable, run a cross-tabulation. Before conducting your analysis, click **Cells** and ask SPSS to generate column percentages. Then click **Statistics** and check *Chi-square* and *Phi and Cramér's V* in the *Nominal* area of the *Statistics* dialog box as shown in Fig. 7.15.

Depending on how the values of the two variables are coded, Cramér's V can range from 0 to +1. If two variables are not at all related to one another, Cramér's V will equal 0; if both variables are perfectly related to one another, Cramér's V will equal +1. The phi coefficient that also appears in the output will have the same magnitude as Cramér's V in the case of a 2×2 table. For larger tables, phi should not be used because it cannot achieve its maximum value. For these tables Cramér's V has an achievable upper value of +1, and therefore should be used.

In our example, if there is no relationship between the sex of the respondent and whether or not he or she had access to a health care plan, then Cramér's V would equal 0. If Cramér's V were equal to or very close to 0, knowing whether the respondent was male or female would not allow us to improve our ability to tell whether or not he or she had a health-care plan. On the other hand, if males always had a plan

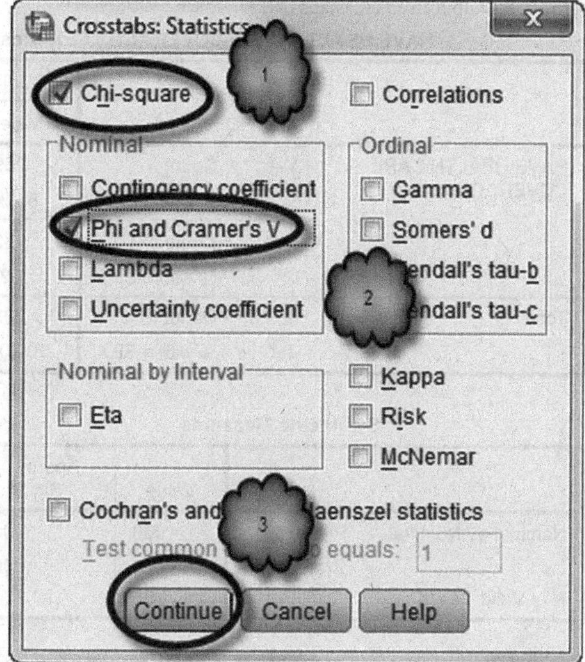

Fig. 7.15 Selecting Cramér's V

and women never did, or if males never had a plan, and women always did, Cramér's V would equal +1. In these cases, knowing the sex of the respondent would always tell us whether or not the respondent had a health care plan.

The output of the cross-tabulation is shown in Table 7.4.

Answer the following questions.

7.5.1 In our sample, were men or women more likely to have a health care plan?

7.5.2 What is the value of Cramér's V?

Testing hypotheses about Cramér's V Recall that sample data are always subject to the effects of chance. As a consequence, we can never be certain that the results we obtained from a given sample give us a true reading of the population from which we drew the sample. For example, the Cramér's V that we calculated in the previous section was based on a sample of New York state residents, not the entire population of people who live in the state. The value of Cramér's V that we computed was true of the sample, but because of chance factors, may not approximate the value of Cramér's V that we would have calculated if we could have interviewed everyone in the state. In fact, it is possible the value of Cramér's V in the population is actually zero. Hence we need to choose between two possibilities: the population value of Cramér's V is equal to zero (the null hypothesis) or the population value of

Table 7.4 Output from crosstabs

HAVE HEALTH CARE COVERAGE * SEX Crosstabulation

			SEX		Total
			Male	Female	
HAVE HEALTH CARE COVERAGE	Yes	Count	2594	4475	7069
		% within SEX	88.8%	92.4%	91.0%
	No	Count	326	370	696
		% within SEX	11.2%	7.6%	9.0%
Total		Count	2920	4845	7765
		% within SEX	100.0%	100.0%	100.0%

Symmetric Measures

		Value	Approx. Sig.
Nominal by Nominal	Phi	-.060	.000
	Cramer's V	.060	.000
N of Valid Cases		7765	

Cramér's *V* is not equal to zero (the alternative hypothesis). To make this choice, we need to know the probability that the value of Cramér's *V* that we calculated based on our sample would have been obtained if the population value was zero, i.e., if the null hypothesis were true.

For each value of Cramér's *V* (and the phi coefficient), SPSS calculates an approximate *p*-value, and labels it *Approx. Sig.* As long as this *p*-value is ≤ 0.05, we can confidently reject the null hypothesis and conclude that the sample value of Cramér's *V* was not solely due to chance, but also a result of a true relationship within the population from which the sample was taken.

Answer the following questions.

7.5.3 In our analysis of the relationship between sex and having a health care plan, what was the *p*-value associated with Cramér's *V*?

7.5.4 Can we reject the null hypothesis that Cramér's *V* is equal to zero? Why or why not?

7.5.5 In the population of New York State residents, can we conclude that women are more likely to have a health care plan?

Comparing values of Cramér's *V* across a categorical variable It is possible that the strength of a relationship between two categorical variables varies across values of a third categorical variable. Consequently, researchers often determine

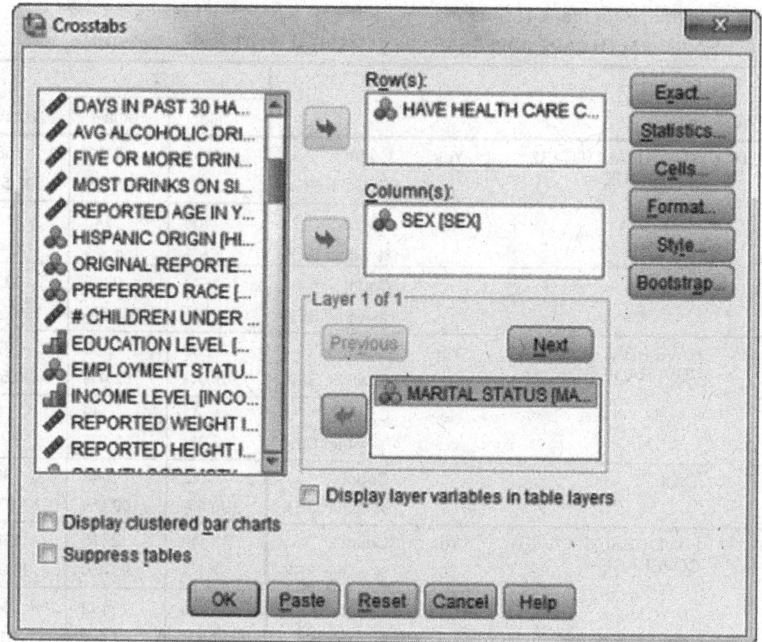

Fig. 7.16 Selecting marital status as a layer variable

whether the value of Cramér's *V* (or whatever measure of association they are using) depends on some other factor. For instance, in our example, we found that women are more likely to have a health care plan than men. This conclusion applies to the population of New York State as a whole, but there might be exceptions. For example, maybe married couples share their spouses' plan, and as a result there is no difference between the percentages of married men and women who have a health care plan. In this section, we determine if the relationship between sex and health coverage depends on whether people are married or divorced.

Begin by checking that the values of the variable, **MARITAL STATUS** [*MARITAL*] (variable 24; 1 = Married, 2 = Divorced, 3 = Widowed, 4 = Separated, 5 = Never married, 6 = A member of an unmarried couple, and 9 = Refused to answer) have been labeled and that the value of 9 has been declared as a missing value. Then use **Data > Select Cases** to restrict our analysis to married and divorced respondents. Then return to the cross-tabulation dialog box that we set up in our previous analysis and move **MARITAL STATUS** to the box labeled *Layer 1 of 1*. The dialog box should now look similar to the one shown in Fig. 7.16.

Be sure that *Phi and Cramér's V* in the *Crosstabs: Statistics* dialog box is still checked. Then click **Continue** and **OK**.

Table 7.5 gives the output that is generated by the above analysis.

Table 7.5 Controlling for marital status

HAVE HEALTH CARE COVERAGE * SEX * MARITAL STATUS Crosstabulation

MARITAL STATUS				SEX		Total
				Male	Female	
Married	HAVE HEALTH CARE COVERAGE	Yes	Count	1466	2122	3588
			% within SEX	93.1%	93.7%	93.5%
		No	Count	108	143	251
			% within SEX	6.9%	6.3%	6.5%
	Total		Count	1574	2265	3839
			% within SEX	100.0%	100.0%	100.0%
Divorced	HAVE HEALTH CARE COVERAGE	Yes	Count	280	593	873
			% within SEX	87.0%	92.4%	90.6%
		No	Count	42	49	91
			% within SEX	13.0%	7.6%	9.4%
	Total		Count	322	642	964
			% within SEX	100.0%	100.0%	100.0%
Total	HAVE HEALTH CARE COVERAGE	Yes	Count	1746	2715	4461
			% within SEX	92.1%	93.4%	92.9%
		No	Count	150	192	342
			% within SEX	7.9%	6.6%	7.1%
	Total		Count	1896	2907	4803
			% within SEX	100.0%	100.0%	100.0%

Symmetric Measures

MARITAL STATUS			Value	Approx. Sig.
Married	Nominal by Nominal	Phi	-.011	.499
		Cramer's V	.011	.499
	N of Valid Cases		3839	
Divorced	Nominal by Nominal	Phi	-.087	.007
		Cramer's V	.087	.007
	N of Valid Cases		964	
Total	Nominal by Nominal	Phi	-.025	.085
		Cramer's V	.025	.085
	N of Valid Cases		4803	

Answer the following questions.

7.5.6 Do the values of Cramér's V vary across marital status?

7.5.7 Among married people within New York State, are men or women more likely to have health coverage?

7.5.8 What about among New York's divorced residents?

7.5.9 Is our earlier conclusion that women are more likely to have health coverage generally true or are there exceptions? Explain.

7.6 Measuring the Strength of the Relationship: Gamma

If both variables are ordinal, researchers are interested in determining not only how strongly the two variables are related but in determining whether the relationship is positive or negative. In a *positive* relationship, increases in one variable tend to be associated with *increases* in the other. In a *negative* relationship, increases in one variable tend to be associated with *decreases* in the other. One measure of association between ordinal variables that measures both strength and direction is called gamma. Gamma can range from − 1 to + 1. The closer gamma is to either extreme, the stronger is the relationship between the two variables. The sign tells the direction of the relationship. If the overall tendency is for an increase in one ordinal variable to be associated with an increase in the other ordinal variable, gamma will be positive. If the overall tendency is for an increase in one ordinal variable to be associated with a decrease in the other ordinal variable, then gamma will be negative.

Gamma is calculated as follows. First, two types of pairs of observations are identified. A pair of observations, call them A and B, is said to be *concordant* if A is higher than B in one variable and A is higher than B in the other variable. A pair of observations is said to be *discordant* if A is higher than B in one variable, but B is higher than A in the other variable. Next, the total number of concordant pairs and the total number of discordant pairs are calculated. Gamma is then computed as the difference between the number of concordant and discordant pairs relative to the number of all pairs which are either concordant or discordant. If there are more concordant pairs than discordant pairs, then gamma will be positive. If there are more discordant pairs than concordant pairs, then gamma will be negative. Gamma will be + 1 if there are no discordant pairs, and gamma will be − 1 if there are no concordant pairs.

We will use gamma to study the relationship between reported health status (good or better health versus fair or poor health) and BMI category (neither overweight nor obese, overweight, obese). We will conduct the analysis on the entire sample.

Begin by returning to the **Data > Select Cases** dialog box. Select *All cases* and click **OK**. Be sure that the value of 9 has been declared as missing for the variable, **HEALTH STATUS** [*@_RFHLTH*] (variable 58; 1 = Good or Better Health, 2 = Fair or Poor Health) and that the value labels have been assigned. Then set up a cross-tabulation with **BODY MASS INDEX-THREE LEVELS CATEGORY** [*@_BMI4CAT*] (variable 79) as the column variable and **HEALTH STATUS** as the row variable. Click **Statistics** and as shown in Fig. 7.17, check *Gamma* in the ordinal area and *Chi-square*.

Click **Continue.** Now click **Cells** to be sure that column percentages have been selected. After clicking **Continue,** run the analysis.

The output that is generated by this analysis is shown in Table 7.6.

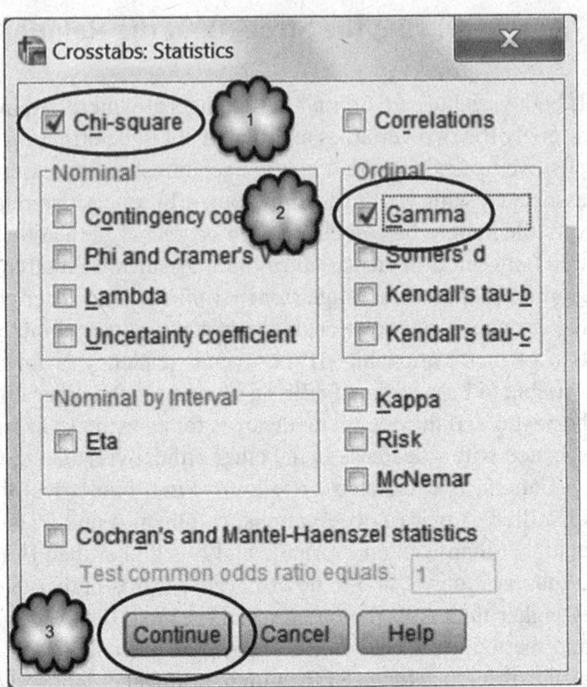

Fig. 7.17 Selecting gamma

Answer the following questions.

7.6.1 Is there a significant relationship between the two variables?
7.6.2 What is the value of gamma?
7.6.3 Is the relationship positive or negative?
7.6.4 What conclusion can we draw about the relationship between BMI category and the reported health for residents of New York state?

7.7 Exercise Questions

1. Using the variables **INCOME CATEGORIES** [*@_INCOMG*](variable 83) and **GENERAL HEALTH** [*GENHLTH*] (variable 3) of the **CDC BRFSS** data set, investigate whether the reported general health of adult residents of New York State is related to their income. Before you begin, declare 7 and 9 as missing values for **GENERAL HEALTH** and 9 for **INCOME CATEGORIES.** Then generate a cross-tabulation between **GENERAL HEALTH** and **INCOME CATEGORIES. INCOME CATEGORIES** will be the explanatory variable so make it the column variable in the cross-tabulation. Include both row and column percentages.

Table 7.6 Analysis with gamma

HEALTH STATUS * BODY MASS INDEX-THREE LEVELS CATEGORY Crosstabulation

			BODY MASS INDEX-THREE LEVELS CATEGORY			
			Neither Overweight nor Obese	Overweight	Obese	Total
HEALTH STATUS	Good or Better Health	Count	2619	2293	1267	6179
		% within BODY MASS INDEX-THREE LEVELS CATEGORY	87.2%	85.0%	74.5%	83.5%
	Fair or Poor Health	Count	384	404	433	1221
		% within BODY MASS INDEX-THREE LEVELS CATEGORY	12.8%	15.0%	25.5%	16.5%
Total		Count	3003	2697	1700	7400
		% within BODY MASS INDEX-THREE LEVELS CATEGORY	100.0%	100.0%	100.0%	100.0%

Chi-Square Tests

	Value	df	Asymp. Sig. (2-sided)
Pearson Chi-Square	133.864[a]	2	.000
Likelihood Ratio	124.733	2	.000
Linear-by-Linear Association	113.060	1	.000
N of Valid Cases	7400		

a. 0 cells (.0%) have expected count less than 5. The minimum expected count is 280.50.

Symmetric Measures

		Value	Asymp. Std. Error[a]	Approx. T[b]	Approx. Sig.
Ordinal by Ordinal	Gamma	.258	.025	9.801	.000
N of Valid Cases		7400			

a. Not assuming the null hypothesis.
b. Using the asymptotic standard error assuming the null hypothesis.

a. Regardless of their reported health, how many respondents reported an annual household income less than US$ 15,000?
b. What percent of the total sample reported an annual household income less than US$ 15,000?
c. Regardless of their reported health, how many respondents reported a household income equal to or greater than US$ 50,000?
d. What percent of the total sample reported an annual household income equal to or greater than US$ 50,000?
e. Of the respondents who reported an annual household income less than US$15,000, what percentage also reported that they were in excellent health?

f. Of the respondents who reported an annual household income equal to or more than US$ 50,000, what percentage also reported that they were in excellent health?
g. Of the respondents who reported an annual household income less than US$ 15 000, what percentage also reported that they were in poor health?
h. Of the respondents who reported an annual household income equal to or more than US$ 50 000, what percentage also reported that they were in poor health?
i. Does it appear that reported general health and income level are related? Defend your answer.

2. Determine if sex and smoking are related. Consider sex the explanatory variable. To conduct this analysis, use the variables **SEX** [*SEX*] (variable 32; 1=Male, 2=Female) and **CURRENT SMOKING STATUS RISK FACTOR** [@_*RFSMOK3*] [variable 64; 1=No (meaning that the respondent was not a smoker at the time of the interview); 2=Yes (the respondent was a smoker); and 9=Do Not Know/Refused to Answer/Missing] in the **CDC BRFSS** data set. Be sure that the values of each variable have been labeled, and declare a value of 9 as missing to limit the analysis to respondents whose smoking status was coded as either No or Yes. Then conduct a cross-tabulation that generates a contingency table with column percentages and that calculates Cramér's *V*.

   a. How many participants were included in the analysis?
   b. What was the value of Cramér's *V*?
   c. According to Cramér's *V*, is there a statistically significant relationship between sex and smoking status? If so, which sex is more likely to smoke?
   d. Create a clustered bar graph of sex and smoking status. Put sex on the *x*-axis and percent (not count) on the *y*-axis. Be sure that the percentages reflect the column percentages of the contingency table.

3. Repeat the above analysis, but this time, determine if emotional support moderates the extent to which sex and smoking are related. To conduct this analysis, recode **HOW OFTEN GET EMOT SUPPORT NEEDED** [*EMTSUPRT*] (variable 49; 1=Always; 2=Usually; 3=Sometimes; 4=Rarely; and 5=Never) into a new variable, **EMOT SUPPORT 3 GROUPS.** For the new variable, instruct SPSS to code those who reported usually or always receiving support as 1, sometimes receiving support as 2, and rarely or never as 3; and to copy the remaining variables (7 and 9) from the old variable to the new one. Then for the new variable, assign value labels (e.g., 1=Usually or Always), and declare 7 and 9 as missing values. Finally, run the cross-tabulation of Question 2 with the new variable as the layer variable.

   a. Enter into Table 7.7 the values of Cramér's *V* for each level of emotional support.
   b. When does the prevalence of smoking significantly differ between men and women?

4. Determine if the overall general health of New York State adults is related to the time since they last had a routine checkup. The relevant variables are **HEALTH**

Table 7.7 Cramér's *V*

Emotional Support	Cramér's *V*
Usually or Always	
Sometimes	
Rarely or Never	

STATUS [*@_RFHLTH*] (variable 58; 1 = Good or Better Health; 2 = Fair or Poor Health; and 9 = Do Not Know/Not Sure/Refused/Missing) and **HOW LONG SINCE LAST ROUTINE CHECKUP** [*CHECKUP*] (variable 10; 1 = Within the Last Year; 2 = Within the Last 2 Years; 3 = Within the Last 5 Years; 4 = Five or More Years Ago; 7 = Do Not Know/Not Sure; 8 = Never; 9 = Refused) in the **CDC BRFSS** data set. Be sure that the value of 9 has been declared as missing for the variable, **HEALTH STATUS,** and that the values of 7 and 9 have been declared as missing for **HOW LONG SINCE LAST ROUTINE CHECKUP**.

In this analysis, we are interested only in those who have had a routine checkup at least once in their lives, so using **Data > Select Cases,** exclude respondents who had never had a checkup.

Then recode **HOW LONG SINCE LAST ROUTINE CHECKUP** into a new variable, **CHECKUP 2 GROUPS**. In this new variable, assign a 1 to those who reported that they had a checkup within the last 2 years and a 2 to those who reported that they had a checkup over 2 years ago.

Next, declare 7 and 9 as missing for the new variable, and assign value labels to the new variable, and if necessary, to the variable, **HEALTH STATUS.**

Now create a contingency table with **HEALTH STATUS** as the explanatory variable and **CHECKUP 2 GROUPS** as the response variable. Include in the analysis column percents. To quantify the degree of relationship between the two variables, ask SPSS to calculate either Cramér's *V* or gamma, whichever you believe is appropriate to the analysis.

a. How many participants are in the analysis?
b. In this analysis, is Cramér's *V* or gamma the appropriate measure of association? Why?
c. Report the value of Cramér's *V* or gamma (whichever statistic you calculated).
d. Based on this statistic, how would you describe the relationship between general health and time since last checkup?

5. Study the clustered bar chart in Fig. 7.18 and the output summarized Table 7.8. These were generated by a cross-tabulation of the CDC data.

   Based on these data, answer the following question: Within the population of male New York State residents, are veterans more or less likely than nonveterans to be heavy drinkers? Explain your answer.

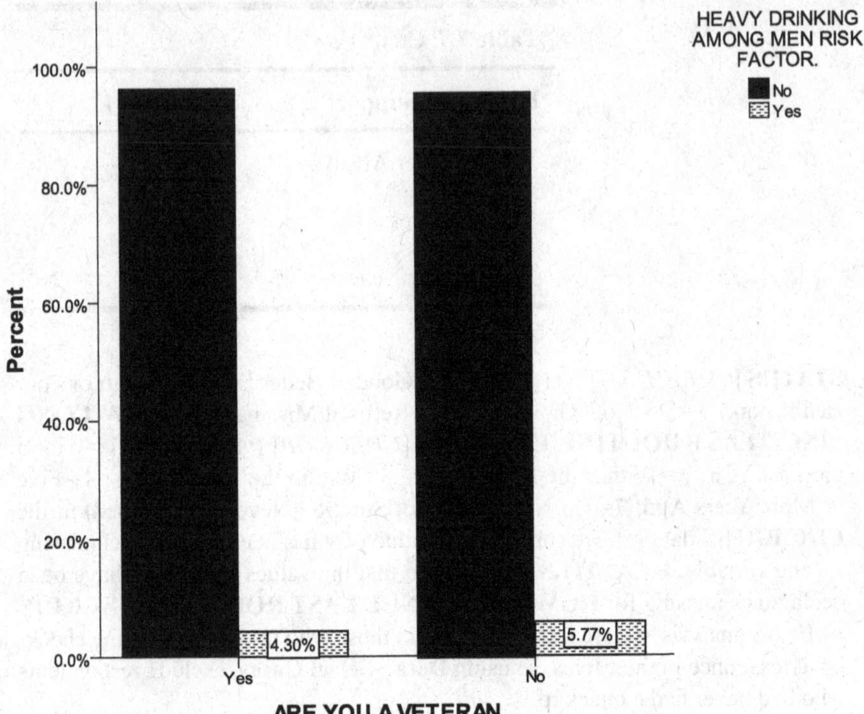

Fig. 7.18 Clustered bar chart (Question 5)

Table 7.8 Output (Question 5)

Symmetric Measures

		Value	Approx. Sig.
Nominal by Nominal	Phi	.029	.123
	Cramer's V	.029	.123
N of Valid Cases		2832	

Data Set and Reference

1. CDC BRFSS.sav obtained from: Centers for Disease Control and Prevention (CDC). Behavioral risk factor surveillance system survey data. Atlanta: US Department of Health and Human Services, Centers for Disease Control and Prevention (2005). Public domain. For more information about the BRFSS, visit http://www.cdc.gov/brfss/. Accessed 16 Nov 2014

Chapter 8
Assessing Screening and Diagnostic Tests

Abstract Clinicians often use screening and diagnostic tests to identify asymptomatic patients, confirm diagnoses or assess treatment effectiveness. The usefulness of these tests depends on their ability to correctly classify patients as having or not having a particular disease. This ability is assessed by determining the extent to which a test's classifications agree with those of a criterion or gold standard. This chapter reviews several measures of agreement, including the test's positive and negative predictive values, its true positive rate or sensitivity, its true negative rate or specificity, and the ratio of its true positive rate to its false positive rate, or likelihood ratio. The chapter concludes with a discussion of how a receiver operating characteristic (ROC) curve is used to evaluate the accuracy of a test that generates a range of quantitative values, and to select a cutoff value that optimizes sensitivity and specificity.

8.1 Overview

In Chap. 6, we learned that prevalence is the proportion of a population that has a given illness. Using this information, clinicians can get an initial sense of the likelihood that an individual patient has a particular disease. However, the accuracy of diagnosis can be greatly improved by including information generated by standardized clinical or laboratory tests. In some cases, a test can establish with great confidence whether or not a patient has a given medical condition. Unfortunately, such tests, referred to as *criterion standards* or *gold standards*, can have significant disadvantages. For example, they may be expensive, invasive, pose serious risks to patients, or cannot be used until after patients have died. Instead of using criterion standards, clinicians often use screening and diagnostic tests. Clinicians use *screening* tests to identify among asymptomatic patients those who have disease in its early stages and *diagnostic* tests to confirm a diagnosis or to track the progress of treatment. Although less accurate than a criterion standard, a good screening or diagnostic test helps clinicians to adjust their initial judgments in the direction of a more accurate assessment of the likelihood that the patient has a given disease.

The results of a screening or diagnostic test are said to be either positive or negative for the presence of disease. A *positive* result means that the test has classified

W. H. Holmes, W. C. Rinaman, *Statistical Literacy for Clinical Practitioners*,
DOI 10.1007/978-3-319-12550-3_8

the patient as having disease. A *negative* result means that the test has classified the patient as being free of disease. For these classifications to be useful to the clinician, they must tend to correctly identify whether or not the patient in fact has the disease. Since the test classifies patients as positive or negative, and since patients either have or do not have the disease, the screening or diagnostic usefulness of the test can be assessed with a 2×2 contingency table. In the last chapter, we learned how to use contingency tables to study the relationship between two categorical variables. In this chapter, we will see how contingency tables can be used to determine how well screening and diagnostic tests detect disease. The categorical variables will be the results of the screening or diagnostic test (positive versus negative) and the disease status of the patient as determined by a criterion test (disease is present versus disease is absent).

8.2 Positive and Negative Predictive Values

One measure of the usefulness of a test is its *positive predictive value* (PPV), the proportion of times a positive test result is followed by a positive result on a criterion test. If a test has a high PPV, then patients who test positive on it will tend to also test positive on the criterion test. Another measure is a test's *negative predictive value* (NPV), the proportion of times a negative test result is followed by a negative result on the criterion test. If a test has a high NPV, then patients who test negative on it will tend to also test negative on the criterion test. In this section, we will determine the PPV and NPV of a screening exam, specifically a digital rectal exam (DRE) that was conducted on 301 men to detect the presence of prostate cancer. These data are stored in the file, **PSA.sav** [1]. Subsequent to the exam, the prostate of each patient was biopsied. The researchers who conducted this study stored the results of the DRE in a variable called **DRE Result** [*dre*] (variable 3; 1=Positive; 2=Negative) and the results of the biopsy in a variable called **Biopsy Result** [*biopsy*] (variable 8, 1=Cancer Present; 2=Cancer Absent). Did the results of the digital exam predict the results of the biopsy?

If we were to answer this question by hand, we would first set up a 2×2 contingency table. Following customary procedures, we would label the two rows with the possible results of the screening test, with the first row consisting of patients who tested positive. We would label the columns with the two possible results of the criterion test, with the first column consisting of patients identified as having the disease. Then we would calculate the PPV of the DRE by computing the proportion of patients who tested positive on the DRE who then tested positive on the biopsy. To do this, we would consult the top row of the contingency table and divide the number of patients who had a positive biopsy result by the total number of patients who tested positive on the DRE. To calculate the NPV of the DRE, we would compute the percentage of patients who tested negative on the DRE who then subsequently tested negative on the biopsy. To do this, we would consult the second row and divide the number of patients who had a negative biopsy result by the total number of patients who tested negative on the DRE.

Table 8.1 Positive and negative predictive values

DRE Result * Biopsy Result Crosstabulation

Positive Predictive Value

			Biopsy Result		
			Cancer Present	Cancer Absent	Total
DRE Result	Positive	Count	68	117	185
		% within DRE Result	36.8%	63.2%	100.0%
	Negative	Count	27	89	116
		% within DRE Result	23.3%	76.7%	100.0%
Total		Count	95	206	301
		% within DRE Result	31.6%	68.4%	100.0%

Negative Predictive Value

Positive Predictive Value **= Number of patients with the disease / Number of patients who tested positive on the screening or diagnostic test = 68/185 = .368.**

Negative Predictive Value **= Number of patients without the disease / Number of patients who tested negative on the screening or diagnostic test = 89/116 = .767.**

To get SPSS to do all of this for us, load the file, **PSA.sav**, and select **Analyze > Descriptive Statistics > Crosstabs**. In the resulting dialog box, move **DRE Result** to the *Row(s)* window, and **Biopsy Result** to the *Column(s)* window. Select **Cells**, check *Row* percentages, and click **Continue** followed by **OK**. This will generate the contingency table that we need.

The contingency table would be similar to the one displayed in Table 8.1.

Answer the following questions:

8.2.1 How many patients tested positive on the DRE?
8.2.2 Of these, how many subsequently tested positive on the biopsy?
8.2.3 What is the positive PPV of the DRE?
8.2.4 If we were to predict that a patient who tested negative on the DRE would also have a negative biopsy, how often would we be correct?

From the first row, we can see that 185 patients tested positive on the DRE. Of these, 68 or 36.8 % subsequently tested positive on the biopsy. Thus, the PPV of the DRE is 0.368. If we were to predict that patients who tested positive on the DRE would subsequently have positive biopsy results, we would be correct about 37 % of the time. From the second row, we can see that 116 patients tested negative on the DRE. Of these, 89 or 76.7 % also tested negative on the biopsy. Thus, the NPV is 0.767. We would be right about 77 % of the time if we were to predict that a patient who tested negative on the DRE would subsequently have a negative biopsy.

Although predictive values are indicators of the ability of a test to detect disease, they are sensitive to the prevalence of the disease within the population to which the test was administered. If the disease is highly prevalent, the PPV will also be high. If the same test were used to detect the disease in a population in which the disease is rare, the PPV would be lower. Consequently, judging a test on the basis of its predictive values requires that prevalence rates be taken into account. This can make comparing the usefulness of various tests difficult if the tests were administered to populations with different prevalence rates. More helpful in evaluating tests are diagnostic statistics that are independent of prevalence. We turn to those statistics in the next section.

8.3 True Positives, True Negatives, False Positives, and False Negatives

A screening or diagnostic test classifies patients as either positive or negative for the presence of disease. If a patient has disease, the test should return a positive result. If a patient does not have disease, the test should return a negative result. Each of these correct classifications is called a *true positive* and a *true negative*, respectively. Conversely, if a patient has disease, the test should not return a negative result, and if a patient does not have disease, the test should not return a positive result. Each of these two errors in classification is called a *false negative* and a *false positive*, respectively. Table 8.2 displays the number of true positives (TP), true negatives (TN), false positives (FP) and false negatives (FN) that occurred in

Table 8.2 Contingency table for computing test accuracy, sensitivity, and specificity

DRE Result * Biopsy Result Crosstabulation

			Biopsy Result		
		Sensitivity	Cancer Present	Cancer Absent	Total
DRE Result	Positive	Count	TP → 68	FP → 117	185
		% within Biopsy Result	71.6%	56.8%	61.5%
	Negative	Count	FN → 27	TN → 89	116
		% within Biopsy Result	28.4%	43.2%	38.5%
Total		Count	95	206	301
		% within Biopsy Result	100.0%	100.0%	100.0%

Specificity

TP = Number of true positives. TN = Number of true negatives.
FP = Number of false positives. FN = Number of false negatives.

***Accuracy* = (TP + TN)/Total number of classifications = 157/301 = .522.**
***Sensitivity* = TP/Number of patients with disease = 68/95 = .716.**
***Specificity* = TN/Number of patients without disease = 89/206 = .432.**

our example. The table displays the same frequency data reported in Table 8.1, but the cell percentages are different as they are calculated within each column instead of within each row. We will discuss those cell percentages in a moment.

The proportion of times a test makes a correct classification is its *accuracy*. Accuracy is calculated by dividing the total number of correct classifications (TP plus TN) by the total number of classifications. As we can see from Table 8.2, the accuracy of the DRE is 68 TP plus 89 TN divided by 301 total classifications, or 157 correct classifications divided by 301 total classifications. This yields an accuracy of 0.522. The DRE correctly classified patients about 52 % of the time.

Accuracy can give a global sense of the usefulness of a test but it does not reveal whether the test is more prone to making false negative errors (not detecting disease when it is present) or false positive errors (detecting disease when none is present). The relative seriousness of the consequences that follow from these errors varies across situations, so clinicians try to use tests that for a given situation commit the more serious error less often while keeping the frequency of the less serious mistake within tolerable levels. For example, if a disease is more likely to be cured if it is treated before patients show symptoms, then it is important that a screening test identify within an asymptomatic population as many patients with the disease as possible, even if this means that more patients who are disease-free will be misdiagnosed as having the disease. In this case, missing a patient who has the disease (a false negative result) would be seen as the more serious error and a screening test that minimizes FN would be preferred. Once patients have been screened, they could then be given a diagnostic test to confirm the presence of the disease. In this case, identifying a patient as having the disease when it is not present (a false positive) would be considered the more serious mistake, and a diagnostic test that minimizes FP would be preferred.

To assess the rate at which a screening or diagnostic test correctly classifies patients, its rates of TP and TN are calculated. The *true positive rate* is the proportion of patients who in fact had the disease for whom the test had returned a positive result. It is calculated by dividing the number of patients who had tested positive on the screening or diagnostic test by the total number of patients who in fact had the disease. Remember that whether or not the patient in fact had the disease is determined by the criterion test. Consequently, we calculate the true positive rate by consulting the first column of our contingency table. The *true negative rate* is the proportion of patients who in fact did not have the disease for whom the screening or diagnostic test returned a negative result. It is calculated by consulting the second column of the contingency table and dividing the number of patients who tested negative on the screening or diagnostic test by the total number of patients who were in fact disease-free.

To get SPSS to do these calculations for us, return to the *Crosstabs* dialog box, click *Cells,* uncheck *Row(s)*, and check *Column(s)*. Click **Continue** and **OK.** The output will include the contingency table displayed in Table 8.2.

Answer the following questions:

8.3.1 What proportion of patients who by biopsy were diagnosed as having prostate cancer had tested positive on the DRE?

8.3.2 What proportion of patients who by biopsy were diagnosed as not having prostate cancer had tested negative on the DRE?

8.3.3 What are the true positive and true negative rates of the DRE?

8.3.4 For which group of patients was the DRE a better measure of the presence or absence of cancer, those who had cancer or those who were cancer-free?

We can see from the first column that 95 patients were by biopsy diagnosed with prostate cancer. Of these, 68 or 71.6 % had tested positive on the DRE. We can see from the second column that 206 patients were by biopsy diagnosed as cancer-free. Of these, 89 or 43.2 % had tested negative on the screening test. Thus, the true positive and true negative rates are 0.716 and 0.432, respectively. If a patient had prostate cancer, the chances were about 72 % that the DRE would detect it. If a patient did not have cancer, the chances were about 43 % that the screening test would classify the patient as cancer-free.

The true positive rate is the proportion of patients with disease who tested positive on the screening or diagnostic test. When cell percentages of the contingency table are calculated within columns, the true positive rate can be found in the first column of the first row. Notice that the two cell percentages in this column account for 100 % of all patients with disease. Who are the patients in the second row of the first column? They are the remaining proportion of patients with disease whose disease was not detected by the test. This proportion is the *false negative rate* and is equal to 1 minus the true positive rate. In our example, the true positive rate was 0.716. As we can see in the second row of the first column, our true positive rate means that the DRE missed $1-0.716$ or 28.4 % of patients who had prostate cancer.

The true negative rate is the proportion of patients without disease who tested negative on the screening or diagnostic test. It can be found in the second row of the second column. Notice that the two cell percentages in the second column account for 100 % of patients who were disease-free. Who are the patients in the first row of the second column? They are the remaining proportion of patients who were cancer-free who were mistakenly diagnosed by the digital exam as having disease. This proportion is the *false positive rate* and is equal to 1 minus the true negative rate. In our example, the true negative rate was 0.432. As we can see in the first row of the second column, this true negative rate means that 56.8 % of cancer-free patients were erroneously diagnosed with cancer by the digital exam.

Recall that the accuracy of the digital exam was 0.522; it correctly classified a little over half of the patients. We now know why: The exam missed about 28 % of the patients who had prostate cancer and falsely detected cancer in about 57 % of those who were cancer-free. The exam made both types of classification mistakes, but was especially susceptible to making false positive errors.

The statistics we have discussed in this section do not depend on the prevalence of disease, but on the ability of a test to detect disease when it is present. Of course, if the disease in question is uncommon, it might be difficult to find enough patients with disease to adequately assess a test intended to detect it. Nevertheless, true and false positive rates and true and false negative rates are characteristics of the test, not of the population that is given the test.

8.4 Sensitivity and Specificity

If patients are given a test that has true positive and true negative rates equal to 1, then they will test positive if and only if they have disease. Such a test would be perfectly sensitive to the presence of the disease and generate a positive result each and every time the disease is present. In addition, a positive result would be specific to the presence of the disease: The test would always "come back" negative unless the disease is present. For this reason, true positive and true negative rates are often referred to as the *sensitivity* and *specificity* of the test, respectively. Sensitivity is equal to the true positive rate and specificity is equal to the true negative rate. (If you have trouble keeping these terms straight, try using the "opposites rule." Sensitivity refers to true **p**ositives while s**p**ecificity refers to true **n**egatives.) In our example, the sensitivity of the DRE was 0.716 and its specificity was 0.432. The digital exam had fairly good sensitivity but much lower specificity: Usually patients with prostate cancer tested positive, so the test was relatively sensitive, but as a high percentage of patients who did not have cancer also tested positive, a positive test result was not specific to the presence of prostate cancer.

Answer the following true or false questions:

8.4.1 The sensitivity and specificity of a test can be determined without giving it to patients who are disease-free.

8.4.2 The false positive rate of a test is equal to 1 minus specificity.

Because the sensitivity of a test is the same as the test's true positive rate, the rate of making FN is equal to 1 minus sensitivity. Because specificity is the same as the test's true negative rate, the rate of making FP is equal to 1 minus specificity. These facts have some interesting implications. First, neither sensitivity nor specificity depends on disease prevalence. They are characteristics of the test, not of the population to which the test was administered, and so are convenient benchmarks for assessing various tests that are administered to different populations. Second, if we know the sensitivity of a test, we can easily calculate the test's false negative rate, and if we know the specificity of a test, we can easily calculate its false positive rate.

Third, the sensitivity of a test does not tell us its specificity as the two statistics are based on separate patients groups: Sensitivity is about patients who have disease and specificity is about patients who are disease-free. A high value of one does not imply a high value of the other. Recall that in our example, sensitivity was relatively high but specificity was relatively low. In fact, it is possible for the sensitivity of a test to equal 1 and specificity to equal 0, and vice-versa. The former would occur if the test classifies all patients, including those without disease, as positive, and the latter if the test classifies all patients, including those with disease, as negative. Consequently, when evaluating a test, both its sensitivity and specificity must be separately computed.

Fourth, to calculate sensitivity and specificity, the test must be administered to patients who have disease and to patients who do not. For example, the usefulness of the DRE in detecting prostate cancer cannot be determined by administering the exam solely to patients with prostate cancer.

8.5 Prior Odds, Posterior Odds, and the Likelihood Ratio

Another statistic that is useful in judging a screening or diagnostic test is its *likelihood ratio*. This statistic compares the probability of testing positive of two patients: one with disease and one who is disease-free. If the sensitivity and specificity of a test are equal to 1, all patients who have the disease will test positive (thanks to perfect sensitivity) but none of patients who are disease-free will (thanks to perfect specificity). The true positive rate will equal 1 and the false positive rate, which, remember, is equal to 1 minus specificity, will equal 0. Consequently, the probability of testing positive for a patient who has disease will equal 1 and the probability of testing positive for a patient without disease will equal 0. The test would be able to discriminate between a patient with disease and a patient without disease 100 % of the time. Screening and diagnostic tests, however, produce one or both types of classifications errors, so they do not allow clinicians to be able to always distinguish between the two types of patients. However, a test does not have to be perfect to be useful. But to be useful, the test must have at least some ability to discriminate between a patient who has disease and a patient who does not. We can tell how well a test can distinguish between patients with and without disease by comparing the true positive rate to the false positive rate. If this comparison is done in terms of the ratio of the true positive rate to the false positive rate, we have the likelihood ratio. A ratio of 1 indicates that the test has no ability to distinguish between patients with and without disease. The higher the ratio, the better the test is at screening or diagnosing disease.

As an example of a test that cannot discriminate, let us imagine that the data from the prostate cancer study were those displayed in Table 8.3.

Answer the following questions about these new data (Table 8.3):

8.5.1 What is the sensitivity or true positive rate of this DRE?

8.5.2 What is the probability that a patient with disease tested positive on the digital exam?

Table 8.3 Contingency table for a screening test with a likelihood ratio of 1

DRE Result * Biopsy Result Crosstabulation

			Biopsy Result		
			Cancer Present	Cancer Absent	Total
DRE Result	Positive	Count	54	117	171
		% within Biopsy Result	56.8%	56.8%	56.8%
	Negative	Count	41	89	130
		% within Biopsy Result	43.2%	43.2%	43.2%
Total		Count	95	206	301
		% within Biopsy Result	100.0%	100.0%	100.0%

Table 8.4 Contingency table for a screening test with a likelihood ratio of 6.216

DRE Result * Biopsy Result Crosstabulation

			Biopsy Result		
			Cancer Present	Cancer Absent	Total
DRE Result	Positive	Count	86	30	116
		% within Biopsy Result	90.5%	14.6%	38.5%
	Negative	Count	9	176	185
		% within Biopsy Result	9.5%	85.4%	61.5%
Total		Count	95	206	301
		% within Biopsy Result	100.0%	100.0%	100.0%

8.5.3 What is the false positive rate?
8.5.4 What is the probability that a patient without disease tested positive on the digital exam?
8.5.5 In this example, is a patient with disease more likely to test positive than a disease-free patient?

We can see from Table 8.3 that the sensitivity of the exam is now 0.568, down from 0.716 in our first example. We can also see that sensitivity is equal to the false positive rate. This means that the probability of a patient testing positive is the same whether or not the patient has prostate cancer. Since both patients are equally likely to test positive, a positive test offers no evidence that the patient has cancer—he is equally likely to be disease-free. So in this example, the likelihood ratio is equal to 1 and a positive test result would be of no help to a clinician trying to decide whether or not the patient has cancer.

Table 8.4 shows the results from the prostate cancer study that might have been obtained if the digital exam had high levels of both sensitivity and specificity.

Answer the following questions about these new data (Table 8.4):

8.5.6 What is the sensitivity or true positive rate of this DRE?

8.5.7 What is the probability that a patient with disease tested positive on the digital exam?

8.5.8 What is the false positive rate?

8.5.9 What is the probability that a patient without disease tested positive on the digital exam?

8.5.10 Is a patient with disease more likely to test positive than a disease-free patient?

We can see from Table 8.4 that the sensitivity of the exam is now 0.905, up from 0.716 in our first example, specificity is now 0.854, up from 0.432, and that the false positive rate is now 0.146, down from 0.568. We can also see that sensitivity is substantially greater than the false positive rate. In fact, it is 6.216 times greater. This means that the probability of a patient testing positive is over six times greater for a patient who has prostate cancer. So in this example, the likelihood ratio is equal to 6.216 and a positive test result is clear evidence of the presence of cancer.

Now let us see how useful the digital exam really was. Recall from Sect. 8.4 that the sensitivity of the digital exam was 0.716 and its specificity was 0.432.

Answer the following questions:

8.5.11 What was the false positive rate of the exam?

8.5.12 What was the likelihood ratio?

8.5.13 What does the likelihood ratio tell us about the value of the exam in detecting prostate cancer?

Prior and posterior odds Unless a test is free of classification errors, the clinician can never be 100% certain that a positive test result means that the patient has disease. But a positive result from a test that has a likelihood ratio greater than 1 should increase the clinician's level of confidence that the patient has disease. The higher the likelihood ratio of the test, the more impact a positive result will have on the clinician's confidence in the diagnosis. One way to think about the impact of a positive test result on diagnosis is to imagine the following scenario.

A clinician who has no information about a patient other than some demographic information is asked to estimate the probability that the patient has a particular disease. To make a judgment, the clinician uses the prevalence of the disease among people who share the patients' demographic profile. This judgment, arrived at prior to obtaining additional information about the patient, is called the *prior* or *pretest probability* of disease. To obtain more information about the patient, the clinician then orders a test which returns a positive result. Based on this finding, the clinician adjusts the prior probability. The clinician's revised judgment of the chances that the patient has the disease is called the *posterior* or *posttest probability*. If the prior and posterior probabilities are expressed as odds, the likelihood ratio of the test that the clinician ordered will indicate the extent to which the prior odds should be adjusted by a positive test result. Specifically,

$$\text{Posterior Odds} = \text{Likelihood Ratio} \times \text{Prior Odds}. \quad (8.1)$$

This relationship between prior and posterior odds is called Bayes' Rule, named after the nineteenth century probability theorist who discovered it. When applied to a medical test, Bayes' Rule tells us that the impact of a positive test result on a clinician's judgment is directly related to the test's likelihood ratio. This makes sense since tests with large likelihood ratios are better able to discriminate between patients with and without disease and so should have a greater impact.

If the prior odds of disease are based on disease prevalence, then Bayes' Rule also tells us that the odds that a patient who has tested positive has the disease are equal to the prevalence of the disease (expressed as odds) times the likelihood ratio of the test. To demonstrate, let us review the three versions of the digital exam data that we have discussed thus far. In each, 95 of 301 patients had prostate cancer. This is a prevalence of 0.316. Assume that these 301 patients were taken at random from a population of men who fit a given demographic profile. Then the prevalence of prostate cancer in that population would be estimated to be 0.316, and the prior probability that any individual in that population has prostate cancer is also 0.316. If a clinician had no information about a patient other than that he is a member of this population, the clinician would estimate the patient's chances of having cancer as 31.6 %. This is equivalent to prior odds of 0.316/0.684 or 0.462.

In our first hypothetical example, displayed in Table 8.3, the likelihood ratio was equal to 1. In this example, the test had no ability to discriminate prostate cancer patients from healthy patients, so a positive result would have no impact on judgment. In our second hypothetical example, displayed in Table 8.4, the likelihood ratio was 6.216. In this example, a positive test result would increase the odds of disease by more than six-fold, so the posterior odds would be 6.216×0.462 or 2.872. These odds are equivalent to a posterior probability of 2.872/(1 + 2.872) or 0.742. Not surprisingly, a positive result from a test as discriminating as the one in our second hypothetical example would have a relatively large impact on diagnosis.

We can see from Table 8.2 that the actual likelihood ratio of the DRE was 0.716/0.568 or 1.26. A man who had prostate cancer would be only 1.26 times more likely to test positive on the digital exam than a man who was disease-free. This means that if a patient were to test positive for prostate cancer, his odds of having the cancer would increase by a factor of only 1.26, and his chances of having the cancer would increase from 31.6 to only 36.8 %. Because the test had limited ability to discriminate prostate cancer patients from healthy patients, the impact of a positive test result on the clinician's judgment would be small.

Calculating posterior probabilities by hand requires converting prior probabilities to odds and then converting posterior odds back to probabilities. A faster way

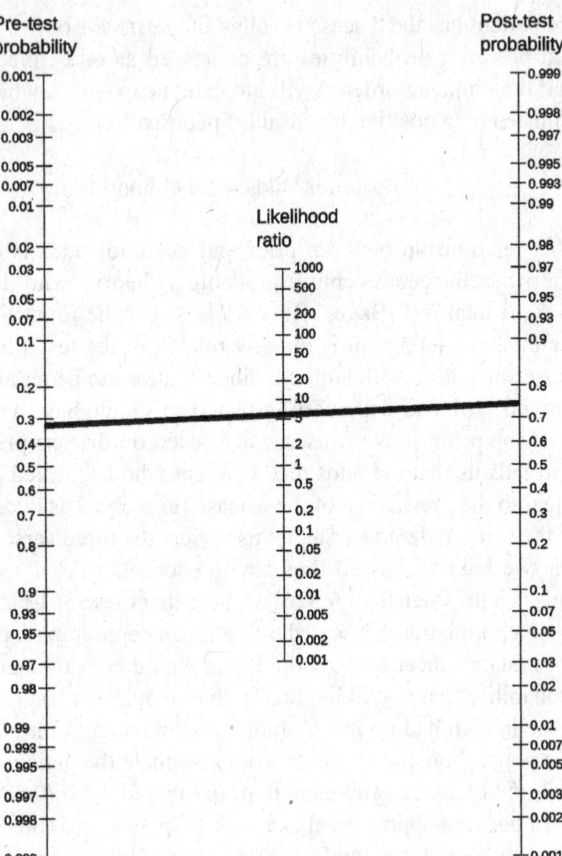

Fig. 8.1 Fagan's Nomogram. (Nomogram template by Mikael Häggström, public domain, Wikipedia Commons, http://commons.wikimedia.org/wiki/File%3AFagan_nomogram.svg)

is to use *Fagan's nomogram*, displayed in Fig. 8.1. To obtain a posterior probability, one draws a straight line from the prior probability value listed on the scale to the left through the appropriate likelihood ratio on the center scale to the posterior probability. The straight line in the nomogram of Fig. 8.1, for example, shows that a prior probability of 0.31 converts to a posterior probability of 0.74 when the test has a likelihood ratio of 6.2.

Before we leave the topic of likelihood ratios, we should point out that the likelihood ratio we have been using always generates a posterior probability that is equal to the PPV, that is, the probability that a patient who tests positive has disease. We should also mention that another version of the likelihood ratio is relevant to the prediction of the probability that a patient does not have disease. This version is sometimes called the *likelihood ratio for a negative result*. It compares as a ratio the proportion of patients without and with disease who test negative. When used with the complement of prevalence (1 minus prevalence), it generates the NPV, that is, the probability that a patient who tests negative does not have the disease.

8.6 The Receiver Operating Characteristic (ROC) Curve

So far we have looked at diagnostic statistics that apply to tests that can return only one of two values. In the last two sections, we will look at how these statistics are applied to tests that generate a range of values that can be arranged along a quantitative scale, such as the prostate-specific antigen (PSA) test which measures the level of prostate-specific antigen, expressed in units of ng/ml. For these tests, it is necessary to determine a *cutoff value.* If patients who have disease tend to have higher test values, then patients whose test values are above the cutoff are classified as positive. If patients who have disease tend to have lower test values, then patients whose test values are below the cutoff are classified as positive. Each of the numerical values generated by the test is a potential cutoff value. From these a cutoff is chosen that most often yields TP and TN.

As an example, return to the **PSA.sav** data file. The file includes the PSA test result for each of the 301 patients. Patients who have prostate cancer tend to have higher PSA scores, so a positive test result will be any PSA score that is above the cutoff. Imagine that we rank order the 301 patients by their PSA scores from the lowest to the highest. We choose a cutoff value and classify all patients whose PSA scores are above the cutoff as positive. In the ideal, every patient with prostate cancer would be above the cutoff and every patient without cancer would be below. This would give us a test with 100 % sensitivity and specificity, respectively. However, in reality, there will be patients who do not have prostate cancer but whose PSA scores will be above the cutoff. These patients will be FP. For these patients, the cutoff was too low. In addition, there will be patients who do have prostate cancer but whose PSA scores will be below the cutoff. These patients will be FN. For these patients, the cutoff was too high. If we have so many FP that the specificity of the test is too low, we could raise the cutoff value so that fewer cancer-free patients with high PSA scores are classified as positive. Unfortunately, raising the cutoff may result in some cancer patients with lower PSA scores no longer being classified as positive, resulting in a decrease in the sensitivity of the test. The challenge then is to choose a cutoff value that strikes the best balance between sensitivity and specificity. This is done by first computing the sensitivity and specificity for each possible test result. In effect, for each possible test value, a 2 × 2 contingency table is constructed in which patients whose scores are equal to or greater than the test value (if patients with disease tend to have higher test scores) or equal to or less than the test value (if patients with disease tend to have lower test scores) are classified as positive, and sensitivity and specificity are calculated in the usual manner. Then the test score that generates the best combination of sensitivity and specificity is chosen to be the cutoff value. This procedure is labor intensive, especially if the test, such as the PSA test, generates a large number of possible values. Fortunately, there is a quicker method. Developed by signal detection theorists, engineers who design machines that detect environmental threats (such as fire or carbon monoxide) quickly without triggering an excessive number of false alarms, this method involves generating what is called a *receiver operating characteristic curve*, or *ROC curve*. In this section, we will learn how to interpret an ROC curve.

Return to the **PSA.sav** data file. Each patient's PSA value is stored in **Prostate-Specific Antigen Level (ng/ml)** [*psa*] (variable 5). Values range from 0.3 to 221.0. The average value was about 8.8. Select **Analyze>ROC Curve** to open the *ROC Curve* dialog. In SPSS, the screening or diagnostic test is referred to as the *test variable,* and the criterion test as the *state variable.* So move **Prostate-Specific Antigen Level (ng/ml)** to the *Test Variable* window and **Biopsy Result** to the *State Variable* window. In the *Value of State Variable,* enter the value of the state variable that indicates that the patient had disease. In the *Display* area, check all of the options. We are now ready to generate the ROC curve, but before we do, click **Options.** By default, SPSS assumes that higher values of the state variable indicate greater probability of disease, as is the case in our example. So in the *Test Direction* area, *Larger test result indicates more positive test* should already have been selected. If lower values had indicated greater probability, we would have selected *Smaller test result indicates more positive test.* While we're here, notice that the confidence interval for the estimate of the area under the curve can be set in the *Confidence level* window. We will leave it at 95 %. Click **Continue** and then **OK.** The steps for assigning test and state variables, and selecting output, test direction and confidence level are displayed in Figs. 8.2 through 8.4.

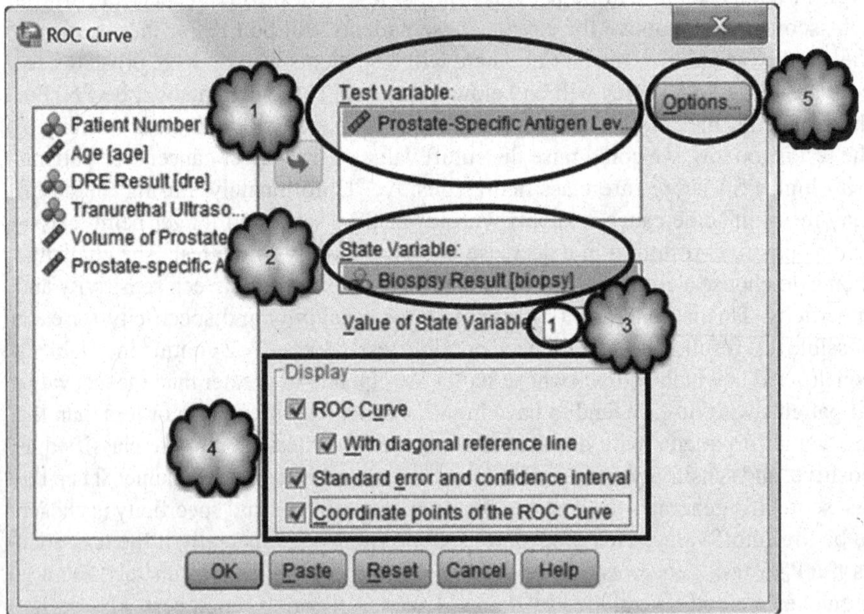

Fig. 8.2 Assigning the test and state variables, selecting output to display, and opening the Options dialog

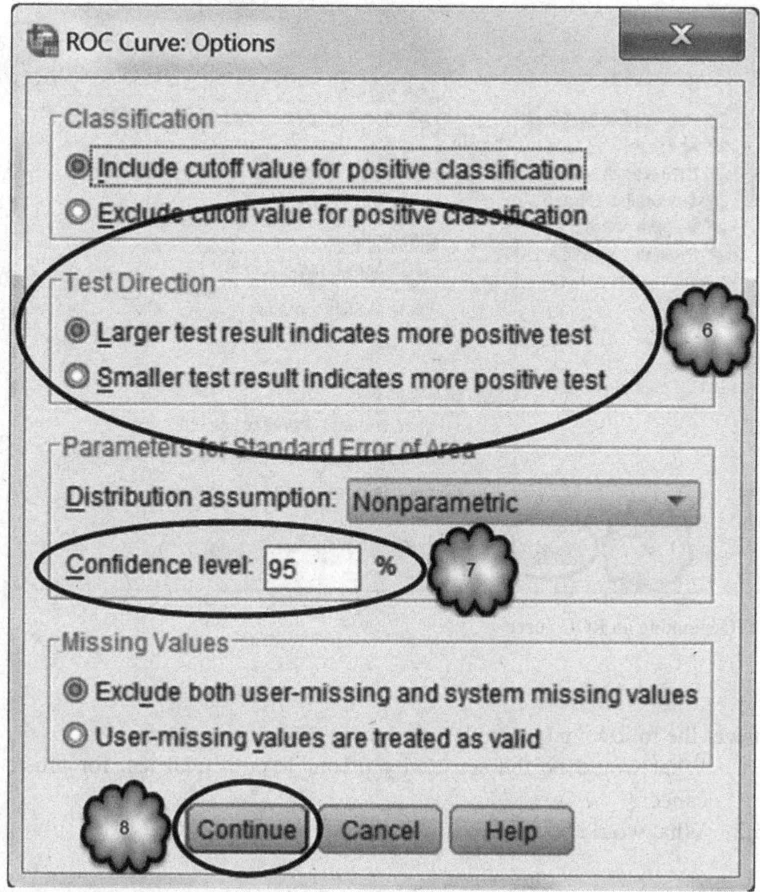

Fig. 8.3 Selecting the test direction and confidence level

The output includes the *Case Processing Summary* displayed in Table 8.5. Using the state variable, the *Summary* displays the number of patients with (95) and without (206) disease.

Figure 8.5 displays the ROC curve. This graph plots the test's false positive and true positive rates generated by each of the possible cutoff points. The false positive rate, or 1 minus specificity, is plotted along the x-axis and the true positive rate, or sensitivity, is plotted along the y-axis. To understand the graph, imagine what would happen if we attempted to diagnose each of the 301 patients in our earlier example on the basis of information that is entirely irrelevant to the question of whether or not cancer is present: the patient's height. Let us assume that our shortest patient is 5 ft, 0 in. tall and our tallest is 6 ft, 3 in. tall. Let us begin by setting the cutoff to a height greater than the height of the tallest person. Say we set it to 6 ft, 4 in. We then classify all patients whose height is above the cutoff as positive for prostate cancer, and plot the resulting sensitivity and false positive rates.

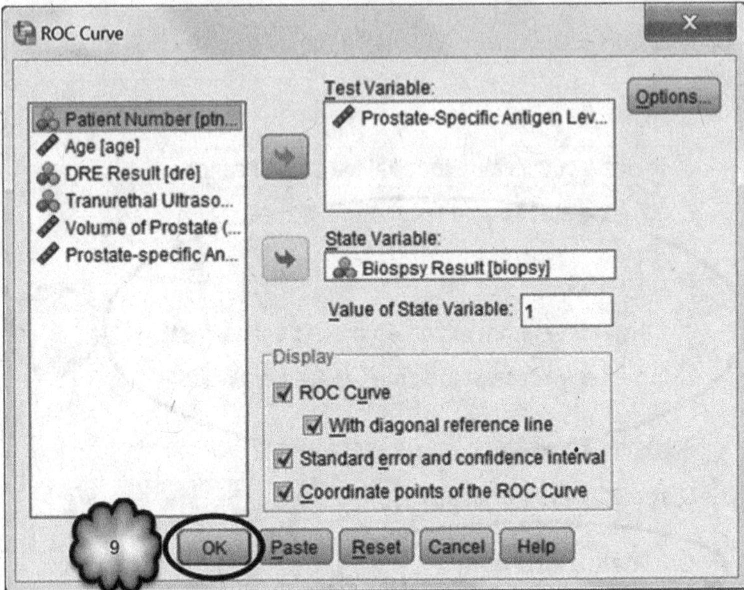

Fig. 8.4 Generating an ROC curve

Answer the following questions:

8.6.1 What would be the sensitivity of our hypothetical test for prostate cancer?

8.6.2 What would be the hypothetical test's specificity?

In setting the cutoff to a level greater than the height of the tallest patient, all of the patients are below the cutoff and so we end up classifying none of them as having prostate cancer. This means that none of the patients who in fact have the cancer

Table 8.5 Case processing summary

Case Processing Summary

Biopsy Result	Valid N (listwise)
Positive[a]	95
Negative	206

Larger values of the test result variable(s) indicate stronger evidence for a positive actual state.

a. The positive actual state is Cancer Present.

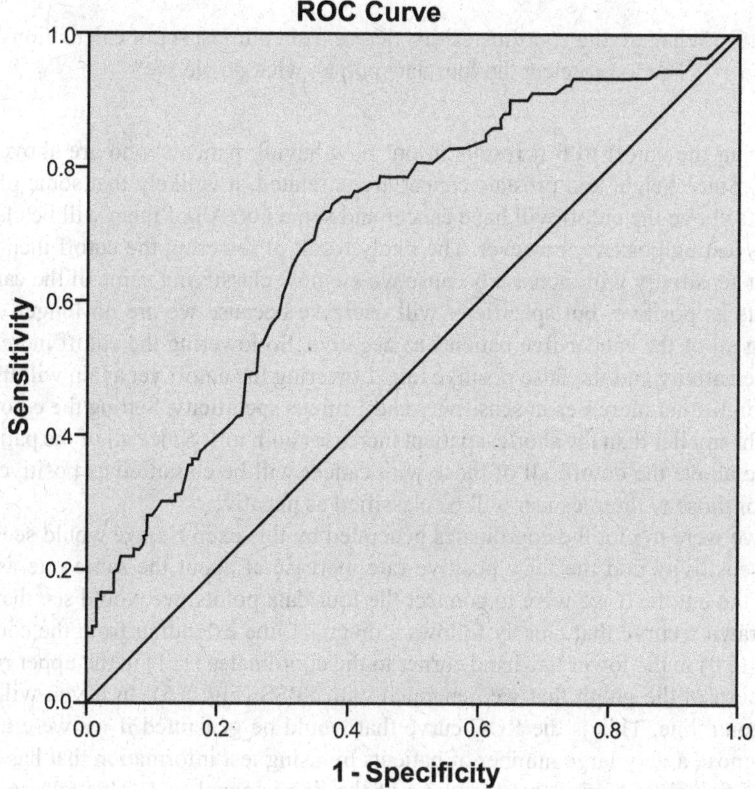

Fig. 8.5 ROC curve displaying the PSA test's true positive rate (sensitivity) as a function of its false positive rate (1 minus specificity)

are correctly diagnosed, yielding a sensitivity of 0, but all of the patients who are cancer-free are classified as negative, yielding a specificity of 1. When we plot the values generated by our cutoff for the false positive rate (which, remember, is equal to 1 minus specificity) and sensitivity, the *x*- and *y*-coordinates are 0 and 0. Our first data point would be in the lower left-hand corner of the graph.

Next we lower the cutoff to 6 ft, classify all patients taller than that as having the cancer, grind out the values for sensitivity and 1 minus specificity and plot them on the graph. We do all of this a third time, but with the cutoff lowered to 5.5 ft.

8.6.3 As we lower the cutoff, what happens to sensitivity?
8.6.4 To specificity?
8.6.5 To the false positive rate?

Finally, we set the cutoff to a value smaller than the height of the shortest person, say, 4 ft, 11 in., repeat our calculations and plot the results. When we're done, we connect the four data points.

8.6.6 What are the coordinates that derive from our last set of calculations?
8.6.7 When we connect the four data points, what do we see?

Lowering the cutoff to 6 ft results in our now having patients who are above the cutoff. Since height and prostate cancer are unrelated, it is likely that some of the patients above the cutoff will have cancer and some not. All of them will be classified as testing positive, however. The likely result of lowering the cutoff then will be that sensitivity will increase because we are now classifying some of the cancer patients as positive, but specificity will decrease because we are no longer classifying all of the cancer-free patients as negative. So lowering the cutoff increases both sensitivity and the false positive rate. Lowering the cutoff yet again will likely result in further increases in sensitivity and 1 minus specificity. Setting the cutoff to a height smaller than the shortest patient increases both to 1: Since all of the patients will be above the cutoff, all of those with cancer will be classified as positive but none of those without cancer will be classified as negative.

If we were to plot the coordinates generated by this exercise, we would see that both sensitivity and the false positive rate increase at about the same rate as we lower the cutoff. If we were to connect the four data points, we would see that we had drawn a curve that closely follows a diagonal line extending from the coordinates (0, 0) in the lower left-hand corner to the coordinates (1, 1) in the upper right.

Return to the graph that we generated with SPSS (Fig. 8.5). In it you will see a diagonal line. This is the ROC curve that would be generated if we were to try to diagnose a very large number of patients by using test information that has zero diagnostic value. Notice that the slope of the line is equal to 1. This tells us that lowering the cutoff has the same impact on sensitivity as it has on the false positive rate. Notice too that the ratio of any pair of coordinates on this line is equal to 1. This ratio is the likelihood ratio. Recall from Sect. 8.5 that a test with no diagnostic value will have a likelihood ratio of 1.

The diagonal line serves as a visual baseline or reference for determining the diagnostic value of a test. The better a test is at distinguishing between patients with and without disease, the further from the diagonal the test's ROC curve will be. Study the ROC curve for the PSA test. The curve begins and ends at or near the (0, 0) and (1, 1) coordinates, as all ROC curves must. As we follow the curve from lower left to upper right, we see that decreasing the cutoff increases sensitivity. Decreasing the cutoff also increases the false positive rate, but not as much. As a result, the curve for a while moves further and further away from the diagonal, showing visually the positive impact that decreasing the cutoff has on the test's diagnostic ability. For example, decreasing the cutoff to what turns out to be a value of about 6 increases sensitivity to about 0.73 while increasing the false positive rate to only about 0.36. Eventually, though, further decreases in the cutoff produce a slower rate of increase in sensitivity relative to the increase in the false positive rate, the diagnostic value of the test declines as the false positive rate catches up to sensitivity, and the curve moves closer and closer to the diagonal.

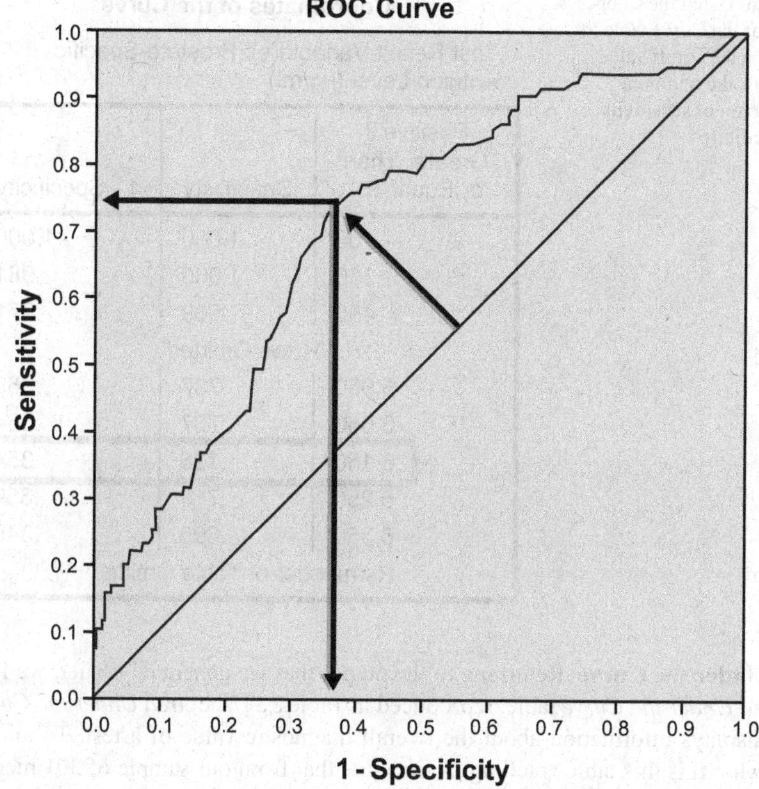

Fig. 8.6 Determining optimal values of sensitivity and specificity from an ROC curve

Visual inspection of an ROC curve helps clinicians to determine the cutoff value that best discriminates between patients with disease and patients without. First the optimal combination of sensitivity and false positive rate is identified. This will be the pair of coordinates that is furthest away from the diagonal along a line perpendicular to the diagonal. These coordinates are then read off from the graph as shown in Fig. 8.6.

The coordinates are about 0.36 for the false positive rate and 0.73 for sensitivity. Now that we know these values, we can determine the cutoff by consulting the *Coordinates of the Curve* table that is included in SPSS output. This table, a fragment of which is reproduced in Table 8.6, presents the cutoffs and the values of sensitivity and 1 minus specificity. SPSS lists the cutoffs in terms of values that lie between actual values. We find the coordinates that are in the neighborhood of 0.73 and 0.36, and determine that the sensitivity and false positive rate that yield the highest likelihood ratio are 0.726 and 0.354. According to the table, these were generated by a cutoff equal to or greater than 6.15. So our cutoff is 6.1. Classifying patients with a PSA value greater than 6.1 generates the optimal combination of sensitivity, which is about 0.73, and specificity, which is about 0.65.

Table 8.6 Using the Coordinates of the Curve table to determine the cutoff value that yields the optimum combination of sensitivity and specificity

Coordinates of the Curve

Test Result Variable(s): Prostate-Specific Antigen Level (ng/ml)

Positive if Greater Than or Equal To[a]	Sensitivity	1 - Specificity
-.700	1.000	1.000
.350	1.000	.981
.450	.989	.971
Rows Omitted		
5.950	.737	.369
6.050	.737	.364
6.150	.726	.354
6.250	.716	.350
6.350	.695	.345
Remainder of Table Omitted		

Area Under the Curve Returning to the output that we generated earlier, we find the *Area Under the Curve* table, reproduced in Table 8.7. The *Area Under the Curve* table displays information about the overall diagnostic value of a test. To understand what it is this table is telling us, imagine that from our sample of 301 men, a patient who has prostate cancer and a patient who does not are selected at random. We are asked to identify which of the two patients has prostate cancer. Say we choose the patient who is taller. What is the probability that we chose correctly? If a man's height is unrelated to whether or not he has prostate cancer, then choosing on the basis of height is equivalent to guessing, and the probability of our choosing correctly would be 0.5. It turns out that the area under an ROC curve is the probability

Table 8.7 Area under the curve and its standard error, *p*-value and 95 % confidence interval

Area Under the Curve

Test Result Variable(s): Prostate-Specific Antigen Level (ng/ml)

Area	Std. Error[a]	Asymptotic Sig.[b]	Asymptotic 95% Confidence Interval	
			Lower Bound	Upper Bound
.707	.032	.000	.645	.770

The test result variable(s): Prostate-Specific Antigen Level (ng/ml) has at least one tie between the positive actual state group and the negative actual state group. Statistics may be biased.
a. Under the nonparametric assumption
b. Null hypothesis: true area = 0.5

of choosing correctly in this situation. Recall that a test that has no diagnostic value produces in the long run the diagonal line in our graph. Notice that the diagonal line divides the area of the graph in half, and so the area under the diagonal is 0.5. According to the *Area Under the Curve* table in Table 8.7, the area under the ROC curve of the PSA test is 0.707. This value means that when deciding which of the two randomly paired patients has prostate cancer, we would choose correctly about 71 % of the time if we select the patient with the higher PSA score.

The 0.707 value is based on a sampling of men and so is subject to sampling variability. The null hypothesis is that if we had administered the PSA test to all men within the population from which our 301 men were drawn, the area under the curve would be 0.5. According to the highly significant *p*-value, however, we can very confidently reject the null hypothesis and conclude that the PSA test discriminates between a patient with cancer and a patient who is cancer-free better than at chance level. The 95 % confidence interval indicates that while the area under the curve in the sample is 0.707, we can be 95 % confident that in the population the area is somewhere between about 0.645 and 0.770.

Comparing the diagnostic value of two or more tests The area under the curve can be used to compare the overall diagnostic value of two or more tests. In the **PSA.sav** file, the variable, **Prostate-specific Antigen Density Level** [*psad*] (variable 7), contains each patient's PSA level relative to the volume (ml) of his prostate gland. Return to the *ROC Curve* dialog box, and as shown in Fig. 8.7, add **Prostate-specific Antigen Density Level** to the *Test Variable* window and click OK.

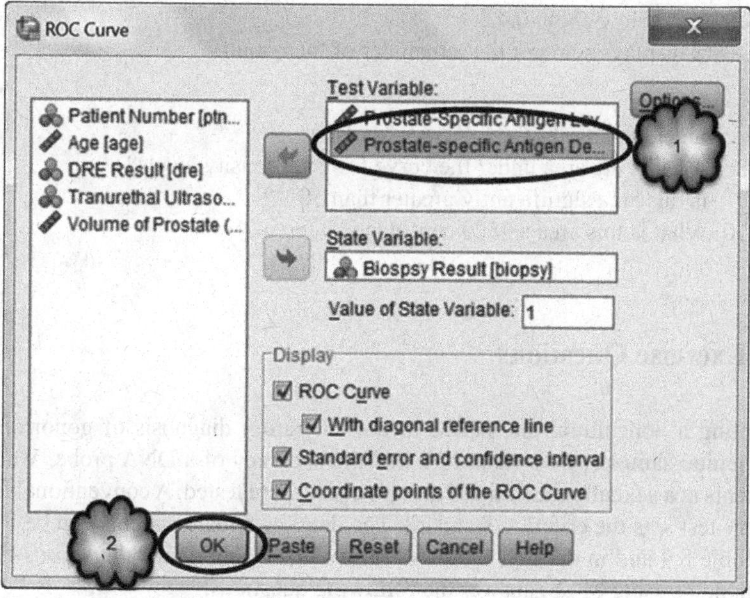

Fig. 8.7 Generating ROC curves to compare the diagnostic value of two tests

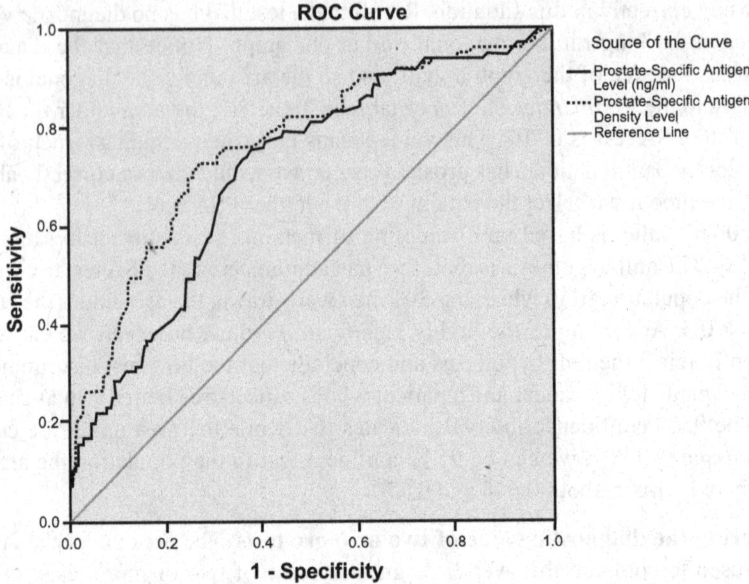

Fig. 8.8 ROC curves of two screening tests

Study the ROC curves of the two tests, shown in Fig. 8.8. (We edited the formatting of the curves a bit so that the two can be more easily distinguished from one another in grayscale.) According to these data, PSA density levels more accurately detect the presence of prostate cancer than do PSA levels, especially when the false positive rate is below about 0.4.

Table 8.8 displays some of the remainder of the output.

Using Table 8.8, answer the following questions:

8.6.8 What is the area under the curve for PSA density levels?

8.6.9 Is this area significantly greater than 50 %?

8.6.10 What is this area's 95 % confidence interval?

8.7 Exercise Questions

1. Wanting a noncultural alternative to the laboratory diagnosis of gonorrhea in urogenital samples, investigators tested the accuracy of a DNA probe. Walk-in patients at a sexually transmitted disease clinic were tested. A conventional laboratory test was the criterion standard. The data for female patients can be found in Table 8.9 and in the file, **Gonorrhea.sav** [2]. Doing your calculations either by hand or using SPSS, answer the following questions:

Table 8.8 Area under the curve of each of two screening tests

Area Under the Curve

Test Result Variable(s)	Area	Std. Error[a]	Asymptotic Sig.[b]	Asymptotic 95% Confidence Interval	
				Lower Bound	Upper Bound
Prostate-Specific Antigen Level (ng/ml)	.707	.032	.000	.645	.770
Prostate-specific Antigen Density Level	.760	.031	.000	.700	.821

The test result variable(s): Prostate-Specific Antigen Level (ng/ml), Prostate-specific Antigen Density Level has at least one tie between the positive actual state group and the negative actual state group. Statistics may be biased.
a. Under the nonparametric assumption
b. Null hypothesis: true area = 0.5

Table 8.9 Culture and DNA probe results

DNA probe result	Laboratory test result (criterion)	
	Positive	Negative
Positive	42	3
Negative	4	155

a. What was the PPV of the DNA probe?
b. What was the sensitivity of the DNA probe?
c. What was the probe's likelihood ratio?
d. What were the prior or pretest odds that a patient had gonorrhea?
e. If a patient tested positive for gonorrhea, what were the posterior or posttest odds that she had the disease?
f. On the nomogram in Fig. 8.9, show how the posterior probability would be found.

2. Researchers asked a radiologist to rate the CT images of 109 patients for neurological disease. Fifty-one of the patients were known to be abnormal. The radiologist made the ratings along a 5-place scale ranging from definitely normal (1) to definitely abnormal (5). The data can be found in the file, **CT Scan.sav** [3]. The data are in summary form; the file lists the number of normal patients whose CT images were definitely normal, the number of normal patients whose images were probably normal, and so on. So before going any further, open the file, select **Data > Weight Cases** and ask SPSS to weight each case by its frequency. The variable, **CT Rating** [*CT_Rating*] (variable 1) contains the radiologist's ratings. The variable, **Disease Status** (variable 2; 0 = normal, 1 = abnormal) is the criterion variable. Construct an ROC curve.
   a. By visual inspection of the curve, what appears to be the optimum combination of sensitivity and specificity of the radiologist's ratings?

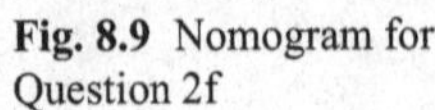

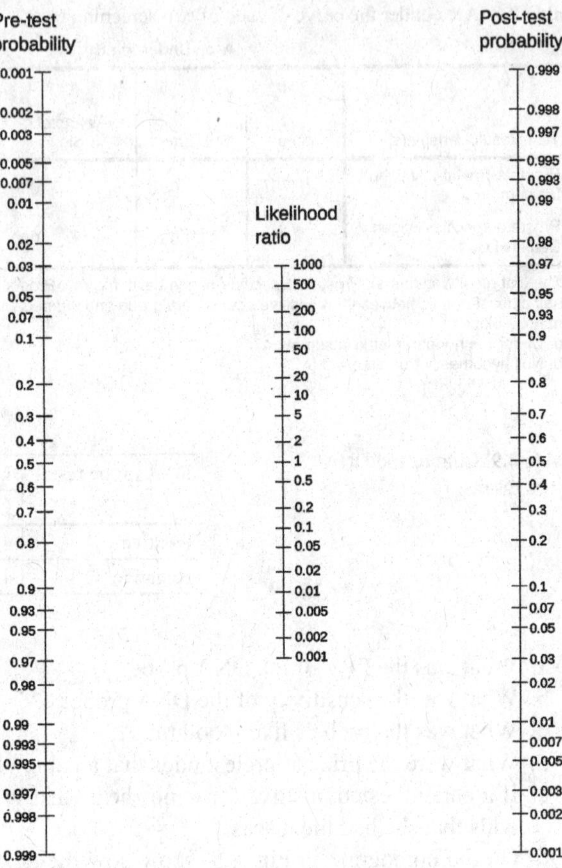

Fig. 8.9 Nomogram for Question 2f

b. What cutoff value should be used to optimize the diagnostic value of the radiologist's ratings? Explain how you arrived at your answer.

3. The file, **Xray.sav** [4], consists of 150 patients who underwent surgery to determine if they had suffered a bone fracture due to disease. The file contains the results of three biochemical tests intended to detect the disease: **BiochemA** [*test1*] (variable 4), **BiochemB** [*test2*] (variable 5), and **BiochemC** [*test3*] (variable 6). The disease status of the patient as determined by the surgery is in **Disease Positive** [*disease*] (variable 7). We wish to know which of the three biochemical tests best detects the presence of the disease.

   a. Figures 8.10 through 8.12 display three pairs of histograms. Each pair shows the distribution of the results of one of the biochemical tests for patients who

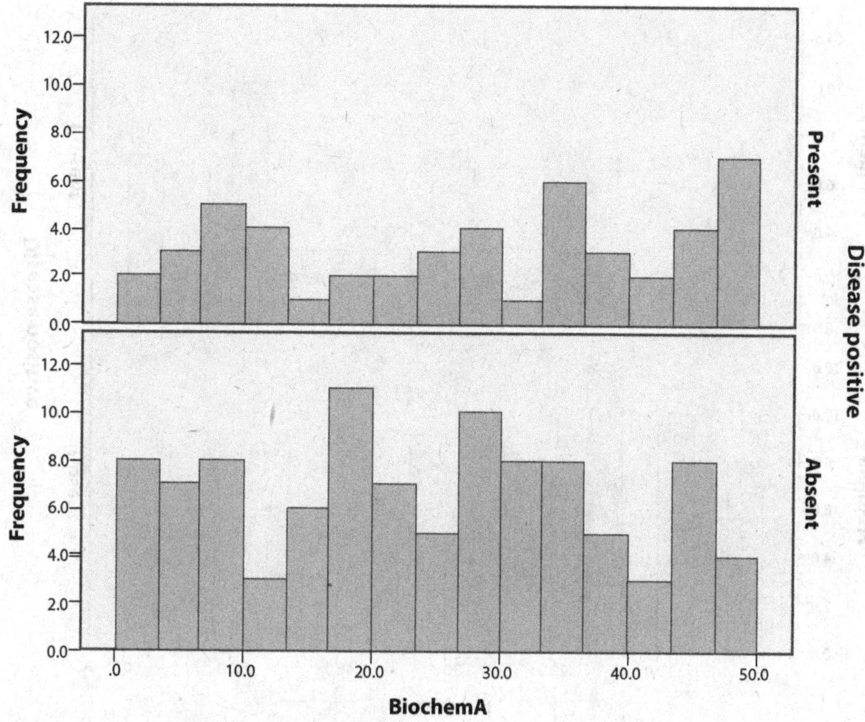

Fig. 8.10. Distribution of biochemical Test A

had the disease (labeled by the researchers as "Disease positive present") and patients who did not have the disease ("Disease positive absent"). Judging from these histograms, which test should best discriminate between patients with disease and disease-free patients? Explain

b. Generate a set of ROC curves that compares the diagnostic performance of these three tests. Based on visual inspection of the ROC curves, which biochemical test best detects this disease? How can you tell from the graph?
c. Focusing on the best of the three tests, what is the area under its curve? Is it significantly different from 50 %?
d. Staying with the best of the three tests, what appears from the graph to be the optimal combination of sensitivity and specificity?
e. If you wanted to use the best of the three tests as a screening tool, would you use the cutoff that generates the optimum level of sensitivity, a level of sensitivity higher than the optimum or a level lower than the optimum? Explain.

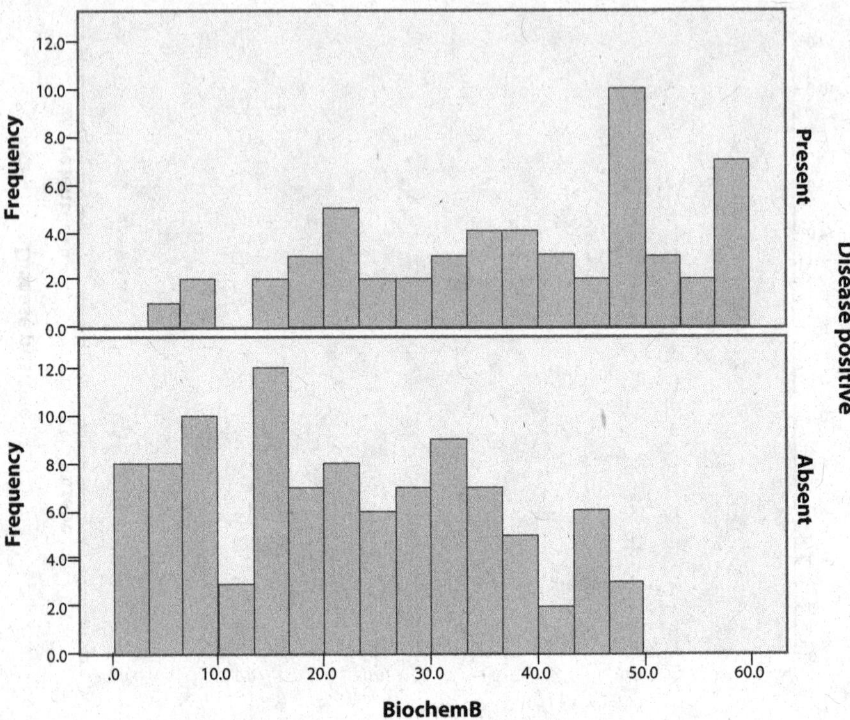

Fig. 8.11 Distribution of biochemical Test B

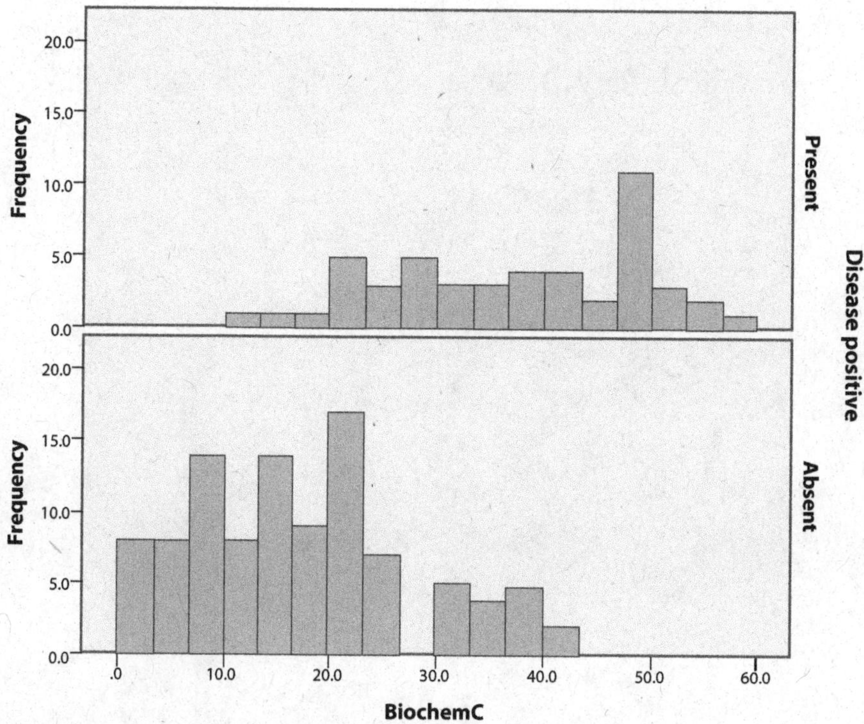

Fig. 8.12 Distribution of biochemical Test C

Data Sets and References

1. PAS.sav obtained from: Riffenburgh, R.H.: Statistics in Medicine, 2nd edn. Elsevier Academic, Burlington (2006). (With the kind permission of the Elsevier Books and Dr. Thomas K. Huisman)
2. Gonorrhea.sav obtained from: Granato, P.A., Franz, M.R.: Evaluation of a prototype DNA probe test for the noncultural diagnosis of gonorrhea. J. Clin. Microbiol. **27**(4), 632–635 (1989). (With the kind permission of the American Society for Microbiology)
3. CT Scan.sav obtained from: Hanley, J.A., McNeil, B.J.: The meaning and use of the area under a Receiver Operating Characteristic (ROC) curve. Radiology **143**(1), 29–36 (1982). (With the kind permission of the Radiological Society of North America)
4. Xray.sav obtained from: Peat, J., Barton, B.: Medical Statistics: A Guide to Data Analysis and Critical Appraisal. Blackwell, Malden (2005). (With the kind permission of John Wiley and Sons)

Chapter 9
Relationships in Quantitative Data

Abstract This chapter investigates assessing relationships between two quantitative variables. Scatter plots are introduced as a graphical way to determine whether a relationship exists between the two variables and assess the shape, direction, and strength of the relationship. When the relationship is linear, the Pearson correlation coefficient is introduced to measure the strength of the relationship. Tests and confidence intervals on the Pearson correlation coefficient are discussed. For nonlinear relationships Spearman's rho is discussed.

9.1 Overview

We learned in Chap. 7 that contingency tables and clustered bar graphs are used to display the relationship between two categorical variables. However, if the variables of interest are quantitative, the relationship between the two can be displayed with a *scatter plot* (also known as a scatter diagram). With this technique, we can determine whether a relationship exists, and if so, whether it is linear or not, whether it is positive or negative, and whether the relationship is weak or strong. In this chapter, we learn about scatter plots. In Chap. 7, we also learned about two statistics that are used to measure the extent to which two categorical variables are related: Cramér's V and gamma. In this chapter, we learn about two statistics that allow us to measure the strength of relationship between two quantitative variables: the *Pearson correlation coefficient* and *Spearman's rho*.

Two quantitative variables are related if, for a given value of one variable, there is a tendency for the second variable to have a certain value. A graphical means for determining if a relationship exists is a scatter plot. Each observational unit has two quantitative measurements taken on it. One is called the explanatory variable, and the other is called the response variable. On an *x*-*y* coordinate system, the explanatory variable forms the horizontal axis, and the response variable forms the vertical axis. The values of the two variables for each observational unit form an (x,y) pair that is plotted. The resulting plot of these points is a scatter plot.

To determine if a relationship exists, we look for a pattern in the scatter plot. If there is no pattern, then we say that the two variables are not related. If there is a pattern, then we can say that the two variables are related. If the pattern seems to

W. H. Holmes, W. C. Rinaman, *Statistical Literacy for Clinical Practitioners*,
DOI 10.1007/978-3-319-12550-3_9

follow a straight line, then we say that the relationship is *linear.* If the pattern is such that an increase in one variable is associated with an increase in the other variable, then we say that the relationship is *positive*. If the pattern reveals that an increase in one variable is associated with a decrease in the other variable, then we say that the relationship is *negative.*

The strength of the relationship is determined by the degree to which the pattern follows a straight line or some sort of curve. If the points follow a line or curve closely, then the relationship is said to be *strong.* As the points follow a line or curve less well, then the relationship is weaker.

9.2 Scatter Plots

In this section, we interpret scatter plots. Begin by loading the data file, **CDC BRFSS.sav [1]**, into SPSS. In order to generate a meaningful scatter plot, it will be necessary to exclude from our analyses answers of "do not know," etc. So declare the values of 7777 and the range 9000–9999 as missing for the variable **REPORTED WEIGHT IN POUNDS** [*WEIGHT2*] (variable 29), and 999 for the variable **REPORTED HEIGHT IN INCHES** [*HTIN3*] (variable 75). (Do not confuse the latter variable with a similar one that is expressed in feet and inches.) Select **Graphs>Chart Builder** and open the *Chart Builder* dialog box. As shown in Fig. 9.1, select *Scatter/Dot* from the *Gallery* and drag the picture of the simple scatter plot (the one in the upper left-hand corner) to the window directly above it. Drag **REPORTED WEIGHT IN POUNDS** to the *Y-Axis* box, and drag **REPORTED HEIGHT IN INCHES** to the *X-Axis* box. It is general practice to put the explanatory variable on the horizontal axis and the response variable on the vertical axis of a scatter plot. Click **OK.**

Study the output, reproduced in Fig. 9.2.

Answer the following questions.

9.2.1 Does a relationship between the two variables seem to exist?
9.2.2 If so, does the relationship appear to be linear?
9.2.3 Does it appear to be positive or negative?
9.2.4 Does the relationship appear to be strong or weak?

Best Fitting Straight Line Although visual inspection of a scatter plot can often reveal whether two variables are linearly related, it is helpful to plot the straight line that best describes that relationship.

Double-click on the scatter plot we just generated to open the *Chart Editor*. As shown in Fig. 9.3, click the *Add Fit Line at Total* icon. SPSS will then display the best fitting straight line. It also displays in the upper right-hand corner of the plot a quantity labeled *R Sq Linear* which we will discuss a bit later. To close Chart Editor,

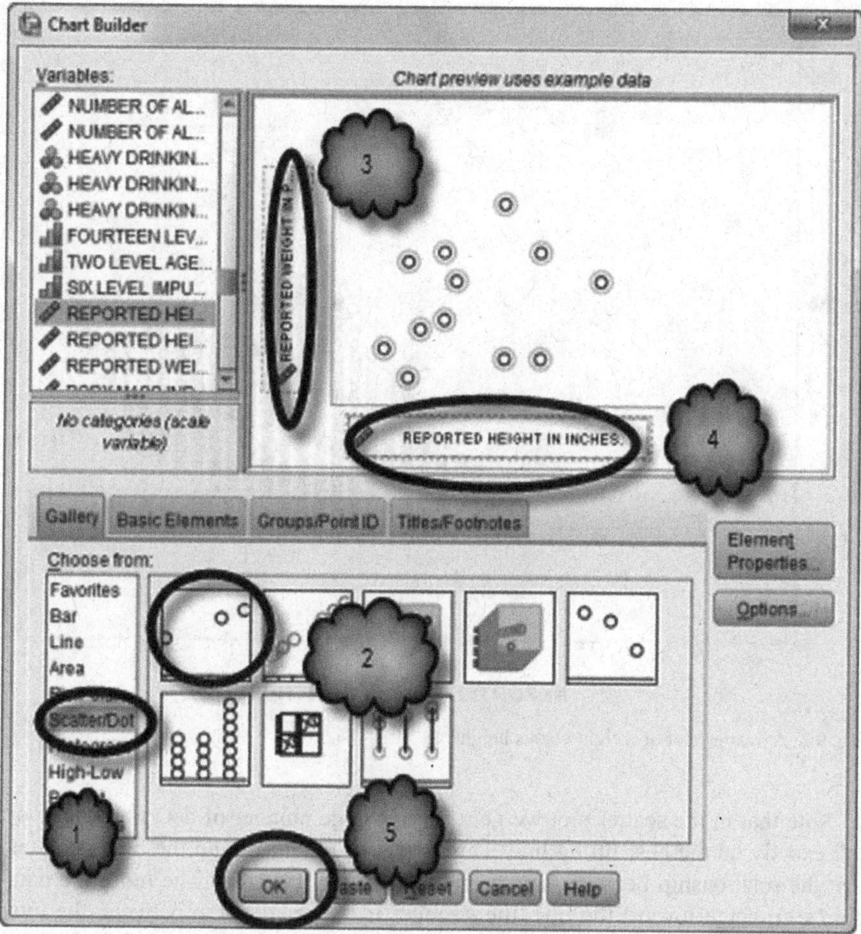

Fig. 9.1 Creating a scatter plot

click **X** in the upper right-hand corner of the editor. The resulting scatter plot is shown in Fig. 9.3.

Assuming that values along the *x*-axis increase from left to right, and values along the *y*-axis increase from bottom to top, a positive relationship will be indicated by a line that extends from the lower left to upper right (i.e., the line will have a positive slope). For negative relationships, the line will extend from upper left to lower right (i.e., the line will have a negative slope). If there is no linear relationship between the two variables, the line will be relatively flat.

9.2.5 What relationship between weight and height is indicated by the best fitting straight line in the scatter plot?

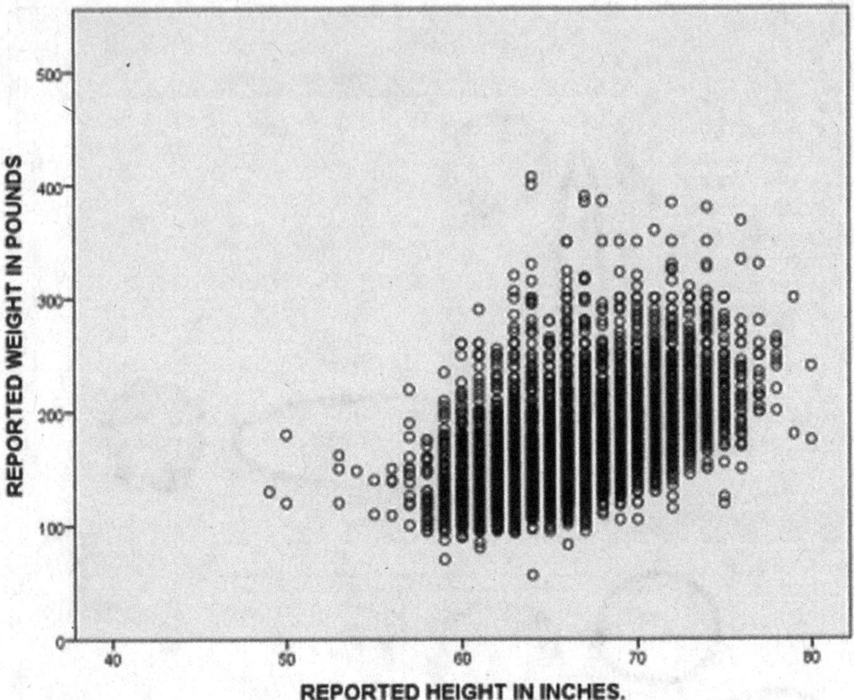

Fig. 9.2 A Scatter plot of weight versus height

Note that in the scatter plot we generated, a large number of data points do not fall exactly on the best fitting line. This scatter of points around the line indicates that the relationship between height and weight is not perfect. The more the data points gravitate toward the line, the stronger is the relationship between the two variables. If the relationship is linear and perfect, all of the points will fall on the line. Finding two variables which are perfectly linearly related to one another is a very rare occurrence.

R Squared: Proportion of Variability in Y Accounted for by Variability in X The fact that the scatter plot does not show a perfect relationship is evidence that factors other than those used to create the scatter plot influence the relationship between them. After all, if values of the *Y* variable were related only to values of the *X* variable and to nothing else, the relationship between the two variables would be perfect and all of the data points would fall on the best fitting line. In the jargon of statisticians, all of the variability in the *Y* scores would be *accounted for* or *explained by* variability in the *X* scores. However, it is rare that the values of any one variable are related only to one other variable. Almost always, the *Y* variable will be related to many variables, not just to the *X* variable.

Weight, for example, is related to height, but it is also related to other factors as well. To fully account for variability in people's weight, one would have to take into

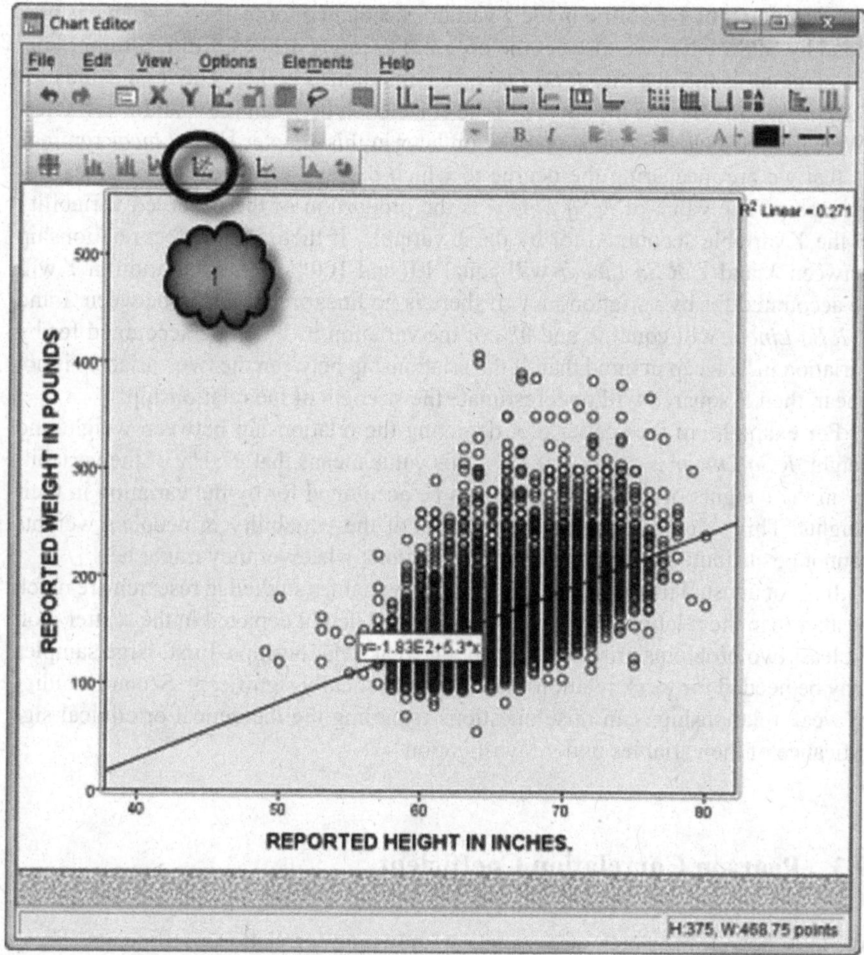

Fig. 9.3 Adding a best fit line to a scatter plot

account not only each person's height but also each person's diet, exercise habits, etc. The more factors we can take into account in addition to height, the more we will be able to account for the variability in people's weight.

In theory, if we could measure every factor that affects the *Y* variable, we could explain 100 % of the variability in that variable. For example, if we could measure every factor that determines weight, we could explain 100 % of the variability in people's weight. However, when we measure only one factor, it is likely that we will be able to account for only a small percentage of the variability in the *Y* variable. For example, knowing the height of each person in a group of people would not allow us to account for all of the variability in their weight. However, knowing people's height will at least allow us to account for some of the variability in their weight.

The amount of variability in the *Y* variable accounted for by the *X* variable is provided by SPSS when we instruct the program to insert the best fitting straight line. This amount is the quantity *R Sq Linear* we mentioned earlier. The *R Sq* stands for *R Squared* and refers to the square of the correlation between the *X* and *Y* variables. (We will take a closer look at correlation later in this chapter.) The *Linear* reminds us that we are measuring the degree to which the two variables have a linear relationship. The value of *R Sq Linear* is the proportion of the observed variability in the *Y* variable accounted for by the *X* variable. If there is a perfect relationship between *X* and *Y*, *R Sq Linear* will equal 1.0 and 100% of the variation in *Y* will be accounted for by variation in *X*. If there is no linear relationship between *X* and *Y*, *R Sq Linear* will equal 0, and 0% of the variation in *Y* will be accounted for by variation in *X*. Keep in mind that, if the relationship between the two variables is not linear, then R squared will underestimate the strength of the relationship.

For example, in the scatter plot depicting the relationship between weight and height, *R Sq Linear* is equal to 0.271. This value means that 27.1% of the variability in the weights of the respondents can be accounted for by the variation in their heights. This value also means that 72.9% of the variability in people's weights cannot be attributed to height but to other factors, whatever they might be.

It is not unusual that relationships between variables studied in research are much weaker than the relationship between weight and height depicted in the scatter plot. At least two problems arise when studying weak relationships. First, large samples may be needed for weak relationships to be statistically significant. Second, studies of weak relationships can raise questions regarding the theoretical or clinical significance of the variables under investigation.

9.3 Pearson Correlation Coefficient

We look now at measures of association known as correlation coefficients. These give a numerical measure of the strength of the relationship between two variables. If both variables under study are quantitative and the relationship is linear, the *Pearson correlation coefficient* is the statistic of choice. We will use this statistic to study the relationship between height and weight.

As shown in Fig. 9.4, select **Analyze>Correlate>Bivariate** to bring up the *Bivariate Correlations* dialog box. Move **REPORTED WEIGHT IN POUNDS** and **REPORTED HEIGHT IN INCHES** into the *Variables* box. Be sure that *Pearson* has been selected in the *Correlation Coefficients* area. As we are dealing with quantitative data, let us generate some means and standard deviations as well. Click **Options** to open the *Bivariate Correlations: Options* dialog box. Check *Means and standard deviations*. Notice that in the *Missing Values* area, *Exclude cases pairwise* has been selected by SPSS. Now click **Continue** (Fig. 9.5).

Before we run the analysis, notice that in the *Tests of Significance* area, *Two-tailed* has been selected. Unless we instruct SPSS to do otherwise, it will conduct a two-tailed test of significance. Now click **OK** and study the output.

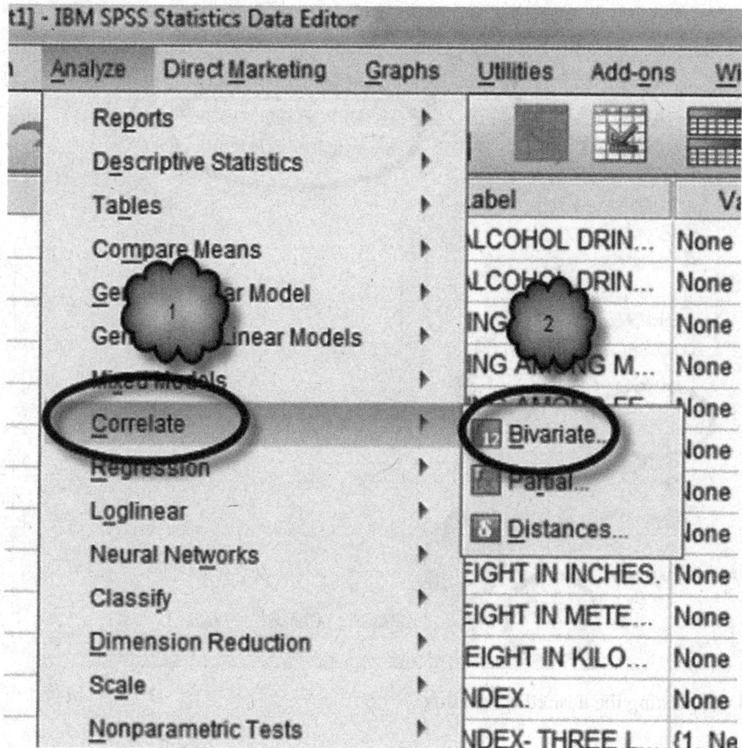

Fig. 9.4 Selecting correlation

The output includes a table, shown in Table 9.1, that displays means and standard deviations of the two variables.

9.3.1 What was the average height and weight of the sample?

The output also includes a table displaying Pearson correlation coefficients. The table, sometimes called a *correlation matrix,* is shown in Table 9.2.

In a matrix, the names of the variables are listed both down the rows and across the columns. The correlation between any two variables listed within the table is displayed in the cell that forms the intersection between the appropriate row and column. The matrix is symmetric, so it does not matter whether you first select the appropriate column and then move down to the appropriate row, or you first select the appropriate row and move across to the appropriate column. In a matrix generated by SPSS, most of the cells also display the *p*-values associated with the correlations and the number of cases that were used in calculating them. The correlation is labeled *Pearson Correlation,* the *p*-value *Sig (2-tailed),* and the sample size, *N.* Let us look at each of these three entries more closely.

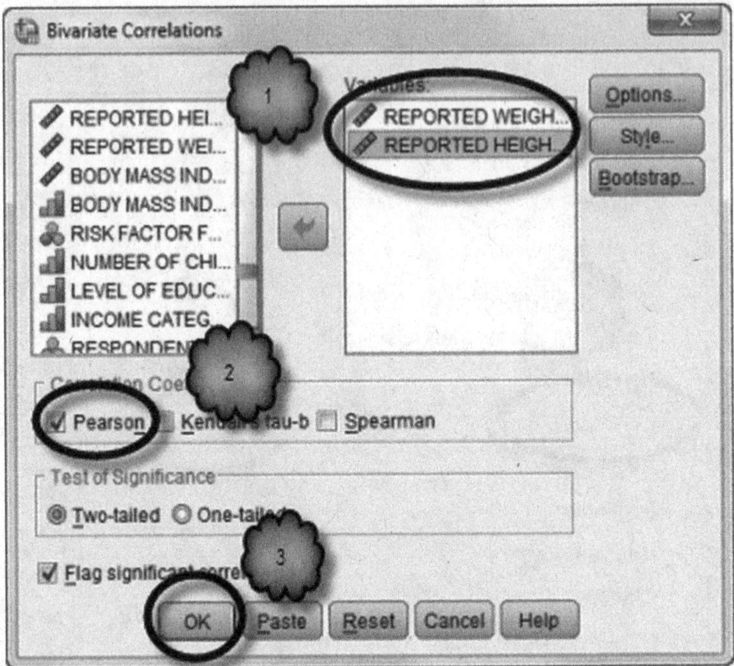

Fig. 9.5 Requesting the desired correlation

Table 9.1 Summary statistics

Descriptive Statistics

	Mean	Std. Deviation	N
REPORTED WEIGHT IN POUNDS	168.18	40.348	7454
REPORTED HEIGHT IN INCHES	66.21	3.949	7718

Table 9.2 Correlation results

Correlations

		REPORTED WEIGHT IN POUNDS	REPORTED HEIGHT IN INCHES
REPORTED WEIGHT IN POUNDS	Pearson Correlation	1	.520**
	Sig. (2-tailed)		.000
	N	7454	7404
REPORTED HEIGHT IN INCHES	Pearson Correlation	.520**	1
	Sig. (2-tailed)	.000	
	N	7404	7718

**. Correlation is significant at the 0.01 level (2-tailed).

Pearson Correlation Pearson correlation coefficients vary from −1 to 0 to+1. The closer the value is to+1 or −1, the stronger is the relationship between the two variables. A positive correlation indicates that increases in one variable are associated with increases in the other, while a negative correlation indicates that increases in one variable are associated with decreases in the other. Note that because the matrix displays the correlations between all possible pairings of the variables in the analysis, the correlation between each variable and itself is also displayed. These values are always equal to 1 and can be found on a diagonal from the uppermost left cell to the lowermost right cell.

***p*-value** Immediately below each of the correlations that do not lie along the diagonal is the *p*-value. As we learned in Chap. 5, a *p*-value is the probability of observing a value of a test statistic that is equal to or greater than the value we computed if the null hypothesis were true. SPSS tests the null hypothesis that the population correlation is zero, that is, that the two variables are uncorrelated. If the *p*-value is ≤ 0.05, we reject the null hypothesis in favor of the alternative hypothesis. If we conduct a two-tailed test, the alternative hypothesis is that the population correlation is not equal to zero. If we conduct a one-tailed test, the alternative hypothesis is either that the population correlation is greater than zero or that the population correlation is less than zero. Recall that by default, SPSS conducts a two-tailed test. We did not ask SPSS to conduct a one-tailed test, so in our analysis the alternative hypothesis is that the population correlation is not equal to zero.

Sample Size The sample sizes displayed in the matrix refer to the numbers of cases upon which the correlations are based. By default, SPSS excludes cases pairwise, that is, it will omit cases with missing data with reference only to the two variables for which it is about to calculate the correlation coefficient. If the analysis involves the calculation of two or more correlations, different correlations may be based on different numbers of cases or on different subsets of cases. If you want to avoid these outcomes, check *Exclude cases listwise* in the *Missing Values* area of the *Bivariate Correlations: Options* dialog box. SPSS will exclude all cases that have missing data on any of the variables involved in the analysis before it calculates the correlations. The resulting correlations will be based on the same subset of cases and will of course have the same sample size. However, the resulting sample size can be appreciably smaller than those that would have been obtained had cases been excluded on a pairwise basis.

Study the correlation matrix and answer the following questions.

9.3.2 What is the value of the Pearson correlation in our analysis?

9.3.3 Would you describe the relationship between weight and height as positive or negative?

9.3.4 Would you describe the relationship between weight and height as weak or strong?

9.3.5 What is the *p*-value associated with the correlation?

9.3.6 What does the *p*-value tell us?

9.3.7 What was the sample size?

Confidence Intervals and Null Hypotheses About Nonzero Values of Population Correlations If we wish to construct a confidence interval for a population correlation or test a null hypothesis that the population correlation is some value other than zero, we need to use a procedure known as *Fisher's Z Transformation,* developed by Ronald A. Fisher. Fisher found that if both variables come from normal populations, then transformation

$$z = \frac{1}{2}\ln\left(\frac{1+r}{1-r}\right) \tag{9.1}$$

where ln is the natural logarithm and r is the sample correlation. If both variables have a normal distribution, Z has a normal distribution. This means that we can use the z transformation to convert the values of the sample correlation and the population correlation posited by the null hypothesis. We can then use the normal distribution to compute a p-value. We can also construct a confidence interval for the converted correlation and transform that interval back to obtain a confidence interval for the population correlation.

These procedures are not built-in features of SPSS. However, we can use a script called **correlation.sbs** to implement them. The script is located in the same place as the scripts we used in Chap. 6.

To illustrate the script, suppose we wish to test whether the population correlation between **REPORTED WEIGHT IN POUNDS** and **REPORTED HEIGHT IN INCHES** is greater than 0.5, and we wish to construct a 99 % confidence interval for this correlation. Select **Utilities>Run Script** and run **correlation.sbs** to open the *Inference for a Population Correlation* dialog box shown below. In the *Sample Correlation* box, enter the Pearson correlation that we obtained earlier (0.52). In the *Test Correlation* box, enter the value of the population correlation being tested in the null hypothesis (0.50). In the *Sample Size* box, enter the size of the sample (7404), and in the *Confidence Level (%)* box, enter in percent the desired confidence level (99) for the Pearson correlation. Click *Greater Than* in the *Alternative* box. The dialog box should look like the one shown in Fig. 9.6.

Click **OK.**

The Z-transformation produces the output shown in Table 9.3.

9.3.8 What is the value of Z for the test?
9.3.9 What is the p-value for the test?
9.3.10 Does the p-value indicate that the population correlation is >0.5?
9.3.11 What is the 99 % confidence interval for the population correlation?
9.3.12 Is it consistent with the test result?

When you opened the dialog box for the script, you may have noticed that the *Test Correlation* box contained a default value of 0, and the *Confidence Level (%)* box contained a default value of 95. If all you want to do is conduct a hypothesis test on

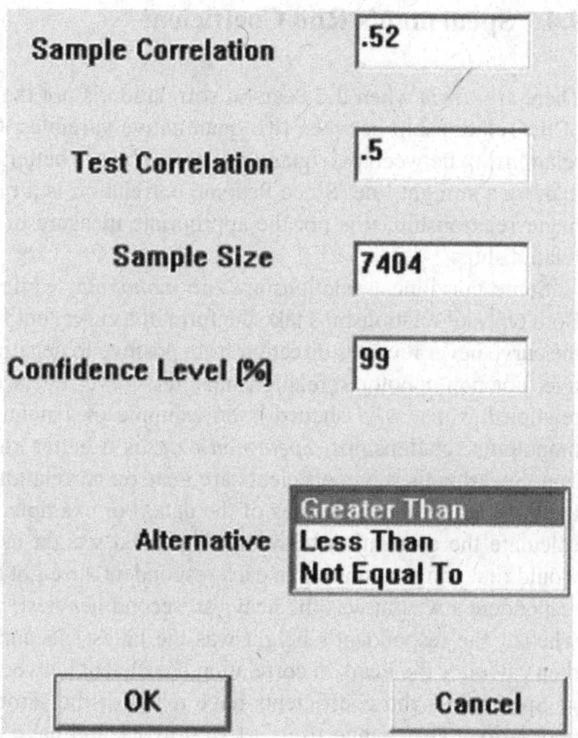

Fig. 9.6 Correlation script dialog box

Table 9.3 Test and confidence interval for a correlation

Test of Correlation = .5 vs. Correlation Greater Than .5

	Sample Corr.	Sample Size	Z	P-value
	.52	7404	2.325673	1.001801E-02

99% Confidence Interval for a Correlation

	N	Sample Corr.	Lower	Upper
	7404	0.52	0.4978159	0.5415041

the population correlation, simply set up the dialog box for the desired test, without specifying a confidence level. If all you want to do is construct a confidence interval for the population correlation, set up the dialog box for the desired confidence interval without specifying a test correlation.

9.4 Spearman's Rho Coefficient

There are times when the Pearson correlation is not the most appropriate measure of the relationship between two quantitative variables. One such time is when the relationship between two quantitative variables is better described by a curve rather than by a straight line. Since Pearson correlation is a measure of the strength of a linear relationship, it is not the appropriate measure of association for curvilinear relationships.

Some curvilinear relationships are *monotonic* while others are *nonmonotonic.* Both types of relationships take the form of a curve, but for monotonic relationships, the curve never reverses direction from positive to negative or from negative to positive. For nonmonotonic relationships, the curve reverses direction at least once. A relationship that is U shaped is an example of a nonmonotonic relationship. For monotonic relationships, *Spearman's rho* is a better choice than Pearson correlation. Spearman's rho coefficients are Pearson correlation coefficients calculated on the basis of the ranked values of the data. For example, if we were to ask SPSS to calculate the correlation between height and weight using Spearman's rho, SPSS would first assign a ranking to each respondent's weight (to indicate whether a given respondent's weight was the heaviest, second heaviest, etc.) and height (to indicate whether the respondent's height was the tallest, second tallest, etc.). SPSS would then calculate the Pearson correlation coefficient between the two sets of rankings.

Spearman's rho coefficients have many of the same properties as the Pearson correlation. They range from −1 to 0 to +1 and have the same meaning. For example, if weight and height were perfectly positively related, the tallest respondent would also be the heaviest, the second tallest would also be the second heaviest, etc., and rho would equal 1. The difference between Pearson and rho coefficients is that if the data follow some sort of nonlinear monotonic curve, the value of the Pearson correlation will underestimate the strength of the relationship. However, be aware that if the curve is *nonmonotonic,* Spearman's rho may also underestimate the strength of the relationship.

Another instance where Pearson correlation would be inappropriate occurs when either of the two variables is not normally distributed. In these circumstances, Spearman's rho is preferred. Whether each of the two variables is normally distributed can be determined by using the techniques explained in Chap. 5.

An Example The file, **Bodymass.sav [2],** contains three BMI scores of each of 20 hospitalized female anorexics: her BMI when she was admitted, her preferred BMI as reported upon admittance, and her BMI at discharge. Let us determine the nature of the relationship between **Preferred body mass** [*Prefer*] (variable 3) and **Body mass at admittance** [*Admit*] (variable 2).

Load the data file. Using **Analyze>Descriptive Statistics>Explore,** conduct tests of normality on each variable. Then using *Chart Builder,* generate a scatter plot of the two variables. Put **Body mass at admittance** on the x-axis.

The results of the tests of normality are shown in Table 9.4, and the scatter plot is shown in Fig. 9.7.

Answer the following questions.

9.4.1 Are both variables normally distributed?

9.4.2 Does the relationship between the two variables appear to be linear or nonlinear?

9.4.3 Does the relationship appear to be monotonic or nonmonotonic?

9.4.4 Which correlation coefficient should we compute: Pearson or Spearman's rho?

Table 9.4 Tests of normality

Tests of Normality

	Kolmogorov-Smirnov[a]			Shapiro-Wilk		
	Statistic	df	Sig.	Statistic	df	Sig.
Body mass at admittance	.097	20	.200*	.967	20	.700
Preferred body mass	.212	20	.019	.889	20	.026

*. This is a lower bound of the true significance.
a. Lilliefors Significance Correction

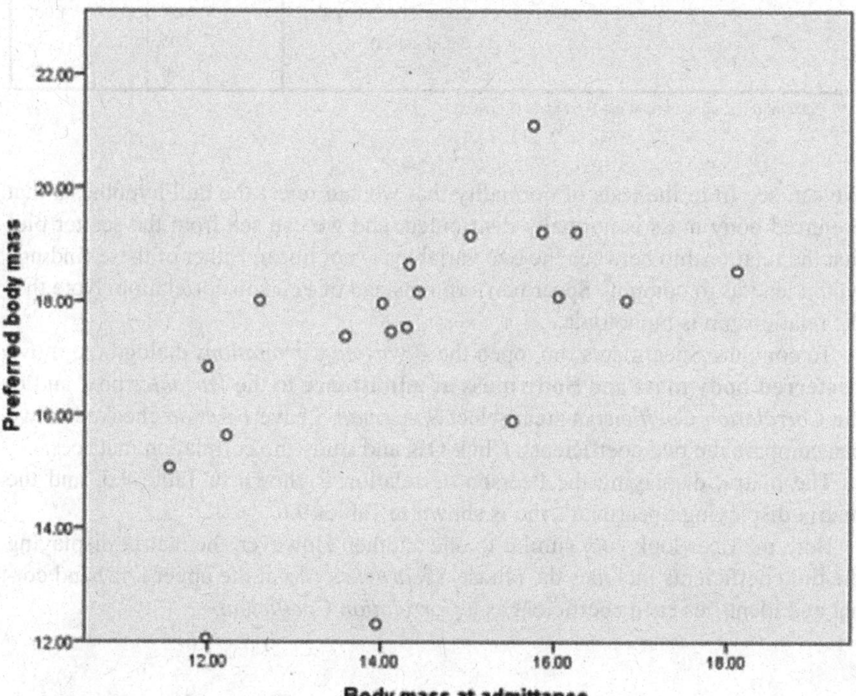

Fig. 9.7 Scatter plot

Table 9.5 Pearson correlation

Correlations

		Preferred body mass	Body mass at admittance
Preferred body mass	Pearson Correlation	1	.572**
	Sig. (2-tailed)		.008
	N	20	20
Body mass at admittance	Pearson Correlation	.572**	1
	Sig. (2-tailed)	.008	
	N	20	20

**. Correlation is significant at the 0.01 level (2-tailed).

Table 9.6 Spearman's rho

Correlations

			Preferred body mass	Body mass at admittance
Spearman's rho	Preferred body mass	Correlation Coefficient	1.000	.742**
		Sig. (2-tailed)	.	.000
		N	20	20
	Body mass at admittance	Correlation Coefficient	.742**	1.000
		Sig. (2-tailed)	.000	.
		N	20	20

**. Correlation is significant at the 0.01 level (2-tailed).

We can see from the tests of normality that we can reject the null hypothesis that preferred body mass is normally distributed, and we can see from the scatter plot that the relationship between the two variables is not linear. Either of these findings would lead us to compute Spearman's rho instead of Pearson correlation. Note that the relationship is monotonic.

To compute Spearman's rho, open the *Bivariate Correlations* dialog box, move **Preferred body mass** and **Body mass at admittance** to the *Variables* box, and in the *Correlation Coefficients* area, select *Spearman.* Leave *Pearson* checked so we can compare the two coefficients. Click **OK** and study the correlation matrices.

The matrix displaying the Pearson correlation is shown in Table 9.5, and the matrix displaying Spearman's rho is shown in Tables 9.6.

Both matrices look very similar to one another. However, the matrix displaying the rho coefficients includes the phrase *Spearman's rho* in the upper left-hand corner and identifies each coefficient as a *Correlation Coefficient.*

Answer the following questions.

9.4.5 What is the value of Spearman's rho?

9.4.6 How confident can we be that the population correlation is not equal to zero?

9.4.7 How does the value of Spearman's rho compare to the value of the Pearson correlation?

9.5 Exercise Questions

1. Open the file, **Framingham.sav [3].** This file contains a subset of data from the Framingham Heart Study, a prospective cohort study of cardiovascular disease among residents of Framingham, Massachusetts. Generate a scatter plot depicting the degree of linear relationship between **Diastolic Blood Pressure** [*dbp*] (variable 3) and **Body Mass Index** [*bmi*] (variable 8). Plot **Diastolic Blood Pressure** on the *y*-axis and **Body Mass Index** on the *x*-axis. After you have generated the scatter plot, insert the best fitting straight line.
2. Which of the following best describes the relationship depicted in the scatter plot between diastolic blood pressure and BMI you generated in question 1? Explain your answer.
   a. There is no relationship.
   b. There is a weak positive relationship.
   c. There is a strong positive relationship.
   d. There is a weak negative relationship.
   e. There is a strong negative relationship.
3. According to the scatter plot you generated in question 1, how much variability in diastolic blood pressure is accounted for by variability in BMI? How do you know?
4. Figure 9.8 shows a set of four scatter plots depicting the relationship between diastolic blood pressure and BMI. These plots were generated in *Chart Builder* by assigning **Gender** [*sex*] (variable 1) as the *Rows Panel* variable and **Coronary Heart Disease** [*chdfate*] (variable 5) as the *Columns Panel* variable. For which group of patients is diastolic blood pressure and BMI most strongly related? How do you know?
   a. Female patients without coronary heart disease
   b. Female patients with coronary heart disease
   c. Male patients without coronary heart disease
   d. Male patients with coronary heart disease
5. This question focuses on the relationship between **Systolic Blood Pressure** [*sbp*] (variable 2) and **Diastolic Blood Pressure** among the entire sample in the **Framingham** data set.

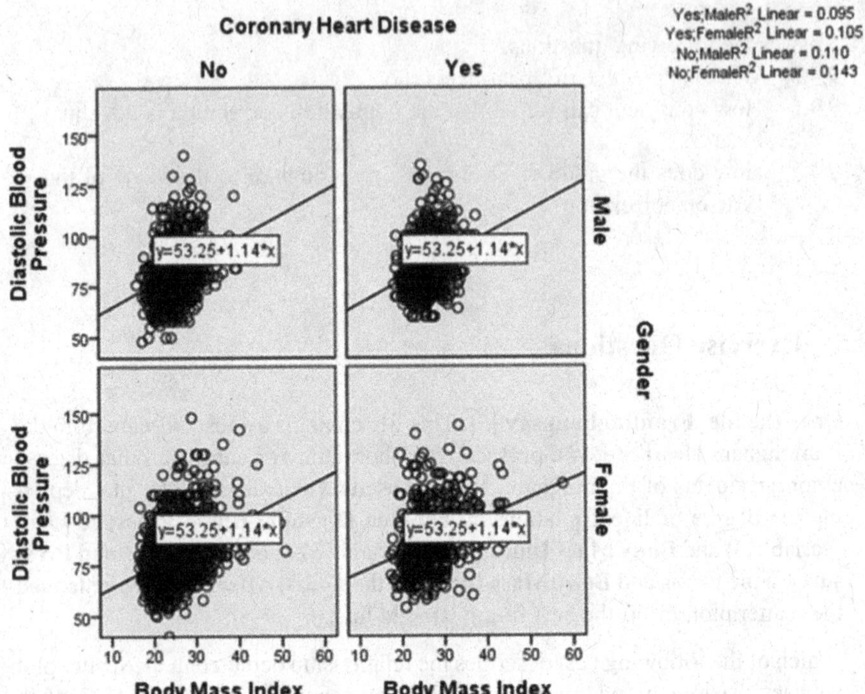

Fig. 9.8 A set of scatter plots of diastolic blood pressure versus body mass index (Question 4)

a. Create a correlation matrix that displays the correlation between systolic and diastolic blood pressure.
b. What is the value of the Pearson correlation between systolic and diastolic blood pressure?
c. What is the sample size upon which the correlation is based?
d. What is the *p*-value for the test of the alternative hypothesis that the correlation between systolic and diastolic blood pressure in the population of Framingham residents is not zero?
e. What is the *p*-value for the test of the alternative hypothesis that the correlation between systolic and diastolic blood pressure in the population of Framingham residents is >0.70? (Hint: You will need to conduct another analysis to answer this question.)
f. What is the 95 % confidence interval for the correlation between systolic and diastolic blood pressure?

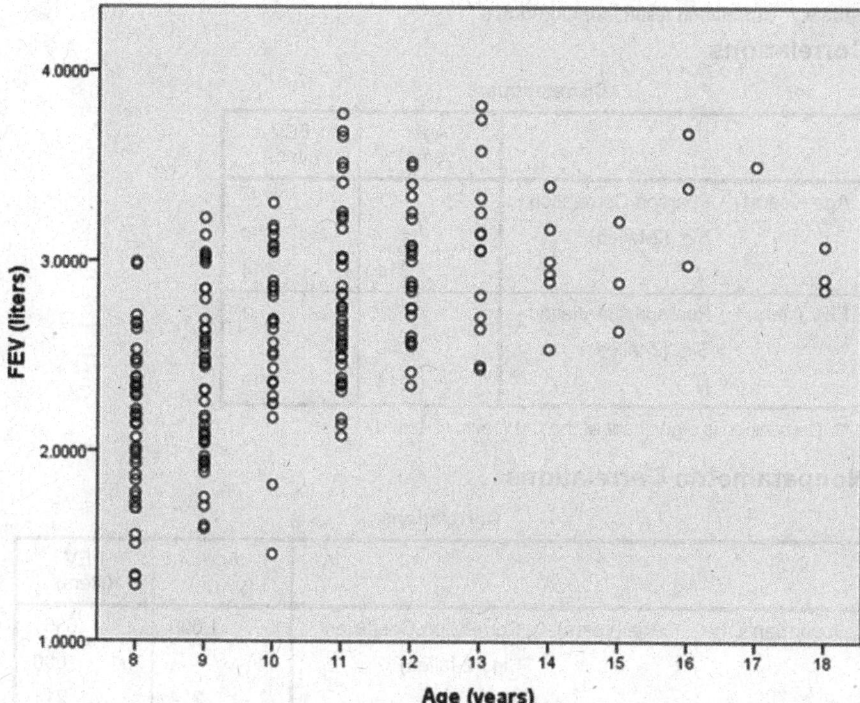

Fig. 9.9 Scatter plot for Question 6

6. Figure 9.9 is a scatter plot of the relationship between forced expiratory volume (FEV) and age for girls between the ages of 8 and 18 who do not smoke. These data are in **FEV.sav** [4]. The values of the Pearson correlation and Spearman's rho coefficients are shown in Table 9.7.

   a. Does the relationship between FEV and age appear to be linear? Is it monotonic? Explain.
   b. What are the two values of the Pearson and Spearman's rho correlations?
   c. What are the p-values for each correlation?
   d. What is the null hypothesis for each correlation?
   e. Can we reject the null hypothesis for each correlation?
   f. Which correlation is the better choice for these data: Pearson or Spearman's rho? Why?

Table 9.7 Correlation results for Question 6

Correlations

Correlations

		Age (years)	FEV (liters)
Age (years)	Pearson Correlation	1	.578**
	Sig. (2-tailed)		.000
	N	214	214
FEV (liters)	Pearson Correlation	.578**	1
	Sig. (2-tailed)	.000	
	N	214	214

**. Correlation is significant at the 0.01 level (2-tailed).

Nonparametric Correlations

Correlations

			Age (years)	FEV (liters)
Spearman's rho	Age (years)	Correlation Coefficient	1.000	.636**
		Sig. (2-tailed)	.	.000
		N	214	214
	FEV (liters)	Correlation Coefficient	.636**	1.000
		Sig. (2-tailed)	.000	.
		N	214	214

**. Correlation is significant at the 0.01 level (2-tailed).

Data Sets and References

1. CDC BRFSS.sav obtained from: Centers for Disease Control and Prevention (CDC): Behavioral Risk Factor Surveillance System Survey Data. US Department of Health and Human Services, Centers for Disease Control and Prevention, Atlanta (2005). Public domain. For more information about the BRFSS, visit http://www.cdc.gov/brfss/. Accessed 16 Nov 2014
2. Bodymass.sav obtained from: Hand, D.J., Daly, F., Lunn, A.D., McConway, K.J., Ostrowski, E.: A Handbook of Small Data Sets. Chapman & Hall, London (1994). (With the kind permission of the Routledge Taylor and Francis Group, and Professor Shelley L Channon).
3. Framingham.sav obtained from: Dupont, W.D.: Statistical Modeling for Biomedical Researchers, 2nd ed. Cambridge University Press, New York (2009). (With the kind permission of Sean Coady, National Heart, Blood, and Lung Institute).
4. FEV.sav obtained from: Rosner, B.: Fundamentals of Biostatistics, 6th ed. Thomson Brooks/Cole, Belmont (2006). With the kind permission of Professor Bernard Rosner. For context, see Tager, I.B., Weiss, S.T., Rosner, B., Speizer, F.E.: Effect of parental cigarette smoking on pulmonary function in children. American Journal of Epidemiology. 110, 15–26 (1979).

Chapter 10
Comparing Means of Independent Samples

Abstract This chapter reviews the independent-samples *t*-test and the one-way analysis of variance, inferential statistics that are commonly used to test null and alternative hypotheses about mean differences among independent populations. Because both procedures assume equal population variances, Levene's test for homogeneity of variances is discussed, as are methods for hypothesis testing when homogeneity of variances cannot be safely assumed. The chapter continues by using a measure of effect size, partial eta squared, to distinguish between statistical and clinical significance, and concludes with a discussion of post hoc multiple comparisons and contrast analysis.

10.1 Overview

Often researchers make two sets of measurements and then, using a test of hypotheses, compare the two sets to determine if the difference observed in the sample measurements is attributable to the population from which the data were drawn. Sometimes the measurements are made of two different groups of participants. For example, the blood pressure of hypertensive patients who had received a new treatment might be compared to that of a group who had received a standard treatment. In this type of study, researchers are said to be comparing two *independent samples*. Sometimes the two sets of observations are made of the same group of participants. For example, the blood pressure of hypertensive patients who had received a new treatment might be compared to the blood pressure of the same group of patients before they had received the treatment. In this type of study, researchers are said to be making *paired comparisons*.

If the observations are quantitative (e.g., blood pressure), researchers can compute the means of the two sets of observations and assess whether the observed difference is significant by using what is known as a *t-test*. If the two sets of observations are made of two different groups (e.g., the mean blood pressure of hypertensive patients receiving a new treatment is to be compared to the mean blood pressure of hypertensive patients receiving a standard treatment), an *independent-samples t-test* will be used. If the two sets of observations are of the same group (e.g., the mean blood pressure of hypertensive patients who had received a new

W. H. Holmes, W. C. Rinaman, *Statistical Literacy for Clinical Practitioners*,
DOI 10.1007/978-3-319-12550-3_10

treatment is to be compared to the mean blood pressure of the same group of patients before they had received the treatment), a *paired-samples t-test* will be used. In this chapter, we focus on comparing independent samples. In the next chapter, we will study paired comparisons.

When comparing independent samples, the observations ideally will have been made within the context of a controlled experiment in which an explanatory variable is manipulated by the researcher to determine its causal impact on a response variable. For example, a new treatment for hypertension might be given to an experimental group of hypertensive patients while a standard treatment is given to a control group of hypertensives. Whether a patient is given the new or standard treatment would be decided at random. In these cases, if the results of a statistical test support the hypothesis that the difference between two sets of observations is attributable to the general population rather than to random sampling variability, a causal relationship between the explanatory and response variables can be established. Often, though, comparisons are made across sets of observations in studies that do not involve manipulation of an explanatory variable. For example, the explanatory variable might be gender, race, age, or economic status, or it might be whether or not participants in the course of their daily lives had been exposed to a risk factor. In these *observational studies,* investigators cannot randomly assign participants to various values of the explanatory variable. Consequently, the results of a hypothesis test reveal only if the difference in the response variable can be confidently attributed to the population from which the sample was taken rather than to sampling variability, but the cause of the difference cannot be established.

An alternative to the *t*-test is a procedure known as *one-way analysis of variance* (*one-way ANOVA*). As with the *t*-test, one-way ANOVA can be used to compare two group means. However, one-way ANOVA can also be used to compare three or more means at one time. In this chapter, we explore one-way ANOVA as a method of comparing two or more means.

In order to conduct a *t*-test or a one-way ANOVA, the response variable must be quantitative. Usually, the explanatory variable is categorical. For example, in a randomized controlled trial of a new hypertensive medication, the explanatory variable might be whether or not hypertensive patients were given the new or standard drug. In an observational study of salt intake and blood pressure, the explanatory variable might be whether or not participants self-report that they avoid salty foods. Sometimes though, the explanatory variable is quantitative. If the explanatory variable is quantitative, its values are few in number, and there are a sufficient number of cases at each of those values to allow for a meaningful comparison of group averages, then a *t*-test or one-way ANOVA might be conducted. Otherwise, the relationship between the explanatory and response variable would be assessed by other techniques. For example, the investigator might calculate the Pearson correlation between the two quantitative variables, or first transform the quantitative explanatory variable into a categorical variable and then conduct the *t*-test or ANOVA if the transformed variable generates two groups or conduct the ANOVA if the transformed variable generates more than two groups.

For example, in a randomized controlled trial, an investigator might determine the relative effect of two different amounts of a new hypertension medication by giving the smaller dose to a group of 50 hypertensive patients and the larger dose to a second group of 50 hypertensives. The investigator would then compare the average blood pressure of both groups by using either a *t*-test or a one-way ANOVA. On the other hand, in an observational study of the relationship between salt intake and blood pressure, an investigator might analyze participants' diets to obtain a quantitative measure of daily salt intake. Since the measure of salt intake would generate a large number of possible values, the investigator would compute the correlation between salt intake and blood pressure, or if the sample size is sufficiently large to allow for a meaningful analysis of group means, transform the amount of daily salt intake into a categorical variable (e.g., by grouping participants in terms of whether their salt intake was in the first, second, third or fourth quartile), and then compare the mean blood pressure of the resulting groups.

As we saw in Chap. 5 and as we will see later in this chapter, it is possible for differences among sets of observations to be statistically significant even if the differences are small. For example, an experimental group of hypertensive patients who received a marginally effective treatment might experience a small yet statistically significant reduction in blood pressure. Therefore, in addition to determining whether differences among groups are statistically significant, researchers conducting experiments will quantify the size of the impact of the causal variable on the response variable, and researchers conducting observational studies will quantify the strength of the relationship between the explanatory and response variables. One method by which to do this is by computing what is called *effect size*. In this chapter, we look at a measure of effect size that can be computed when a one-way ANOVA is used.

10.2 Comparing Two Means: The Independent-Samples t-Test

In this section, we demonstrate how two means are compared when using the independent-samples *t*-test. The two means will be the average body mass index (BMI) values of male and female residents of NY.

Load the data file, **CDC BRFSS.sav** [1], into SPSS. As shown in Figs. 10.1, 10.2, 10.3 and 10.4, select **Analyze** > **Compare Means** > **Independent-Samples T-Test** to open the *Independent-Samples T-Test* dialog box. Move **BODY MASS INDEX** [*BMI*] (variable 107) into the *Test Variable(s)* box and **SEX** [*SEX*] (variable 32) into the *Grouping Variable* box. You will notice that *Sex(?,?)* is displayed in the *Grouping Variable* box. The question marks indicate that you need to define what value of the grouping variable corresponds to the first group and what value corresponds to the second group. To do this, click **Define Groups** to open the *Define Groups* dialog box. Type "1" in the *Group 1* box, and "2" in the *Group 2* box.

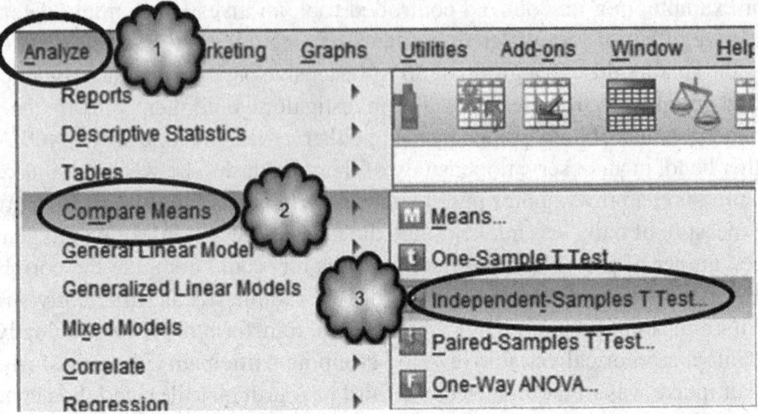

Fig. 10.1 Opening the Independent-Samples T-Test dialog

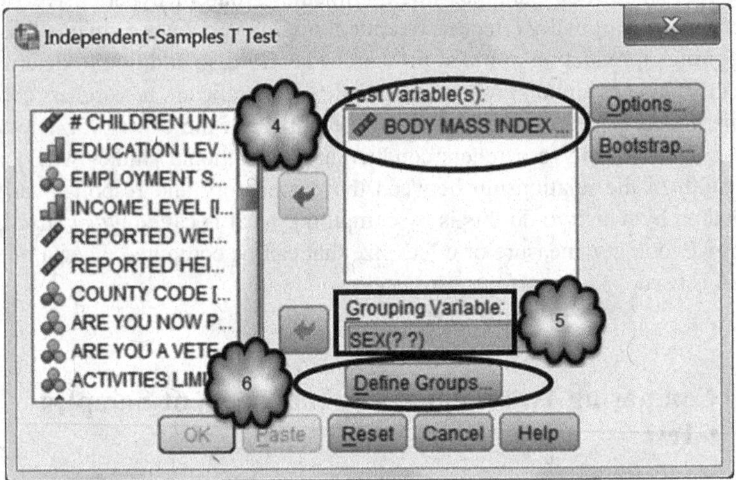

Fig. 10.2 Selecting the test and grouping variables and opening the Define Groups dialog

(Do not include the quotation marks.) Typing in these numbers will tell SPSS which values of **SEX** we wish to use. Of course, there are only the two values, but we have to tell SPSS anyway. Click **Continue** and then **OK**.

The output of the *t*-test consists of two tables. The first is Table 10.1, *Group Statistics*. It displays some descriptive statistics.

Fig. 10.3 Defining groups

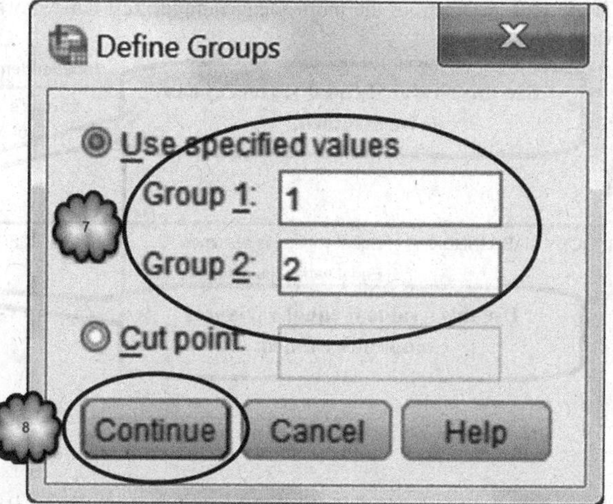

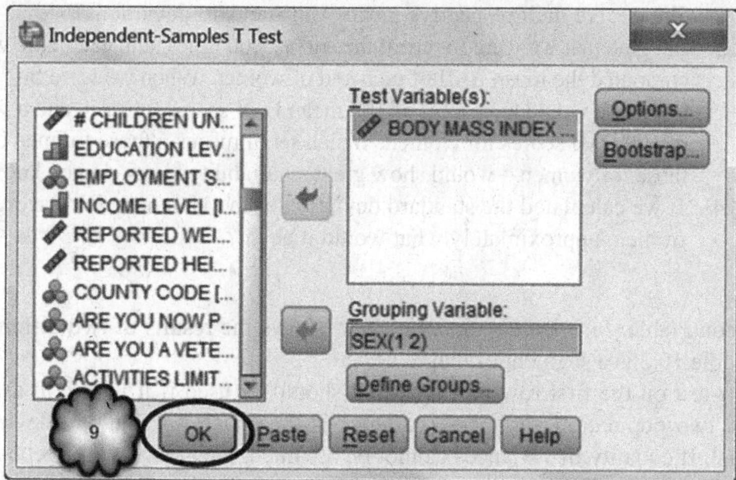

Fig. 10.4 Executing the independent-samples t-test

Table 10.1 Group statistics generated by an independent-samples t-test

Group Statistics

	SEX	N	Mean	Std. Deviation	Std. Error Mean
BODY MASS INDEX	Male	2883	27.4496	4.85540	.09043
	Female	4534	26.5124	5.95192	.08839

Table 10.2 Segment of the Indpendent-Samples Test table showing Levene's test for equality of variances

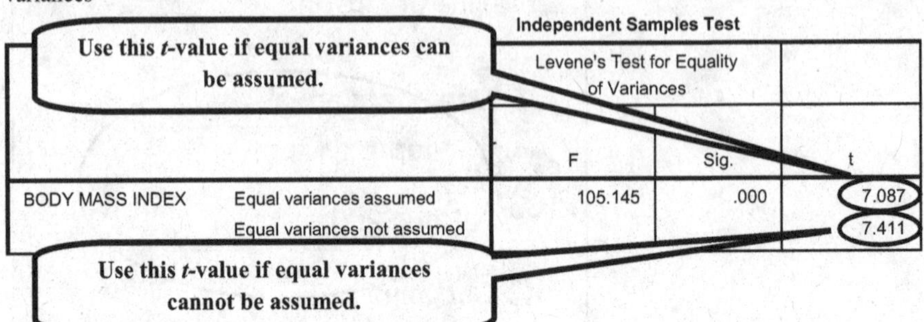

Independent Samples Test

		Levene's Test for Equality of Variances		
		F	Sig.	t
BODY MASS INDEX	Equal variances assumed	105.145	.000	7.087
	Equal variances not assumed			7.411

Study the Group Statistics table and answer the following questions.

10.2.1 How many men were included in the analysis? Women?

10.2.2 What were their respective means and standard deviations?

10.2.3 Imagine that we were to repeat the survey 100 times, and each time we computed the mean BMI of men and of women. When we were finished, we would have a set of 100 mean BMI scores for men, and a set of 100 BMI scores for women. Which set of means—those for men or those for women—would show greater variability? How do you know?

10.2.4 If we calculated the standard deviation of the 100 mean BMI scores of men, approximately what would it equal?

The second table, *Independent-Samples Test,* shows the results of two different *t*-tests. Table 10.2 is a segment of that table.

The *t*-test on the first row of Table 10.2 should be used if it is safe to assume that the two population variances (variance is the square of standard deviation) are equal. If equality of variances cannot be assumed, the *t*-test on the second row should be used. To make this determination, researchers refer to the results of what is known as *Levene's test.* For this test, the null hypothesis is that the two population variances are equal, and the alternative hypothesis is that they are not equal. The *p*-value for this test appears in the *Sig.* box in the *Levene's Test for Equality of Variances* area. It has the same interpretation as the other *p*-values we have encountered.

10.2.5 Were the two sample standard deviations equal?

10.2.6 If not, what does the *p*-value for Levene's test lead us to conclude about whether or not this difference can be attributed to the populations?

10.2.7 What is the *p*-value?

10.2.8 Is the difference in sample variances significant at the 0.05 level?

Table 10.3 Results of the independent-samples t-test

Independent Samples Test

		t	df	Sig. (2-tailed)
BODY MASS INDEX	Equal variances assumed	7.087	7415	.000
	Equal variances not assumed	7.411	6973.107	.000

If the difference in sample variances is significant at the 0.05 level, we conclude that the difference in the variances of the BMI scores of the 7000 or so men and women in our *sample* was due to a difference in the variance of BMI scores of the millions of men and women in the *population* from which the sample was taken. Otherwise, we conclude that the difference in the variances of the BMI scores of the 7000 or so men and women in our sample was due just to chance, and that there is *no* difference in the variance of BMI scores of the millions of men and women in the population from which the sample was taken.

10.2.9 Based on the results of Levene's test, which version of the independent-samples *t*-test should we use to decide whether or not the difference in sample means is significant?

Now we are ready to determine if the data support the null hypothesis that the mean BMI of men is the same as the mean BMI of women or the alternative hypothesis that the mean BMI of men differs from the mean BMI of women. Table 10.3 is that portion of the *Independent-Samples Test* that displays the results of the independent-samples *t*-test.

Using the appropriate row of the table, find the *t-value*. This value is in the column labeled *t*, and is calculated using a formula that uses three properties of the data: the size of the difference between the two group means (the sample mean from group 2 is subtracted from the sample mean from group 1), the variability of the scores within each group, and the number of observations in each group. The result is the *t*-value. In our example, what is the *t*-value? Be sure to be reading from the appropriate row.

Values of *t* can be either positive or negative, depending on the direction of the difference between the two means. If the sample mean from group 1 is greater than the sample mean from group 2, the *t*-value will be positive. If the sample mean from group 1 is less than the sample mean from group 2, the *t*-value will be negative. If the two sample means are equal, the *t*-value will equal zero. Does your observed *t*-value indicate that the difference between the two sample mean BMI scores is positive, negative or zero?

Table 10.4 Mean difference, and its standard error and 95 % confidence interval

		t-test for Equality of Means			
				95% Confidence Interval of the Difference	
		Mean Difference	Std. Error Difference	Lower	Upper
BODY MASS INDEX	Equal variances assumed	.93720	.13224	.67797	1.19643
	Equal variances not assumed	.93720	.12645	.68932	1.18509

Before the *p*-value is calculated, the number of *degrees of freedom* is computed. There is a different formula for each of the two versions of the *t*-test. Degrees of freedom reflect sample size. The larger the sample, the greater is the number of degrees of freedom.

10.2.10 What are the degrees of freedom in our example for the *t*-test that is appropriate for this situation? Look in the column labeled *df*.

The number of degrees of freedom and the *t*-value are then used to calculate the *p*-value. The *p*-value is the probability of observing a value of *t* as or more extreme under the assumption that the null hypothesis—the two population means BMI scores are equal—is true. The *p*-values will decrease as *t* increases or the number of degrees of freedom increases. When both are large, *p*-values are quite small, often less than 0.001.

What is the *p*-value in our example? To find out, read from the table in the column labeled *Sig. (2-tailed)*. The term *2-tailed* indicates that this is the *p*-value for the alternative hypothesis that the two population means are not equal to each other. Do the data support the null or the alternative hypothesis? That is, can we say that the difference is statistically significant?

The rest of the output in *Independent-Samples Test* provides information regarding the construction of a 95 % confidence interval for the difference between the two population means (the mean for group 2 subtracted from the mean for group 1). This information is displayed in Table 10.4. The table displays the size of the difference between the two means in our sample (found in the column labeled *Mean Difference*), the standard error of the difference (found under *Std. Error Difference*), and the 95 % confidence interval of the difference, with its lower and upper values.

To see if you understand these statistics, answer the following questions.

10.2.11 Does the confidence interval indicate that the population mean BMI for men is greater than the population mean BMI for women? Less than? Neither? Why?

10.2.12 Can we be sure this conclusion is correct? Why or why not?

10.3 Comparing Two Means: One-way Analysis of Variance

An alternative to the independent-samples *t*-test is known as *one-way analysis of variance,* or *one-way ANOVA*. In addition to comparing two means, one-way ANOVA can be used to compare three or more group means at the same time. For example, we might wish to compare the mean blood pressure of hypertensive patients who were given a new drug with that of patients who were kept on standard drug treatment with that of patients who were given an alternative to a drug treatment, say, an exercise and diet regimen. The *t*-test cannot handle more than two means at a time, so in this case, one-way ANOVA would be the test of choice. Later in this chapter, we will look at how the ANOVA approaches the analysis of three or more means.

One-way ANOVA can be used to compare two means when it may be safely assumed that the population variances are equal. Earlier, we saw that the variances in BMI varied significantly across gender. Because it is not appropriate to use the standard one-way ANOVA in this example, we will change our example and look at the relationship between BMI and coronary heart disease. On average, who has the larger BMI: patients who have coronary heart disease or patients who do not? To answer this question, we will analyze data from the Framingham Heart Study, a prospective cohort study of cardiovascular disease.

Open the file, **Framingham.sav** [2]. This file consists of a sample of 4699 men and women whose cardiovascular health was monitored for an average of about 22 years. As shown in Figs. 10.5, 10.6, 10.7 and 10.8, select **Analyze > Compare Means > One-Way ANOVA** to open the *One-Way ANOVA* dialog box. Move **BODY MASS INDEX** [*bmi*] (variable 8) into the *Dependent List* box and **Coronary Heart Disease** [*chdfate*] (variable 5; 0 = No; 1 = Yes) into the *Factor* box. Click **Options** to

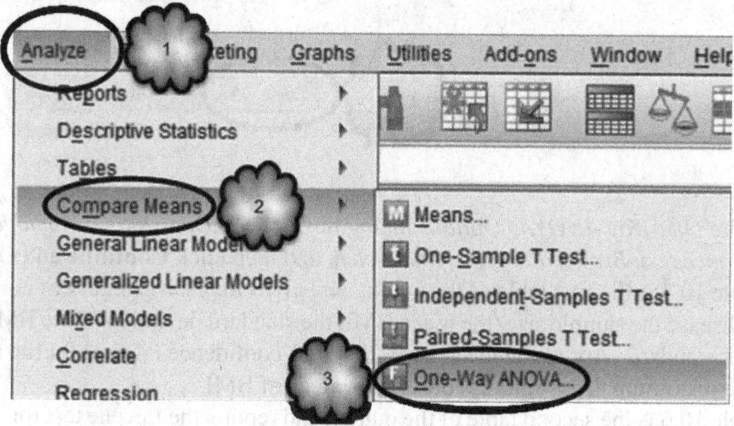

Fig. 10.5 Opening the One-Way ANOVA dialog

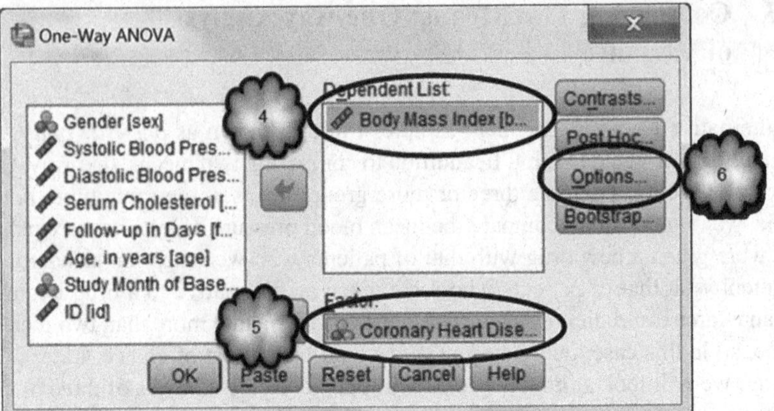

Fig. 10.6 Selecting the dependent variable and factor, and opening the Options dialog

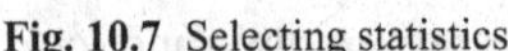

Fig. 10.7 Selecting statistics

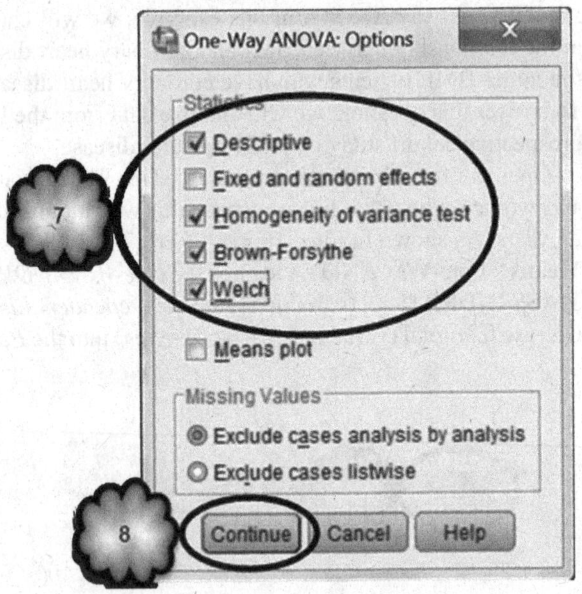

open the *One-Way ANOVA: Options* dialog box. Check *Descriptive, Homogeneity of variance test, Brown–Forsythe, and Welch,* and then click **Continue** and **OK**.

Table 10.5 is the first table of the output, and gives for each category of coronary heart disease the sample size, the mean BMI, the standard deviation of the BMI values, the standard error of the mean BMI, the 95 % confidence interval for the mean, and the maximum and minimum observed values of BMI.

Table 10.6 is the second table of the output, and reports the Levene test for equality of variances of the BMI values in the two disease categories. The null hypothesis

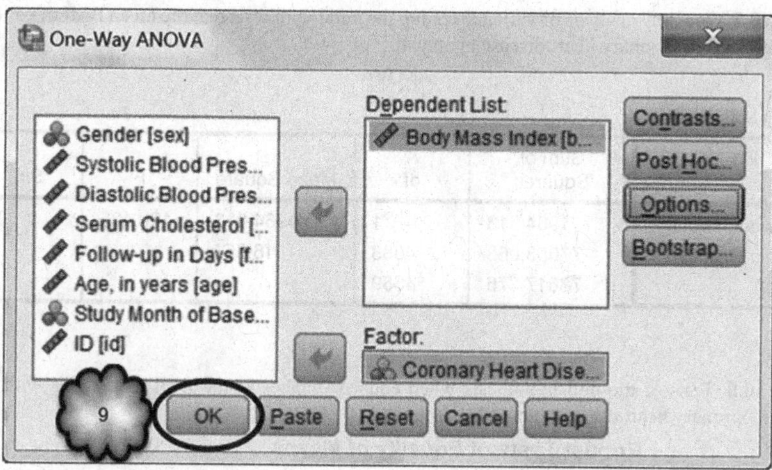

Fig. 10.8 Executing a one-way ANOVA

Table 10.5 Descriptive statistics generated by a one-way ANOVA on the BMI of patients with and wthout coronary heart disease (rows labelled yes and no, respectively)

Descriptives

Body Mass Index

	N	Mean	Std. Deviation	Std. Error	95% Confidence Interval for Mean		Minimum	Maximum
					Lower Bound	Upper Bound		
No	3218	25.19	4.010	.071	25.06	25.33	16	51
Yes	1472	26.59	4.116	.107	26.38	26.80	17	58
Total	4690	25.63	4.095	.060	25.51	25.75	16	58

Table 10.6 Levene test of the homegeneity of variances in the BMI of patients with and without conronary heart disease

Test of Homogeneity of Variances

Body Mass Index

Levene Statistic	df1	df2	Sig.
.006	1	4688	.937

is that the two population variances are equal, and the alternative hypothesis is that the two population variances differ.

If the Levene test indicates that it is safe to assume that the two variances are equal, then it is appropriate to use the F statistic given in the *ANOVA* table shown in Table 10.7 to test whether or not the group means are equal. The null hypothesis is that the group means are equal, and the alternative hypothesis is that the group means are not the same.

Table 10.7 One-way analysis of variance testing the null hypothesis that the mean BMI of patients with and wthout coronary heart disease are equal

ANOVA

Body Mass Index

	Sum of Squares	df	Mean Square	F	Sig.
Between Groups	1964.313	1	1964.313	120.135	.000
Within Groups	76653.063	4688	16.351		
Total	78617.376	4689			

Table 10.8 Tests of the null hypothesis when equal variances in the BMI of patients with and without coronary heart disease cannot be assumed

Robust Tests of Equality of Means

Body Mass Index

	Statistic[a]	df1	df2	Sig.
Welch	117.810	1	2785.143	.000
Brown-Forsythe	117.810	1	2785.143	.000

a. Asymptotically F distributed.

Table 10.8 is the last table of the output, and gives the results of the Welch test and the Brown–Forsythe test for equality of group means. These tests are appropriate when the Levene test indicates that it is not safe to assume that the two variances are the same. Again, the null hypothesis is that the group means are equal, and the alternative hypothesis is that the group means differ.

Values of t, F, and the Welch and the Brown–Forsythe statistics have several common characteristics. Each of the four statistics is a ratio in which the numerator reflects the size of the difference between the two group means, and the denominator reflects the variability of the scores within each group and the size of the sample. In addition, larger values of each of the four statistics result in smaller p-values. However, F ratios and the Welch and Brown–Forsythe statistics can never be negative. They begin at 0 and go up from there. A value of 0 results when the sample means are equal, giving evidence that there is no difference between the population means. In the case of testing the difference between two group means, you may note that the value of the F ratio is equal to the square of the value of the t-test statistic when the two population variances are equal.

As is the case with the t-value, the calculations of the F ratio and the Welch and Brown–Forsythe statistics have degrees of freedom associated with them. However, unlike the t-value, each of the latter three statistics has two values for the degrees of freedom, one associated with the numerator of the statistic and one associated with the denominator of the statistic. For the F ratio, the numerator degrees of freedom are equal to the number of group means being tested minus 1, while the denominator degrees of freedom have the same value as those for the equal variances *t*-test. The numerator degrees of freedom for the Welch and the Brown–Forsythe statistics are the same as that of the *F* ratio, but there is a rather complicated formula for arriving at the degrees of freedom for the denominator.

The value of the *F* ratio, the Welch statistic or the Brown–Forsythe statistic, and its associated degrees of freedom are used to compute a *p*-value. If we can assume equal variances, the *p*-value associated with the *t*-test will be the same as that for the one-way ANOVA. In this situation, whether we conduct a *t*-test or a one-way ANOVA, we will come to the same conclusion as to whether the difference between the two group means was statistically significant.

Study the output in Tables 10.5, 10.6, 10.7 and 10.8, and answer the following questions.

10.3.1 What is the mean BMI of patients who have coronary heart disease?

10.3.2 What is the mean BMI of patients who do not have coronary heart disease?

10.3.3 What test or tests of equality of means should we use with these data? Why?

10.3.4 What is the value of the test statistic that compares the two means?

10.3.5 What is the *p*-value associated with the test statistics that compares the two means?

10.3.6 Can we confidently conclude that in the population of Framingham residents, coronary heart disease and BMI are related? Why or why not?

10.4 Effect Size

Large values of *t* or one-way ANOVA statistics occur when the difference between the two sample means is large, the variability of scores within each of the two groups is small, or when the number of scores in each group is large. Since large values of these statistics are associated with small *p*-values, and since statistically significant results are usually desirable, researchers will often conduct studies in such a way as to maximize the average difference in scores between the two groups under study, minimize the variability of scores within each group, and maximize the size of the sample.

For example, in an experimental investigation of whether a newly developed hypertensive drug reduces blood pressure, a researcher might maximize the difference between the average blood pressure of the experimental and control groups by administering to the experimental group as large a dose of the new drug as is safely possible. To minimize the variability of blood pressure readings in each of the two groups, the researcher would take care to measure blood pressure at the same time of day each day, and in the same way with the same equipment. To maximize sample size, the researcher would recruit large numbers of patients.

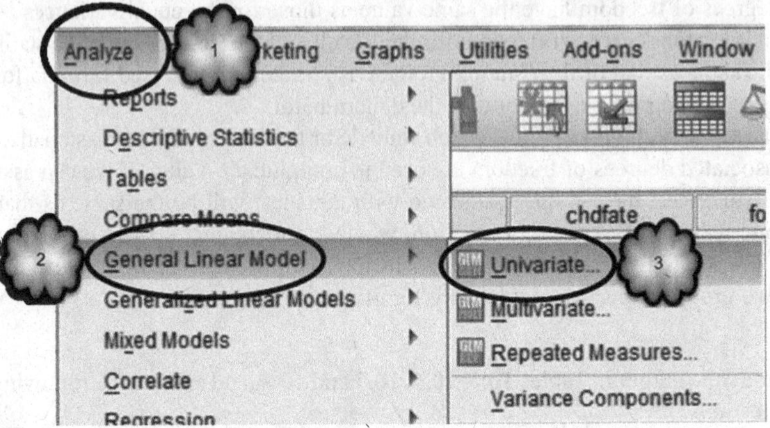

Fig. 10.9 Opening the Univariate dialog

It should be pointed out that there are cases when a tiny and clinically unimportant difference between two group means can still result in a significant *p*-value. For example, the impact on blood pressure of a newly developed drug may be statistically significant but perhaps only because the researcher recruited a very large number of patients. The impact of the drug might be quite small, so small as to have little or no clinical or practical significance. So, not only will researchers look for statistical significance but they will also use a *measure of effect size* to determine if the difference between the means is meaningful. These statistics gauge whether a statistically significant difference between two groups reflects a weak, moderate or strong relationship between the two variables under investigation. These measures involve taking into account the size of the difference between the means of the two groups, the variability of the scores within each group and the size of the sample. The details of these measures vary from one to the other, but all quantify the strength of relationship between two variables.

Partial eta squared In this section, we use a measure of effect size called *partial eta squared* to determine the strength of relationship between sex and BMI. In the exercise questions, we leave it to you to determine the strength of relationship between coronary heart disease and BMI in our Framingham data set. Partial eta squared varies from 0 to 1. The closer the value of partial eta squared is to 0, the weaker is the relationship between the two variables. The closer the value is to 1, the stronger is the relationship.

In order to compute partial eta squared with SPSS, we need to use an alternative procedure to conducting the one-way analysis of variance. Return to the Centers for Disease Control and Prevention (CDC) data set. As shown in Figs. 10.9, 10.10 and 10.11, select **Analyze** > **General Linear Model** > **Univariate** to open the *Univariate* dialog box. Move **BODY MASS INDEX** [*BMI*] (variable 107) to the *Dependent Variable* box and **SEX** [*SEX*] (variable 32) to the *Fixed Factor(s)* box. To obtain the value for partial eta squared and the group means, click **Options** to bring

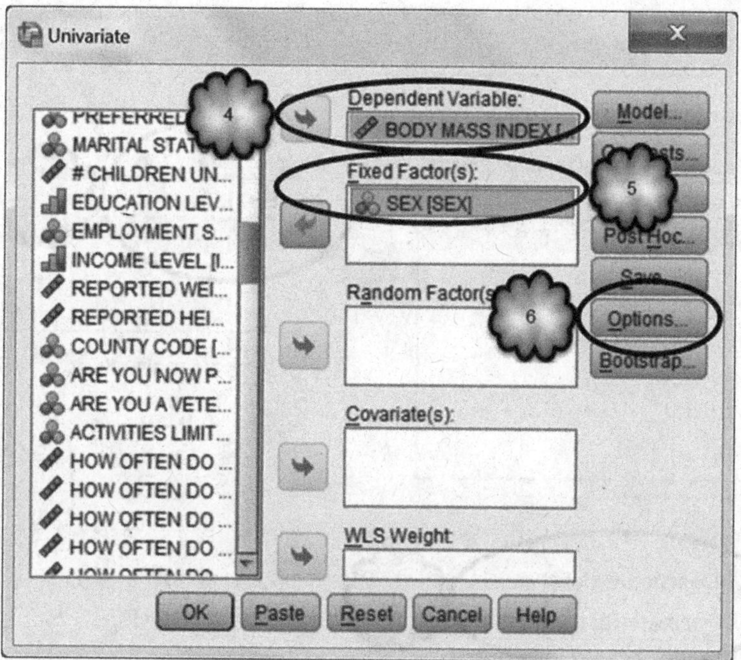

Fig. 10.10 Selecting the dependent variable and factor, and opening the Options dialog

up the *Univariate: Options* dialog box. Move **(OVERALL)** and **SEX** to the *Display Means for* box, and check *Descriptive statistics* and *Estimates of effect size* in the *Display* area. Click **Continue** and then **OK** (Fig. 10.12).

The output includes Table 10.9, which displays sample sizes, and Table 10.10, which displays means and standard deviations. The sample sizes, means, and standard deviations should be identical to those generated by the *t*-test we conducted in Sect. 10.2 and displayed in Table 10.1.

What is different in the output is the content of a third table, Table 10.11. This table is called *Tests of Between-Subjects Effects,* and displays the test statistic and the measure of effect size.

To find the test statistic, that is, the *F* ratio, first locate the column labeled *F* in the table. Then read down the column until you encounter the *F* ratio that is found in the row labeled with the name of the factor of interest, in our example, *SEX*. Once you have found the *F* ratio, the *p*-value associated with it can be found in the *Sig.* column in that row. This *p*-value is based on the assumption that the variances in BMI are the same for each sex.

10.4.1 What is value of the *F* ratio?
10.4.2 What is the *p*-value?

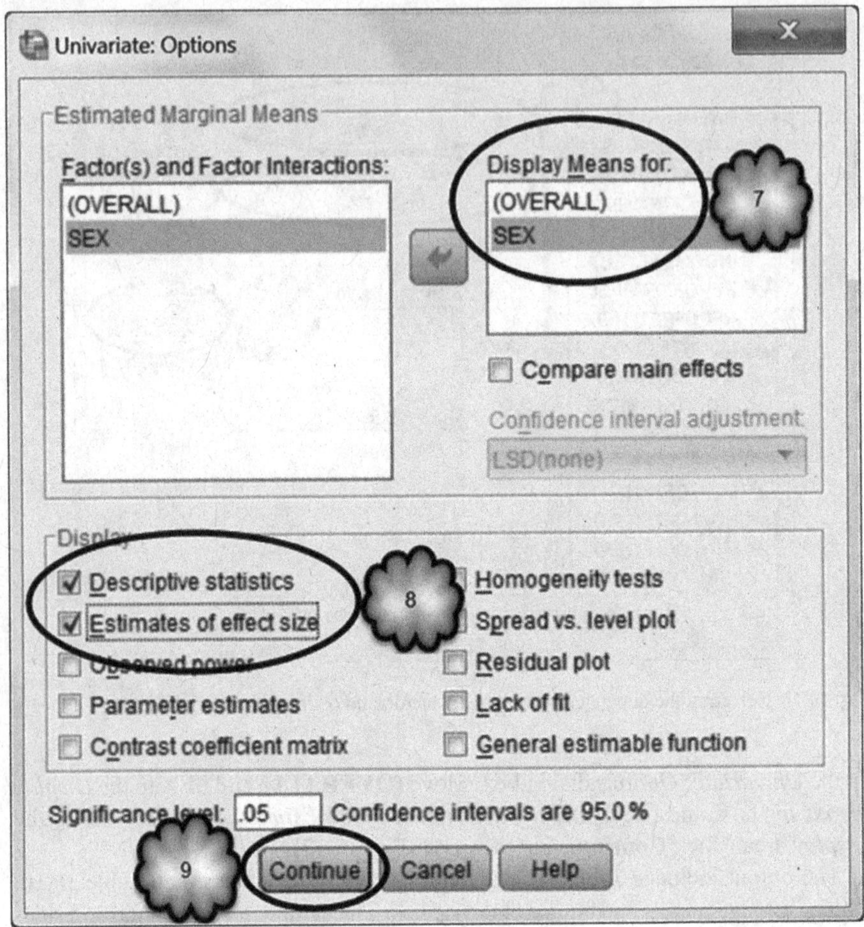

Fig. 10.11 Selecting output to be displayed

To determine the values for degrees of freedom associated with the *F* ratio, look in the *df* column of the table. The entry in the row corresponding to the factor of interest (*sex* in this example) gives the numerator degrees of freedom. The denominator degrees of freedom can be found by continuing down the *df* column to the row labeled *Error*.

10.4.3 What are the numerator and denominator degrees of freedom?

To find the value of partial eta squared, look in the last column of the table in the row corresponding to the factor of interest, in our case, *SEX*.

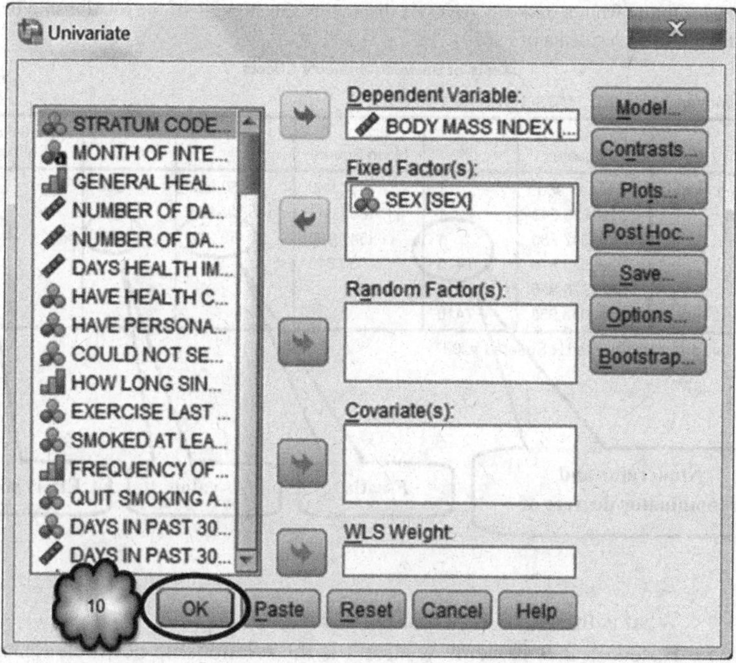

Fig. 10.12 Using the Univariate dialog to execute a one-way ANOVA

Table 10.9 Sample sizes of male and female residents of NY

Between-Subjects Factors

		Value Label	N
SEX	1	Male	2883
	2	Female	4534

Table 10.10 Descriptive statistics of the BMI of male and female residents of NY

Descriptive Statistics

Dependent Variable: BODY MASS INDEX

SEX	Mean	Std. Deviation	N
Male	27.4496	4.85540	2883
Female	26.5124	5.95192	4534
Total	26.8767	5.56992	7417

Table 10.11 Output from a one-way ANOVA displaying the strength of the relationship between sex and BMI among residents of NY

Tests of Between-Subjects Effects

Dependent Variable: BODY MASS INDEX

Source	Type III Sum of Squares	df	Mean Square	F	Sig.	Partial Eta Squared
Corrected Model	1547.980[a]	1	1547.980	50.227	.000	.007
Intercept	5131835.343	1	5131835.343	166513.056	.000	.957
SEX	1547.980	1	1547.980	50.227	.000	.007
Error	228525.978	7415	30.819			
Total	5587776.825	7417				
Corrected Total	230073.958	7416				

a. R Squared = .007 (Adjusted R Squared = .007)

> 10.4.4 What is the value of partial eta squared?
> 10.4.5 Based on that value, how strong is the relationship between sex and BMI?

Statistical Significance and Effect Size We can now put together two important concepts: statistical significance and effect size.

> 10.4.6 Based on your analysis of the CDC data, would you say that there is or is not a difference between the population mean BMIs of men and women?
> 10.4.7 If you say that there is a difference, would you say that it is small, moderate, or large?

Remember, a statistically significant relationship between two variables does not necessarily mean that the relationship is a powerful one. The relationship between sex and BMI is a case in point. Although the mean BMI of men was significantly different from the mean BMI of women, sex and BMI were only weakly related. In fact, the effect size is tiny, suggesting that the difference in BMI between the two sexes may have little or no practical or clinical significance.

10.5 Comparing More than Two Means

As we noted earlier in this chapter, ANOVA is typically used when one wishes to compare three or more means. In this section, we explore how ANOVA can be used for this purpose. As an example, we study the average BMI of four groups

Table 10.12 Descriptive statistics of the BMI of NY residents of varying levels of education

Descriptives

BODY MASS INDEX

	N	Mean	Std. Deviation	Std. Error
Did not graduate High School	584	28.2939	5.72488	.23690
Graduated High School	2096	27.6262	5.90429	.12897
Attended College or Technical School	1708	27.2022	5.86608	.14194
Graduated from College or Technical School	3002	25.8973	4.93031	.08998
Total	7390	26.8786	5.56995	.06479

Table 10.13 Levene's test of homogeneity of variances in the BMI of NY residents of varying levels of education

Test of Homogeneity of Variances

BODY MASS INDEX

Levene Statistic	df1	df2	Sig.
21.902	3	7386	.000

of respondents in the CDC data set: those who did not graduate from high school, those who graduated from high school, those who attended college or technical school, and those who graduated from college or technical school.

Begin by declaring cases that have values for the variable, **LEVEL OF EDUCATION COMPLETED** [*@_EDUCAG*] (variable 82), equal to 9 as missing. Then select **Analyze > Compare Means > One-Way ANOVA** to open the one-way ANOVA dialog box. Move **LEVEL OF EDUCATION COMPLETED** to the *Factor* box, and **BODY MASS INDEX** (variable 107) to the *Dependent List* box. In the *Options* dialog box, be sure that the statistics *Descriptive, Homogeneity of variance test, Brown–Forsythe,* and *Welch* have been selected. Now run the analysis.

As we saw in Sect. 10.3, the output consists of a table of descriptive statistics. Table 10.12 displays the sample sizes, means, standard deviations, and standard errors from this table. The output also consists of Levene's test for equality of variances (Table 10.13), the ANOVA table (Table 10.14) and the results of the Brown–Forsythe and Welch tests of the equality of means when equality of variances cannot be assumed (Table 10.15).

Table 10.14 One-way analysis of variance testing the null hypothesis that the mean BMI of NY residents of varying levels of education are equal

ANOVA

BODY MASS INDEX

	Sum of Squares	df	Mean Square	F	Sig.
Between Groups	5410.714	3	1803.571	59.515	.000
Within Groups	223827.831	7386	30.304		
Total	229238.544	7389			

Table 10.15 Tests of the null hypothesis when equal variances in the BMI of NY residents of varying levels of education cannot be assumed

Robust Tests of Equality of Means

BODY MASS INDEX

	Statistic[a]	df1	df2	Sig.
Welch	62.811	3	2252.593	.000
Brown-Forsythe	56.333	3	3942.539	.000

a. Asymptotically F distributed.

However, the analysis we conducted in Sect. 10.3 compared two sample means, the average BMI of males and the average BMI of females. Our analysis here compares four sample means: the average BMI of respondents who did not graduate from high school, the average BMI of high school graduates, the average BMI of those who attended college or technical school, and the average BMI of college or technical school graduates.

Recall that the null hypothesis tested by ANOVA is that the population means are equal, and that the alternative hypothesis is that the population means are not equal. In the present example, the null hypothesis is that within the population of NY residents, the mean BMIs of those who did not finish high school, of high school graduates, of those who did not finish college or technical school, and of college graduates are all the same. The alternative hypothesis is that the population means of these four groups are not all the same.

Study the four group means and the associated tests of the equality of those means, and answer the following questions.

10.5.1 If we assume that the variances in BMI of the four population groups are equal, what is the value of the test statistic that tests the null hypothesis?

10.5.2 If we assume that the population variances are equal, what is the probability that we would obtain a test statistic that is equal to or greater than the value we obtained if the null hypothesis is true?

> 10.5.3 Can we safely assume that the population variances are equal? Why or why not?
>
> 10.5.4 If we cannot safely assume that the variances are equal, can we reject the null hypothesis that the four population means are equal? Why or why not?

In this example, even if we cannot assume that the population variances are the same, we can confidently reject the null hypothesis in favor of the alternative hypothesis that in the population of NY residents, the mean BMI scores of these four education groups are not the same. It is important to point out, however, that the null hypothesis states that the population means are equal, and that the alternative hypothesis states that the population means are not equal. By rejecting the null hypothesis, we are concluding that the four population means are not equal. However, we are not stating that all four means are different from one another. All we know at this point is that at least one of the four population means differs from at least one other. We will have to conduct some additional analyses to find out which of the four means differs significantly from which of the others.

You might be thinking at this point that the next step is to conduct a series of *t*-tests on every possible pair of means to determine which pairings yield *p*-values ≤ 0.05. Unfortunately, a problem with this approach is that the probability that at least one of the comparisons will be significant will be greater than the alpha level set for each comparison. That is, after we have completed all of our *t*-tests, our Type I error rate, the rate at which we rejected a true null hypothesis, will be 5%. In our example, for instance, we have four mean BMIs. A set of four means allows for as many as six pairings (the mean BMI of the first group versus the mean of the second, the mean of the first versus the mean of the third, the mean of the first versus the mean of the fourth, the mean of the second versus the mean of the third, and so on). If we were to compare one and only one pair of means, and if we were to set alpha to 0.05, the probability that we would reject the null hypothesis when it is in fact true would be 0.05. However, if we were to conduct *t*-tests on two or more pairings, and set alpha to 0.05 for each comparison, the probability of making a Type I error on at least one of those comparisons will be greater than 0.05.

When conducting multiple comparisons of group means, it is necessary that we use statistical techniques that are designed to keep the overall probability of making a Type I error at the desired alpha level (e.g., 0.05). There are many such techniques. Some, called *post hoc comparisons,* conduct a series of comparisons, each involving two group means. In our example, we might compare the mean BMI of each group against the mean BMI of each of the other three. Other techniques, called *contrasts,* can compare the means of subsets of groups. For instance, in our example, we could compare the mean BMI of the three groups of respondents who did not graduate from college with the mean BMI of college graduates.

Post hoc comparisons We will turn our attention first to two examples of post hoc comparisons: Bonferroni and Tamhane's T2. The former is used when equality of variances can be assumed; the latter when equality of variances cannot be assumed.

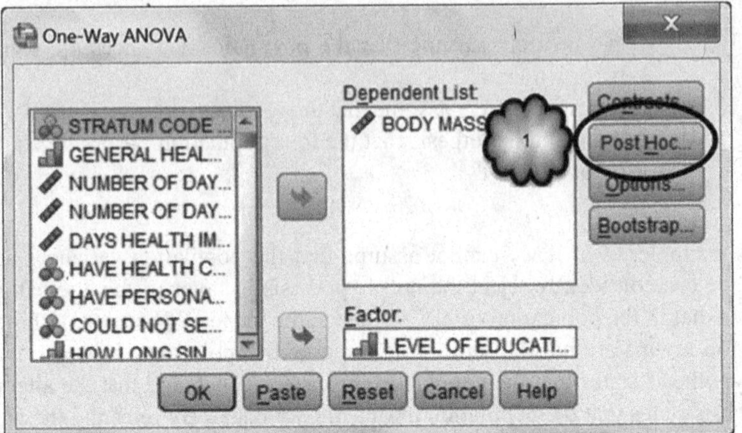

Fig. 10.13 Opening the one-way ANOVA: Post Hoc Multiple Comparisons dialog

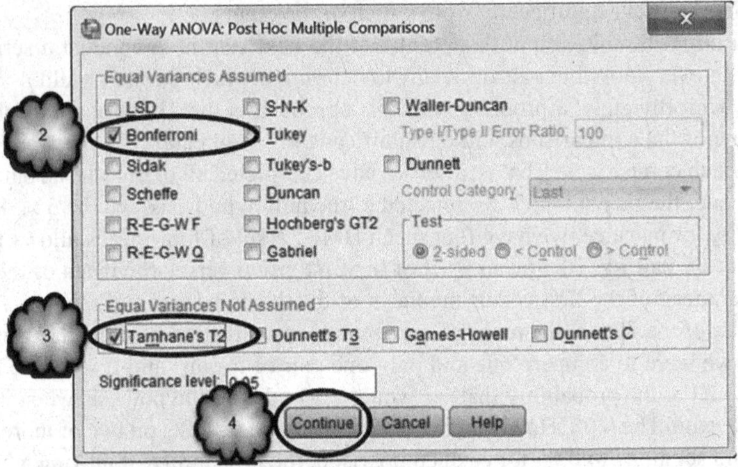

Fig. 10.14 Selecting Bonferroni and Tamhane's T2

Although equality of variances cannot be assumed in our example, we will include the Bonferroni test here to show you how to use it, and because it is frequently used by researchers when equality of variances can be assumed.

Return to the *One-Way ANOVA* dialog box. As shown in Figs. 10.13, 10.14 and 10.15, click **Post Hoc** to open the *One-Way ANOVA: Post Hoc Multiple Comparisons* dialog box. Select Bonferroni and Tamhane's T2 under *Equal Variances Assumed* and *Equal Variances Not Assumed,* respectively. Click **Continue** and then **OK.**

The output consists of the information that we generated earlier plus a table called, *Multiple Comparisons*. This table, a fragment of which is shown in Table 10.16, displays the results of the Bonferroni and Tamhane's T2 analyses.

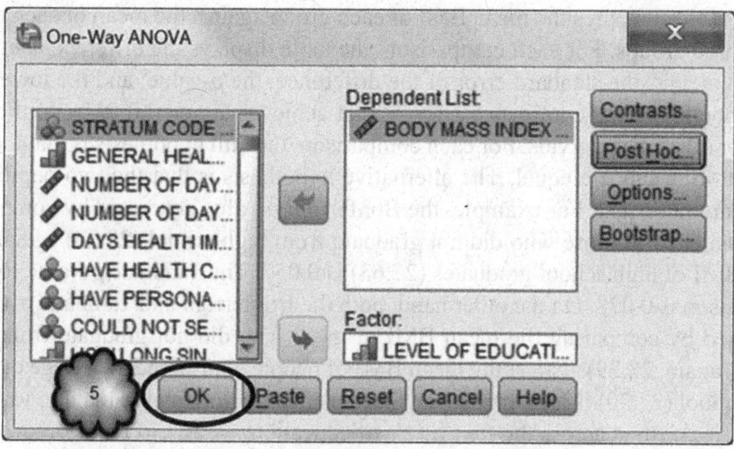

Fig. 10.15 Executing the one-way ANOVA with post hoc multiple comparisons

Table 10.16 Bonferroni and Tamhane's T2 post hoc multiple comparisons

Multiple Comparisons

Dependent Variable: BODY MASS INDEX

	(I) LEVEL OF EDUCATION COMPLETED	(J) LEVEL OF EDUCATION COMPLETED	Mean Difference (I-J)	Std. Error	Sig.
Bonferroni	Did not graduate High School	Graduated High School	.66771	.25758	.057
		Attended College or Technical School	1.09170*	.26388	.000
		Graduated from College or Technical School	2.39657*		.000
Tamhane	Did not graduate High School	Graduated High School	.66771	.26973	.078
		Attended College or Technical School	1.09170*	.27617	.000
		Graduated from College or Technical School	2.39657*		.000

Bonferroni *p*-values generated by comparing the mean BMI of New Yorkers who did not graduate from high school against the BMI means of the other

Tamhane *p*-values generated by comparing the mean BMI of New Yorkers who did not graduate from high school against the BMI means of the other three

*. The mean difference is significant at the 0.05 level.

The table compares the mean BMI of each group against the mean of each of the other three groups. For each comparison, the table displays the difference between the two means, the standard error of the difference, the *p*-value, and the lower and upper bounds of the confidence interval that achieves an overall 95 % confidence level for all of the intervals. For each comparison, the null hypothesis is that the two population means are equal. The alternative hypothesis is that the two population means are not equal. For example, the Bonferroni *p*-value generated by comparing the mean BMI of those who did not graduate from high school (28.29) against the mean BMI of high school graduates (27.63) is 0.057. The Tamhane *p*-value for this comparison is 0.078. On the other hand, both the Bonferroni and Tamhane *p*-values generated by comparing the mean BMI of those who did not graduate from high school (again, 28.29) against the mean BMI of people who attended college or technical school (27.20) is less than 0.001. Because we cannot assume that the variance in BMI is constant across the four levels of education, we would focus on the Tamhane findings, but as it turned out, both types of post hoc comparisons happened to lead to same results: We reject the null hypothesis for the second comparison but not for the first.

Answer the following questions.

10.5.5 According to the Bonferroni test, does the mean BMI of those who did not graduate from high school significantly differ from the mean BMI of college or technical school graduates?

10.5.6 According to the Bonferroni test, what is the standard error of the difference between the mean BMI of those who did not graduate from high school and the mean BMI of those who attended college or technical school?

10.5.7 Do either of the answers to the previous questions differ if one uses the Tamhane's T2 test?

Contrasts Sometimes it is useful to conduct a *contrast analysis* by which we compare the mean of a subset of groups against the mean of another subset of groups. In our example, we might wish to know if the mean BMI of those with at least some post-high school education differs from the rest of the population. To find out, we could compare the mean BMI of two subsets of groups. One group would consist of those who either attended college or technical school or who graduated from college or technical school. The second group would consist of those who attended high school or graduated from high school. In this section, we carry out this contrast.

Return to the *One-Way ANOVA* dialog box. Click **Contrasts** to open the *One-Way ANOVA: Contrasts* dialog box. To conduct a contrast, we must assign a number to each of the four groups of respondents. These numbers are called *coefficients* and will indicate to SPSS the comparison or contrast we wish to generate. Certain rules must be followed when assigning coefficients. First, groups assigned the same coefficient are allocated to the same subset. Second, the sum of the coefficients should be equal to zero. Third, groups that are to be excluded from an analysis should be assigned coefficients equal to zero. Fourth, coefficients are entered into SPSS one at a time and in the ascending order of the values of the variable that defines the groups that are being compared.

In our example, we wish to group together respondents who either attended high school or graduated from high school. Therefore, we will assign those two groups the same coefficient. Although we could use any number, we will use "1." The remaining groups (those who attended college or technical school or who graduated from college or technical school) will be assigned their own coefficient. Since the sum of the coefficients should equal zero, we will assign "− 1" to those two groups. We will use all four groups, so none of the groups will be assigned a zero coefficient.

The variable, **LEVEL OF EDUCATION COMPLETED,** has four values ranging from 1 to 4, where 1 represents those who attended high school, 2 represents those who graduated from high school, 3 represents those who attended college or technical school, and 4 those who graduated from college or technical school. Therefore, the first coefficient we enter into SPSS will be assigned to those who attended high school, the second coefficient to high school graduates, and so on. As a result, the sequence by which we will enter the four coefficients into SPSS will be 1, 1, − 1, and − 1.

Enter each of the coefficients, one at a time and in the correct sequence, into the *Coefficients* area of the *One-Way ANOVA: Contrasts* dialog box. To do this, enter the first coefficient (1) into the *Coefficients* box, and then click **Add**. Repeat for the remaining three coefficients. When you have finished, you will see a column of the four coefficients in the box to the right of the **Add** button. Click **Continue.** The steps for setting up a contrast are depicted in Figs. 10.16 and 10.17.

Back in the *One-Way ANOVA* dialog box, click **OK** to conduct the analysis. In addition to the information that we have already discussed, the output will contain a *Contrast Coefficients* table, reproduced in Table 10.17. This table displays the four coefficients that we assigned.

The output will also contain a *Contrast Tests* table, reproduced in Table 10.18. This table tells us whether the two means were significantly different as determined by a *t*-test.

Two values of *t* are reported, one under the assumption of equal variances, the other when this assumption is not made. The null hypothesis is that the population means of the two groups are equal. The alternative hypothesis is that the population means of the two groups are not equal.

10.5.8 Is the mean BMI of those who had at least some college or technical school experience significantly different from the mean BMI of those who did not attend college or technical school?

10.5.9 Does your answer depend on whether or not we assume that the population variances are equal?

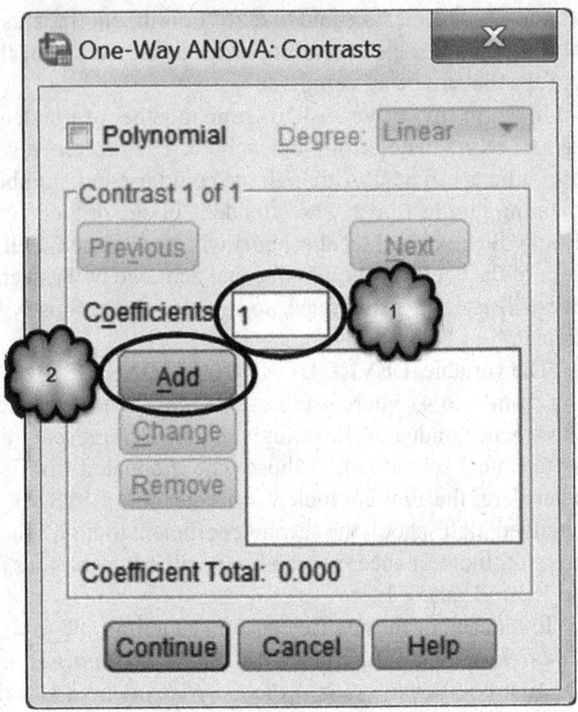

Fig. 10.16 Adding the first of four contrast coefficients

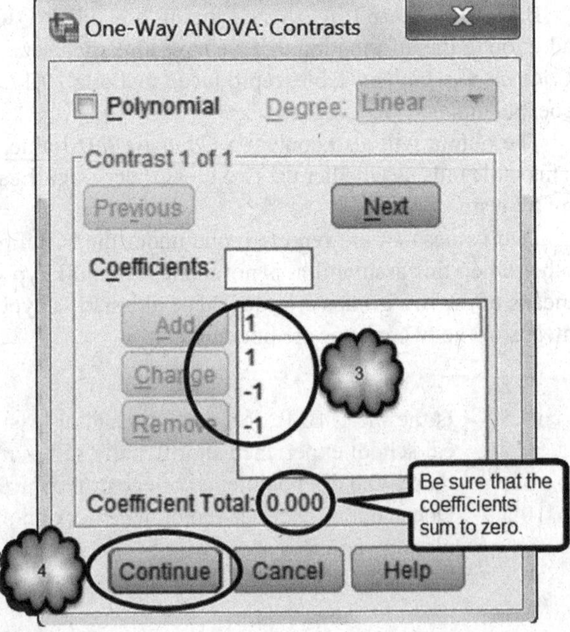

Fig. 10.17 Four contrast coefficients to test the mean BMI of New Yorkers with no more than a high school education against the mean BMI of New Yorkers with at least some postsecondary education

Table 10.17 The four contrast coefficients

Contrast Coefficients

Contrast	LEVEL OF EDUCATION COMPLETED: Did not Graduate High School	Graduated High School	Attended College or Technical School	Graduated from College or Technical School
1	1	1	-1	-1

Table 10.18 Contrast testing the mean BMI of New Yorkers with no more than a high school education against the mean BMI of New Yorkers with at least some postsecondary education

Contrast Tests

		Contrast	Value of Contrast	Std. Error	t	df	Sig. (2-tailed)
BODY MASS INDEX	Assume equal variances	1	2.8206	.30690	9.191	7386	.000
	Does not assume equal variances	1	2.8206	.31780	8.875	1760.526	.000

10.6 Exercise Questions

1. Using the CDC data set, conduct a *t*-test for independent samples to determine if the number of minutes of weekly vigorous physical activity in which people engage varies between those who are overweight or obese and those who are neither overweight nor obese. Number of minutes is stored in the variable, **MINUTES OF VIGOROUS PHYSICAL ACTIVITY** [@*_VIGPAMN*] (variable 95). BMI categories are stored in the variable, **RISK FACTOR FOR OVERWEIGHT OR OBESE** [@*_RFBMI4*] (variable 80; 1 = No, 2 = Yes).
   a. What was the average number of minutes of vigorous activity for those who were neither overweight nor obese (people coded as "No")?
   b. What was the average number of minutes of vigorous activity for those who were either overweight or obese?
   c. What is the numerical difference between the two averages?
   d. Can we assume that the variance in the number of minutes of vigorous activity is the same across the two BMI categories? Why or why not?
   e. How many degrees of freedom are associated with the *t*-value that would be appropriate to use in the analysis?
   f. Do the data indicate that you can reject the null hypothesis that the two population mean number of minutes differ? Why or why not?
2. Conduct a one-way ANOVA to determine if on average the number of minutes of weekly vigorous activity varies among three groups: those who are neither overweight nor obese, those who are overweight, and those who are obese. BMI category is stored in the variable, **BODY MASS INDEX-THREE LEVELS CATEGORY** [@*_BMI4CAT*] (variable 79). Be sure that 9 is declared as a

Table 10.19 Descriptive Statistics

BMI category	Mean	Standard deviation
Neither overweight nor obese		
Overweight		
Obese		

missing value for the BMI variable. Include in your analysis Bonferroni or Tamhane T2 tests, whichever is more appropriate.

a. Complete the table of descriptive statistics (Table 10.19).
b. Should we use one of the robust tests of equality of means to test the null hypothesis that the three population means are equal? Why or why not?
c. How many numerator degrees of freedom are associated with the test statistic that we should use?
d. Do the data indicate that the three population means differ across the three BMI categories?
e. Which post hoc test is more appropriate for these data, Bonferroni or Tamhane? Why?
f. Which of the following statements is supported by the analysis. On average, minutes of weekly vigorous activity differed significantly between:

    i. People who were neither overweight nor obese and people who were overweight.
    ii. People who were neither overweight nor obese and people who were obese.
    iii. People who were overweight and people who were obese.

3. Using a contrast, determine if the mean BMI of college and technical school graduates is significantly different from the mean BMI of the remainder of the sample. Educational level is stored in **LEVEL OF EDUCATION COMPLETED** [@_*EDUCAG*] (variable 82). Be sure that 9 has been declared as missing.

    a. What are the values of the contrast coefficients?
    b. What are the degrees of freedom associated with this contrast if equal variances cannot be assumed?
    c. What is the *t*-value associated with this contrast if equal variances cannot be assumed?
    d. Can we reject the null hypothesis that the mean BMI of college and technical school graduates is equal to the mean BMI of the rest of the population?

4. Using the Framingham data set and partial eta squared, determine the strength of relationship between **Body Mass Index** [*bmi*] (variable 8) and **Gender** [*sex*] (variable 1) and between **Body Mass Index** and **Coronary Heart Disease** [*chdfate*] (variable 5).

Table 10.20 Test of homogeneity of variances for Question 5

Test of Homogeneity of Variances

	Levene Statistic	df1	df2	Sig.
Prostate-Specific Antigen Level (ng/ml)	38.905	1	299	.000
Log PSA	1.350	1	299	.246

Table 10.21 One-way analysis of variance for Question 5

ANOVA

		Sum of Squares	df	Mean Square	F	Sig.
Prostate-Specific Antigen Level (ng/ml)	Between Groups	6349.643	1	6349.643	23.899	.000
	Within Groups	79440.520	299	265.687		
	Total	85790.163	300			
Log PSA	Between Groups	7.310	1	7.310	37.141	.000
	Within Groups	58.846	299	.197		
	Total	66.155	300			

a. Is gender significantly related to BMI? How do you know?
b. Is coronary heart disease significantly related to BMI?
c. What are the values of partial eta squared for the relationships between BMI and gender, and BMI and coronary heart disease?
d. Does BMI seem to be more strongly related to gender or to coronary heart disease?

5. A researcher wished to know whether average PSA levels differ between patients with prostate cancer and patients without. Suspecting that the variance in PSA scores could not be assumed to be equal across the two groups, she performed a log transformation and included log PSA values in her one-way ANOVA. The software that she used did not include robust tests of equality of means, but it did generate Tables 10.20 and 10.21. Which *F* ratio should she report? Why?

6. Using the Sit-and-Reach Test, a team of physician assistant students measured the flexibility of three groups of collegiate athletes: football players, male athletes playing a sport other than football, and female athletes playing any sport [3]. The *F* ratio was significant so the researchers conducted post hoc comparisons. Tables 10.22 and 10.23 are fragments of the output generated by a one-way ANOVA.

   After inspecting these results, the team conducted a contrast in which they compared the mean flexibility of both groups of male athletes against the mean flexibility of the female athletes. The results are displayed in Table 10.24.

Table 10.22 Descriptive statistics for Question 6

Flexibility

	N	Mean	Std. Deviation	Std. Error
Football Players	96	33.0862	7.36286	.75147
Males Playing Another Sport	30	31.9704	8.99715	1.64265
Female Athletes	24	37.6088	6.93294	1.41518
Total	150	33.5867	7.81231	.63787

Table 10.23 Post hoc multiple comparisons for Question 6

Multiple Comparisons

Dependent Variable: Flexibility

Tamhane

(I) Group	(J) Group	Mean Difference (I-J)	Std. Error	Sig.
Football Players	Males Playing Another Sport	1.11586	1.80638	.903
	Female Athletes	-4.52257*	1.60232	.023
Males Playing Another Sport	Football Players	-1.11586	1.80638	.903
	Female Athletes	-5.63843*	2.16818	.036
Female Athletes	Football Players	4.52257*	1.60232	.023
	Males Playing Another Sport	5.63843*	2.16818	.036

*. The mean difference is significant at the 0.05 level.

Table 10.24 Contrast tests for Question 6

Contrast Tests

		Contrast	Value of Contrast	Std. Error	t	df	Sig. (2-tailed)
Flexibility	Assume equal variances	1	-10.1610	3.50921	-2.896	147	.004
	Does not assume equal variances	1	-10.1610	3.35767	-3.026	41.746	.004

a. According to the post hoc comparisons, was the average flexibility of the two groups of male athletes significantly different?
b. What conclusion should we draw from the contrast?

Data Sets and References

1. CDC BRFSS.sav obtained from: Centers for Disease Control and Prevention (CDC): Behavioral Risk Factor Surveillance System Survey Data. US Department of Health and Human Services, Centers for Disease Control and Prevention, Atlanta (2005). Public domain. For more information about the BRFSS, visit http://www.cdc.gov/brfss/. Accessed 16 Nov 2014
2. Framingham.sav obtained from: Dupont, W.D.: Statistical Modeling for Biomedical Researchers, 2nd edn. Cambridge University Press, New York (2009). (With the kind permission of Sean Coady, National Heart, Blood, and Lung Institute)
3. From: Barker, S., Jerome, J., Woods, D., Zaika, C., Brown, R.G., Holmes, W.H.: The Sit and Reach Test as a Measure of Flexibility for Predicting Lower Extremity Injury in Division III Athletes. Unpublished data. Le Moyne College, Syracuse (2010)

[illegible]

a. [illegible] Discuss [illegible]
b. What considerations should we [illegible]?

Data Sets and References

[illegible]

Chapter 11
Comparing Means of Related Samples

Abstract This chapter reviews the paired-samples *t*-test and the repeated measures analysis of variance (ANOVA). These are inferential statistics commonly used to test the difference between the means of populations that are related to each other, such as the means of a quantitative measurement taken of the same group of participants on two or more occasions. Because the ANOVA assumes the presence of a condition known as sphericity, the chapter also reviews Mauchly's test of sphericity and methods for hypothesis testing when sphericity cannot be assumed.

11.1 Overview

In the previous chapter, we considered analyses that compare quantitative measurements taken from independent groups of participants. The procedures were the independent samples *t*-test when there were two groups and the one-way ANOVA when there were three or more groups. There are, however, many situations when it is more desirable to take multiple measurements on the same participant. For example, the blood pressure of hypertensive patients who had received a new treatment might be compared to the blood pressure of the same group of patients before they had received the treatment. In this type of study, researchers are said to be using a *paired comparisons* analysis. Sometimes three or more sets of observations are made of the same group of participants. In this type of study, researchers are said to be using a *repeated measures* analysis.

Ideally, the observations will have been made within the context of a controlled experiment or randomized controlled trial. This type of study can determine the causal impact of an explanatory variable on a response variable. In such experiments, the advantage of paired comparisons and repeated measures analyses is that, because the measurements are being made on the same subject, any differences detected across those measurements can be more confidently attributed to the explanatory variable under investigation rather than to some patient-related factor that might have been confounded with the treatment.

For example, imagine that we conduct a parallel-groups trial in which we give a new treatment for hypertension to one group of patients and a standard treatment to another. Imagine further that because of genetic factors, the blood pressure of some

W. H. Holmes, W. C. Rinaman, *Statistical Literacy for Clinical Practitioners*,
DOI 10.1007/978-3-319-12550-3_11

of our patients is innately higher than some of the others. To control for these genetic factors, we randomly decide which patient receives which treatment. We find that the posttreatment average blood pressure of the patients given the new treatment is lower than that of the patients given the standard treatment. We also find that the results of a *t*-test for independent samples support the hypothesis that this difference can be generalized to the population from which the patients were taken, that is, the difference between the average blood pressure of the two groups was not due solely to chance. In this situation, we could be confident that the difference in average blood pressure between the two groups was not due to differences between the two groups in their genetic makeup. But we could not be certain. Despite the random assignment of the patients to the two treatment groups, it would still be possible that, just by chance, the genetic makeup of the two treatment groups differed, and differed enough to cause the observed difference in their average blood pressure readings.

Now imagine that we conduct a crossover trial in which we give each patient the standard treatment and after some specified period of time measure his or her blood pressure. We then give each patient the new treatment and after the same specified amount of time has passed, take his or her blood pressure again. We compare the two blood pressure readings of each patient and discover that on average, the blood pressure reading following the new treatment is lower. We also find that the results of a statistical test allow us to generalize our findings to the population from which the sample of patients was taken. In this situation, both treatment groups consisted of the same set of patients, so we could be certain that genetic factors were not responsible for our observed difference in blood pressure between the new and standard treatments.

Although experiments can generate confident cause-and-effect conclusions, it is often necessary in medical research to make comparisons across multiple measurements that were taken outside the context of an experiment. For example, we might conduct a prospective cohort study of air traffic controllers to see if hypertension is associated with long-term exposure to stress. Here, the results of a hypothesis test would still reveal if any increases in the response variable (in our example, blood pressure) can be confidently generalized to the population from which the sample was taken, but we would not be able to establish with confidence that the cause of the increase was our explanatory variable (long-term exposure to stress).

In this chapter, we study two statistical tests that are used when researchers compare measurements of a quantitative response variable taken from the same set of participants on two or more occasions. If two measurements are taken, a paired comparisons analysis is carried out by conducting a *paired-samples t-test:* The difference between the two measurements on each subject is calculated, the mean difference across all subjects is computed, and the resulting sample of differences is subjected to the one-sample *t*-test from Chap. 5. When there are three or more quantitative measurements taken on the same group of subjects, a repeated measures analysis is carried out by conducting a *repeated measures analysis of variance* (also known as a *repeated measures ANOVA*) to compare the means of these multiple measurements. This analysis is analogous to how we used one-way ANOVA to compare the means of three or more independent groups in the previous chapter.

We will begin with the paired-samples *t*-test and compare the severity of headaches experienced by patients before and after acupuncture. We will then repeat the analysis using the repeated measures procedure.

11.2 Paired-Samples *T*-Test

The file, **Acupuncture.sav** [1], consists of data from 401 male and female patients who suffered from chronic headache. For 4 weeks prior to the beginning of the study, patients rated the severity of their headaches along a scale ranging from "No headache" to "Intense, incapacitating headache." From these ratings, a baseline measure of headache severity was computed, such that the higher the rating, the more severe the headache. Each patient was then randomly assigned to one of two conditions: Acupuncture and Control. Patients assigned to the acupuncture group were referred by their general practitioners to acupuncturists who offered weekly sessions for a period of 3 months. Patients in the control group were not referred. Three months (3-month follow-up) and again 12 months (1-year follow-up) later, a second and third measure of headache severity was obtained. We will use a paired-samples *t*-test to compare the baseline and 3-month follow-up ratings of headache severity provided by the patients who were referred to acupuncture treatment.

Begin by loading the file. The group to which each patient was assigned is stored in the variable, **Group** [*group*] (variable 6; 0=Control; 1=Acupuncture). We want to focus on the acupuncture group, so use **Select>Cases** to filter out the control cases. Then select **Analyze>Compare Means>Paired-Samples T-Test** to bring up the *Paired-Samples T-Test* dialog box. Move **Headache Severity at Baseline** [*hs0*] (variable 7) to the *Variable 1* box of the *Paired Variables* window. This can be done either by selecting the variable and clicking the right-pointing arrow or by dragging the variable. Now move the second variable, **Headache Severity at 3 Month Follow-up** [hs3] (variable 8) to the *Variable 2* box. Click **OK**. These steps are shown in Figs. 11.1, 11.2 and 11.3 and 11.4.

Much of the output is presented in Tables 11.1 and 11.2.

As you can see, the output is somewhat different from that of an independent-samples *t*-test. For example, there is no test to determine if the variances of the two populations of scores are significantly different. Since the paired-samples *t*-test begins by subtracting the value of one variable from that of the other variable to get a single sample of differences, we have only one set of scores: the differences between the two variables.

Although the output is not displayed exactly as is the output from an independent-samples *t*-test, you should be able to answer the following questions:

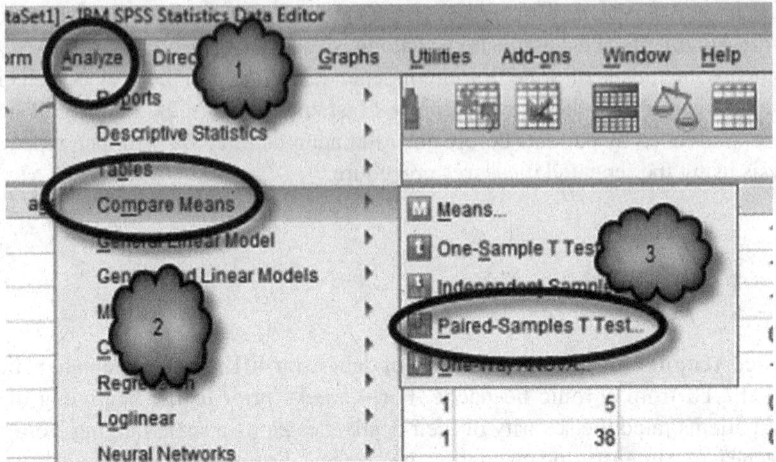

Fig. 11.1 Selecting the paired-samples t-test

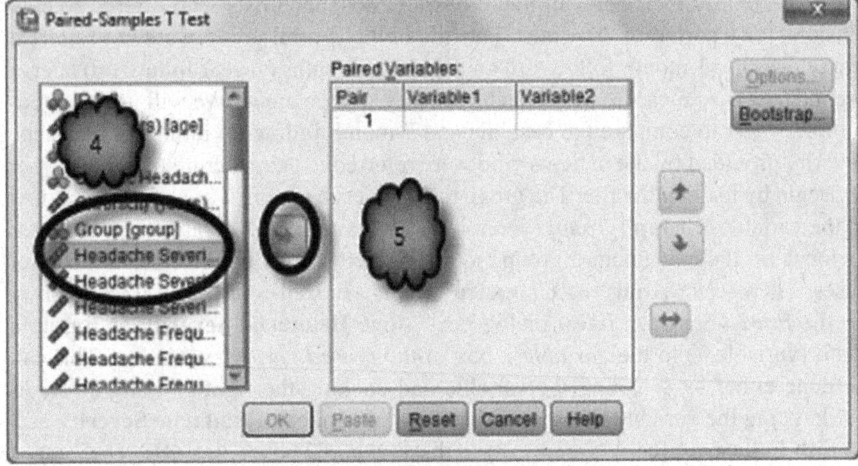

Fig. 11.2 Selecting baseline headache severity

11.2.1 What is the sample size?
11.2.2 What is the average severity rating at baseline? At 3-month follow-up?
11.2.3 What is the average difference in the two sets of ratings?
11.2.4 What is the null hypothesis?
11.2.5 What is the alternative hypothesis? How do you know?
11.2.6 Were the two set of ratings significantly different?

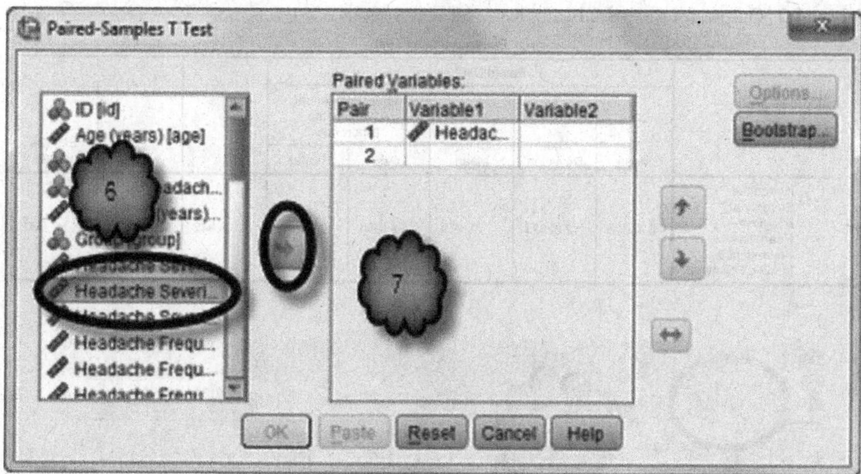

Fig. 11.3 Selecting 3-month headache severity

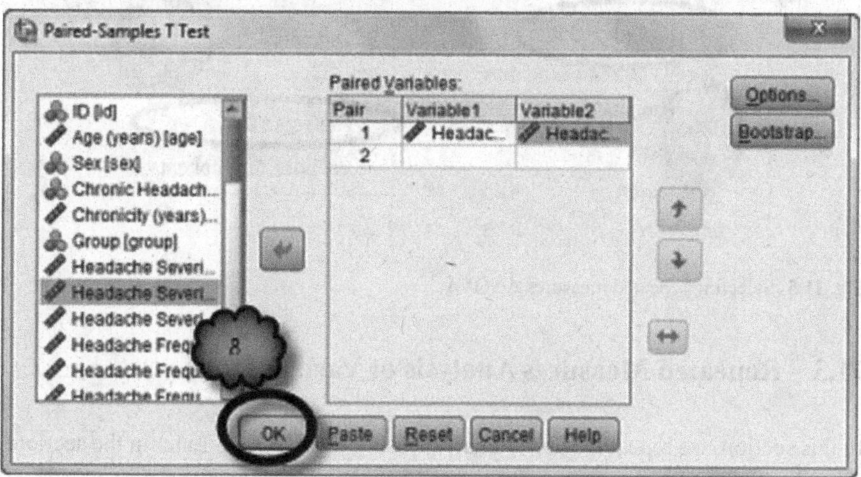

Fig. 11.4 Conducting the analysis

Table 11.1 Summary statistics

Paired Samples Statistics

		Mean	N	Std. Deviation	Std. Error Mean
Pair 1	Headache Severity at Baseline	25.5058	173	15.31463	1.16435
	Headache Severity at 3 Months Follow-up	19.05	173	15.651	1.190

Table 11.2 Output for the paired-samples t-test

Paired Samples Test

		Paired Differences					t	df	Sig. (2-tailed)
		Mean	Std. Deviation	Std. Error Mean	95% Confidence Interval of the Difference Lower	Upper			
Pair 1	Headache Severity at Baseline - Headache Severity at 3 Months Follow-up	6.45376	12.22871	.92973	4.61860	8.28891	6.942	172	.000

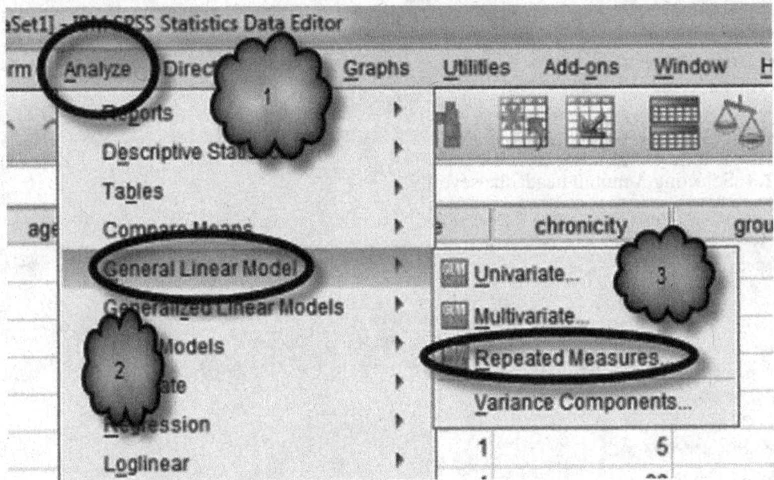

Fig. 11.5 Selecting repeated measures ANOVA

11.3 Repeated Measures Analysis of Variance

In this section, we repeat the above analysis using the ANOVA. Later in the section, we will compare three means.

Comparing Two Means Remember that when we make a pair-wise comparison, we are comparing the scores of one group with a second set of scores from the same set of participants. Therefore, we cannot use the same ANOVA that is used as an alternative to the independent-samples *t*-test. Instead, we must use an ANOVA that is an alternative to the paired-samples *t*-test. In the language of analysis of variance, we need to conduct what is called a *repeated measures ANOVA*. The term "repeated measures" denotes that two or more measurements were taken of each case, i.e., each participant was measured more than once.

As shown in Figs. 11.5, 11.6, 11.7, 11.8, 11.9 and 11.10, select **Analyze > General Linear Model > Repeated Measures** to open the *Repeated Measures Define Factor(s)* dialog box. Type a name for our repeated measures variable into the box labeled, *Within-Subject Factor Name*. For example, you could type in "Time" (no

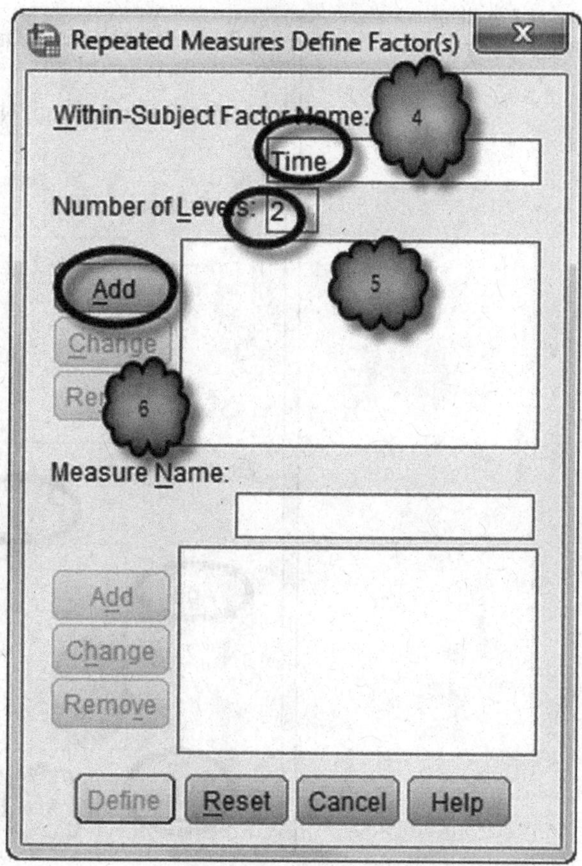

Fig. 11.6 Creating a within factor

quotation marks) to indicate that we are making a comparison over time. In the *Number of Levels* box, enter the number of levels or values of the repeated measures factor. We have two values—baseline and 3-month follow-up—so enter "2" (again no quotation marks). Click the **Add** button in the *Number of Levels* area. Next, enter into the *Measure Name* box a name of the variable that was assessed. The severity of each patient's headache was measured, so you might type "Severity" into the box. Click **Add** in the *Measure Name* area. Now click **Define** to bring up the *Repeated Measures* dialog box. In the Repeated Measures dialog box, highlight **Headache Severity at Baseline** and move it into the *Within-Subjects Variable* window by clicking the right-pointing arrow or by dragging the variable over. Then move **Headache Severity at 3-Month Follow-up** into the same window. Now click **Options** to bring up the *Repeated Measures: Options* dialog box. Move the entries *(OVERALL)* and *Time* from the *Factor(s) and Factor Interactions* box on the left to the *Display Means for* box on the right. This will tell SPSS to print the overall mean and the means for the two groups of data (that is, the mean headache severity at baseline and the mean headache severity at 3-month follow-up). In the *Display* area, select *Descriptive statistics* so we can generate standard deviations and such. Click **Continue** and then **OK**.

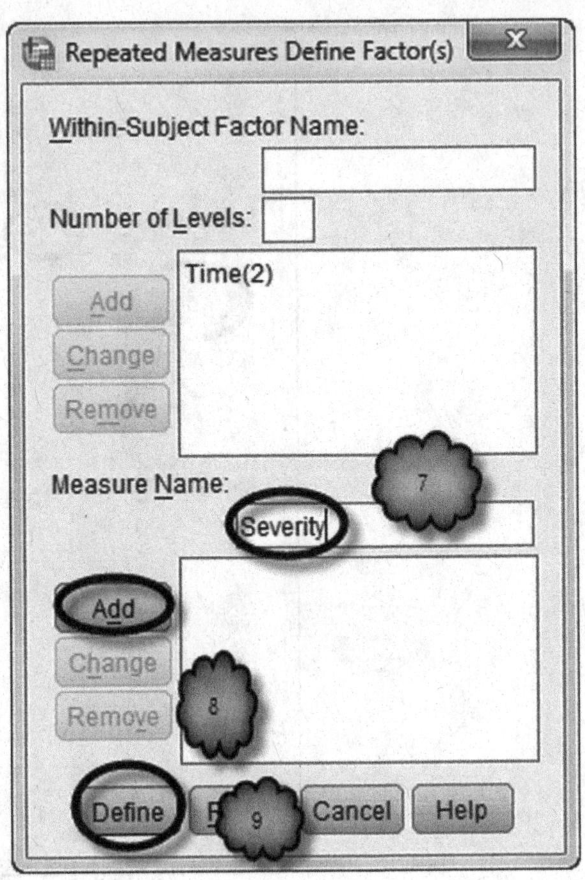

Fig. 11.7 Adding a measure name

Output from a repeated measures ANOVA can be complex, but fortunately, we need be concerned with only a subset of it, reproduced in Tables 11.3, 11.4, 11.5 and 11.6.

Table 11.3, titled *Descriptive Statistics,* reports the means, standard deviations and sample size of the repeated measurements.

Table 11.4, titled *2. Time,* reports means, standard errors, and confidence intervals of the repeated measures variable, in our case, *Time*.

11.3.1 How do the values of the statistics in the above tables compare to those in Sect. 11.2?

The *Mauchly's Test of Sphericity* table shown in Table 11.5 gives the results of a test of sphericity. Roughly speaking, sphericity is analogous to the requirement in one-way ANOVA that every group has the same variance. The null hypothesis is

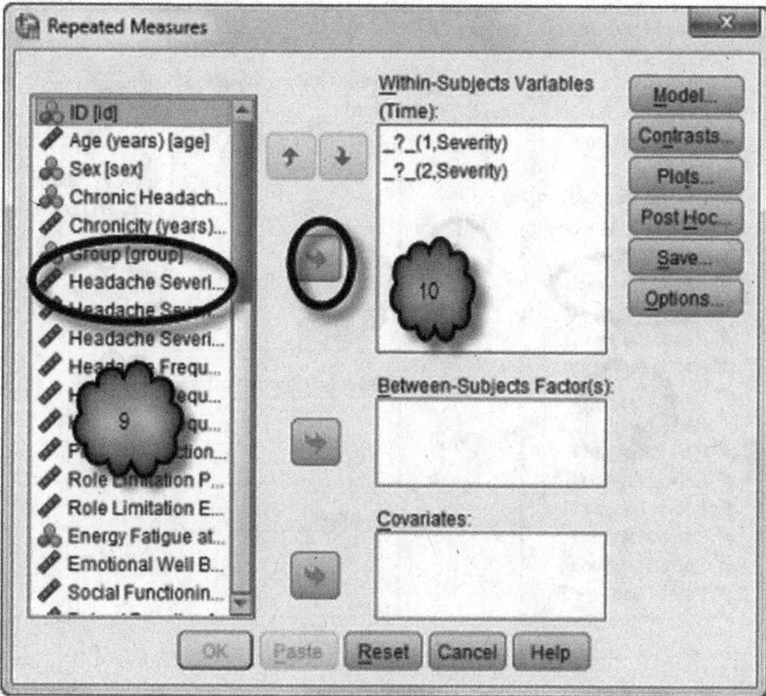

Fig. 11.8 Selecting the first within-subjects variable

that there is sphericity, and the alternative hypothesis is that sphericity is not present. If the test is significant, one of the adjustments—Greenhouse-Geisser, Hyunh-Feldt, or Lower-bound—in the *Tests of Within-Subjects Effects* table has to be used. Sphericity is relevant when the repeated measures factor has three or more values. As we have only two values (baseline and 3-month follow-up), we can move on.

In the *Tests of Within-Subjects Effects* table, shown in Table 11.6, we find the *F* ratio, the degrees of freedom, and the *p*-value. These statistics are interpreted in the same way as those of ANOVA tables we have encountered before.

11.3.2 What is the *F* ratio?
11.3.3 What are the degrees of freedom associated with the *F* ratio?
11.3.4 What is the *p*-value?

Comparing More than Two Means Repeated measures ANOVA can be used to compare three or more measurements on subjects. Just as we could view one-way ANOVA as an extension of the independent samples *t*-test to more than two independent samples, we can view repeated measures ANOVA as an extension of the paired-samples *t*-test to more than two measurements. Also, as with one-way

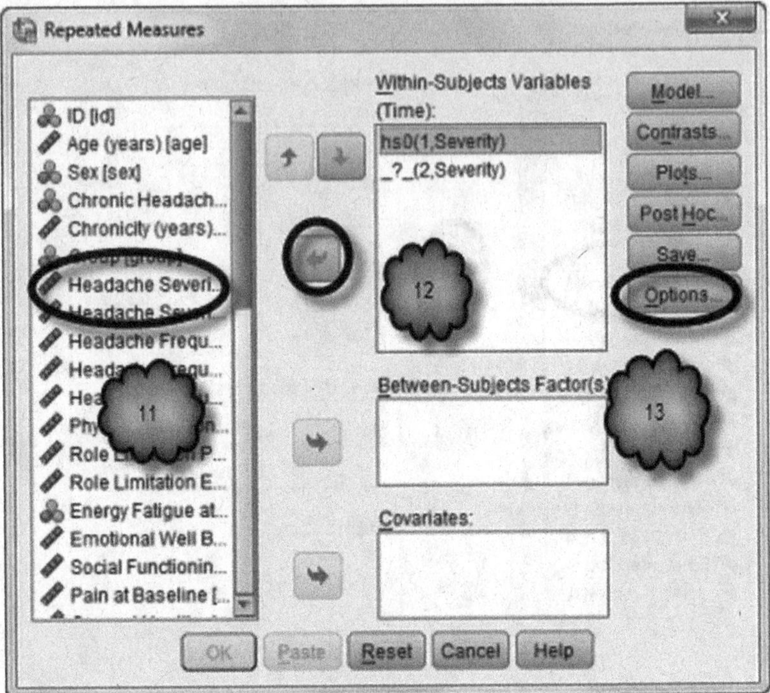

Fig. 11.9 Defining the second within-subjects variable and selecting Options

ANOVA, when we determine that there is a difference in treatment levels we can conduct multiple comparisons to try to ascertain how the treatment levels differ. To demonstrate, we will once again analyze the headache severity ratings of the acupuncture study, but this time we will include ratings from the 1-year follow-up.

Return to the *Repeated Measures Define Factor(s)* dialog box. In this analysis, we are adding a third measurement—severity ratings at 1-year follow-up. These data are stored in the variable, **Headache Severity at 1-Year Follow-up** [*hs12*] (variable 9). So first we need to tell SPSS that we now have three levels of our *Time* factor. To do this, highlight *Time(2),* change the *Number of Levels* from 2 to 3, and click **Change**. To add the third measurement to the analysis, click **Define** to open the *Repeated Measures* dialog box and move **Headache Severity at 1-Year Follow-up** to the *Within-Subjects Variable* window. Because we now are comparing three means, we may want to conduct a multiple comparisons analysis, so click **Options,** check *Compare main effects* and select *Bonferroni* in the *Confidence interval adjustment* box. Click **Continue.**

When measurements are taken over time from the same set of participants, it is often useful to display the means of each of those measurements in a graph called a *means plot.* We could construct such a graph with *Chart Builder* but we can also

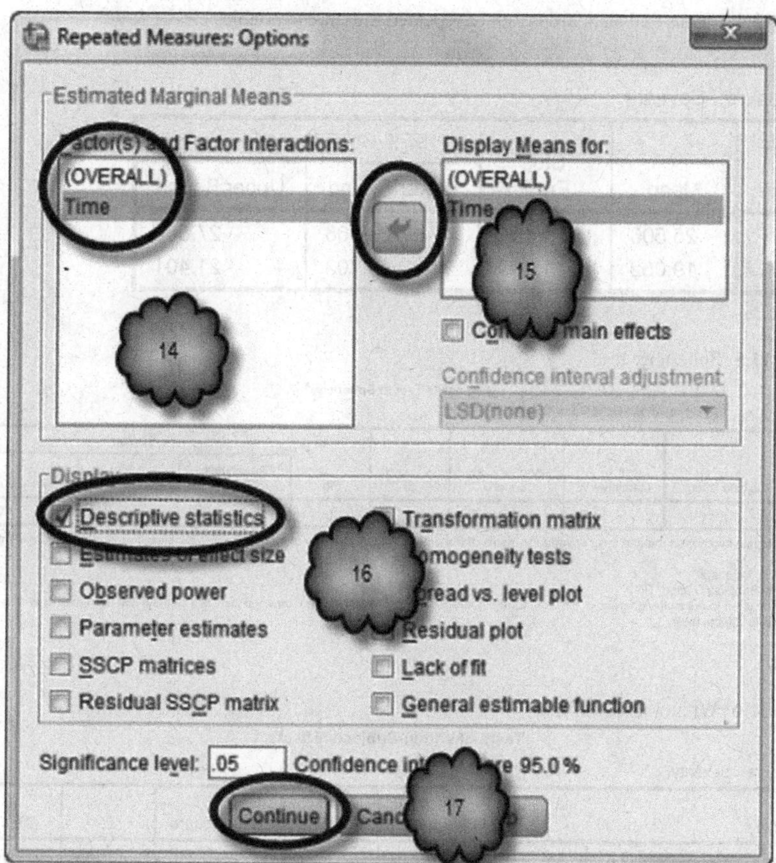

Fig. 11.10 Generating descriptive statistics

Table 11.3 Descriptive statistics

Descriptive Statistics

	Mean	Std. Deviation	N
Headache Severity at Baseline	25.5058	15.31463	173
Headache Severity at 3 Months Follow-up	19.05	15.651	173

do so from within the ANOVA dialog boxes. Back in the *Repeated Measures* dialog box, click **Plots,** move **Time** to the *Horizontal Axis* window, click **Add** and then **Continue.** Click **OK** to conduct the analysis. These steps are shown in Figs. 11.11, 11.12, 11.13 and 11.14.

Table 11.4 Means and standard errors of repeated measures variables

2. Time

Measure: Severity

Time	Mean	Std. Error	95% Confidence Interval	
			Lower Bound	Upper Bound
1	25.506	1.164	23.208	27.804
2	19.052	1.190	16.703	21.401

Table 11.5 Sphericity test

Mauchly's Test of Sphericity[a]

Measure: Severity

Within Subjects Effect	Mauchly's W	Approx. Chi-Square	df	Sig.	Epsilon[b]		
					Greenhouse-Geisser	Huynh-Feldt	Lower-bound
Time	1.000	.000	0	.	1.000	1.000	1.000

Tests the null hypothesis that the error covariance matrix of the orthonormalized transformed dependent variables is proportional to an identity matrix.

a. Design: Intercept
Within Subjects Design: Time

b. May be used to adjust the degrees of freedom for the averaged tests of significance. Corrected tests are displayed in the Tests of Within-Subjects Effects table.

Table 11.6 Within-subjects tests

Tests of Within-Subjects Effects

Measure: Severity

Source		Type III Sum of Squares	df	Mean Square	F	Sig.
Time	Sphericity Assumed	3602.810	1	3602.810	48.185	.000
	Greenhouse-Geisser	3602.810	1.000	3602.810	48.185	.000
	Huynh-Feldt	3602.810	1.000	3602.810	48.185	.000
	Lower-bound	3602.810	1.000	3602.810	48.185	.000
Error(Time)	Sphericity Assumed	12860.551	172	74.771		
	Greenhouse-Geisser	12860.551	172.000	74.771		
	Huynh-Feldt	12860.551	172.000	74.771		
	Lower-bound	12860.551	172.000	74.771		

The interpretation of the repeated measures output, shown in Tables 11.7, 11.8, 11.9 and 11.10, is the same as the interpretation of the output we saw earlier in this chapter.

The *Pair-wise Comparisons* output shown in Table 11.11 is similar to the multiple comparisons output we studied in the preceding chapter, and is interpreted in the same manner.

The means plot displays the three mean ratings across the three points in time. The values of the means are plotted along the y-axis. The points in time (baseline, 3-months follow-up and 1-year follow-up) are plotted along the x-axis from left to right (Fig. 11.15).

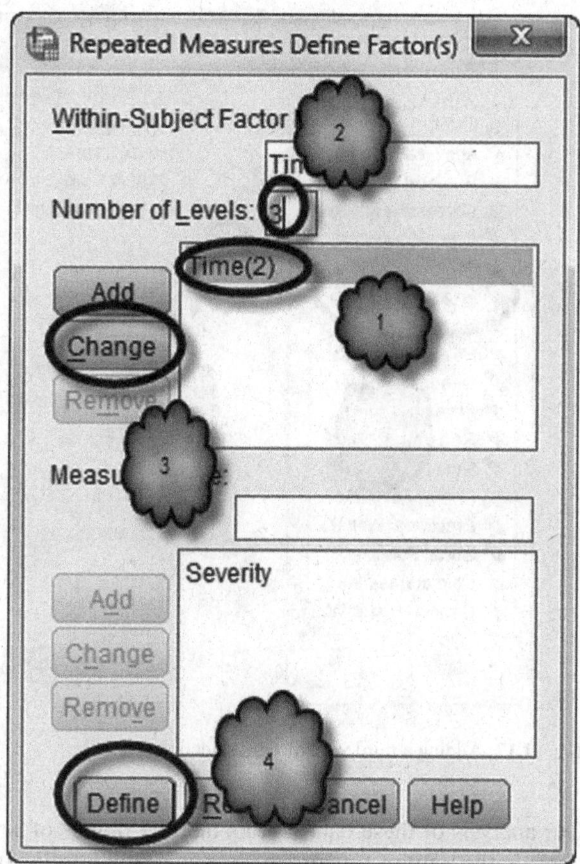

Fig. 11.11 Changing the number of levels

Study the output and answer the following questions:

11.3.5 Is Mauchly's Test of Sphericity significant?

11.3.6 Will you need to adjust for lack of sphericity?

11.3.7 Regarding the mean severity ratings at baseline, 3-month follow-up and 1-year follow-up, what are the null and alternative hypotheses?

11.3.8 What is the *F* ratio?

11.3.9 What are the numerator and denominator degrees of freedom associated with the *F* ratio?

11.3.10 What is the *p*-value?

11.3.11 Can we reject the null hypothesis in favor of the alternative?

11.3.12 What does the means plot tell us about how the ratings of severity changed over time?

11.3.13 According to the pair-wise comparisons, can we confidently conclude that for the population of patients who suffer from chronic headache and who are referred to acupuncture for treatment, headache severity will be less at 1-year follow-up than at 3-month follow-up? Why or why not?

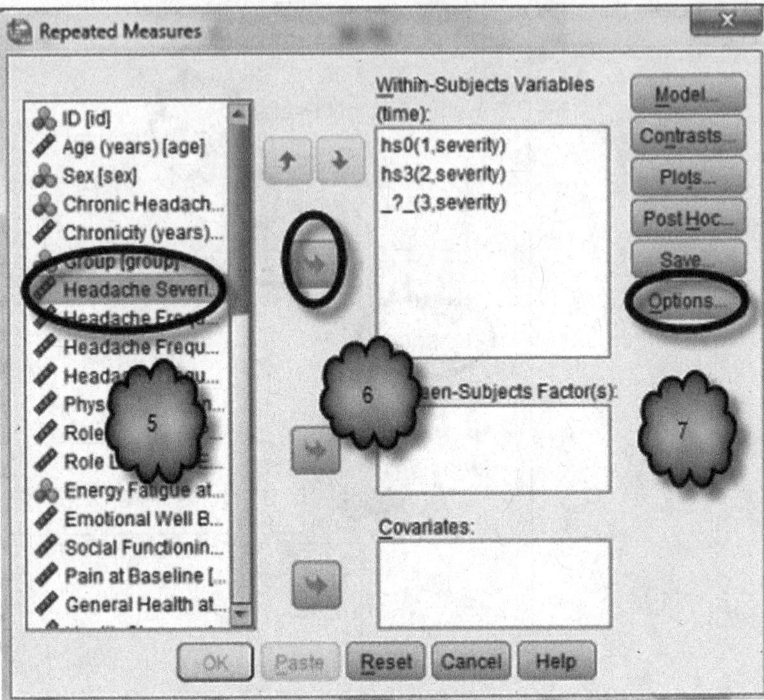

Fig. 11.12 Adding a third variable and selecting Options

Our analysis of these data reveals that the ratings of severity provided by the patients in the acupuncture group were at 3-month follow-up significantly lower than the ratings they provided at the beginning of the study. Because the 3-month follow-up ratings were obtained after the patients had received a series of acupuncture sessions, it would be tempting to conclude that the acupuncture treatment was responsible for the decline in reported severity. However, before we can draw this conclusion, we should consider the possibility that those severity ratings might have declined over time even if the patients had not received acupuncture. To evaluate this possibility, we will need to determine whether the control patients also reported a decline in severity. One way to do this is to repeat our analysis on control patients. We will leave this analysis to you as an exercise. Another would be to include all patients in the analysis—those who had acupuncture and those who did not—and determine in a single analysis whether control patients also reported a decline in severity at 3 months, and if so, whether the decline was significantly less than that reported by the patients who had undergone acupuncture treatment. Such an analysis would require what is called a *two-way analysis of variance,* the topic of the next chapter.

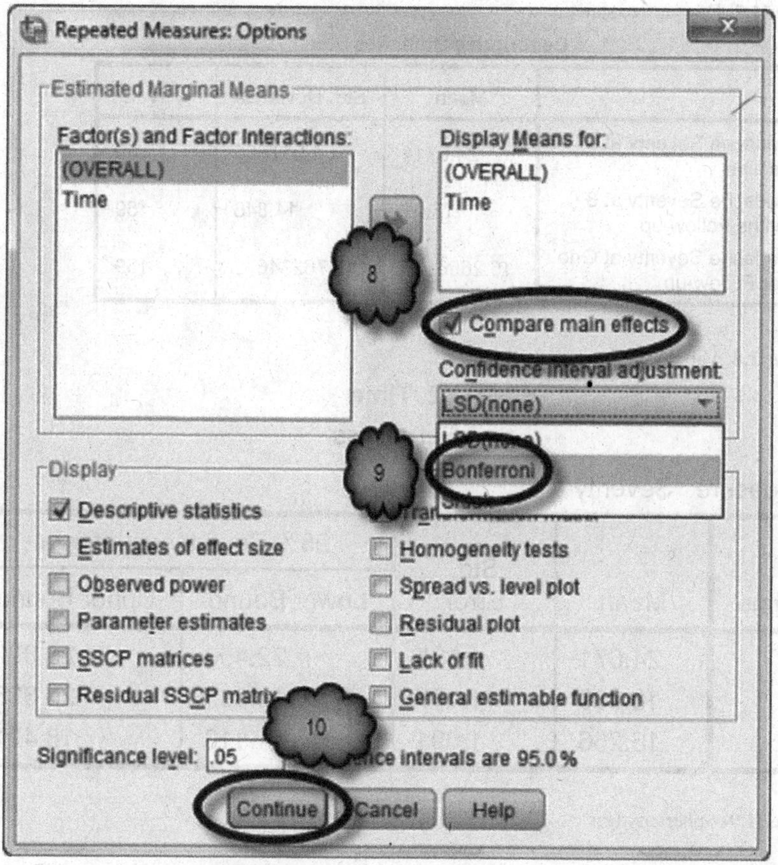

Fig. 11.13 Selecting Bonferroni multiple comparisons

Fig. 11.14 Requesting plots

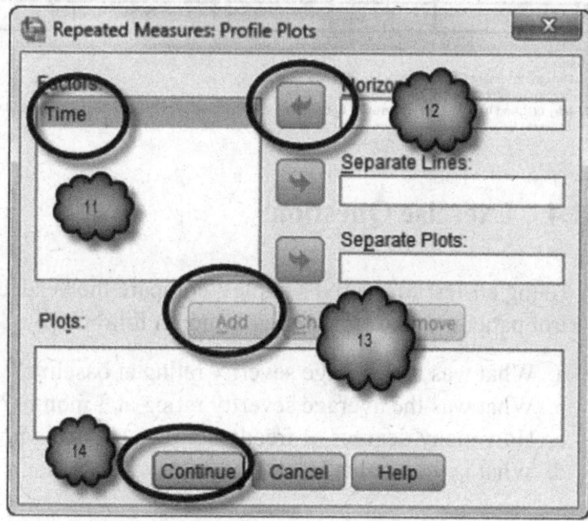

Table 11.7 Descriptive statistics

Descriptive Statistics

	Mean	Std. Deviation	N
Headache Severity at Baseline	24.6714	14.17965	159
Headache Severity at 3 Months Follow-up	18.01	14.846	159
Headache Severity at One Year Follow-up	16.2656185	13.76234672	159

Table 11.8 Variable estimates

2. Time

Estimates

Measure: Severity

Time	Mean	Std. Error	95% Confidence Interval	
			Lower Bound	Upper Bound
1	24.671	1.125	22.450	26.892
2	18.009	1.177	15.684	20.335
3	16.266	1.091	14.110	18.421

Table 11.9 Sphericity test

Mauchly's Test of Sphericity[a]

Measure: Severity

Within Subjects Effect	Mauchly's W	Approx. Chi-Square	df	Sig.	Epsilon[b]		
					Greenhouse-Geisser	Huynh-Feldt	Lower-bound
Time	.992	1.204	2	.548	.992	1.000	.500

Tests the null hypothesis that the error covariance matrix of the orthonormalized transformed dependent variables is proportional to an identity matrix.

a. Design: Intercept
Within Subjects Design: Time

b. May be used to adjust the degrees of freedom for the averaged tests of significance. Corrected tests are displayed in the Tests of Within-Subjects Effects table.

11.4 Exercise Questions

1. Using a *t*-test for paired samples, compare the headache severity ratings of control patients at baseline and at 3-month follow-up.

   a. What was the average severity rating at baseline?
   b. What was the average severity rating at 3 months?
   c. How many degrees of freedom are associated with the *t*-value?
   d. What is the *t*-value?

Table 11.10 Within-subjects tests

Tests of Within-Subjects Effects

Measure: Severity

Source		Type III Sum of Squares	df	Mean Square	F	Sig.
Time	Sphericity Assumed	6258.206	2	3129.103	40.887	.000
	Greenhouse-Geisser	6258.206	1.985	3153.014	40.887	.000
	Huynh-Feldt	6258.206	2.000	3129.103	40.887	.000
	Lower-bound	6258.206	1.000	6258.206	40.887	.000
Error(Time)	Sphericity Assumed	24183.854	316	76.531		
	Greenhouse-Geisser	24183.854	313.604	77.116		
	Huynh-Feldt	24183.854	316.000	76.531		
	Lower-bound	24183.854	158.000	153.062		

Table 11.11 Pair-wise comparisons

Pairwise Comparisons

Measure: Severity

(I) Time	(J) Time	Mean Difference (I-J)	Std. Error	Sig.[b]	95% Confidence Interval for Difference[b] Lower Bound	Upper Bound
1	2	6.662*	.939	.000	4.391	8.933
	3	8.406*	1.011	.000	5.960	10.851
2	1	-6.662*	.939	.000	-8.933	-4.391
	3	1.744	.993	.243	-.658	4.146
3	1	-8.406*	1.011	.000	-10.851	-5.960
	2	-1.744	.993	.243	-4.146	.658

Based on estimated marginal means

*. The mean difference is significant at the .05 level.

b. Adjustment for multiple comparisons: Bonferroni.

e. What is the p-value?
f. Were the ratings of severity on average statistically significantly lower at 3 months?

2. Using a one-way repeated measures ANOVA, compare the headache severity ratings of control patients at baseline, 3-month follow-up, and 1-year follow-up. Include a multiple comparisons analysis and a plot of the three means.

   a. What are the means for each of the severity measurements?
   Baseline: __________
   3-month follow-up: __________
   12-month follow-up: __________

   b. Will you need to adjust for lack of sphericity? Why or why not?
   c. What is the value of the F ratio that compares the three mean severity ratings?

Profile Plots

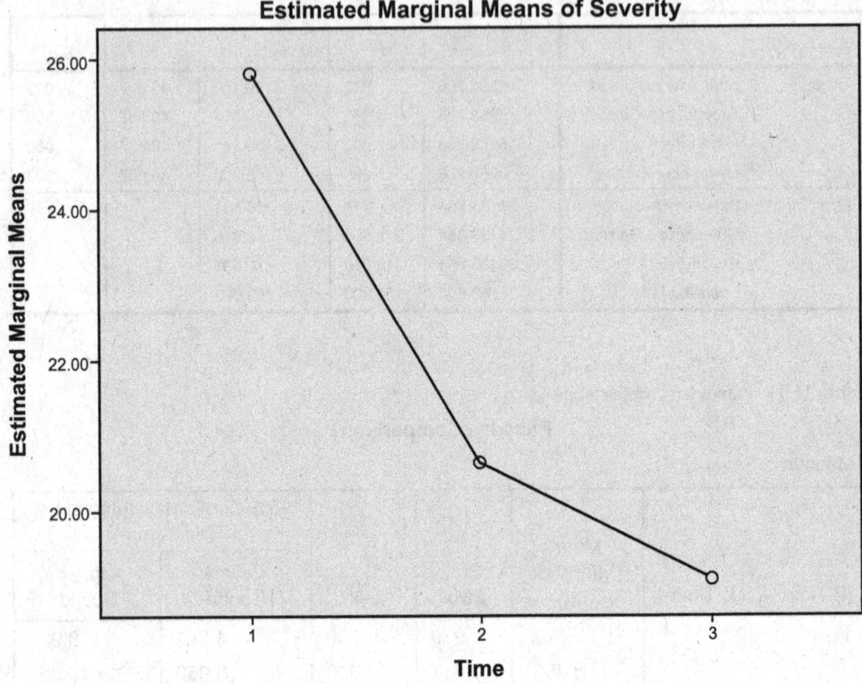

Fig. 11.15 Profile plot

d. What are the numerator and denominator df that are associated with this *F* ratio?
df_n: ___________
df_d: ___________

e. According to the multiple comparisons analysis, was the mean severity rating at 12 months significantly different from the mean severity rating at baseline?

f. Complete the following table:

Mean headache severity ratings			
	Time		
Group	Baseline	3-month follow-up	12-month follow-up
Acupuncture			
Control			

Table 11.12 Output for Question 4

Descriptive Statistics

	Mean	Std. Deviation	N
Body mass at admittance	14.4270	1.78327	20
Preferred body mass	17.3130	2.22382	20
Body mass at discharge	17.7280	3.65422	20

Table 11.13 Output for Question 4

Mauchly's Test of Sphericity[a]

Measure: BMI

Within Subjects Effect	Mauchly's W	Approx. Chi-Square	df	Sig.	Epsilon[b]		
					Greenhouse-Geisser	Huynh-Feldt	Lower-bound
Type_of_BMI	.549	10.807	2	.005	.689	.725	.500

Tests the null hypothesis that the error covariance matrix of the orthonormalized transformed dependent variables is proportional to an identity matrix.
a. Design: Intercept
Within Subjects Design: Type_of_BMI
b. May be used to adjust the degrees of freedom for the averaged tests of significance. Corrected tests are displayed in the Tests of Within-Subjects Effects table.

g. Does it appear from the table that acupuncture reduces headache severity at 3 months? Why or why not?

3. The past two chapters introduced you to two versions of the t-test: independent samples and paired samples.

   a. Which of these two tests should be used to compare the mean severity ratings at 3 months of the acupuncture and control groups? Why?
   b. Conduct the analysis. What is the t-value?
   c. Were the mean severity ratings of the two groups at 3 months significantly different?

4. The file **Bodymass.sav** [2] contains body mass data on 20 anorexia patients. Each patient was measured on admittance, assigned a preferred body mass, and measured body mass on discharge. These data were analyzed with a repeated measures ANOVA. Multiple comparisons were included. Study the output, reproduced in Tables 11.12, 11.13, 11.14 and 11.15.

   a. Do you need to adjust for the lack of sphericity? Why or why not?
   b. What is the value of the F ratio?
   c. Is the F ratio statistically significant?
   d. What do the pair-wise comparisons show about the differences among preferred body mass, body mass at admittance, and body mass on discharge?

Table 11.14 Output for Question 4

Tests of Within-Subjects Effects

Measure: BMI

Source		Type III Sum of Squares	df	Mean Square	F	Sig.
Type_of_BMI	Sphericity Assumed	129.319	2	64.659	12.244	.000
	Greenhouse-Geisser	129.319	1.378	93.846	12.244	.001
	Huynh-Feldt	129.319	1.450	89.158	12.244	.001
	Lower-bound	129.319	1.000	129.319	12.244	.002
Error(Type_of_BMI)	Sphericity Assumed	200.673	38	5.281		
	Greenhouse-Geisser	200.673	26.182	7.665		
	Huynh-Feldt	200.673	27.559	7.282		
	Lower-bound	200.673	19.000	10.562		

Table 11.15 Output for Question 4

Pairwise Comparisons

Measure: BMI

(I) Type_of_BMI	(J) Type_of_BMI	Mean Difference (I-J)	Std. Error	Sig.[b]	95% Confidence Interval for Difference[b]	
					Lower Bound	Upper Bound
1	2	-2.886*	.423	.000	-3.998	-1.774
	3	-3.301*	.804	.002	-5.411	-1.191
2	1	2.886*	.423	.000	1.774	3.998
	3	-.415	.871	1.000	-2.702	1.872
3	1	3.301*	.804	.002	1.191	5.411
	2	.415	.871	1.000	-1.872	2.702

Based on estimated marginal means

*. The mean difference is significant at the .05 level.

b. Adjustment for multiple comparisons: Bonferroni.

Data Sets and References

1. Acupuncuture.sav obtained from: Vickers, A.J., Rees, R.W., Zollman, C.E., et al.: Acupuncture for chronic headache in primary care: large, pragmatic, randomised trial. BMJ. (2004). doi: 10.1136/bmj.38029.421863.EB. (With the kind permission of Professor Andrew J. Vickers)
2. Bodymass.sav obtained from: Hand, D.J., Daly, F., Lunn, A.D., McConway, K.J., Ostrowski, E.: A Handbook of Small Data Sets. Chapman & Hall, London (1994). (With the kind permission of the Routledge Taylor and Francis Group, and Professor Shelley L Channon)

Chapter 12
Analysis of Variance with Two Factors

Abstract Previous chapters have presented statistical techniques for studying the relationship between a response variable and a single explanatory variable. The remaining chapters discuss techniques that investigate the relationship between a response variable and two or more explanatory variables, and that determine whether the impact of one explanatory variable varies across values of a second. In this chapter, two-way analysis of variance, also known as two-way ANOVA, is reviewed. This technique is appropriate when the response variable is quantitative, and is used to test null hypotheses about the main effects of two categorical explanatory variables, and the interaction effect between them. Three examples of two-way ANOVA are discussed: one in which both explanatory variables are independent groups, one in which both are repeated measures, and one in which one variable is independent groups and one is repeated measures.

12.1 Overview

As we saw in the last chapter, in many circumstances researchers wish to compare the means of three or more groups. If the measurements are quantitative, a one-way analysis of variance (ANOVA) is often employed. Unlike the independent samples *t*-test, one-way ANOVA can accommodate more than two means at a time. For example, the blood pressure means of three groups of hypertensive patients—those who had received a new treatment, had received a standard treatment, or had received no treatment—could be compared in a single analysis.

In addition to being able to compare several means simultaneously, ANOVA can also assess the effects of two or more categorical factors in a single analysis, and whether the effect of a factor changes across values of another. For example, a *two-way ANOVA* could assess whether blood pressure was significantly related to the sex of hypertensive patients who had participated in a clinical trial of a new treatment, whether the treatment significantly reduced their blood pressure, and whether the benefit of the treatment was significantly greater for men or women. If race were added to this analysis, a *three-way ANOVA* could be employed to study the individual and combined effects of race, sex, and treatment.

W. H. Holmes, W. C. Rinaman, *Statistical Literacy for Clinical Practitioners*,
DOI 10.1007/978-3-319-12550-3_12

Ideally, the observations will have been made within the context of a controlled experiment in which two or more causal factors were manipulated by the researcher. In these cases, if the results of an ANOVA reveal significant differences across groups, then causality can be established. Often, though, comparisons are made across factors that cannot be manipulated (e.g., gender, race, prior exposure to a risk factor). In these cases, the results of an ANOVA reveal only if differences across groups are statistically significant. The cause of the differences cannot be established.

In theory, there is no limit to the number of factors that can be included in an ANOVA. However, experiments that include a large number of factors can be very expensive and time consuming to conduct. Moreover, the relationships among a large number of factors can be quite complex and difficult to understand. Consequently, researchers seldom conduct an ANOVA that includes more than a handful of factors.

In this chapter, we will focus on the two-way ANOVA. In our first analysis, both factors will be independent groups. In the second analysis, both will be repeated measures. In the third, we will conduct a two-way ANOVA with one independent groups factor and one repeated measures factor.

12.2 ANOVA with One Independent Groups Factor

Before we conduct an ANOVA with two independent groups factors, let us take another look at the one-way ANOVA. Recall that the one-way ANOVA has one independent groups factor. In this section, we will ascertain whether the body mass index (BMI) of female respondents between the ages of 35 and 54, inclusive, is related to engagement in physical activity. Note that in the analysis, we will have a quantitative response variable and a categorical explanatory variable. Note also that an independent-samples *t*-test would be appropriate as an alternative to the ANOVA in this situation as we will be comparing the means of two groups. In this instance, though, we will choose the ANOVA so as to facilitate our later discussion of two-way ANOVA.

Load the data file, **CDC BRFSS.sav** [1]. Begin by assigning labels to the values of the variable, **NO PHYSICAL ACTIVITY OR EXERCISE RISK FACTOR** [*@_RFNOPA*] (variable 102; 1 = Engaged in Physical Activity, 2 = Did not Engage in Physical Activity), and declare the value of 9 as missing. Next, label two of the values of the variable, **SIX LEVEL IMPUTED AGE CATEGORY** [*@_AGE_G*] (variable 74) as follows: 3 = 35 to 44 and 4 = 45 to 54. Then, using **Data > Select Cases**, select female respondents who belong to either the 35 to 44 or 45 to 54 age category. Respondents' sex is stored in **SEX** [*SEX*] (variable 32; 1 = Male, 2 = Female).

SPSS offers two procedures that will carry out an ANOVA involving one independent groups factor. One procedure, called *One-Way ANOVA*, can be used only when there is one explanatory factor and the factor is independent groups. The second procedure, called *General Linear Model* (GLM) is much more flexible.

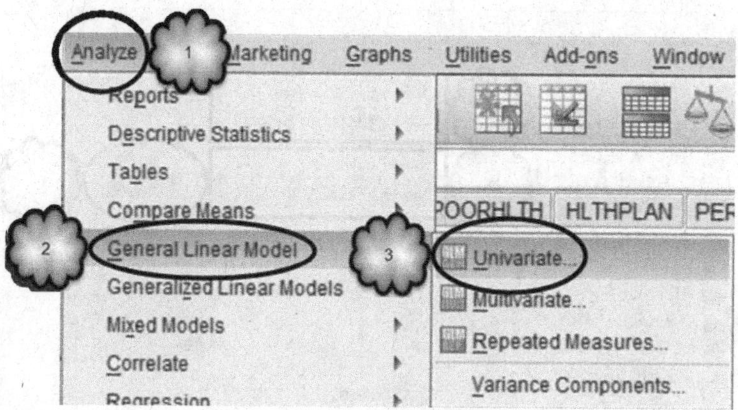

Fig. 12.1 Opening the Univariate dialog

For example, GLM can conduct an ANOVA with two or more factors and the factors can be either independent groups or repeated measures. We will use GLM in this chapter.

As shown in Figs. 12.1 and 12.2, select **Analyze > General Linear Model > Univariate** to bring up the *Univariate* dialog box. Move **BODY MASS INDEX** [*BMI*] (variable 107) into the *Dependent Variable* box. Now move **NO PHYSICAL ACTIVITY OR EXERCISE RISK FACTOR** into the *Fixed Factor(s)* box.

We will want to create a *means plot* so as shown in Fig. 12.2, click **Plots** to bring up the *Univariate: Profile Plots* dialog box. Then as shown in Fig. 12.3, move the physical activity variable into the *Horizontal Axis* box, click **Add,** followed by **Continue**.

Next, we will want to generate some descriptive statistics and an effect size analysis, so in the *Univariates* dialog, click **Options** to bring up the *Univariate: Options* dialog box shown in Fig. 12.4. Move *(OVERALL)* and the physical activity variable to the *Display Means for* box, and check *Descriptive statistics* in the *Display* area. Click **Continue.** Back in the *Univariates* dialog, **click OK.**

Study the resulting output reproduced in Tables 12.1 and 12.2, and Fig. 12.5. The output should have a familiar look, thanks to Chap. 10.

Answer the following questions regarding the null hypothesis that the population BMI means of the two physical activity groups are equal:

12.2.1 What is the mean BMI for each of the two physical activity groups?
12.2.2 Are these means accurately reflected in the means plot?
12.2.3 What is the value of the *F* ratio?
12.2.4 What are the numerator and denominator degrees of freedom?
12.2.5 What is the *p*-value?
12.2.6 Do the data indicate that BMI is related to physical activity for female residents of NY state who are between the ages of 35 and 54?

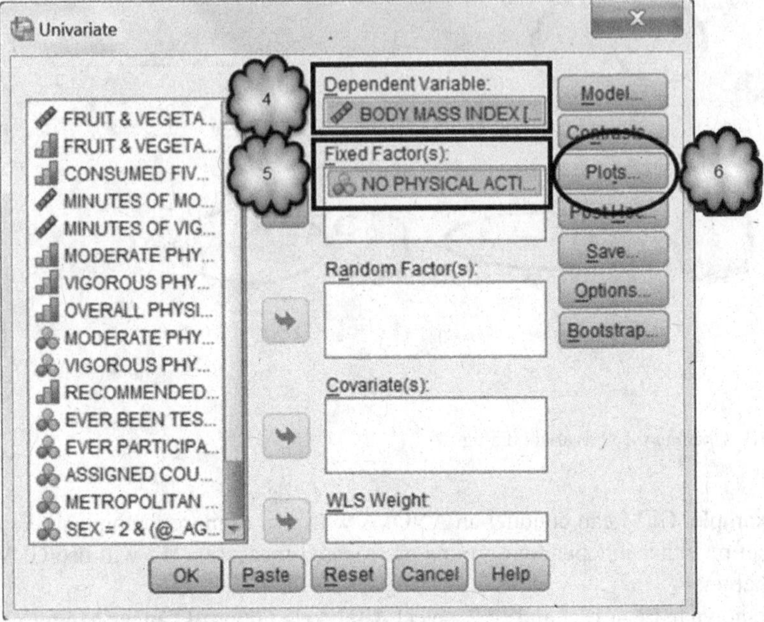

Fig. 12.2 Selecting the dependent variable and fixed factor, and opening the Univariate: Profile Plots dialog

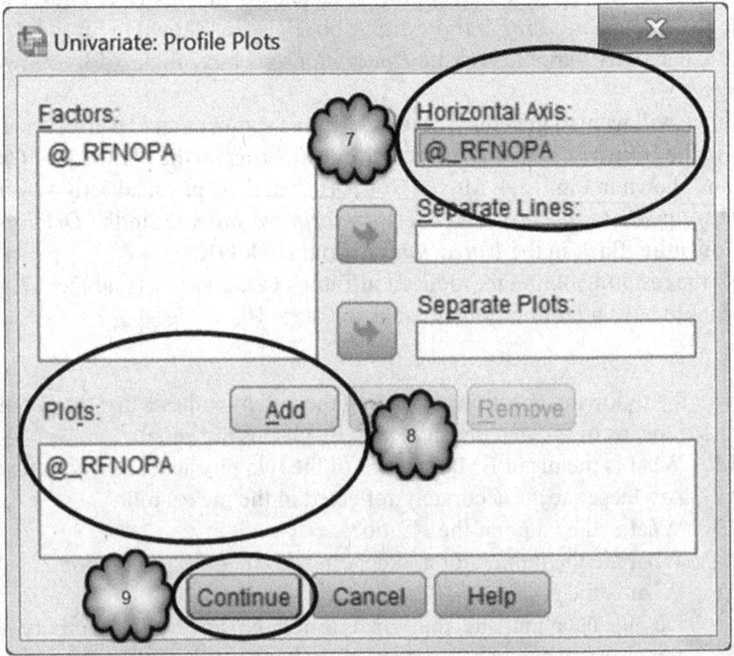

Fig. 12.3 Requesting a means plot of the main effect of physical activity

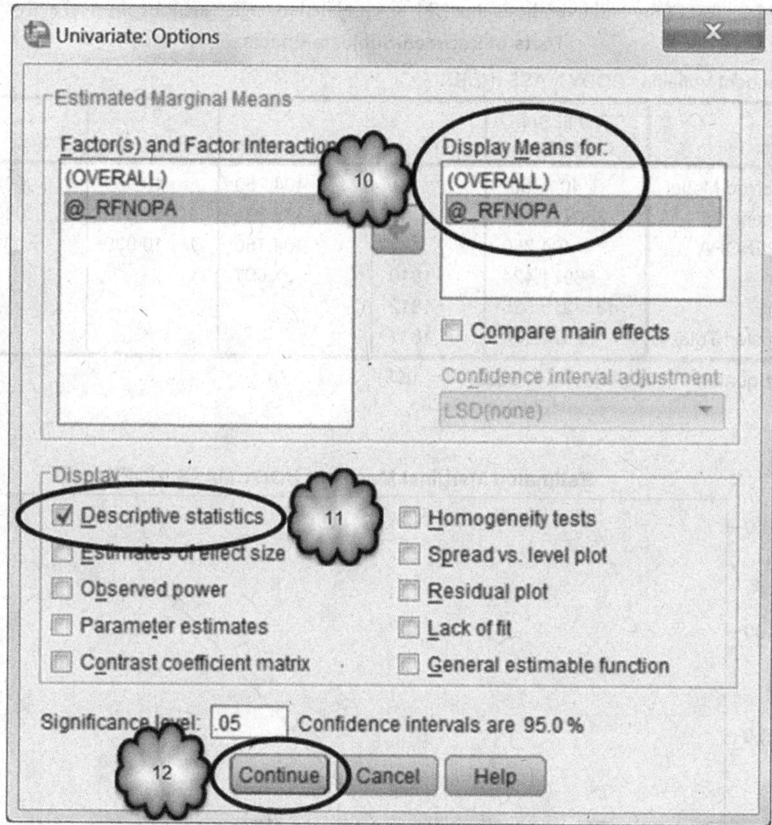

Fig. 12.4 Requesting tables displaying the overall mean, the means of the main effect of age, and descriptive statistics

Table 12.1 Descriptive statistics for no physical activity or exercise risk factor

2. NO PHYSICAL ACTIVITY OR EXERCISE RISK FACTOR

Dependent Variable: BODY MASS INDEX

NO PHYSICAL ACTIVITY OR EXERCISE RISK FACTOR	Mean	Std. Error	95% Confidence Interval	
			Lower Bound	Upper Bound
Engaged in Physical Activity	26.336	.149	26.045	26.628
Did not Engage in Physical Activity	28.112	.516	27.100	29.124

Table 12.2 Test of the null hypothesis that BMI is unrelated to engagement in physical activity

Tests of Between-Subjects Effects

Dependent Variable: BODY MASS INDEX

Source	Type III Sum of Squares	df	Mean Square	F	Sig.
Corrected Model	404.750[a]	1	404.750	10.939	.001
Intercept	380472.394	1	380472.394	10282.819	.000
@_RFNOPA	404.750	1	404.750	10.939	.001
Error	66971.424	1810	37.001		
Total	1337213.025	1812			
Corrected Total	67376.174	1811			

a. R Squared = .006 (Adjusted R Squared = .005)

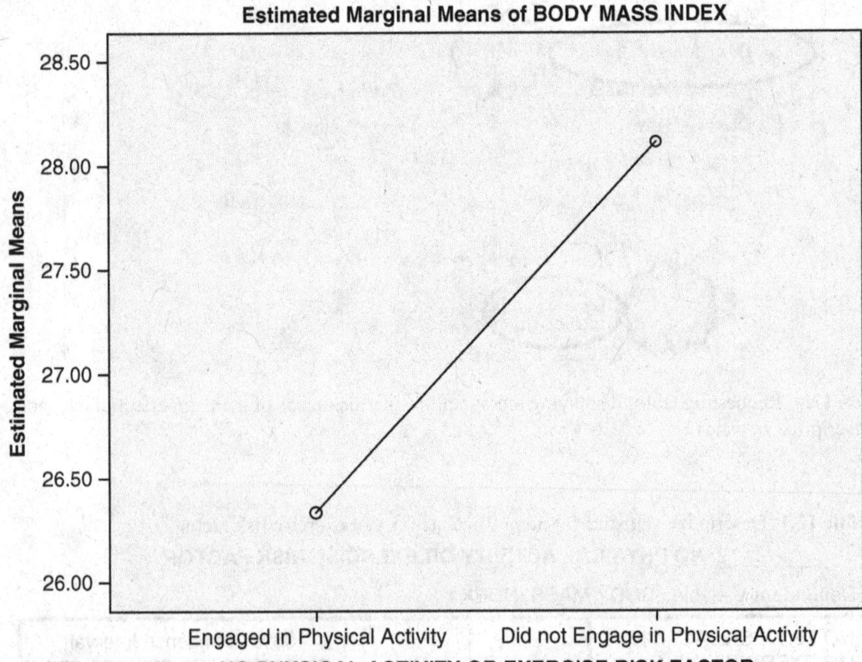

Fig. 12.5 Means plot of the main effect of physical activity on body mass index

12.3 ANOVA with Two Independent Groups Factors

In the previous section, we saw that BMI was significantly related to engagement in physical activity. In the jargon of the ANOVA, we found what is called a significant *main effect* of physical activity. In this section, we will see if BMI is also

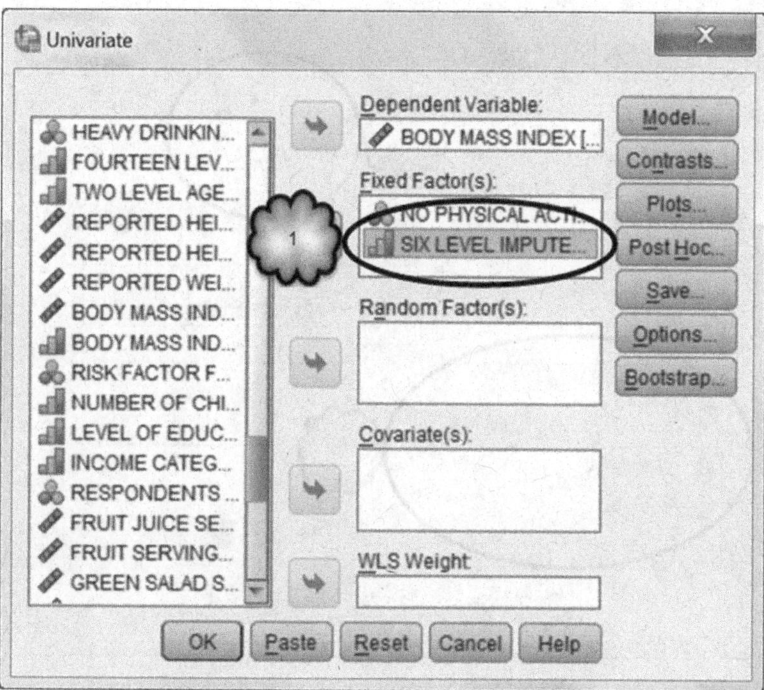

Fig. 12.6 Adding age category as a second factor to the analysis of variance

related to respondents' age category. That is, we will see if there is also a significant main effect of age category. In addition, we will see whether the relationship between physical activity and BMI depends upon the respondents' age category. In the jargon of ANOVA, we will see if there exists a significant *interaction effect* between physical activity and age category.

Before we begin, notice that by adding a second factor to our analysis, we will now have a two-way ANOVA. The term "two-way" indicates that we are categorizing participants in two ways—by whether or not they engaged in physical activity and by their age category. Notice too that our second factor is independent groups. So we will be carrying out a two-way ANOVA in which both factors are independent groups variables.

Return to the *Univariate* dialog box, and as shown in Fig. 12.6, move **SIX LEVEL IMPUTED AGE CATEGORY** into the *Fixed Factor(s)* box to tell SPSS that we wish to add age category as a factor. Remember that earlier we used **Select Cases** to limit the analysis to two age categories, women between the ages of 35 and 44 and women between the ages of 45 and 54.

In the previous analysis, we asked SPSS to plot the mean BMI of those who had engaged in physical activity and the mean BMI of those who had not. Recall that these two means were significantly different. The resulting plot, therefore, displayed a significant main effect of physical activity. Now let us add a plot for the

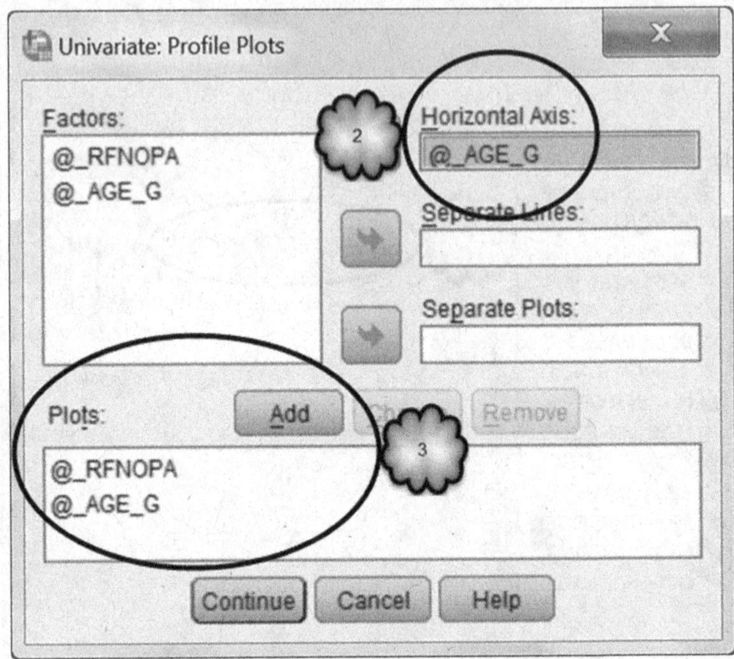

Fig. 12.7 Adding a request for a means plots of the main effect of age category

age variable. This plot will show the mean BMI of each of the two age groups and indicate whether there is a main effect of age category. We will also create what is known as an *interaction plot* to see whether there is an interaction effect involving physical activity and age category, that is, if the relationship between physical activity and BMI varies with age category.

To generate these graphs, click **Plots** in the *Univariate* dialog box. As shown in Fig. 12.7, move **SIX LEVEL IMPUTED AGE CATEGORY** to the *Horizontal Axis* box, and click **Add**. This plot will display the mean BMI of the two age categories. Next, as shown in Fig. 12.8, move the physical activity variable to the *Horizontal Axis* box and **SIX LEVEL IMPUTED AGE CATEGORY** to the *Separate Lines* box. Click **Add**. This plot will display the mean BMI of four independent groups: women who were between the ages of 35 and 44 who had engaged in physical activity, women who were between the ages of 35 and 44 who had not, women between the ages of 45 and 54 who had engaged in physical activity, and women between the ages of 45 and 54 who had not. Now click **Continue** to get back to the *Univariate* dialog box.

Back in the *Univariate* dialog, click **Options.** As shown in Fig. 12.9, add the age variable and its interaction with physical activity to the *Display Means for* box. Click **Continue** followed by **OK** to run the analysis.

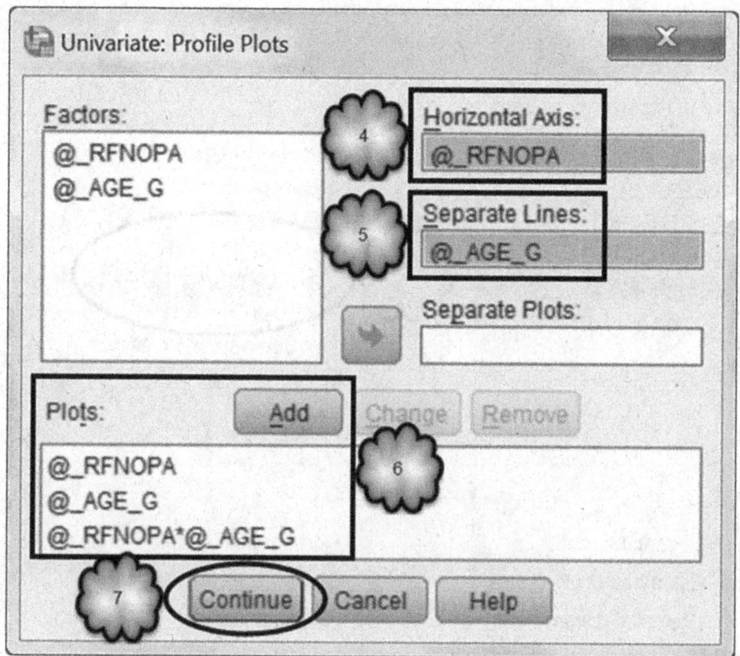

Fig. 12.8 Adding a request for a means plot of the interaction effect between physical activity and age category

Main Effects The output has much the same look as before, but now there is more of it as a result of adding a second factor to the analysis. The output begins with information about sample sizes, shown in Table 12.3.

Table 12.4 displays the mean BMI of the 1673 women who had engaged in physical activity and the mean BMI of the 139 women who had not. Figure 12.10 is the plot of those two means. This information is relevant to the main effect of physical activity.

Table 12.5 displays the mean BMI of the 849 women between the ages of 35 and 44, and the mean BMI of the 963 women between the ages of 45 and 54. Figure 12.11 is the plot of those two means. This information is relevant to the main effect of age category.

Judging by the output thus far, it appears that both physical activity and age category are related to BMI. However, these findings may have been due to random sampling variability. So for each of two main effects we observed in our sample, we need to determine the probability that it would occur if there is no such effect in the population of NY state women. To do this, we refer to the *p*-value of each main effect. To find these values, we would consult the table labeled, *Tests of Between-Subjects Effects*, shown in Table 12.6.

This table is similar to the one we created when we conducted our one-way ANOVA earlier in the chapter, but it now includes the *F* ratio, degrees of freedom,

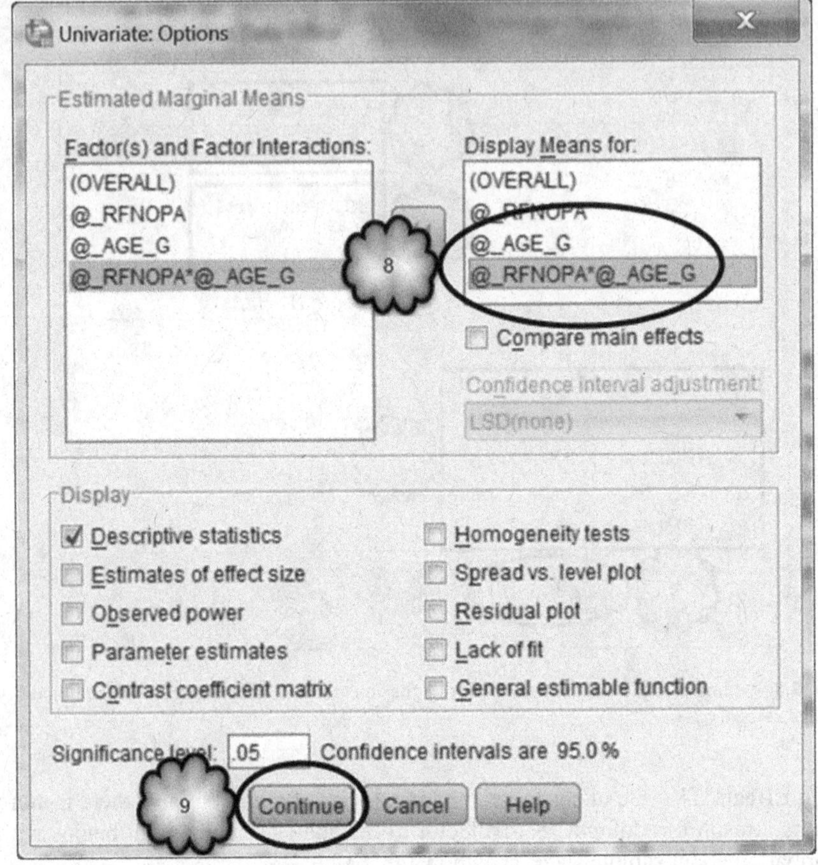

Fig. 12.9 Adding a request for tables displaying the means of the main effect of age category and the interaction effect between physical activity and age category

and *p*-value associated with not only the relationship between physical activity and BMI but with the relationship between age category and BMI as well.

12.3.1 Do the data indicate that the population BMI means differ across the two physical activity groups?
12.3.2 Did we find a significant main effect of physical activity?
12.3.3 Do the data indicate that the population BMI means differ across the two age groups?
12.3.4 Did we find a significant main effect of age category?

Table 12.3 Sample sizes of the independent groups factors

Between-Subjects Factors

		Value Label	N
NO PHYSICAL ACTIVITY OR EXERCISE RISK FACTOR	1	Engaged in Physical Activity	1673
	2	Did not Engage in Physical Activity	139
SIX LEVEL IMPUTED AGE CATEGORY	3	35 to 44	849
	4	45 to 54	963

Table 12.4 Means of the main effect of physical activity on BMI

2. NO PHYSICAL ACTIVITY OR EXERCISE RISK FACTOR

Dependent Variable: BODY MASS INDEX

NO PHYSICAL ACTIVITY OR EXERCISE RISK FACTOR	Mean	Std. Error	95% Confidence Interval	
			Lower Bound	Upper Bound
Engaged in Physical Activity	26.335	.149	26.044	26.626
Did not Engage in Physical Activity	27.578	.541	26.517	28.640

Interaction Effect The inclusion of age as a second factor results in output that tells us whether the relationship between physical activity and BMI varies according to the age category of the participant. When the strength or direction of a relationship between one factor and a response variable depends on the values of a second factor, an *interaction effect* between the two factors is said to be present. To determine whether there is an interaction effect, we can inspect the mean BMI values of each of the four groups of women, and compare the difference between the two mean BMI values of the women between the ages of 35 and 44 who had and had not engaged in physical activity with the difference between the two mean BMI values of the women between the ages of 45 and 54 who had and had not engaged in physical activity. Tables 12.7 and 12.8 display this information. Table 12.7 highlights the BMI means of the two physical activity groups for women between 34 and 44, while Table 12.8 highlights the BMI means of women between 45 and 54.

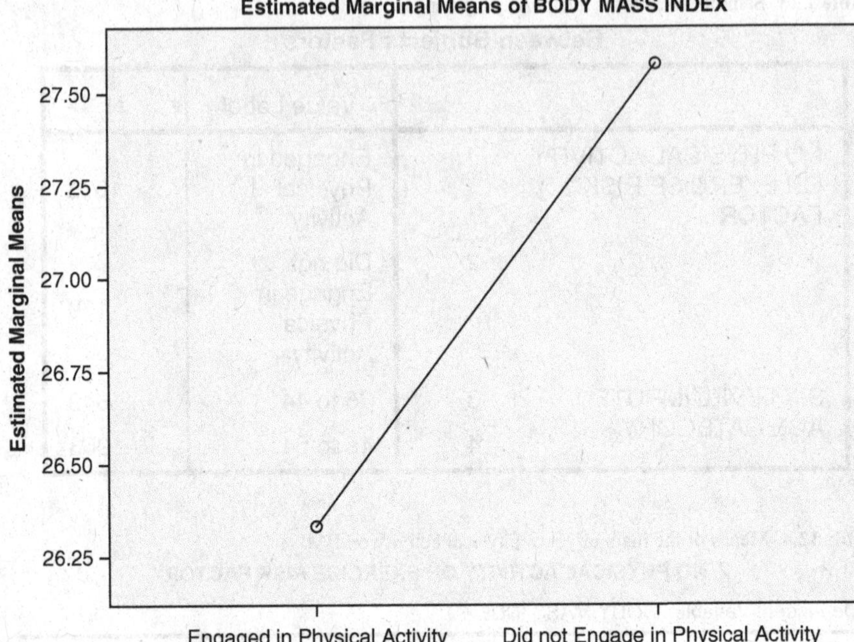

Fig. 12.10 Means plot of the main effect of physical activity on BMI

Table 12.5 Means of the main effect of age category on BMI

3. SIX LEVEL IMPUTED AGE CATEGORY

Dependent Variable: BODY MASS INDEX

SIX LEVEL IMPUTED AGE CATEGORY	Mean	Std. Error	95% Confidence Interval	
			Lower Bound	Upper Bound
35 to 44	26.076	.451	25.192	26.961
45 to 54	27.837	.334	27.181	28.493

Answer the following questions:

12.3.5 Judging from the 4 BMI means, which age group seems to benefit from engagement in physical activity?

12.3.6 Does the pattern of the 4 BMI means suggest an interaction effect between engagement in physical activity and age category?

We see that for the younger group of women, those who had engaged in physical activity and those who had not had about the same average BMI, but that for the older women, those who had engaged in physical activity had an average BMI substantially lower than those who had not engaged in physical activity.

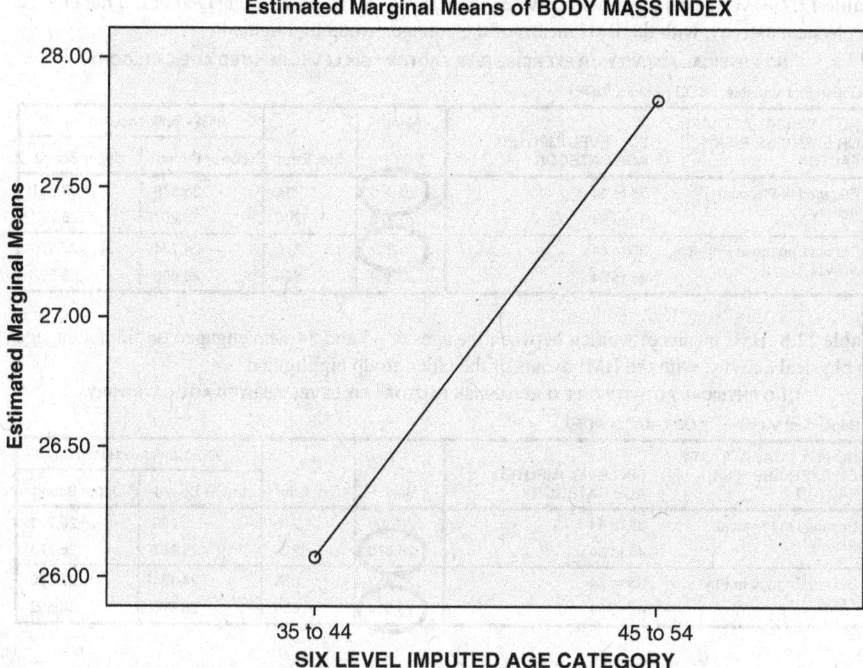

Fig. 12.11 Means plot of the main effect of age category on BMI

Table 12.6 Tests of the null hypotheses that BMI is unrelated to physical activity or age category

Tests of Between-Subjects Effects

Dependent Variable: BODY MASS INDEX

Source	Type III Sum of Squares	df	Mean Square	F	Sig.
Corrected Model	781.212[a]	3	260.404	7.070	.000
Intercept	339780.242	1	339780.242	9224.762	.000
@_RFNOPA	180.745	1	180.745	4.907	.027
@_AGE_G	362.417	1	362.417	9.839	.002
@_RFNOPA * @_AGE_G	334.322	1	334.322	9.077	.003
Error	66594.962	1808	36.833		
Total	1337213.025	1812			
Corrected Total	67376.174	1811			

a. R Squared = .012 (Adjusted R Squared = .010)

Comparing the effect of physical activity on the average BMI of older women to the effect of physical activity on the average BMI of younger women is made easier by inspecting the interaction plot that displays these four means. Study this display, shown in Fig. 12.12. (We modified the formatting of the figure slightly to better distinguish in grayscale the two age categories.) Note whether the relationship between

Table 12.7 BMI means of women between the ages of 35 and 54 who engaged or did not engage in physical activity, with the BMI means of the younger group highlighted

4. NO PHYSICAL ACTIVITY OR EXERCISE RISK FACTOR * SIX LEVEL IMPUTED AGE CATEGORY

Dependent Variable: BODY MASS INDEX

NO PHYSICAL ACTIVITY OR EXERCISE RISK FACTOR	SIX LEVEL IMPUTED AGE CATEGORY	Mean	Std. Error	95% Confidence Interval	
				Lower Bound	Upper Bound
Engaged in Physical Activity	35 to 44	26.300	.214	25.879	26.721
	45 to 54	26.370	.206	25.967	26.773
Did not Engage in Physical Activity	35 to 44	25.852	.876	24.134	27.570
	45 to 54	29.304	.636	28.056	30.552

Table 12.8 BMI means of women between the ages of 35 and 54 who engaged or did not engage in physical activity, with the BMI means of the older group highlighted

4. NO PHYSICAL ACTIVITY OR EXERCISE RISK FACTOR * SIX LEVEL IMPUTED AGE CATEGORY

Dependent Variable: BODY MASS INDEX

NO PHYSICAL ACTIVITY OR EXERCISE RISK FACTOR	SIX LEVEL IMPUTED AGE CATEGORY	Mean	Std. Error	95% Confidence Interval	
				Lower Bound	Upper Bound
Engaged in Physical Activity	35 to 44	26.300	.214	25.879	26.721
	45 to 54	26.370	.206	25.967	26.773
Did not Engage in Physical Activity	35 to 44	25.852	.876	24.134	27.570
	45 to 54	29.304	.636	28.056	30.552

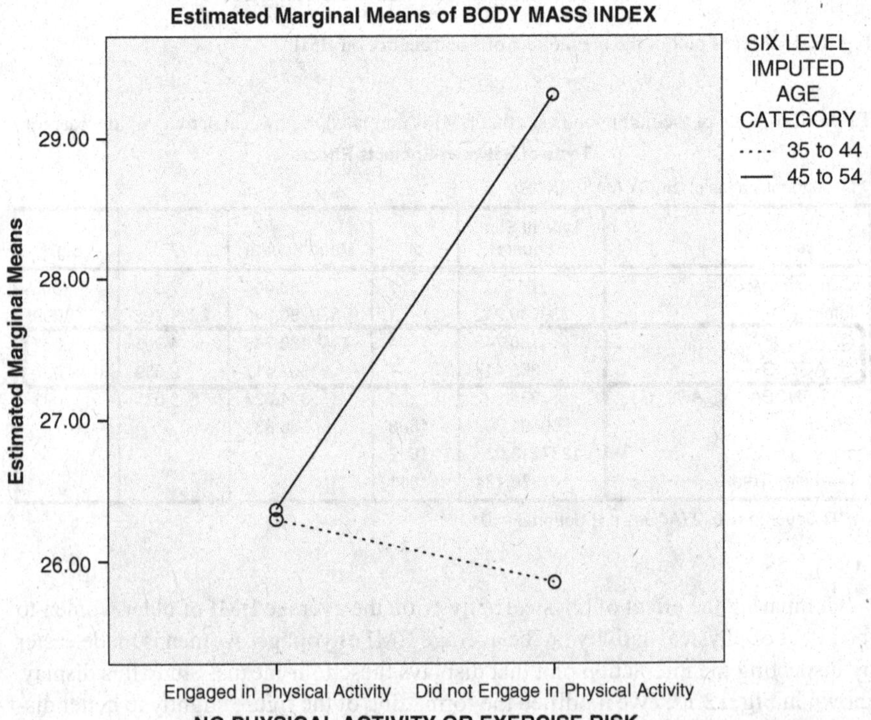

Fig. 12.12 Means plot of the interaction effect between physical activity and age category on BMI

Table 12.9 Test of the interaction effect between physical activity and age category on BMI

Tests of Between-Subjects Effects

Dependent Variable: BODY MASS INDEX

Source	Type III Sum of Squares	df	Mean Square	F	Sig.
Corrected Model	781.212[a]	3	260.404	7.070	.000
Intercept	339780.242	1	339780.242	9224.762	.000
@_RFNOPA	180.745	1	180.745	4.907	.027
@_AGE_G	362.417	1	362.417	9.839	.002
@_RFNOPA * @_AGE_G	334.322	1	334.322	9.077	.003
Error	66594.962	1808	36.833		
Total	1337213.025	1812			
Corrected Total	67376.174	1811			

a. R Squared = .012 (Adjusted R Squared = .010)

physical activity and BMI seems to differ across the two age categories. To be sure that you understand the graph, see if you can find in the graph each of the four means singled out in Tables 12.7 and 12.8.

The graph tells us that the relationship between whether or not women were physically active and their BMI depended on the age category of the women. In the language of ANOVA, we can say that engagement in physical activity appears to *interact* with age.

As you may have guessed from the interaction plot, an interaction effect is evidenced by the lack of parallelism between the lines displayed in the graph. However, as with any sample result, the lack of parallelism in our sample may have been due to random sampling variability and not to an interaction in the population. Consequently, we need to test the null hypothesis that there is no interaction in the population against the alternative hypothesis that there is an interaction. In other words, we need to determine the probability that the sample interaction effect would have occurred if there were no interaction effect in the population.

We can discover this probability by consulting the row in the *Tests of Between-Subjects Effects* table, displayed in Table 12.9. If we consult the row labeled *@_RFNOPA*@_AGE_G*, we will find the *F*-ratio for the interaction effect and its associated *p*-value.

Answer the following questions:

12.3.7 Was the interaction effect between physical activity and age category statistically significant?

12.3.8 Can we reject the null hypothesis that in the population from which the sample was taken, physical activity benefits both age groups equally?

According to Table 12.9, the probability that the interaction we observed in our sample would have occurred if there is no interaction in the population is 0.003.

This probability tells us that it is highly unlikely that we would have observed in our sample the interaction between physical activity and age category if there were no such interaction in the population of NY state women. Therefore, from our sample, we can infer with great confidence that the relationship between physical activity and BMI for female residents of NY depends on whether they are 35–44 years of age or 45–54 years of age.

The existence of a significant interaction effect forces us to be cautious about how we interpret the separate effects of each of the factors involved in the interaction, that is, how we interpret the main effects. For example, consider again the plot of the main effect of physical activity, shown in Fig. 12.10. This graph compares the mean BMI of those who had been physically active with those who had not, regardless of their age category. Our inspection of the interaction plot, reproduced in Fig. 12.12, tells us that we would be mistaken if we were to conclude that the main effect of physical activity describes equally well the relationship between physical activity and BMI for both age groups.

12.4 ANOVA with Two Repeated Measures Factors

In the preceding analysis, we conducted a two-way ANOVA in which each factor formed independent groups. In the next two sections, you will learn how to interpret a two-way ANOVA when at least one of the factors is repeated measures. We will begin with a study that used two repeated measures factors.

The file, **Blood.sav** [2], consists of systolic and diastolic blood pressures (mm Hg) of 15 hypertensive patients who had been given the drug, captopril. Each patient's blood pressure was measured twice, immediately before and 2 h after the drug was administered. Let us investigate the effects of this drug on blood pressure.

We will begin by studying the structure of the data file, reproduced in Fig. 12.13. Note that, as usual, each row contains the data from each participant. In this data set, the first variable refers to patient number (1 through 15), and the next four variables contain the blood pressure readings. Note the ordering of the last four columns: The researchers chose to enter the systolic readings before the diastolic, and for each type of blood pressure, the before reading prior to the after reading.

We will determine if systolic blood pressure was greater than diastolic (which of course it should have been), whether blood pressure dropped significantly after the drug was given, and whether the drug had the same effect on systolic and diastolic blood pressure. In the language of ANOVA, we will see if there was a significant main effect of type of blood pressure (systolic vs. diastolic), a significant main effect of time of measurement (before vs. after), and a significant interaction effect between time of measurement and type of blood pressure.

As with our earlier two-way ANOVA, the outcome variable is quantitative and the explanatory variables are categorical. But this time both explanatory factors are repeated measures. This is because each patient had both types of blood pressure readings taken at both points in time. Consequently, we will be conducting a two-way repeated measures ANOVA.

	Patient	SystolicBefore	SystolicAfter	DiastolicBefore	DiastolicAfter
1	1	210	201	130	125
2	2	169	165	122	121
3	3	187	166	124	121
4	4	160	157	104	106
5	5	167	147	112	101
6	6	176	145	101	85
7	7	185	168	121	98
8	8	206	180	124	105
9	9	173	147	115	103
10	10	146	136	102	98
11	11	174	151	98	90
12	12	201	168	119	98
13	13	198	179	106	110
14	14	148	129	107	103
15	15	154	131	100	82

Fig. 12.13 Blood.sav data set

Select **Analyze>General Linear Model > Repeated Measures** to bring up the *Repeated Measures Define Factor(s)* dialog box. In the *Within-Subject Factor Name* box, we will enter a name for the repeated measures factor, *Type of Blood Pressure*. To minimize typing time and output space, just enter the word, *Type*. In the *Number of Levels* box, enter 2, and then click **Add.** Now enter the second repeated measures factor, *Time of Measurement*, by entering the word, *Time,* into the *Within-Subject Factor Name* box. In the *Number of Levels* box, enter 2, and then click **Add.** In the *Measure Name* box, enter the name of our response variable, *Blood Pressure,* by entering the word, *Pressure*. Click **Add.** These steps are shown in Figs. 12.14, 12.15, 12.16, and 12.17.

At this point, we have told SPSS to execute an ANOVA with two repeated measures factors we have called *Type* and *Time* on an response variable we have called *Pressure* We have also told SPSS that each of the two factors has two values. SPSS will therefore expect that there will be a column of data for each of the four combinations of the values of the two factors. Our next step is to tell SPSS which column of data corresponds to which combination of the values of the factors.

As shown in Fig. 12.17, click **Define** to bring up the *Repeated Measures* dialog displayed in Fig. 12.18. Here, we will match up each relevant column of data listed in the window to the left to each of the combinations of the values of the factors, *Type* and *Time*, listed in the *Within-Subjects Variables* window to the right.

Let us look more closely at the *Within-Subjects Variables* window. Note that the names of the repeated measures factors, *Type* and *Time*, are listed in parentheses just above the window. The factors are listed in the order we entered them in the previous dialog box. *Type* is listed first, *Time* second. Below the names of the factors and also within parentheses are two digits, 1 and 2, followed by the name of

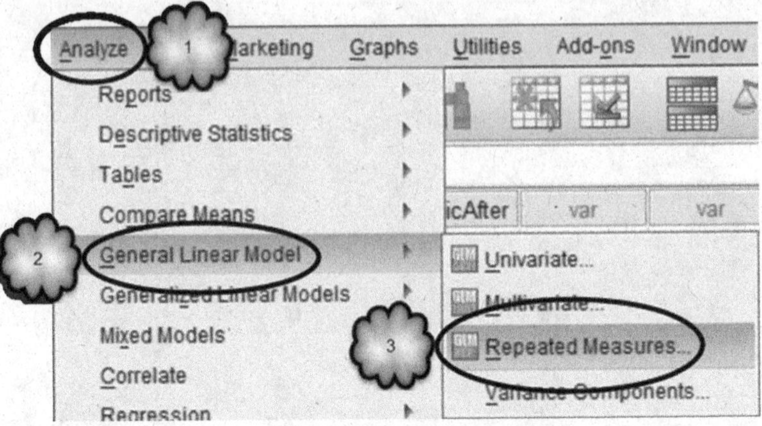

Fig. 12.14 Opening the Repeated Measures Define Factor(s) dialog

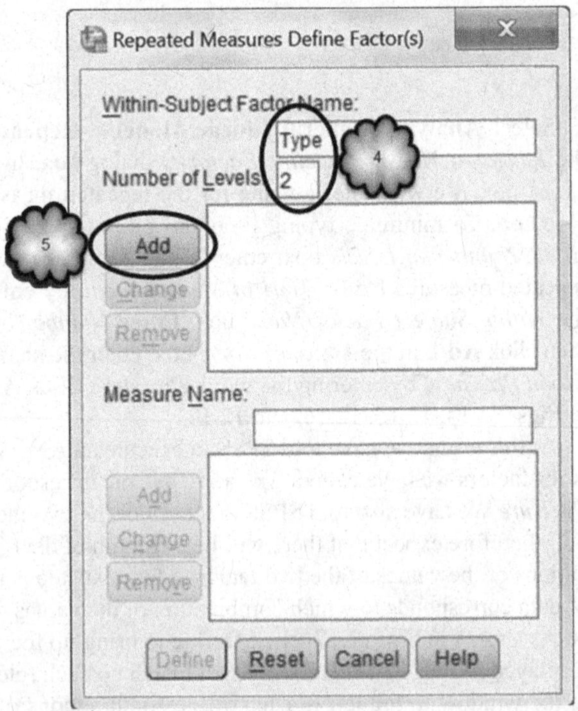

Fig. 12.15 Defining type of blood pressure as a repeated measures factor

our response variable, that is, *(1,1,Pressure)*, *(1,2,Pressure)* and so on. Recall that each factor has two levels: *Systolic* and *Diastolic* for the factor, *Type*; and *Before* and *After* for the factor, *Time*. For each pair of digits, the first number refers to one of the two levels of the first factor, *Type*; and the second number refers to one of the two values of the second factor, *Time*.

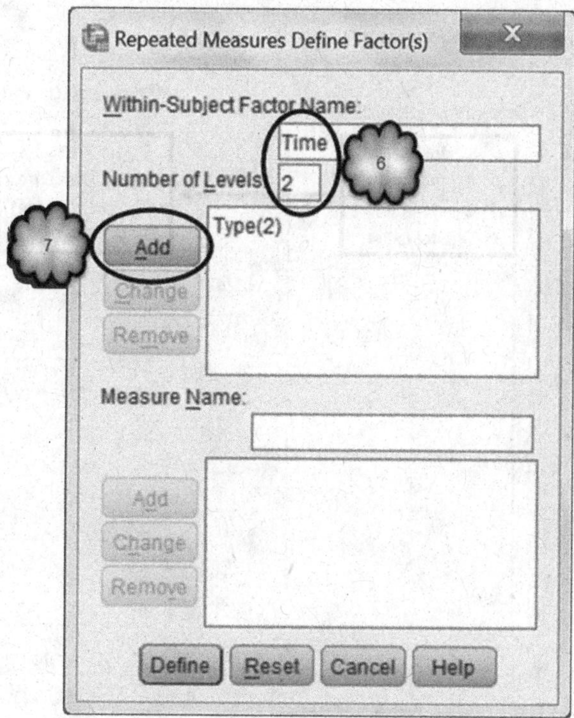

Fig. 12.16 Defining time of measurement as a repeated measures factor

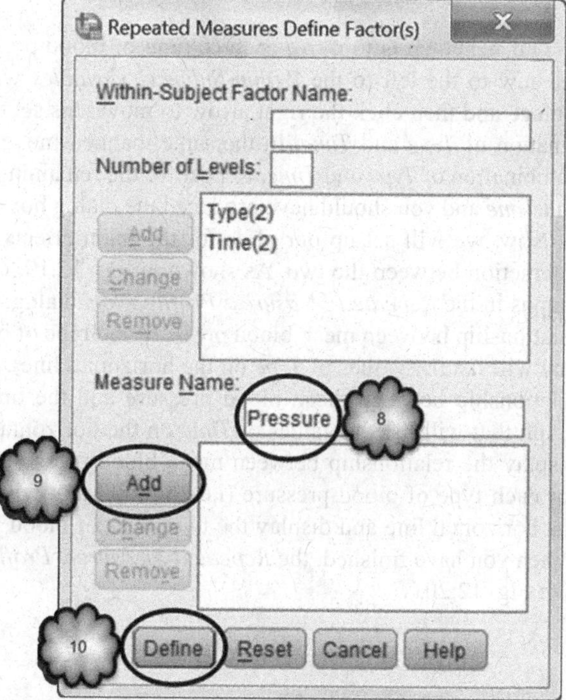

Fig. 12.17 Naming the response variable and opening the Repeated Measures dialog

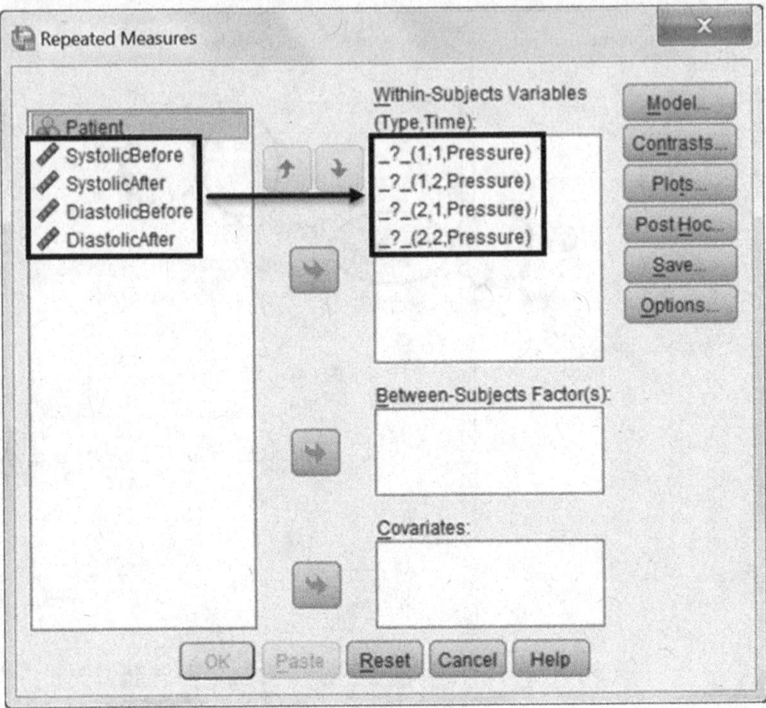

Fig. 12.18 Repeated measures dialog

Our next step is to move each column of blood pressure readings listed in the window to the left to the *Within-Subjects Variables* window. Highlight **Systolic: Before** and then click the right arrow to move this set of readings to the 1,1 combination of *Type* and *Time*. In the same manner, move **Systolic: After** to the 1,2 combination of *Type* and *Time*. Repeat for the remaining two combinations of *Type* and *Time* and you should have produced the dialog box shown in Fig. 12.19.

Now, we will set up our plots for the main effects of *Type* and *Time* and the interaction between the two. As shown in Fig. 12.19, click **Plots** and create three graphs in the *Repeated Measures: Profile Plots* dialog: one which will display the relationship between mean blood pressure and type of blood pressure (i.e., a graph that will list the values of *Type* on the horizontal line), one which will display the relationship between mean blood pressure and the time of measurement (i.e., a graph that will list the values of *Time* on the horizontal line), and one which will display the relationship between mean blood pressure and time of measurement for each type of blood pressure (i.e., a graph that will list the values of *Time* on the horizontal line and display the two types of blood pressure as separate lines). When you have finished, the *Repeated Measures: Profile Plots* dialog should look like Fig. 12.20.

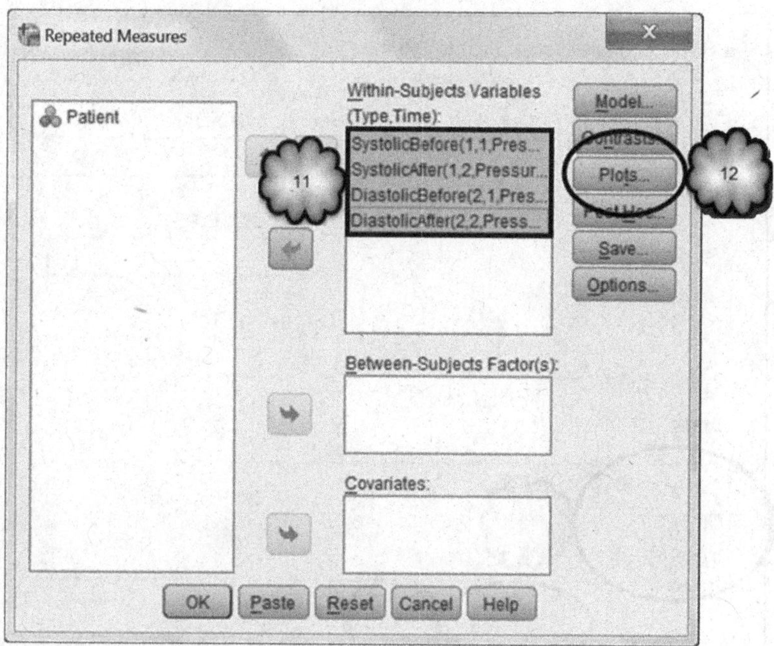

Fig. 12.19 Selecting the variables corresponding to the four combinations of the repeated measures factors, and opening the Repeated Measures: Profile Plots dialog

Click **Continue** to return to the *Repeated Measures* dialog, and then **Options** to open the *Repeated Measures: Options* dialog. Tell SPSS to display means for all factors and factor interactions. Then select *Descriptive statistics*. When you have finished, the *Options* dialog should look like the one in Fig. 12.21. Click **Continue** to return to the *Repeated Measures* dialog box, and **OK** to run the analysis.

Main Effects The output should have a familiar look, thanks to our review of one-way repeated measures ANOVA in Chap. 11. This time though we have descriptive statistics, means plots, and *F*-ratios relevant to the investigation of two main effects instead of just one, and for the investigation of an interaction effect.

Let us begin our study of the output with a trivial question: Was systolic blood pressure significantly different from diastolic? Inspection of the means displayed in Table 12.10 or of the corresponding means plot in Fig. 12.22 tells us not surprisingly that on the average, systolic blood pressure was greater than diastolic.

To determine whether these two means were significantly different, that is, to determine whether there was a significant main effect of type of blood pressure, we do what we had done in Chap. 11—we consult the table labeled *Tests of Within-Subjects Effects.* We find the row labeled *Type* and its corresponding *F*-ratio, degrees of freedom, and *p*-value. That row can be found in Table 12.11.

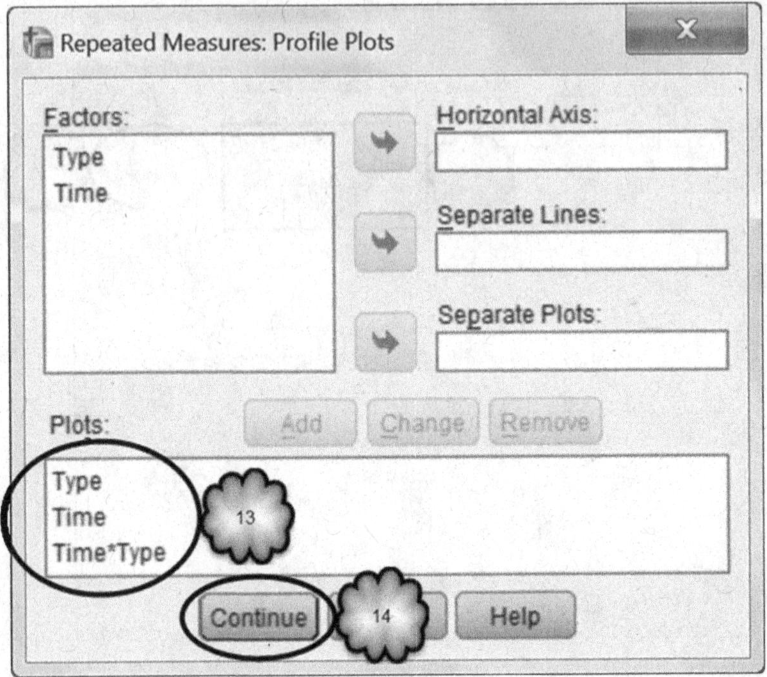

Fig. 12.20 Requesting means plots of the main effects of type of pressure and time of measurement, and of the interaction between type of pressure and time of measurement

Answer the following questions:

12.4.1 What was the value of the F-ratio?

12.4.2 What were the numerator and denominator degrees of freedom associated with the F-ratio?

12.4.3 What was the p-value associated with the F-ratio?

12.4.4 Can we reject the null hypothesis that in the population from which the sample was taken, mean systolic and diastolic blood pressures are equal?

12.4.5 In this analysis, we do not have to be concerned about whether we can assume sphericity. Why?

According to the table, mean systolic blood pressure was significantly different from mean diastolic blood pressure. That is, a significant main effect of type of blood pressure was found.

Now let us focus on whether the drug seemed to have an effect on blood pressure. Inspection of Table 12.12 or of the corresponding means plot in Fig. 12.23 tells us that blood pressure declined following administration of the drug.

To determine whether these two means were significantly different, that is, to determine whether there was a significant main effect of type of blood pressure, we

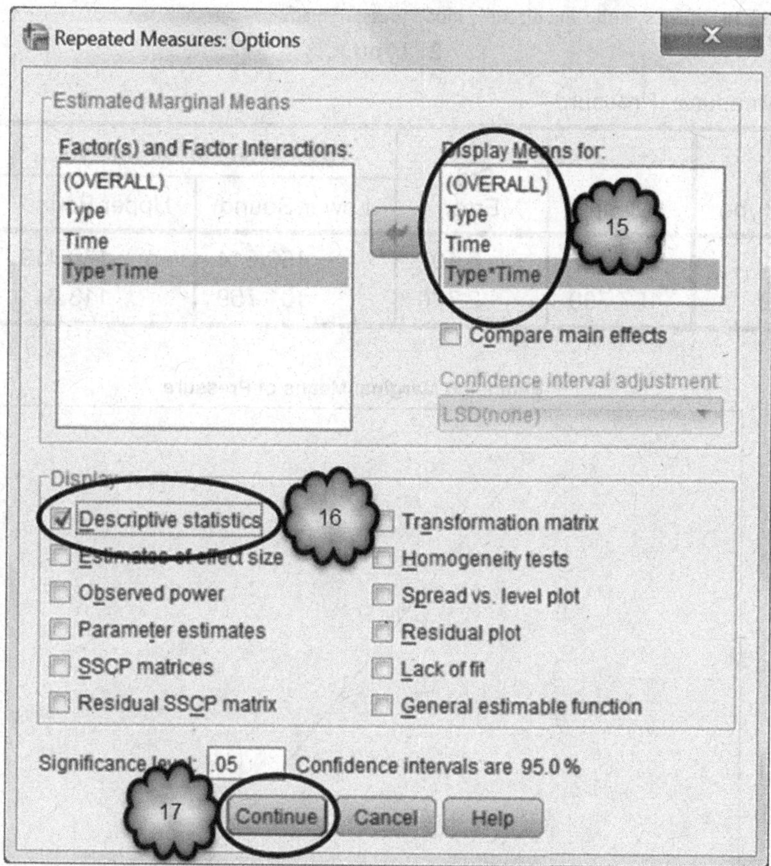

Fig. 12.21 Requesting tables displaying the overall mean, the means of the main and interaction effects, and descriptive statistics

consult the row labeled *Time* in the *Tests of Within-Subjects Effects* table. That row can be found in Table 12.13.

> Answer the following questions:
> 12.4.6 Were the two means displayed in Table 12.13 significantly different?
> 12.4.7 Does the analysis support the conclusion that captopril reduces blood pressure?

Interaction Effect Our last finding has to do with whether the relationship between time of measurement and blood pressure depended on the type of blood pressure measured. Inspection of the means found in Table 12.14 or of the corresponding interaction plot of Fig. 12.24 suggests that although both types of blood pressure declined after administration of the drug, the decline was somewhat greater for systolic pressure.

Table 12.10 Mean systolic and diastolic blood pressure readings

2. Type

Measure: Pressure

Type	Mean	Std. Error	95% Confidence Interval	
			Lower Bound	Upper Bound
1	167.467	5.107	156.514	178.419
2	107.700	2.770	101.759	113.641

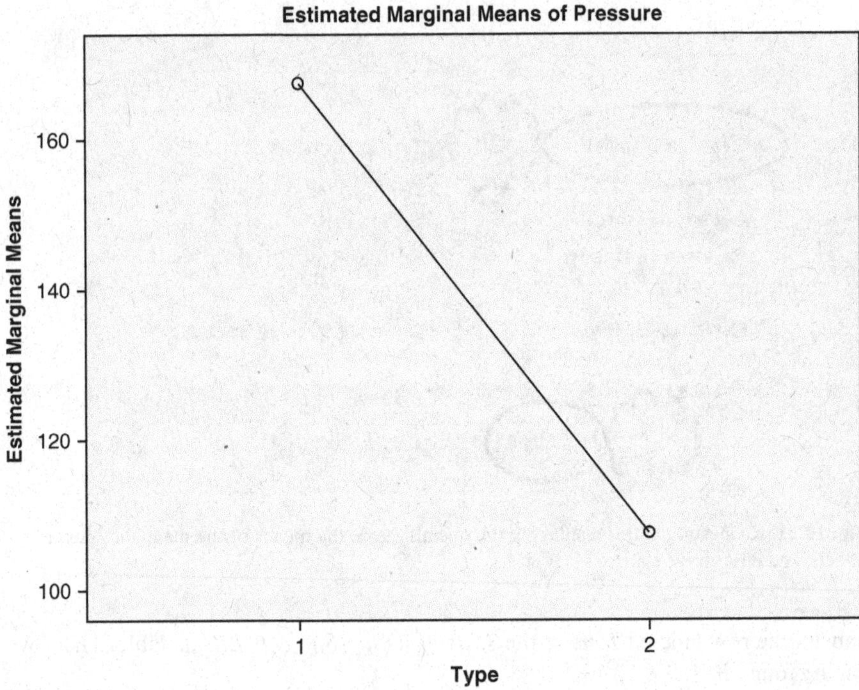

Fig. 12.22 Means plot of the main effect of type of blood pressure: systolic (Type = 1) versus diastolic (Type = 2)

To determine whether there was a significant interaction effect between the type of blood pressure and the time of measurement, we consult the row labeled *Time * Type* in *Tests of Within-Subjects Effect.* That row is included in Table 12.15.

Answer the following questions:

12.4.8 Was the interaction effect statistically significant?

12.4.9 Can we reject the null hypothesis that captopril reduces systolic and diastolic blood pressure equally?

Table 12.11 Test of the null hypothesis that the population systolic and diastolic blood pressure means are equal

Tests of Within-Subjects Effects

Measure: Pressure

Source		Type III Sum of Squares	df	Mean Square	F	Sig.
Type	Sphericity Assumed	53580.817	1	53580.817	240.856	.000
	Greenhouse-Geisser	53580.817	1.000	53580.817	240.856	.000
	Huynh-Feldt	53580.817	1.000	53580.817	240.856	.000
	Lower-bound	53580.817	1.000	53580.817	240.856	.000
Error(Type)	Sphericity Assumed	3114.433	14	222.460		
	Greenhouse-Geisser	3114.433	14.000	222.460		
	Huynh-Feldt	3114.433	14.000	222.460		
	Lower-bound	3114.433	14.000	222.460		

Table 12.12 Mean blood pressure readings before (Time = 1) and after (Time = 2) administration of captopril

3. Time

Measure: Pressure

Time	Mean	Std. Error	95% Confidence Interval	
			Lower Bound	Upper Bound
1	144.633	3.694	136.710	152.557
2	130.533	3.852	122.271	138.795

As usual, the existence of a significant interaction forces us to be careful when we interpret the main effects. As we can see by comparing Figs. 12.23 and 12.24, the main effect of time of measurement (mean blood pressure before vs. mean blood pressure after; Fig. 12.23) somewhat underestimates the drug's effect on systolic blood pressure and somewhat overestimates the drug's effect on diastolic blood pressure (Fig. 12.24).

12.5 ANOVA with One Independent Groups and One Repeated Measure Factor

As our last example of a two-way ANOVA, we will return to a study that we encountered in the previous chapter: the effects of acupuncture on severity of chronic headaches. In this study, 401 male and female patients who suffered from chronic headache were randomly assigned to one of two conditions: Acupuncture and Control. Patients assigned to the acupuncture group were referred by their general practitioners to acupuncturists who offered weekly sessions for a period of 3 months.

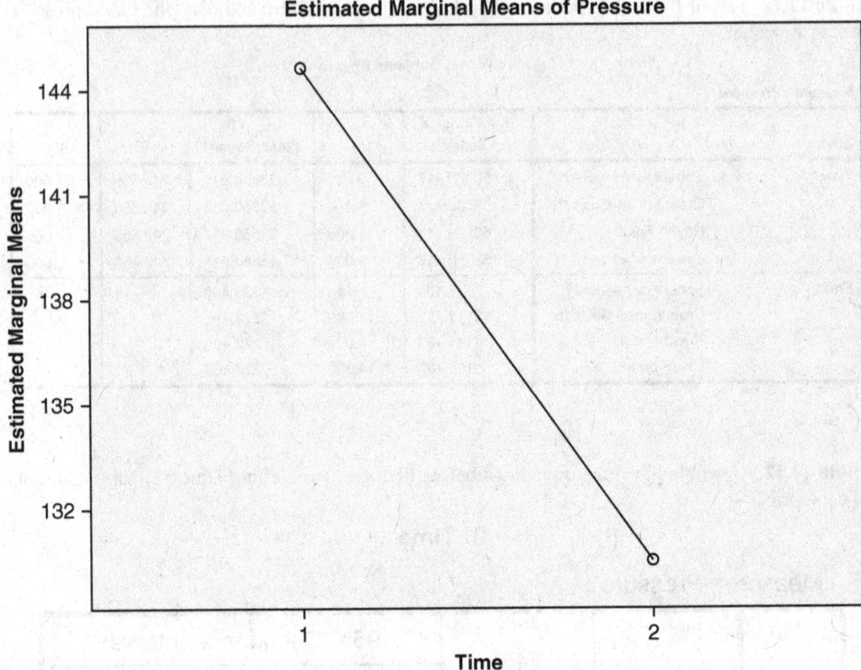

Fig. 12.23 Means plot of the main effect of time of measurement on blood pressure: before (Time=1) and after (Time=2) administration of captopril

Table 12.13 Test of the null hypothesis that the population blood pressure means before and after administration of captopril are equal

Tests of Within-Subjects Effects

Measure: Pressure

Source		Type III Sum of Squares	df	Mean Square	F	Sig.
Time	Sphericity Assumed	2982.150	1	2982.150	46.179	.000
	Greenhouse-Geisser	2982.150	1.000	2982.150	46.179	.000
	Huynh-Feldt	2982.150	1.000	2982.150	46.179	.000
	Lower-bound	2982.150	1.000	2982.150	46.179	.000
Error(Time)	Sphericity Assumed	904.100	14	64.579		
	Greenhouse-Geisser	904.100	14.000	64.579		
	Huynh-Feldt	904.100	14.000	64.579		
	Lower-bound	904.100	14.000	64.579		

Patients in the control group were not referred. Three months (3-month follow-up) and again 12 months (1-year follow-up) later, the severity of the patients' headaches was assessed and compared to their baseline severity ratings obtained at the beginning of the study.

Table 12.14 Mean systolic (Type = 1) and diastolic (Type = 2) blood pressures before (Time = 1) and after (Time = 2) administration of captopril

4. Type * Time

Measure: Pressure

Type	Time	Mean	Std. Error	95% Confidence Interval	
				Lower Bound	Upper Bound
1	1	176.933	5.310	165.545	188.322
	2	158.000	5.165	146.922	169.078
2	1	112.333	2.704	106.534	118.133
	2	103.067	3.242	96.114	110.020

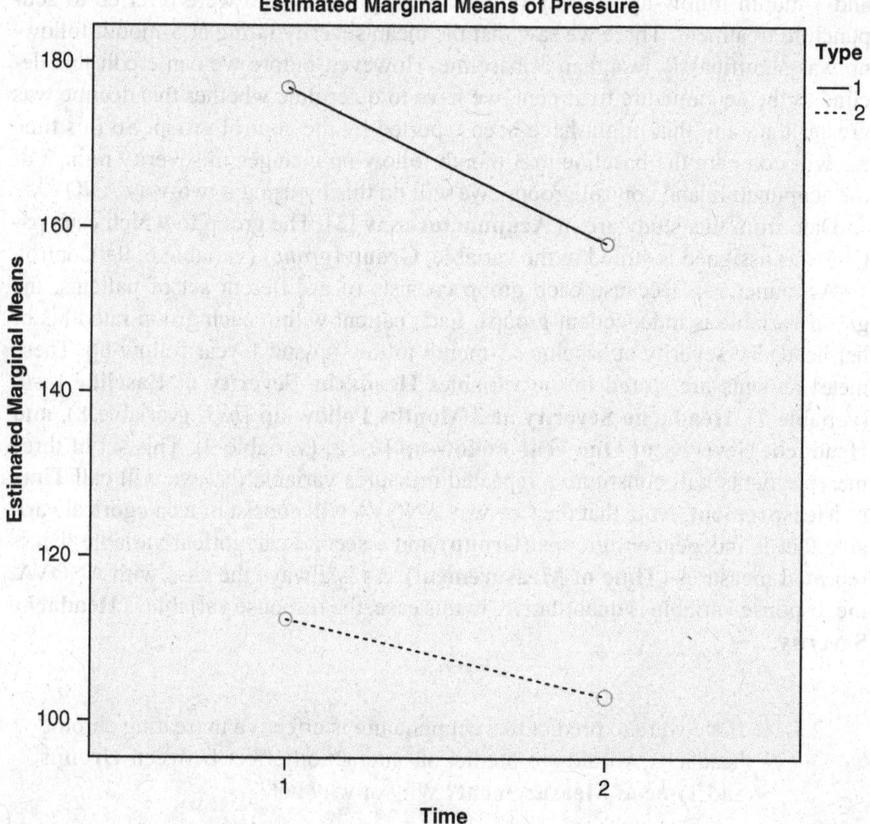

Fig. 12.24 Means plot of systolic (Type = 1) and diastolic (Type = 2) blood pressures before (Time = 1) and after (Time = 2) administration of captopril

Table 12.15 Test of the null hypothesis that the effects of captopril on systolic and diastolic blood pressures are equal

Tests of Within-Subjects Effects

Measure: Pressure

Source		Type III Sum of Squares	df	Mean Square	F	Sig.
Type * Time	Sphericity Assumed	350.417	1	350.417	26.399	.000
	Greenhouse-Geisser	350.417	1.000	350.417	26.399	.000
	Huynh-Feldt	350.417	1.000	350.417	26.399	.000
	Lower-bound	350.417	1.000	350.417	26.399	.000
Error(Type*Time)	Sphericity Assumed	185.833	14	13.274		
	Greenhouse-Geisser	185.833	14.000	13.274		
	Huynh-Feldt	185.833	14.000	13.274		
	Lower-bound	185.833	14.000	13.274		

In the previous chapter, we used a paired-samples *t*-test to compare the baseline and 3-month follow-up severity ratings of the patients who were referred to acupuncture treatment. There we saw that the mean severity rating at 3-month follow-up was significantly less than at baseline. However, before we can credit this decline to the acupuncture treatment, we have to determine whether this decline was greater than any that might have been reported by the control group. So this time we will compare the baseline to 3-month follow-up changes in severity ratings of the acupuncture and control groups. We will do this by using a two-way ANOVA.

Data from this study are in **Acupuncture.sav** [3]. The group to which each patient was assigned is stored in the variable, **Group** [*group*] (variable 6; 0=Control, 1=Acupuncture). Because each group consists of a different set of patients, the group variable is independent groups. Each patient within each group rated his or her headache severity at baseline, 3-month follow-up and 1-year follow-up. These measurements are stored in the variables **Headache Severity at Baseline** [*hs0*] (variable 7), **Headache Severity at 3 Months Follow-up** [*hs3*] (variable 8), **and Headache Severity at One Year Follow-up** [*hs12*] (variable 9). This set of three measurements will constitute a repeated measures variable that we will call **Time of Measurement**. Note that the two-way ANOVA will consist of a categorical variable that is independent groups **(Group)** and a second categorical variable that is repeated measures **(Time of Measurement)**. As is always the case with ANOVA, the response variable is quantitative. In this case, the response variable is **Headache Severity**.

12.5.1 If we were to predict that acupuncture is effective in treating chronic headache, would we predict an interaction effect between **Groups** and **Time of Measurement**? Why or why not?

Load the data file, **Acupuncture.sav**. Because our analysis will include a repeated measures factor, select **Analyze > General Linear Model > Repeated Measures**

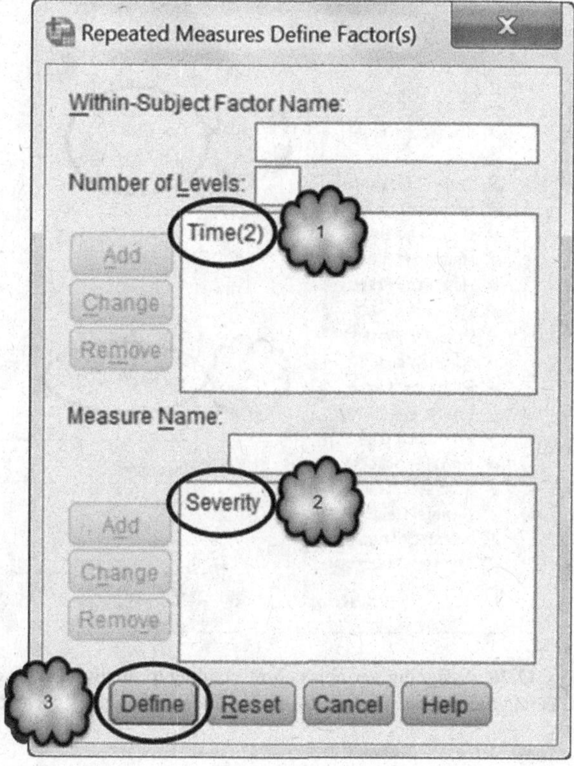

Fig. 12.25 Defining the repeated measures factor, naming the response variable, and opening the Repeated Measures dialog

to bring up the now familiar *Repeated Measures Define Factor(s)* dialog box. Assign a name to the repeated measures factor—the name *Time* will do—and tell SPSS that it has two levels. Then assign a *Measure Name.* This is our response variable. *Severity* will do. When you have finished, the dialog box should look similar to the one in Fig. 12.25.

As shown in Fig. 12.25, click **Define** to bring up the *Repeated Measures* dialog box. Move the baseline and 3-month follow-up variables to the *Within-Subjects Variables* window.

At this point, you have told SPSS that you wish to conduct an ANOVA on a response variable called *Severity*, that the ANOVA has one explanatory factor, *Time*, and that the factor is repeated measures and has two values. If we were to run the analysis now, we would generate a one-way repeated measures ANOVA. But we want a two-way ANOVA. What's missing?

We need to tell SPSS that there is a second factor, **Group,** and that the second factor is independent groups. To do this, move *Group* into the window labeled *Between-Subjects Factor(s)* by selecting it and clicking the right pointing arrow to the left of the *Between-Subjects Factor(s)* window. Now the dialog box should look like the one in Fig. 12.26.

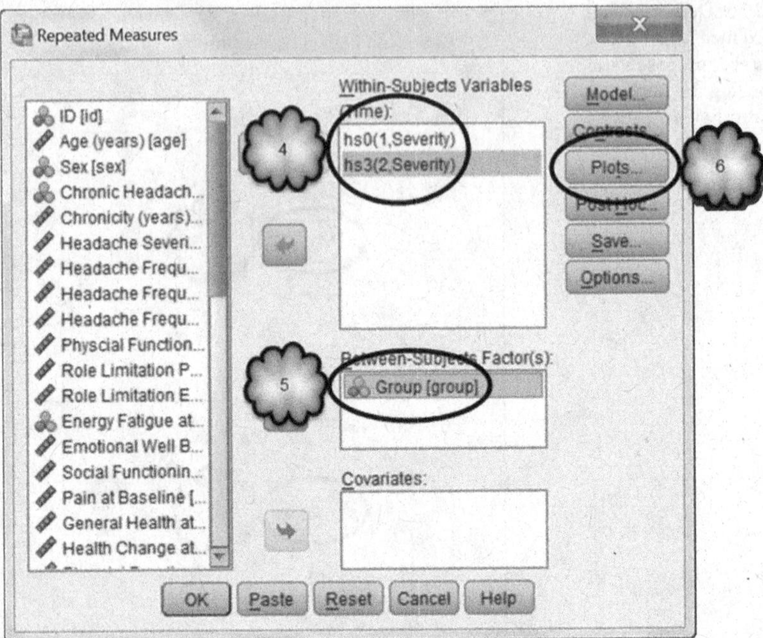

Fig. 12.26 Assigning variables corresponding to the two values of the repeated measures factor, selecting the independent groups factor, and opening the Repeated Measures: Profile Plots dialog

Next, click **Plots** and tell SPSS to plot the main effects of *Time* and *Group* and the interaction between the two factors. For the interaction plot, put *Time* on the *X*-axis. When you're done, the Profile Plots dialog should look like Fig. 12.27. Click **Continue.**

Back in the *Repeated Measures* dialog, click **Options** and instruct SPSS to generate descriptive statistics for all of the variables, as shown in Fig. 12.28. Click **Continue** and then **OK** to run the analysis.

The layout of the output is the same as with the analyses of Sects. 12.3 and 12.4 in that the output provides information about two factors. For example, the output will display the means that correspond to the four combinations of the two factors (Table 12.16), and a means plot of those means (Fig. 12.29). This time, though, one of the factors is independent groups and the other repeated measures. Consequently, to see if the study generated a significant main effect of *Group*, inspect the table labeled *Tests of Between-Subjects Effects* (Table 12.17). To see if the study generated a significant main effect of *Time* or a significant interaction between *Group* and *Time*, inspect the table labeled *Test of Within-Subjects Effects* (Table 12.18).

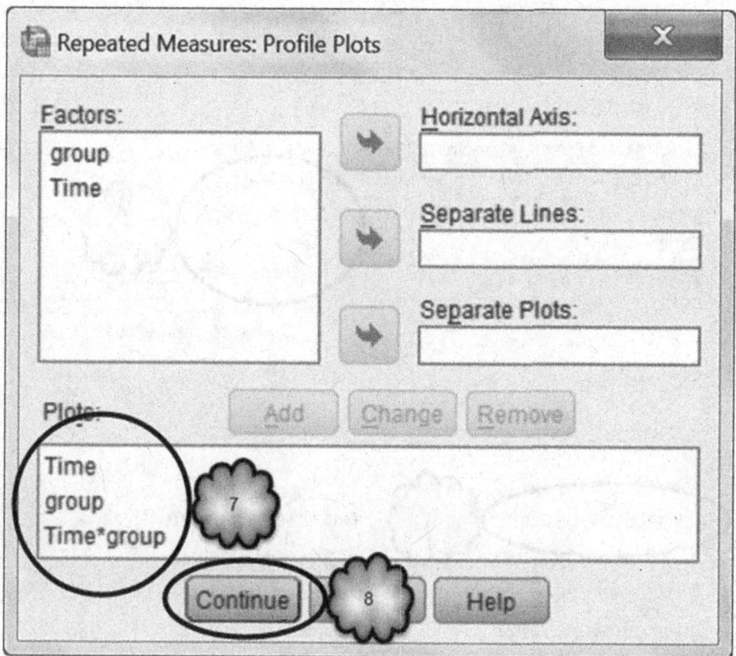

Fig. 12.27 Requesting means plots of the main effects of time of measurement and group, and of the interaction effect between the two factors

Study the output, remembering that higher severity ratings indicate greater headache severity. Then answer the following questions:

12.5.2 What was the *p*-value for the main effect of Group?

12.5.3 Was the mean severity rating at 3-month follow-up significantly less than the mean severity rating at baseline?

12.5.4 What was the mean headache severity rating of the acupuncture group at 3-month follow-up?

12.5.5 Did the acupuncture group experience an average change in severity at 3-month follow-up that was significantly different from the average change experienced by the control group?

12.5.6 What was the *p*-value for the interaction effect?

12.5.7 Do the statistical results of this study support the hypothesis that acupuncture reduces headache severity? Why or why not?

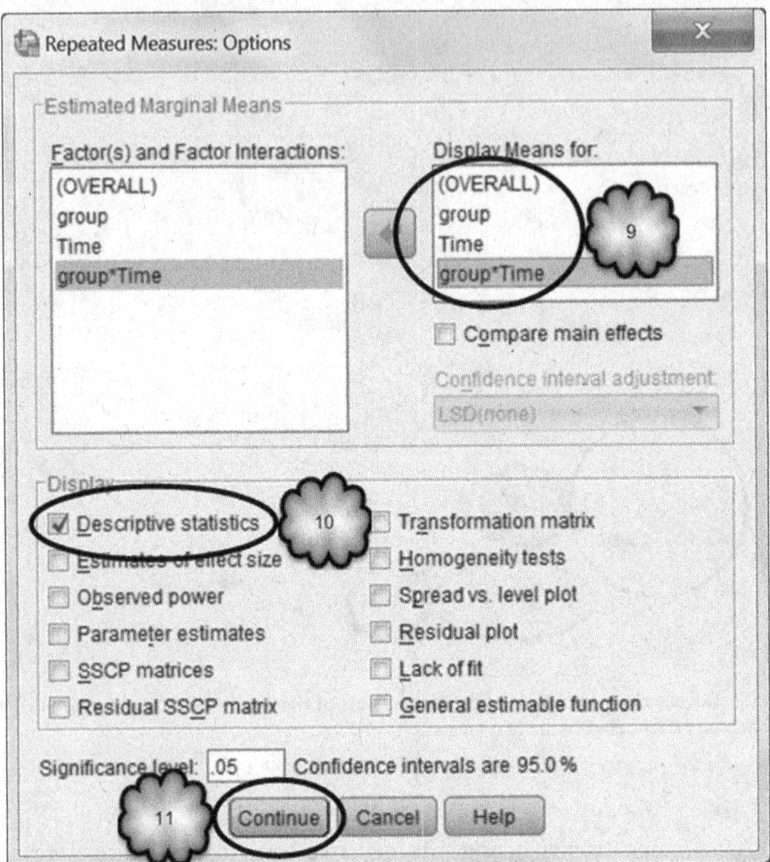

Fig. 12.28 Requesting tables displaying the overall mean, the means of the main and interaction effects, and descriptive statistics

Table 12.16 Mean headache severity ratings of the control and acupuncture groups at baseline (Time = 1) and 3-month follow-up (Time = 2)

4. Group * Time

Measure: Severity

Group	Time	Mean	Std. Error	95% Confidence Interval	
				Lower Bound	Upper Bound
Control	1	27.225	1.283	24.701	29.750
	2	24.477	1.341	21.839	27.116
Acupuncture	1	25.506	1.207	23.131	27.880
	2	19.052	1.261	16.571	21.533

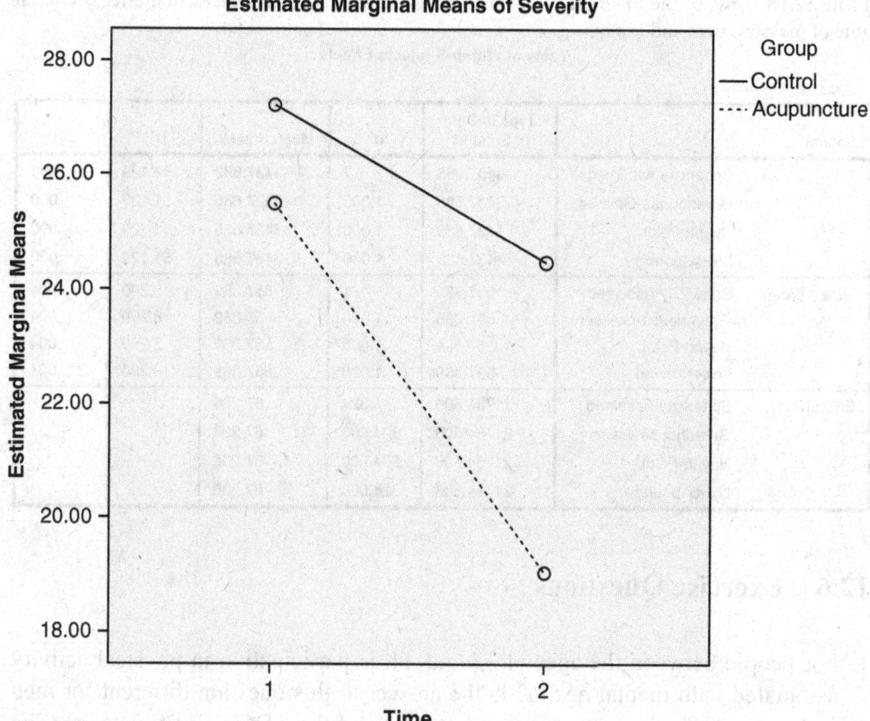

Fig. 12.29 Means plot of the headache severity ratings of the control and acupuncture groups at baseline (Time = 1) and 3-month follow-up (Time = 2)

Table 12.17 Test of the main effect of group

Tests of Between-Subjects Effects

Measure: Severity
Transformed Variable: Average

Source	Type III Sum of Squares	df	Mean Square	F	Sig.
Intercept	376171.096	1	376171.096	817.759	.000
group	2072.390	1	2072.390	4.505	.035
Error	149040.813	324	460.003		

Table 12.18 Tests of the main effect of time of measurement and the interaction effect between time of measurement and group

Tests of Within-Subjects Effects

Measure: Severity

Source		Type III Sum of Squares	df	Mean Square	F	Sig.
Time	Sphericity Assumed	3437.685	1	3437.685	51.129	.000
	Greenhouse-Geisser	3437.685	1.000	3437.685	51.129	.000
	Huynh-Feldt	3437.685	1.000	3437.685	51.129	.000
	Lower-bound	3437.685	1.000	3437.685	51.129	.000
Time * group	Sphericity Assumed	557.389	1	557.389	8.290	.004
	Greenhouse-Geisser	557.389	1.000	557.389	8.290	.004
	Huynh-Feldt	557.389	1.000	557.389	8.290	.004
	Lower-bound	557.389	1.000	557.389	8.290	.004
Error(Time)	Sphericity Assumed	21784.506	324	67.236		
	Greenhouse-Geisser	21784.506	324.000	67.236		
	Huynh-Feldt	21784.506	324.000	67.236		
	Lower-bound	21784.506	324.000	67.236		

12.6 Exercise Questions

1. For people between the ages of 35 and 44, is participation in physical activity associated with mental health? Is the answer to this question different for men and women? To find out, a researcher analyzed the CDC BRFSS data set. The results of the analysis are displayed in Figs. 12.30 and 12.31, and in Table 12.19.
   a. What is the response variable?
   b. Is the response variable categorical or quantitative?
   c. What are the explanatory variables?
   d. Are the explanatory variables independent groups or repeated measures factors?
   e. Ignoring gender, was mental health significantly related to physical activity?
   f. Report the values of the F-ratio, degrees of freedom, and p-value associated with the main effect of physical activity.
   g. Describe the main effect of physical activity.
   h. Does the relationship between physical activity and mental health differ significantly for men and women? What was the p-value associated with this finding?
   i. Describe the interaction effect between physical activity and sex.

2. Using a crossover design, a researcher gave five patients two drugs in tablet form. Drug A was given first. After a washout out period, each patient was given Drug B. For each drug, the researcher measured the level of antibiotic blood serum present at four points in time following ingestion: 1 h, 2 h, 3 h and 6 h. The data are in the file, **Groups.sav** [4]. Conduct a two-way ANOVA.
   a. What is the response variable? Is it categorical or quantitative?
   b. What are the explanatory variables? Are they independent groups or repeated measures factors?

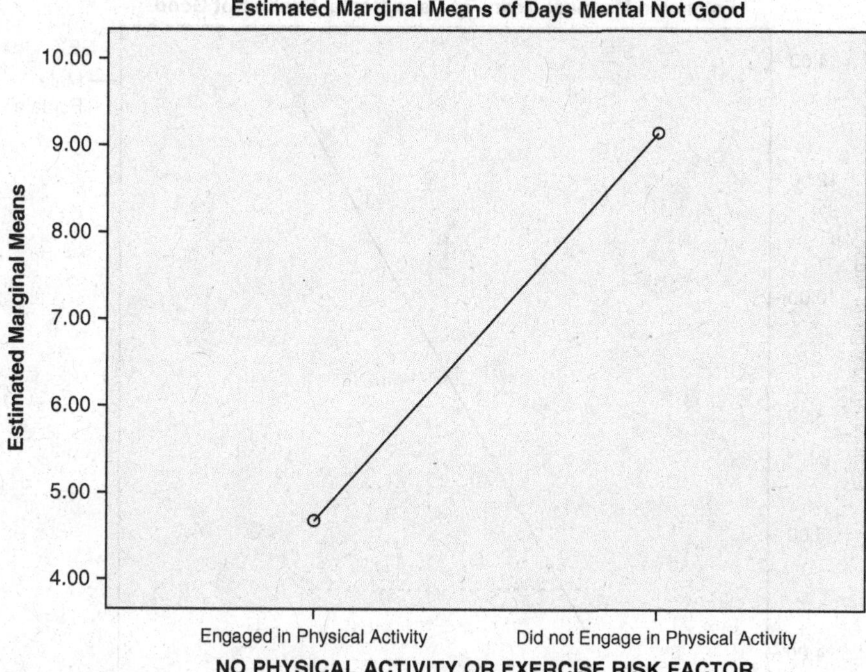

Fig. 12.30 Means plot of the relationship between reported number of days during the past month mental health was "not good" and physical activity (Question 1)

c. Fill in the empty 15 cells of Table 12.20 with the appropriate means.
d. Did the two drugs differ significantly in the overall amount of antibiotic blood serum they produced? What is the *p*-value associated with this finding?
e. Did the number of hours following ingestion produce a significant main effect? What are the values of the means associated with this effect?
f. Did the effect of the number of hours following ingestion significantly depend on which drug had been ingested? What is the *p*-value associated with the answer to this question?
g. When you answered questions 2e and 2f, did you have to take into account the results of the Mauchly's Test of Sphericity? Why or why not?

3. Return to the acupuncture data and include the 1-year follow-up measurement in the analysis.
   a. If we were to predict that acupuncture is effective in treating chronic headache, would we predict an interaction effect between groups and time of measurement? Why or why not?
   b. Did the mean severity ratings at baseline, 3-month follow-up, and 1-year follow-up significantly differ? What is the *p*-value associated with this main effect?
   c. What was the *p*-value for the main effect of Group?

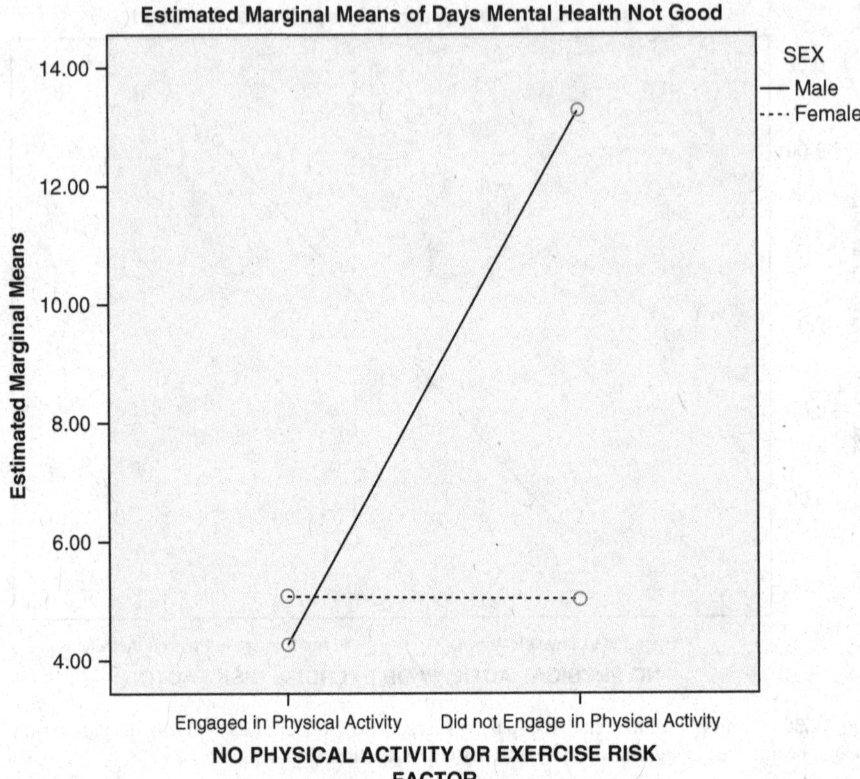

Fig. 12.31 Means plot of the relationship between reported number of days during the past month mental health was "not good" and physical activity for men and women (Question 1)

Table 12.19 Tests of the main and interaction effects (Question 1)

Tests of Between-Subjects Effects

Dependent Variable: Days Mental Health Not Good

Source	Type III Sum of Squares	df	Mean Square	F	Sig.
Corrected Model	2757.973[a]	3	919.324	6.325	.000
Intercept	15553.614	1	15553.614	107.015	.000
SEX	1118.256	1	1118.256	7.694	.006
@_RFNOPA	1621.658	1	1621.658	11.158	.001
SEX * @_RFNOPA	1664.158	1	1664.158	11.450	.001
Error	216848.946	1492	145.341		
Total	256897.000	1496			
Corrected Total	219606.919	1495			

a. R Squared = .013 (Adjusted R Squared = .011)

Table 12.20 Mean antibiotic blood serum

	Hours following ingestion				
Drug	1	2	3	6	Across hours
Drug A					
Drug B					
Across Drugs					

d. Did the decline in severity from baseline to 1-year follow-up differ across the acupuncture and control groups? What is the *p*-value associated with this finding?

e. Do the statistical results of this study support the hypothesis that acupuncture reduces headache severity? Why or why not?

Data Sets and References

1. CDC BRFSS.sav obtained from: Centers for Disease Control and Prevention (CDC). Behavioral Risk Factor Surveillance System Survey Data. US Department of Health and Human Services, Centers for Disease Control and Prevention, Atlanta (2005). Public domain. For more information about the BRFSS, visit http://www.cdc.gov/brfss/. Accessed 16 Nov 2014
2. Blood.sav obtained from: Hand, D.J., Daly, F., Lunn, A.D., McConway, K.J., Ostrowski, E.: A Handbook of Small Data Sets. Chapman & Hall, London (1994). With the kind permission of the Routledge Taylor and Francis Group, and Professor Graham A. MacGregor. For context, see MacGregor, G.A., Markandu, N.D., Roulston, J.E., Jones, J.C.: Essential hypertension: effect of an oral inhibitor of angiotensin-converting enzyme. Br. Med. J. **2**, 1106–1109 (1979)
3. Acupuncture.sav obtained from: Vickers, A.J., Rees, R.W., Zollman, C.E., et al.: Acupuncture for chronic headache in primary care: large, pragmatic, randomised trial. BMJ. (2004). doi:10.1136/bmj.38029.421863.EB. (With the kind permission of Professor Andrew J. Vickers)
4. Groups.sav obtained from: Hand, D.J., Daly, F., Lunn, A.D., McConway, K.J., Ostrowski, E.: A Handbook of Small Data Sets. Chapman & Hall, London (1994). (With the kind permission of Professor David J. Hand)

Chapter 13
Simple Linear Regression

Abstract The principle of least squares is introduced to determine the best fitting straight line. The coefficient of determination is discussed as a measure of how well the straight line fits the data. Estimation and testing of the slope and intercept coefficients is introduced. Confidence intervals on the predictions made by the regression line are discussed. Finally, residual analysis is presented.

13.1 Overview

In Chap. 9, we considered measuring the strength of relationship between two quantitative variables by using the Pearson correlation coefficient. There we learned that a correlation of +1 indicates that two quantitative variables have a perfect linear relationship with a positive slope, a value of −1 indicates a perfect linear relationship with a negative slope, and that correlations with a magnitude near zero indicate a very weak linear relationship. When the variables do exhibit a linear relationship, researchers often would like to know the equation of the straight line that describes the relationship. The equation of a straight line has the following form:

$$y = a + bx \tag{13.1}$$

In the equation, b represents the slope (the change in y for a one unit increase in x) and a represents the y-intercept (the value of y when x equals 0). In this context, the y variable is often called the *dependent variable* and the x variable is often called the *independent variable*. Once researchers have the equation of this line, it can be used to make predictions of y for a given value of x.

Before trying to determine the slope and intercept of the straight line, researchers first create a *scatter plot* to see if the relationship between the two variables is linear. If the relationship is linear, then researchers use a method, known as *least squares*, to find the slope and intercept that "best" describes the linear relationship seen in the data.

The straight line equation describes a linear relationship observed in a sample of data. If the sample had been taken at random from a larger population, the sample's slope and intercept will be affected by random sampling variability. In other words, if

W. H. Holmes, W. C. Rinaman, *Statistical Literacy for Clinical Practitioners*,
DOI 10.1007/978-3-319-12550-3_13

another random sample were to be taken, the values of its slope and intercept would likely be at least a little different from those of the first sample. Because of this random variability, the values of the slope and intercept of a given sample may not be indicative of those of the population. Moreover, the predictions of *y* based on the sample will likely not be the same as those based on another sample randomly drawn from the same population. Consequently, after determining the best fitting straight line for a sample of data, researchers construct confidence intervals (CIs) for the population slope and intercept, test hypotheses regarding their values, and construct CIs for predictions generated by the equation of that line. In this chapter, we will review these procedures. In the next chapter, we will apply these techniques to situations in which predictions of the dependent variable are based on two or more independent variables.

13.2 Describing the Best Fitting Straight Line

In this chapter, we will use data from a study of the pulmonary function of 654 boys and girls between the ages of 3 and 19. The data file includes the forced expiratory volume (FEV) of each child, that is, the amount of air (measured in liters) each child exhaled forcefully in one second. The age, height, and sex of the child, and whether the child was a smoker or nonsmoker are also recorded. We will focus on predicting the FEV of nonsmokers between the ages of 9 and 14. We will begin our study by creating a scatter plot to determine if there appears to be a linear relationship between FEV and age.

Scatter Plots As we saw in Chap. 9, a graphical means for determining if a relationship exists between a quantitative explanatory variable and a quantitative response variable is a scatter plot. In the context of regression, the explanatory variable is called the independent variable and the response variable is called the dependent variable. In our example, age will be the independent variable and FEV will be the dependent variable.

On an *x-y* coordinate system, the independent variable forms the horizontal axis, and the dependent variable forms the vertical axis. The values of the two variables for each case form an (*x*,*y*) pair that is plotted. The resulting plot of these points is a scatter plot. We then look at the pattern of the plotted points to determine the degree to which the two variables are related and whether or not the relationship appears to be linear. The degree to which the plot follows some sort of a curve will show the *strength* of the relationship. The more the points follow a curve, the stronger is the relationship. If the curve shows that there is a tendency for *x* and *y* to both increase, the relationship is said to be *positive*. If the curve shows that there is a tendency for *y* to decrease as *x* increases, the relationship is said to be *negative*. If the points follow a curve that is a straight line, then the relationship is said to be *linear*, otherwise it is said to be *non-linear*.

Open the file, **FEV.sav** [1]. This file consists of the following variables: **Age (years)** [*Age*] (variable 1), **FEV (liters)** [*FEV*] (variable 2), **Height (inches)** [*Height*] (variable 3), **Sex** [*Sex*] (variable 4; 0 = female, 1 = male), and **Smoking Status** [*Smoke*] (variable 5; 0 = nonsmoker, 1 = smoker). We wish to focus on nonsmokers who are between the ages of 9 and 14, inclusive, so begin by selecting cases of nonsmokers within this age range. There are 348 of them distributed across the six age groups. Chapter 2 explains how to use **Data > Select Cases** to choose cases in SPSS.

To draw the scatter plot, we will follow the same procedure we followed in Chap. 9. Select **Graphs > Chart Builder**, select *Scatter/Dot* from the *Gallery*, and drag the picture of the simple scatter plot (the one in the upper left corner) to the empty window above it. Drag the independent variable, **Age (years)** [*Age*] (variable 1) to the *x-Axis* box, and drag the dependent variable, **FEV (liters)** [*FEV*] (variable 2) to the *y-Axis* box. When you are finished, the dialog box should look like the one shown in Fig. 13.1.

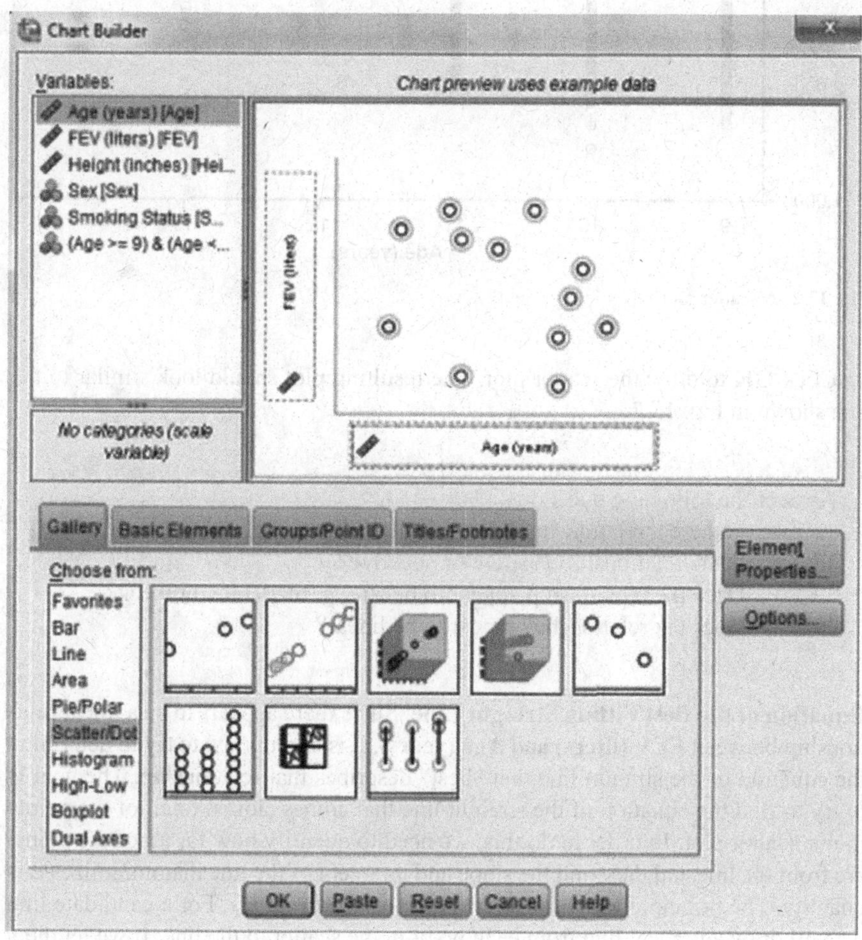

Fig. 13.1 Requesting a scatter plot

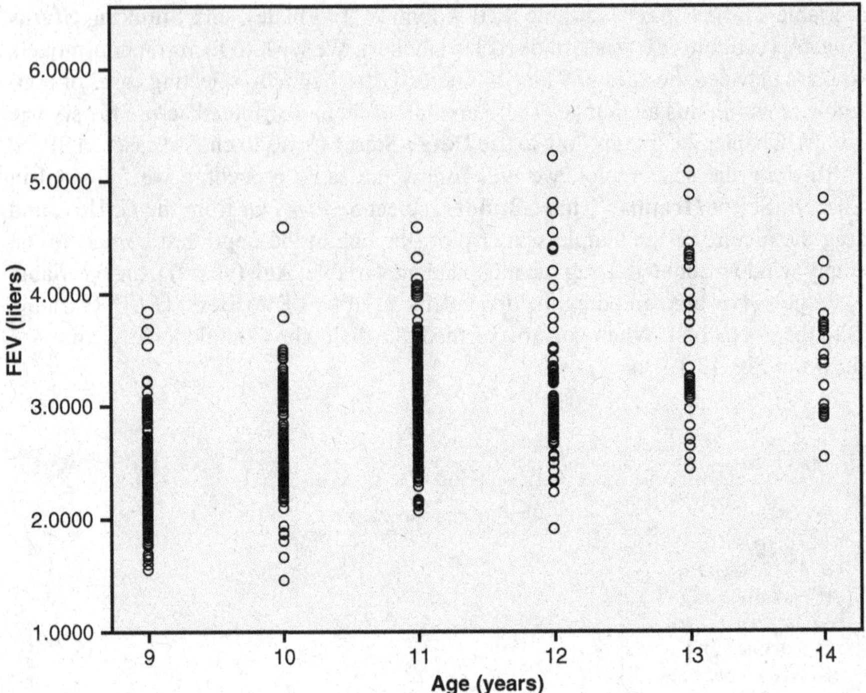

Fig. 13.2 A scatter plot

Click **OK** to draw the scatter plot. The resulting plot should look similar to the one shown in Fig. 13.2.

Answer the following questions.

13.2.1 Is there a relationship between **FEV (liters)** and **Age (years)**?

13.2.2 Is the relationship positive or negative?

13.2.3 Does the relationship appear to be strong, moderate, or weak?

13.2.4 Does the relationship appear to be linear?

Equation of the Best Fitting Straight Line Since there appears to be a linear relationship between **FEV (liters)** and **Age (years)**, it is appropriate to try to determine the equation of the straight line that "best" describes that relationship. The goal is to try to find the equation of the straight line that comes closest to all of the points in our scatter plot. In order to do this, we need to quantify how far all of the points are from the line and then find the slope and intercept of the line that minimizes this quantity. The principle we will use is known as *least squares*. For a candidate line we will draw a vertical line from each point in the scatter to the line. If we let the y

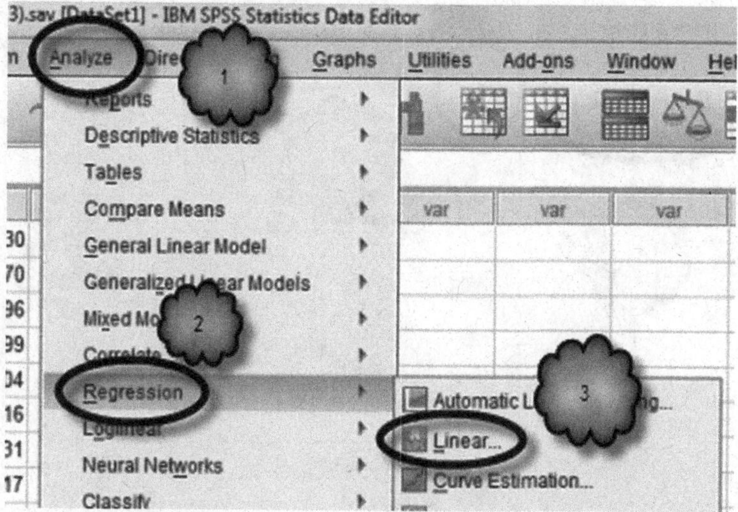

Fig. 13.3 Selecting a linear regression

value of where one of these verticals intercepts the candidate line be denoted by $\hat{y}$, the distance from the point to the line would be $y - \hat{y}$. This quantity is known as a *residual.* We calculate the residual for each point in the data. These residuals are then squared and the squares are summed to obtain what is known as the *residual sum of squares*,

$$\sum (y - \hat{y})^2 \tag{13.2}$$

The slope and intercept of the straight line that minimizes the residual sum of squares are known as the *least squares estimates* (i.e., they make the residual sum of squares have its least value). The equation of the straight line that uses the slope and intercept obtained in this manner is known as the *least squares fit* or the *least squares regression line* for the data. The equation of the least squares line will be

$$\hat{y} = a + bx \tag{13.3}$$

SPSS can compute the slope and intercept for the least squares regression line. As shown in Figs. 13.3, 13.4, 13.5, and 13.6, select **Analyze>Regression>Linear** to bring up the *Linear Regression* dialog box. Place the independent (x) variable, **Age (years)**, in the *Independent(s)* box, and place the dependent (y) variable, **FEV (liters)**, in the *Dependent* box. Click **OK** to run the regression.

The output will contain a number of items. We will explain them eventually, but for now we are interested in determining the equation of the least squares regression line. The slope and intercept of that line are found in the *Coefficients* table shown in Table 13.1.

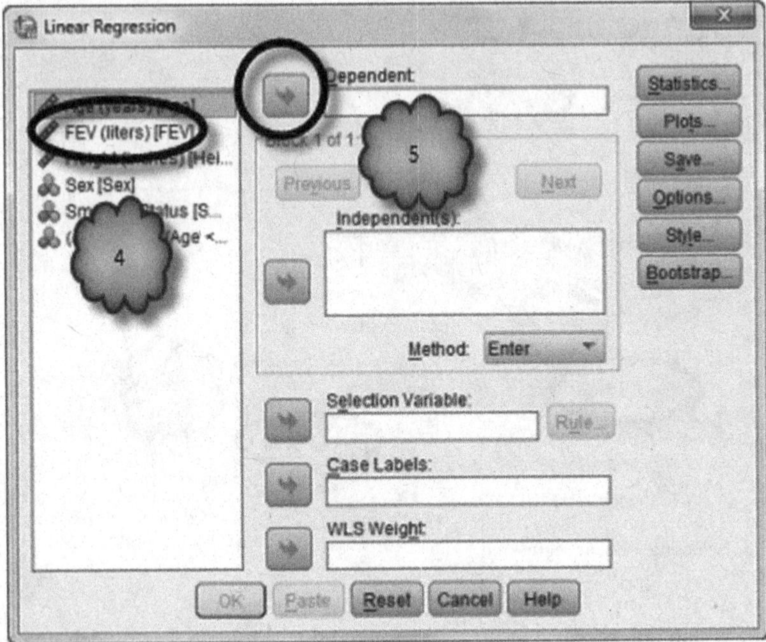

Fig. 13.4 Selecting the dependent variable

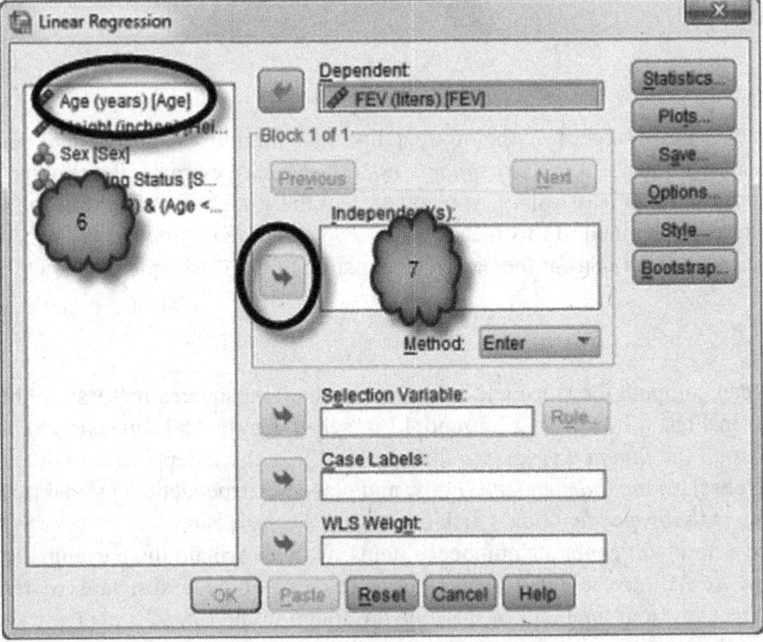

Fig. 13.5 Selecting the independent variable

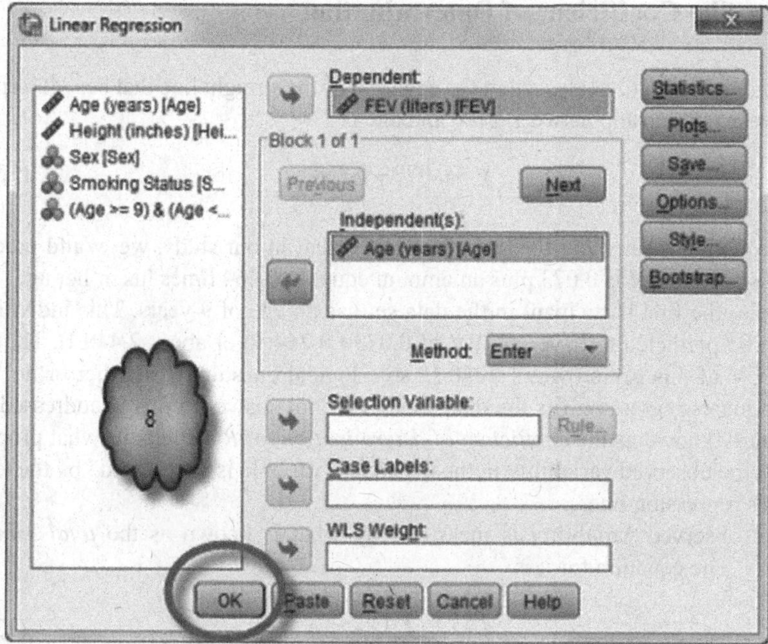

Fig. 13.6 Performing the analysis

Table 13.1 Coefficients table

Coefficients[a]

Model		Unstandardized Coefficients		Standardized Coefficients	t	Sig.
		B	Std. Error	Beta		
1	(Constant)	.073	.229		.317	.751
	Age (years)	.264	.021	.557	12.472	.000

a. Dependent Variable: FEV (liters)

They are in the column labeled *B* in the *Unstandardized Coefficients* area. The value in the row labeled (*Constant*) is the intercept, and the value in the row with the name of the independent variable is the slope. Notice that the slope is positive, indicating that the relationship between the two variables is positive.

13.2.5 What is the value of the y-intercept?
13.2.6 What is the slope of the line?
13.2.7 What is the equation of the least squares regression line?

13.3 The Coefficient of Determination

We can see from our analysis that the equation of the straight line that best describes the linear relationship between FEV and age is

$$\hat{y} = 0.073 + 0.264x \tag{13.4}$$

This equation means that for any given individual in our study, we would predict that his or her FEV is 0.073 plus an amount equal to 0.264 times his or her age. For example, the first participant in the data set has an age of 9 years. This individual would be predicted to have an FEV of 0.073+0.264(9) or about 2.449 L. The actual FEV of this person was 1.7080 L, so a logical question is whether or not the least squares regression fits the data well. A partial answer to this is addressed by a quantity known as the *coefficient of determination,* or R^2. It tells us what proportion of the observed variability in the dependent variable is "explained" by the least squares regression line.

The observed variability is measured by what is known as the *total sum of squares.* The equation for it is

$$TSS = \sum (y_i - \overline{y})^2 \tag{13.5}$$

This variability reflects the extent to which values of the dependent variable vary around the mean of those values. If we had no information about a sample other than the mean, we would use the mean as our estimate of the value of the dependent variable for each individual. For example, the mean FEV of our 348 children is 2.89683 L. If this is all we know about them, then our best guess of the FEV of each of the 348 children would be 2.89683 L. Consequently, TSS also indicates the extent to which using the mean to predict individual values of the dependent variable would be off the mark. It turns out that this sum of squares can be broken into the sum of two other sums of squares, called the *regression sum of squares, RSS,* and the *residual or error sum of squares, ESS.* The equation looks like

$$\underset{\text{TSS}}{\sum (y_i - \overline{y})^2} = \underset{\text{RSS}}{\sum (\hat{y}_i - \overline{y})^2} + \underset{\text{ESS}}{\sum (y_i - \hat{y}_i)^2} \tag{13.6}$$

In the equation, y_i is the actual FEV of a given child, $\overline{y}$ is the mean FEV of the sample, and $\hat{y}_i$ is the predicted value of FEV for that child. You will note that the residual sum of squares is the quantity that the least squares method tries to minimize. The regression sum of squares is referred to as the *amount of the variability in y that is "explained" by the regression line*, and the residual sum of squares is the *amount of the variability in y that is "unexplained" by the regression line.* Therefore, the proportion of the total variability in *y* that is "explained" by the regression will be the ratio RSS/TSS. This quantity is the coefficient of determination, or R^2. Since it

Table 13.2 Model summary

Model Summary

Model	R	R Square	Adjusted R Square	Std. Error of the Estimate
1	.557[a]	.310	.308	.5795303

a. Predictors: (Constant), Age (years)

is a proportion, its range of possible values is from 0 to 1. A value of 1 indicates a perfect fit to the data. That is, the data follow a straight line exactly. A value of 0 indicates that the independent variable is of absolutely no help in predicting the value of the dependent variable. We would be no better off than if we had used the mean of the sample to make our estimates. We put the term "explained" in quotes to emphasize that "explained" in this context does not imply a cause-and-effect relation between the independent and dependent variables.

In SPSS, the coefficient of determination for a regression can be found in the *Model Summary* table under *R Square.* This table is shown in Table 13.2. The *Model Summary* table also contains *R* which is the positive square root of the coefficient of determination; *Adjusted R Square,* which will be discussed in the next chapter, and *Std. Error of the Estimate*, which will be discussed in the next section. Study the output and answer the following questions.

13.3.1 What is the value of R^2?
13.3.2 What is the quality of the fit?

The value of R^2 tells us that the regression line fits the data reasonably well, accounting for 31 % of the variability in FEV. We saw in Chap. 9 that we can ask SPSS to draw the best fitting straight line through the points in a scatter plot by double clicking the plot and clicking the *Add Fit Line at Total* icon. Doing this with the scatter plot we generated earlier in this chapter allows us to visualize the goodness of fit of the regression line. The plot is shown in Fig. 13.7.

We can see from the plot that the data show a weak to moderate tendency to gravitate around the regression line. Notice the value of R^2 linear in the upper right-hand corner of the graph. This is the coefficient of determination. Its value will match the value displayed in the *Model Summary* table.

Let us take a closer look at the regression line. In the scatter plot in Fig. 13.7, the *x*-axis has been extended leftward to its zero point. We did this to show the intercept of the regression line.

The regression line consists of the predicted values of FEV across the values of age. The strength of the relationship between FEV and age is indicated by how closely these predicted values match actual values. For example, as we saw earlier,

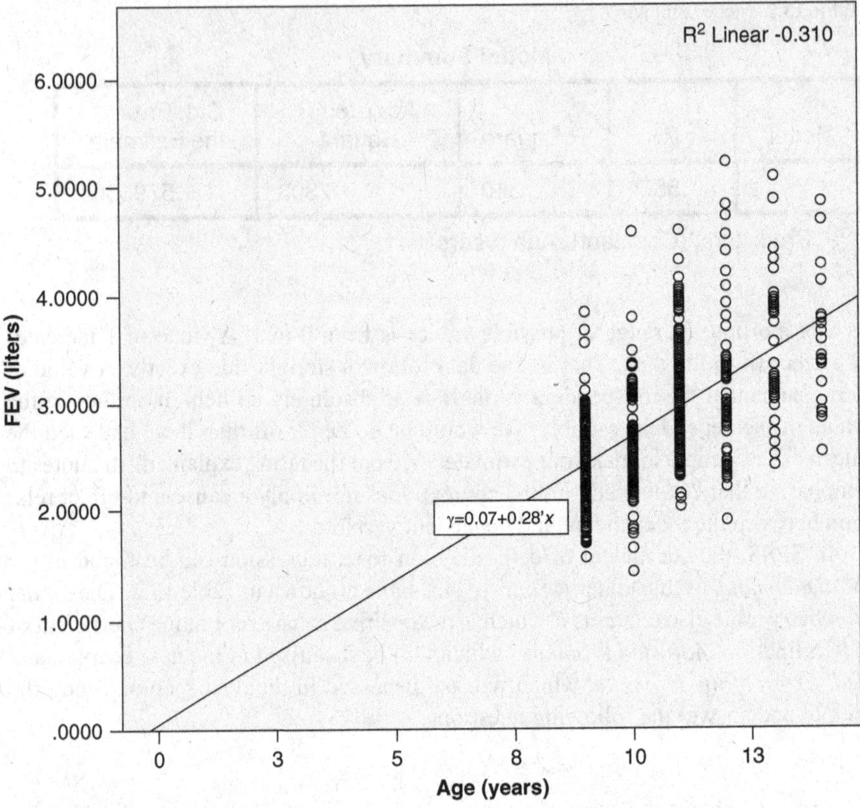

Fig. 13.7 Scatter plot with regression line

the participant who had an age of 9 years would be predicted to have an FEV of about 2.449 L. This child's actual FEV was 1.7080 L, so the predicted value falls short of the actual value by a residual of about of −0.741 L. Another 9-year old had an actual FEV of 2.9880 L. In fact, most of the 9-year olds in the sample had an actual FEV different from the predicted value of 2.449 L. These relationships are displayed in the plot shown in Fig. 13.8. The boxed points are the actual FEV values, and the arrow shows the predicted FEV value (or what we referred to as $\hat{y}$ in the equations above).

There are 348 people in the sample. If we were to square all 348 residuals and then sum them, the result would be the residual or error sum of squares, ESS. Recall that this quantity is equal to 1 minus the coefficient of determination. Thus, our analysis tells us that the straight line that best describes the relationship between FEV and age cannot account for 69.9% of the variability in FEV values. On the other hand, our analysis also tells us that taking into account the linear relationship between FEV and age greatly improves our ability to make accurate estimates of FEV beyond that which we would have been able to make by using the mean of the sample.

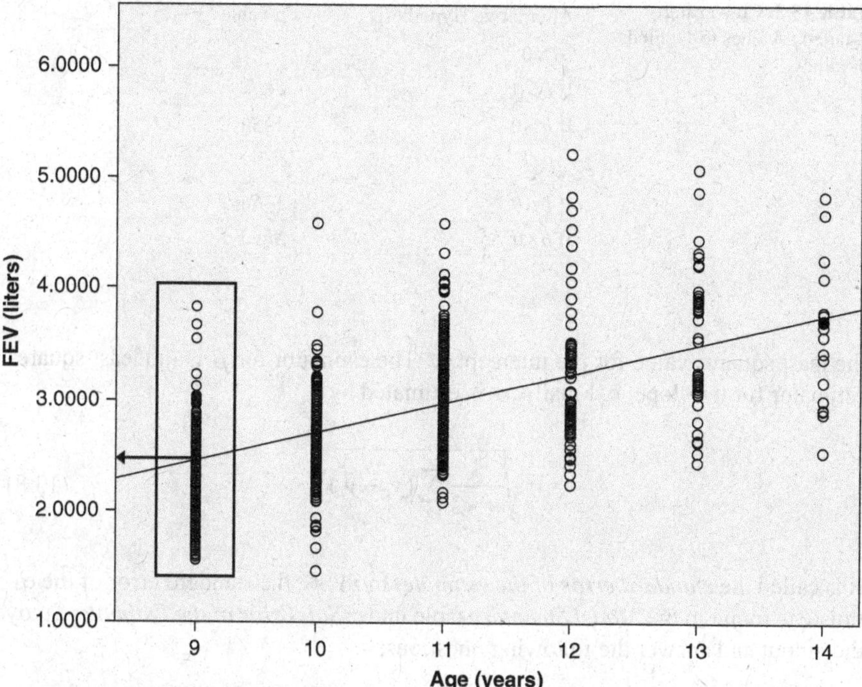

Fig. 13.8 Illustrating errors

13.4 Estimating and Testing Population Coefficients

Estimation If the data used to get the least squares regression line are a random sample from a larger population, we would like to know whether or not the results are indicative of a true linear relationship in the population. In order to do this, we need a model for the population that would produce a scatter plot such as we observed in the sample. That means that we will need a straight line that follows the trend in the data. In addition, we need some randomly generated values that produce the scatter about this line. In order to obtain this, the so-called *classical regression model* looks like the following:

$$y_i = \alpha + \beta x_i + \varepsilon_i \tag{13.7}$$

where y_i is an actual value of y, α is the population y-intercept, β is the population slope, x_i is a known, fixed value of x, and ε_i is a random value that is assumed to have a normal distribution with a mean of 0 and a standard deviation of σ. Thus, the parameters of the model are α, β, and σ. Since we do not know the values of these parameters, we need to use our sample data to estimate them. The estimator for α is

Table 13.3 Converting 2-tailed *p*-values to 1-tailed *p*-values

Alternative Hypothesis	*p*-value
$\beta > 0$	
If $b > 0$	*Sig/2*
If $b \leq 0$	1–*Sig/2*
$\beta < 0$	
If $b > 0$	1–*Sig/2*
If $b \leq 0$	*Sig/2*

the least squares value for the intercept, *a*. The estimator for β is the least squares estimator for the slope, *b*. Finally, σ is estimated by

$$s = \sqrt{\frac{1}{n-2}\sum(y_i - \hat{y}_i)^2} \tag{13.8}$$

It is called the *standard error of the estimate.* In SPSS, the standard error of the estimate is found in the *Model Summary* table under *Std. Error of the Estimate.* Study the output and answer the following questions:

13.4.1 What is the value of the estimate for α?
13.4.2 What is the value of the estimate for β?
13.4.3 What is the value of the estimate for σ?

Testing Hypotheses with the t Distribution Our next step is to determine whether or not the regression equation on our data is indicative of a true linear relationship between the independent and dependent variables in the population from which the data were drawn. To do this, we will test the null hypothesis that the population slope, β, is equal to 0. The alternative hypothesis can be either that the population slope is positive, or that the population slope is negative, or that the population is not equal to 0. SPSS conducts this test in two different ways. We will discuss the first in this section and address the second method in the next section. The first uses a test statistic that has a *t* distribution. The value of the test statistic and the *p*-value for the two-sided alternative hypothesis can be found in the *Coefficients* table in the columns labeled *t* and *Sig.* In the row for the independent variable, the value of the test statistic is in the *t* column and the two-tailed *p*-value is in the *Sig.* column. As usual, small *p*-values correspond to evidence against the null hypothesis. You will note that if you divide the value in the *B* column by the value in the *Std. Error* column you get the *t* value to within rounding. If the alternative hypothesis is one-sided, the two-sided *p*-value is obtained as described in Table 13.3. *Sig.* is the two-tailed *p*-value from the *Coefficients* table.

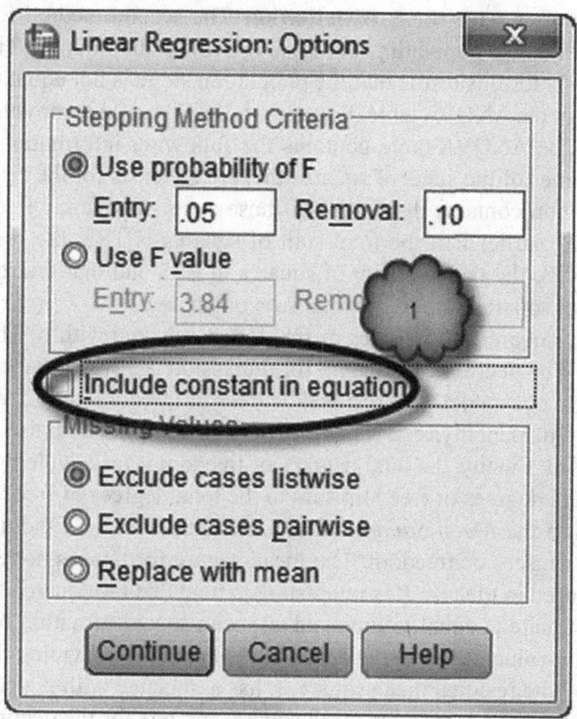

Fig. 13.9 Fitting a regression with an intercept of 0

In the row labeled (*Constant*) the *t* value and the *p*-value are for the two-sided test that the population intercept, α, is equal to 0. If the *p*-value for this test is large (usually greater than 0.1), you might want to consider fitting a model where the intercept is set to 0. This is done by clicking **Options** in the regression main dialog box to bring up the dialog box shown in Fig. 13.9. Unchecking *Include constant in equation* will do a least squares fit with *a* set to 0.

Study the Coefficients table shown in Sect. 13.2 (Table 13.1) and answer the following questions:

13.4.4 What is the *t* value for testing the null hypothesis that the population slope is 0?

13.4.5 What is the two-sided p-value for this test?

13.4.6 What should you conclude regarding the population slope?

13.4.7 What is the *t* value for testing the null hypothesis that the population intercept is 0?

13.4.8 What is the two-sided *p*-value for this test?

13.4.9 What should you conclude regarding the population intercept?

Testing Hypotheses with the F Distribution The second method for testing the null hypothesis that the population slope is 0 uses the *F* distribution. The only alternative hypothesis for this test is that the population slope is not equal to 0. The test is summarized in the ANOVA table. Recall that ANOVA is an acronym for ANalysis Of VAriance. The ANOVA table contains the following information. The *Model* contains the names of the sums of squares that are the basis for the *F* test. The *Sum of Squares* column contains the values of those sums of squares. Recall from our discussion of R^2 earlier that the total sum of squares is TSS, the regression sum of squares is RSS, the residual sum of squares in ESS and that the regression and residual sums of squares sum to the total sum of squares.

Each sum of squares has degrees of freedom associated with it. They appear in the *df* column. The degrees of freedom for regression is 1, the number of independent variables in our model. The residual degrees of freedom in $n-2$, where n is the sample size. Coincidentally, $n-2$ is number of degrees of freedom used in the *t* tests we just discussed. Finally, the total degrees of freedom is $n-1$. Note that the regression and residual degrees of freedom sum to the total degrees of freedom.

The entries in the *Mean Square* column are arrived at by dividing the sum of squares by its degrees of freedom. The mean square for total is not computed because it is not used in the test. It is interesting to note that the square of the standard error of the estimate is equal to the residual mean square to within rounding. The entry in *F* is the value of the test statistic. It is obtained by dividing the regression mean square by the residual mean square. It has associated with it a pair of degrees of freedom, one for the numerator mean square, and one for the denominator mean square. The numerator degrees of freedom are always listed first, followed by the denominator degrees of freedom. Large values of *F* indicate evidence against the null hypothesis. The entry in *Sig.* is the *p*-value for the *F* test. As usual, the smaller the *p*-value, the greater is the strength of evidence against the null hypothesis.

At this point, it is logical to ask why we need two different tests for determining whether or not the population slope is 0. We really do not. It turns out that the *t* and *F* tests are equivalent only in regression models with a single independent variable. In the next chapter, we shall see that the *F* test is different from the *t* test when we consider models with two or more independent variables. To see that the *t* and *F* tests are equivalent in this setting note that the *F* value is the square of the *t* value for testing the slope to within rounding.

Table 13.4 is the ANOVA table reproduced from the output.

13.4.10 What is the value of the regression sum of squares?
13.4.11 What is the value of the residual sum of squares?
13.4.12 What are the degrees of freedom for the regression sum of squares?
13.4.13 What are the degrees of freedom for the residual sum of squares?
13.4.14 Verify that each mean square is obtained by dividing the sum of squares by its corresponding degrees of freedom.

Table 13.4 Regression ANOVA table

ANOVA[a]

Model		Sum of Squares	df	Mean Square	F	Sig.
1	Regression	52.242	1	52.242	155.550	.000[b]
	Residual	116.206	346	.336		
	Total	168.448	347			

a. Dependent Variable: FEV (liters)
b. Predictors: (Constant), Age (years)

13.4.15 Verify that the value of the *F* statistic is the ratio of the regression mean square divided by the residual mean square?
13.4.16 What is the *p*-value for this test?
13.4.17 Based on this *p*-value does it appear that the population slope coefficient is 0? Why or why not.

Confidence Intervals There are times when you want to construct CIs for the population slope and intercept. These CIs have the same interpretation as CIs we have encountered in previous chapters. That is, a 95 % CI means that 95 % of all possible intervals will contain the population parameter of interest. SPSS can construct CIs for the population slope and intercept. In the main regression dialog box click **Statistics** to bring up the dialog box shown in Fig. 13.10.

In the *Regression Coefficient* area check *Confidence intervals*. Enter the desired confidence level, in percent, in the *Level(%)* box. For our example, use a 95 % confidence level. Click **Continue** and **OK** to run the regression in the usual manner. The requested CIs will be appended on the right-hand side of the *Coefficients* table in the output, as shown in Table 13.5.

Study the output shown in Table 13.5 and answer the following questions.
13.4.18 What is the 95 % CI for the population slope?
13.4.19 What is the 95 % CI for the population intercept?
13.4.20 Are these CIs consistent with the results of the t tests reported in the table?

13.5 Prediction Intervals

The regression equation we obtained was based on the sample of 348 subjects. If we were to collect another sample of 348 subjects we would obtain a different regression equation. The predictions for values of the dependent variable using the

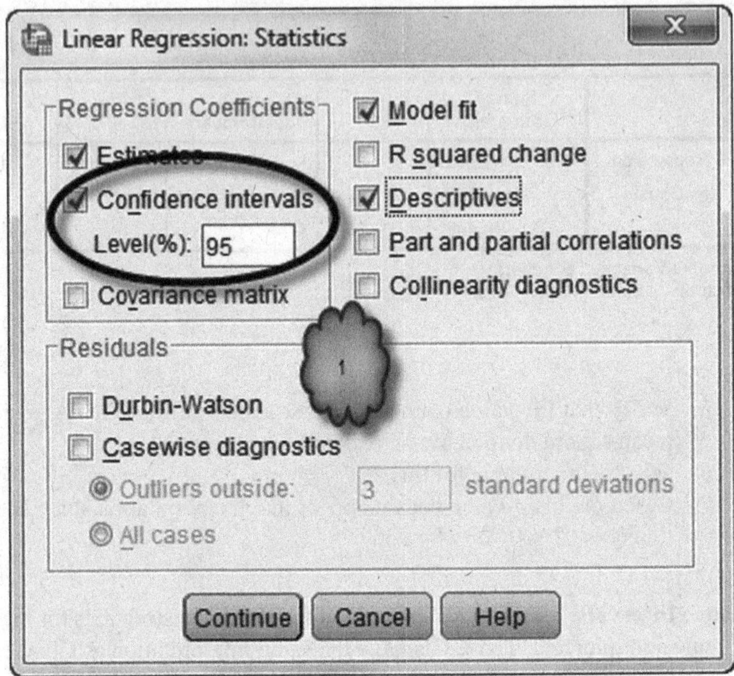

Fig. 13.10 Requesting confidence intervals

Table 13.5 Confidence intervals

Coefficients[a]

Model		Unstandardized Coefficients		Standardized Coefficients	t	Sig.	95.0% Confidence Interval for B	
		B	Std. Error	Beta			Lower Bound	Upper Bound
1	(Constant)	.073	.229		.317	.751	-.377	.522
	Age (years)	.264	.021	.557	12.472	.000	.222	.305

a. Dependent Variable: FEV (liters)

second regression equation would differ from those obtained using the first regression equation. So, in addition to making point predictions for the dependent variable, we would like to construct CIs for the predictions. Such intervals are known as *prediction intervals*. There are two types of prediction intervals depending on how you interpret what the regression equation predicts. The value of the dependent variable that the regression predicts can represent the *mean* value of the dependent variable for that value of the independent variable. The other possibility is that the value of the dependent variable that the regression equation predicts represents the value of the next *individual* having that value of the independent variable. Clearly, we are more confident in the accuracy of predicting a mean compared to an individual. This is reflected in the fact that prediction intervals for means are narrower than prediction intervals for individuals. It is up to the investigator to interpret whether the predictions represent means or individuals. SPSS allows for both possibilities.

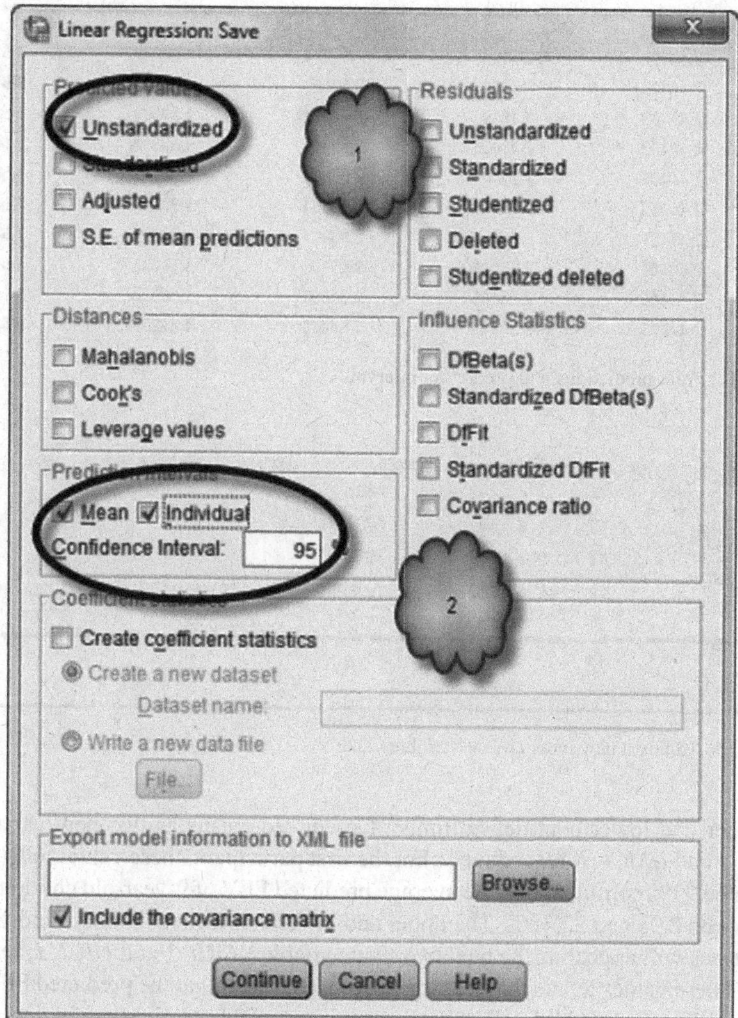

Fig. 13.11 Requesting point predictions and prediction intervals

To construct prediction intervals for values of the independent variable in the data set, click **Save** in the main regression dialog box to bring up the dialog box shown in Fig. 13.11. To compute and save the point predictions check *Unstandardized* in the *Predicted Values* area. To obtain the prediction intervals check *Mean* and *Individual* in the *Prediction Intervals* area. Enter the desired confidence level, in percent, in the *Confidence Interval* box. Click **Continue** and run the regression in the usual manner.

The various predictions and CIs will be appended to the data set as new columns of data. Predictions and CIs for the first 10 participants are shown in Fig. 13.12.

The point predictions appear in a new variable, labeled *PRE_1*. For the first participant, the model predicts an FEV of 2.444. The next two columns present

PRE_1	LMCI_1	UMCI_1	LICI_1	UICI_1
2.44403	2.35005	2.53801	1.30032	3.58774
2.44403	2.35005	2.53801	1.30032	3.58774
2.44403	2.35005	2.53801	1.30032	3.58774
2.44403	2.35005	2.53801	1.30032	3.58774
2.44403	2.35005	2.53801	1.30032	3.58774
2.44403	2.35005	2.53801	1.30032	3.58774
2.44403	2.35005	2.53801	1.30032	3.58774
2.44403	2.35005	2.53801	1.30032	3.58774
2.44403	2.35005	2.53801	1.30032	3.58774
2.44403	2.35005	2.53801	1.30032	3.58774

Fig. 13.12 Point predictions and prediction intervals

	Age	FEV	Height	Sex	Smoke	filter_$
649	18	4.2200	68.0	1	0	0
650	18	4.0860	67.0	1	1	0
651	18	4.4040	70.5	1	1	0
652	19	5.1020	72.0	1	0	0
653	19	3.5190	66.0	0	1	0
654	19	3.3450	65.5	0	1	0
655	15	.	.	.	.	1

Fig. 13.13 Adding a new independent variable value

the upper and lower confidence limits of predicted means as two new variables, *LMCI_1* and *UMCI_1*, respectively. For the first participant, these values tell us that we can be 95 % confident that the average predicted FEV of 9-year-old children will be between 2.35 and 2.538 L. The upper and lower confidence limits for individual predictions will appear as the next two new variables, *LICI_1* and *UICI_1*, respectively. These values tell us that we can be 95 % confident that the predicted FEV for any given 9-year-old child will be between 1.3 and 3.59 L. Notice that for any given value of age, the CI for predicting an individual child's FEV is wider than the CI for predicting the mean FEV.

Often, we will want to make point predictions or get prediction interval limits for values of the independent variable that are not in the data set. To do this, we enter the desired value(s) for the independent variable to the bottom of the data set, leave the dependent variable empty, and run the regression saving the predicted values and the prediction intervals. To see how this works, enter a value of 15 in case 655 of **Age (years)** and a value of 1 in **filter_$**, as shown in Fig. 13.13.

Compute the regression saving the unstandardized predicted values and 95 % prediction intervals for both the mean and individuals. This will produce a second set of predictions and CIs for all of the individuals, and for the new entry. Each of the second set of variables will have "_2" attached to the variable names. See Fig. 13.14.

It is probably not obvious from looking at the values that are stored in the Data View, but predictions intervals get wider as we move from the center of the data to

PRE_2	LMCI_2	UMCI_2	LICI_2	UICI_2
.	.	.	.	.
.	.	.	.	.
.	.	.	.	.
.	.	.	.	.
.	.	.	.	.
.	.	.	.	.
4.02505	3.83693	4.21317	2.86978	5.18031

Fig. 13.14 A new set of predictions and prediction intervals

extremities. This reflects the fact that predictions are more accurate in the center of the data set than they are at the end points. Making predictions beyond the endpoints of the data should be made with care as you need to make the assumption that the pattern of the relationship that you see in the data does not change for values of the independent variable larger or smaller than the largest or smallest value in the data. It is a little hard to see, but the scatter plot shown in Fig. 13.15 shows the predicted values for the dependent variable and the two sets of prediction intervals. The uppermost and lowermost lines are the prediction interval for individuals. The next two are the prediction interval for means. The center line shows the point predictions. If you look closely, you can see that, as we move from the center of the data, the upper and lower confidence limits get farther apart.

Answer the following questions:

13.5.1 What was the point prediction for a value of **Age** of 15?

13.5.2 What are the upper and lower 95 % prediction limits when we interpret the predicted value to be a mean for a 9-year old?

13.5.3 What is the width of this interval?

13.5.4 What are the upper and lower 95 % prediction limits when we interpret the predicted value to be an individual for a 9-year old?

13.5.5 What is the width of this interval?

13.5.6 Which prediction interval is wider?

13.6 Residual Analysis

The validity of the t tests, the F test, the CIs of the population slope and intercept, and the prediction interval we have been discussing depends on the regression model requirements that there is a linear relationship between the independent and dependent variables, and that the error terms have a normal distribution with a mean of 0 and a standard deviation that is constant for all values of the independent variable. We need to verify that these conditions have been met. This is done by examining the residuals that result from the least squares curve fit. Recall that the residual for the ith case is $y_i - \hat{y}_i$. These are the estimates for the value of the error

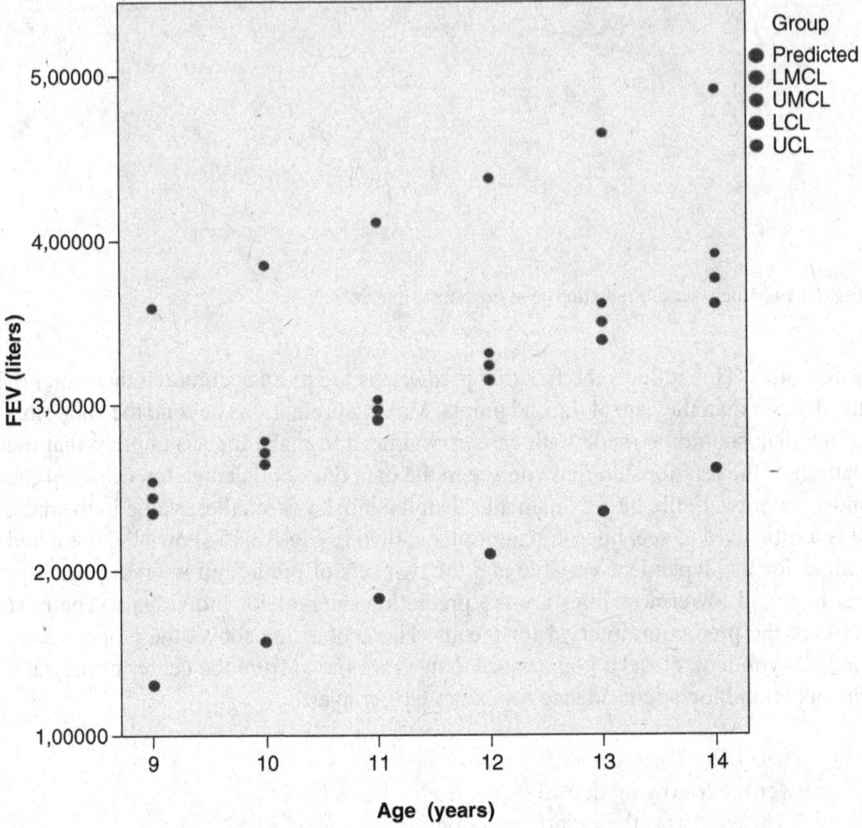

Fig. 13.15 Plot of prediction intervals

term. If the relationship between the independent and dependent variables is linear, the data points should be randomly scattered about the regression line. If the error terms have the same standard deviation, the distance the data points are from the regression line should not show a tendency to get closer or farther from the regression as the value of the independent variable increases.

These properties can be investigated by examining a scatter plot of the residuals versus the predicted values of the dependent variable. Such a scatter plot is known as a *residual plot.* If there is a linear relationship between the independent and dependent variables and the error terms have a constant standard deviation, the residual plot should show a random scatter with no discernable pattern or a tendency to show a wider or narrower dispersion as you move from left to right. Whether or not the error terms have a normal distribution can be assessed by examining a normal probability plot of the residuals. As was the case with the normal probability plots we saw in Chap. 5, if the residuals show a relatively random scatter about the straight line that is drawn, then it is safe to assume that the error terms have a normal distribution.

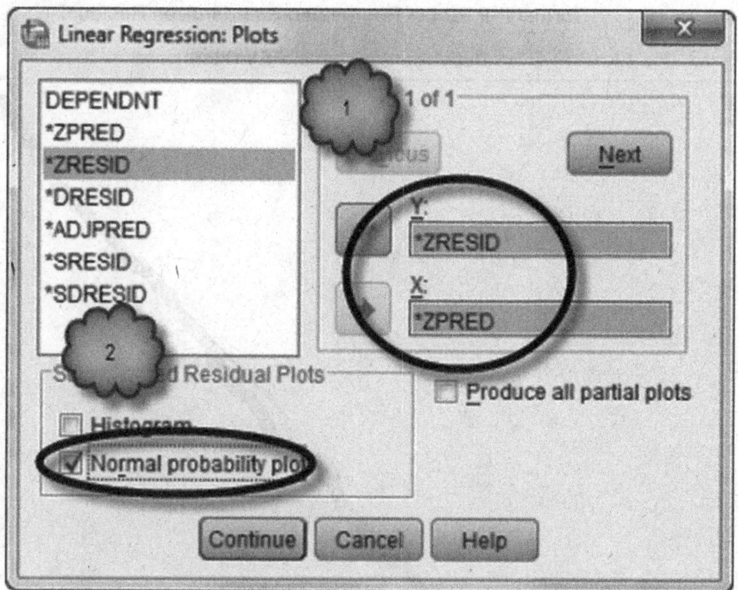

Fig. 13.16 Requesting residual plots

These plots can be obtained in SPSS by clicking **Plots** in the main regression dialog box to bring up the dialog box shown in Fig. 13.16.

The residual plot is obtained by placing *ZRESID* in the *Y* box and *ZPRED* in the *X* box. The leading *Z* means that the residuals and predicted values have been transformed to have a mean of 0 and a standard deviation of 1. The normal probability plot is obtained by checking *Normal probability plot* in the *Standardized Residual Plots* area. When the dialog box has been set up as shown in Fig. 13.16, click **Continue** and run the regression in the usual manner. The requested plots will be drawn in an output window, and are shown in Figs. 13.17 and 13.18.

Study the output and answer the following questions:

13.6.1 Does the residual plot have a random pattern with relatively constant dispersion about 0?

13.6.2 Does the normal probability plot reveal a pattern that is consistent with a normal distribution?

13.6.3 Does the regression model requirement of a linear relationship between the independent and dependent variables appear to have been met?

13.6.4 Do the regression model requirements that the error terms have a normal distribution with a constant standard deviation appear to be met?

13.6.5 Are the results of the *t* tests, the *F* test, the CIs on the population slope and intercept, and the prediction intervals reliable?

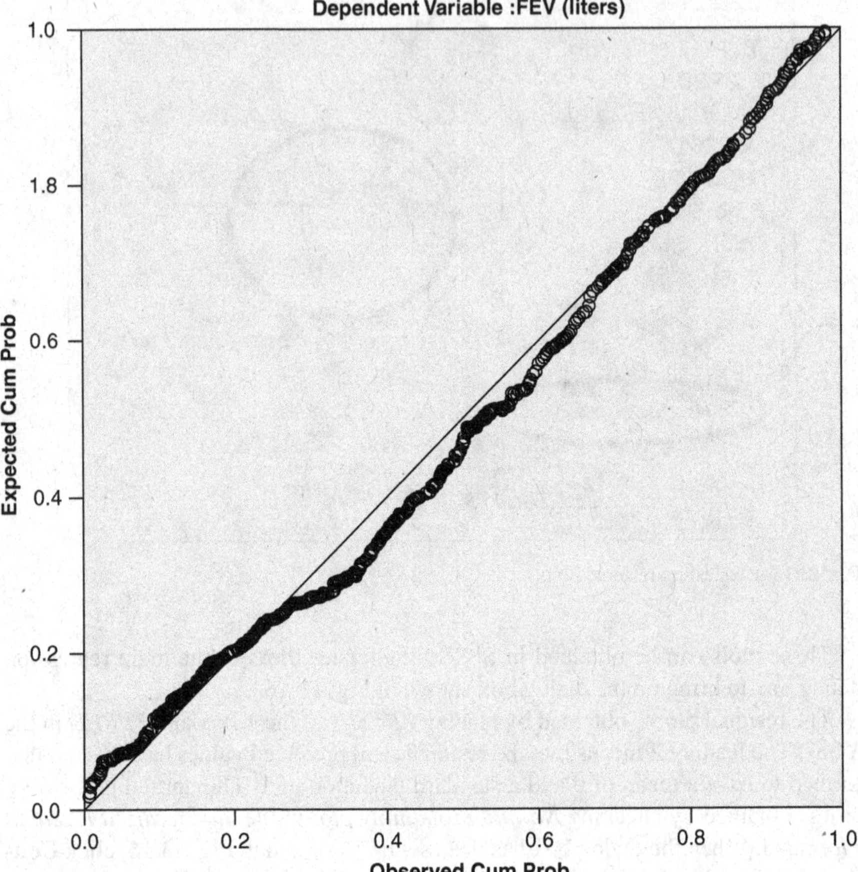

Fig. 13.17 Normal probability plot of residuals

13.7 Exercise Questions

1. Figure 13.19 is a scatter plot of the relationship between diastolic blood pressure and BMI of patients participating in the Framingham heart study. The plot displays the best fitting straight line. Load the data file **Framingham.sav** [2] and conduct a regression on these data.

   a. Report the equation of the best fitting straight line.
   b. According to the value of the slope, how much does diastolic blood pressure increase for every increase of one unit of BMI?
   c. What is the value of the coefficient of determination?
   d. What does the value of the coefficient of determination that you just reported tell us about the relationship between diastolic blood pressure and BMI?

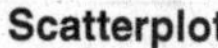

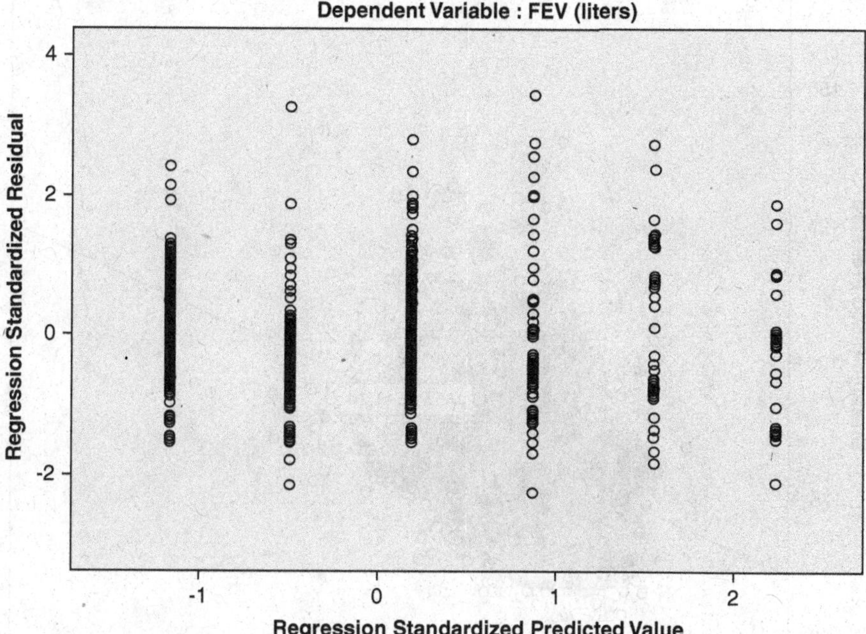

Fig. 13.18 Scatter plot of residuals

e. What is the predicted diastolic blood pressure of an individual patient with a BMI of 30?
f. What would be the 95 % CI for this prediction?

2. Tables 13.6 and 13.7 show some of the output generated by the analysis in Question 1 above.
   a. What is the value of the *t* test for the population slope?
   b. What is the two-sided *p*-value?
   c. What should you conclude regarding whether or not the population slope is 0?
   d. What is the value of the *F*-ratio?
   e. What are the degrees of freedom for the numerator and the denominator?
   f. What is the *p*-value associated with the *F*-ratio?
   g. What should you conclude from this *p*-value?
3. Imagine that we conduct a regression analysis on the Framingham data set to determine the relationship between BMI and age for men. The resulting coefficients are displayed in Table 13.8. Can we conclude from Table 13.8 that BMI and age are related? Why or why not?
4. The regression analysis of Question 3 generated the plots shown in Figs. 13.20 and 13.21.

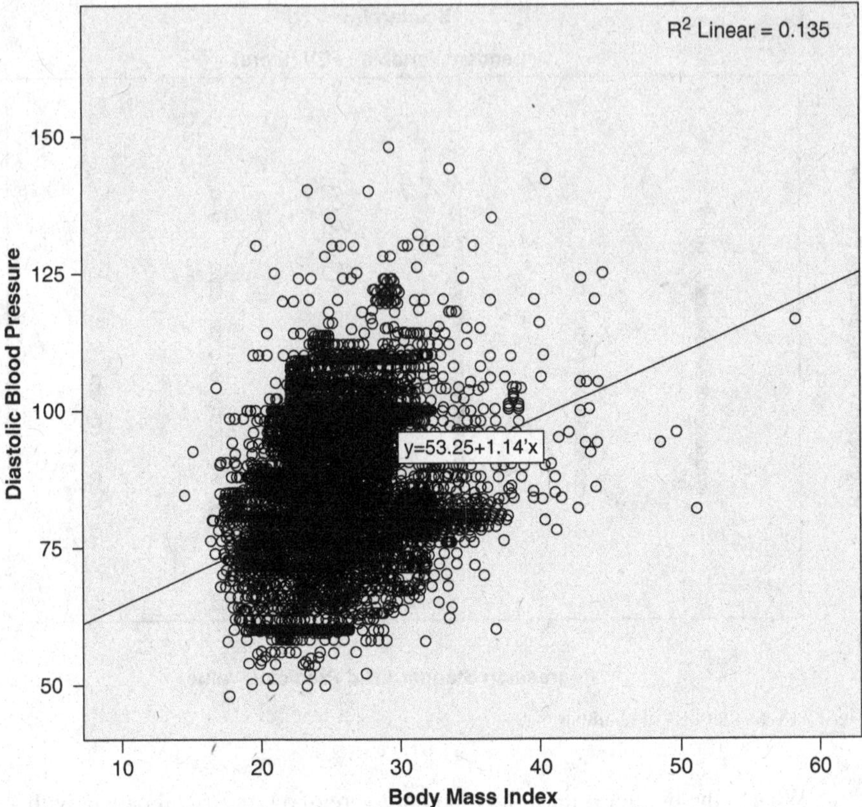

Fig. 13.19 Scatter plot for Question 1

Table 13.6 Output for Question 2

ANOVA[a]

Model		Sum of Squares	df	Mean Square	F	Sig.
1	Regression	102595.981	1	102595.981	731.391	.000[b]
	Residual	657610.220	4688	140.275		
	Total	760206.201	4689			

a. Dependent Variable: Diastolic Blood Pressure
b. Predictors: (Constant), Body Mass Index

Table 13.7 Output for Question 2

Coefficients[a]

Model		Unstandardized Coefficients		Standardized Coefficients	t	Sig.
		B	Std. Error	Beta		
1	(Constant)	53.249	1.096		48.566	.000
	Body Mass Index	1.142	.042	.367	27.044	.000

a. Dependent Variable: Diastolic Blood Pressure

Table 13.8 Coefficients table for Question 3

Coefficients[a,b]

Model		Unstandardized Coefficients		Standardized Coefficients	t	Sig.
		B	Std. Error	Beta		
1	(Constant)	25.381	.412		61.623	.000
	Age, in years	.012	.009	.031	1.410	.159

a. Gender = Male
b. Dependent Variable: Body Mass Index

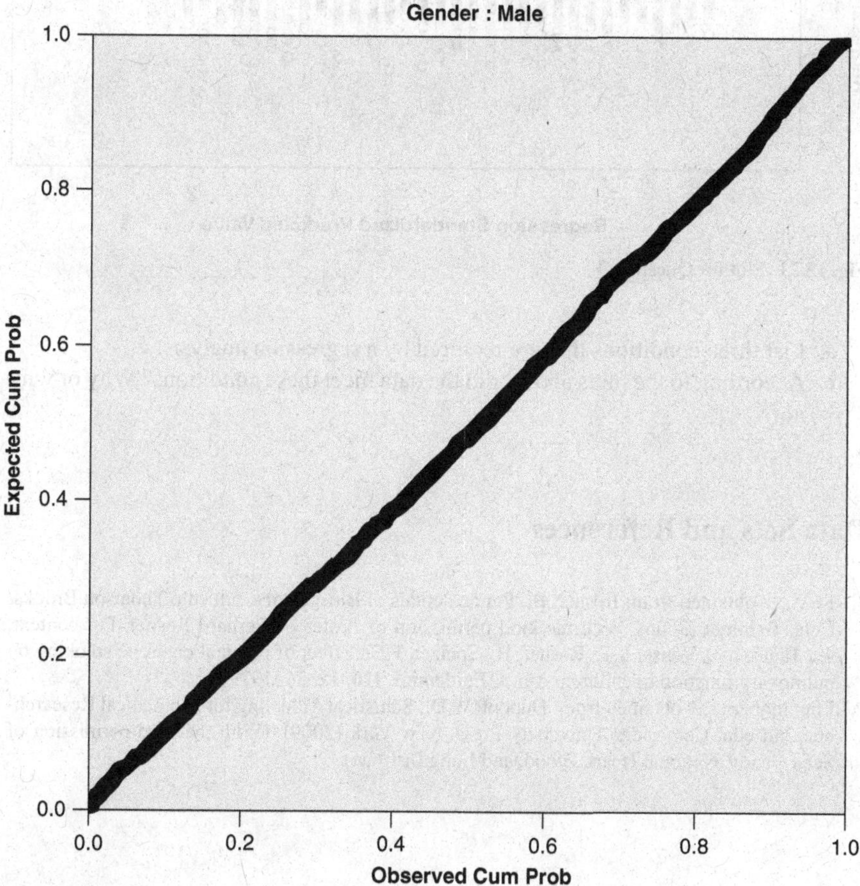

Fig. 13.20 Plot for Question 4

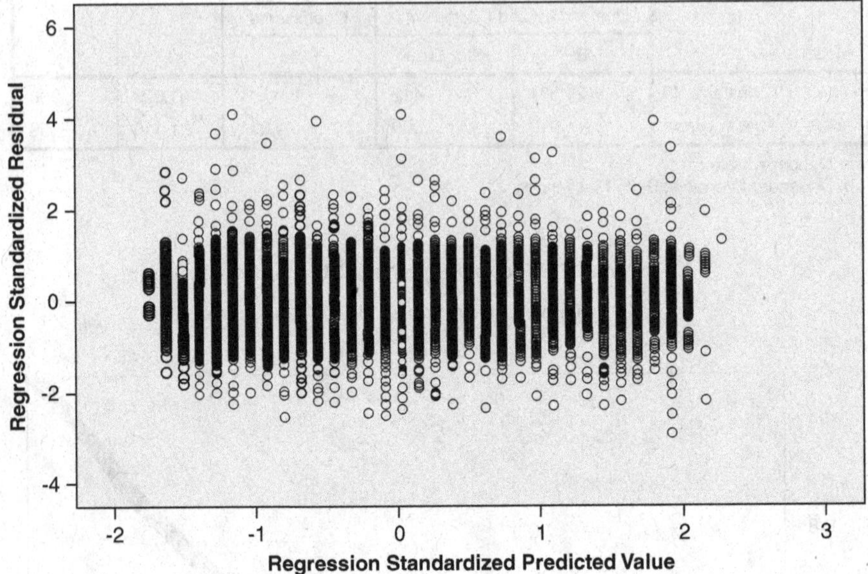

Fig. 13.21 Plot for Question 4

a. List three conditions that are required by a regression analysis.
b. According to the plots above, did the data meet these conditions? Why or why not?

Data Sets and References

1. FEV.sav obtained from: Rosner, B.: Fundamentals of Biostatistics, 6th edn. Thomson Brooks/Cole, Belmont (2006). With the kind permission of Professor Bernard Rosner. For context, see Tager, I.B., Weiss, S.T., Rosner, B., Speizer, F.E.: Effect of parental cigarette smoking on pulmonary function in children. Am. J. Epidemiol. **110**, 15–26 (1979)
2. Framingham.sav obtained from: Dupont, W.D.: Statistical Modeling for Biomedical Researchers, 2nd edn. Cambridge University Press, New York (2009). (With the kind permission of Sean Coady, National Heart, Blood, and Lung Institute)

Chapter 14
Multiple Linear Regression

Abstract This chapter provides an overview of multiple linear regression, a statistical technique that predicts values of a quantitative dependent variable from values of two or more independent variables. By including more than one independent variable, a multiple linear regression can often account for more variability in the dependent variable than can a simple regression, can assess the relationship between the dependent variable and an independent variable after controlling for the presence of other independent variables, and can determine whether the effect of an independent variable varies across levels of another. Topics reviewed include the multiple correlation coefficient, adjusted R^2,interpreting and testing unstandardized and standardized slope coefficients, using categorical and dummy variables as predictors, and testing for the presence of interaction effects.

14.1 Overview

In the previous chapter, we saw how to use a scatter plot to judge whether a straight line describes the relationship between two quantitative variables, how to ascertain the equation of the straight line that best describes the relationship, and how to use that equation to predict the values of a dependent variable from the values of an independent variable. We also saw that when two variables are not perfectly related, the data points will scatter around the best fitting straight line rather than falling on it, and the predicted values will often not match actual values exactly. In clinical research, two variables are rarely perfectly related, so predictions rarely exactly coincide with actual values. To improve the accuracy of prediction, researchers can employ not just one independent variable but a set of two or more variables that are linearly related to the dependent variable. The logic here is that the dependent variable is likely to be a function of a number of factors, not just one, and therefore predictions of the dependent variable will be more accurate if these additional factors are taken into account. In this chapter, we look at a statistical technique that yields a prediction equation that allows researchers to predict values of a dependent variable from values of two or more independent variables. The technique is called *multiple linear regression*.

W. H. Holmes, W. C. Rinaman, *Statistical Literacy for Clinical Practitioners*,
DOI 10.1007/978-3-319-12550-3_14

The prediction equation in a multiple regression analysis takes the following form:

$$\hat{y} = a + b_1 x_1 + b_2 x_2 + \ldots + b_k x_k, \tag{14.1}$$

where $\hat{y}$ is the predicted value of the dependent variable, x_1, x_2, and x_k are the values of each of k independent variables, a is the *intercept,* and b_1, b_2, and b_k are the *slope coefficients.* The values of the intercept and slope coefficients are computed so that the sum of the squared differences between the predicted and actual values of y is as small as possible. That is, the intercept and slope coefficients are *least squares estimates* that minimize the residual sum of squares. The relationship between each independent variable and the dependent variable is assumed to be linear, and as is the case with simple regression, the residuals are assumed to be normally distributed. Both of these assumptions can be checked in the manner explained in the previous chapter.

Often the independent variables are related not only to the dependent variable but to one another. When independent variables correlate with one another, information about the dependent variable that one predictor provides is to some extent redundant with the information provided by the other predictors. This overlap in information provided by the independent variables can affect the predictive value of one or more of the variables. Slope coefficients generated by a regression analysis take the interrelationships among the independent variables into account. Consequently, slope coefficients reflect the degree to which an independent variable is related to the dependent variable after the impact of the remaining predictors has been taken into account or *statistically controlled.*

Factors that are correlated with both the independent and dependent variables but which are not taken into account are called *confounding variables*. Ideally, potential confounding variables are taken into account while the study is in progress through *experimental control.* That is, in the context of an experiment or randomized controlled trial, the dependent variable is measured after all potential confounding variables have been accounted for by either holding them constant or by randomly assigning participants to experimental conditions. However, in clinical research, it is often necessary to collect data outside the context of an experiment. In these cases, after the data have been collected, multiple regression analysis might be used to adjust for the presence of confounding variables. Note however that statistical control can be used only for confounding variables of which we are aware and for which we have measurements.

In this chapter, we use data from a study of the pulmonary function of 654 boys and girls between the ages of 3 and 19. The data file includes the forced expiratory volume (FEV) of each child, that is, the amount of air (measured in liters) each child exhaled forcefully in one second. The age, height, and sex of the child and whether the child was a smoker or nonsmoker are also recorded. We focus on predicting the FEV of nonsmokers between the ages of 9 and 14. In so doing, we learn how to conduct a multiple regression analysis, how to determine whether the inclusion of additional independent variables improved prediction, and how to interpret slope coefficients. As we did in the previous chapter, we also learn how to determine whether the relationships between

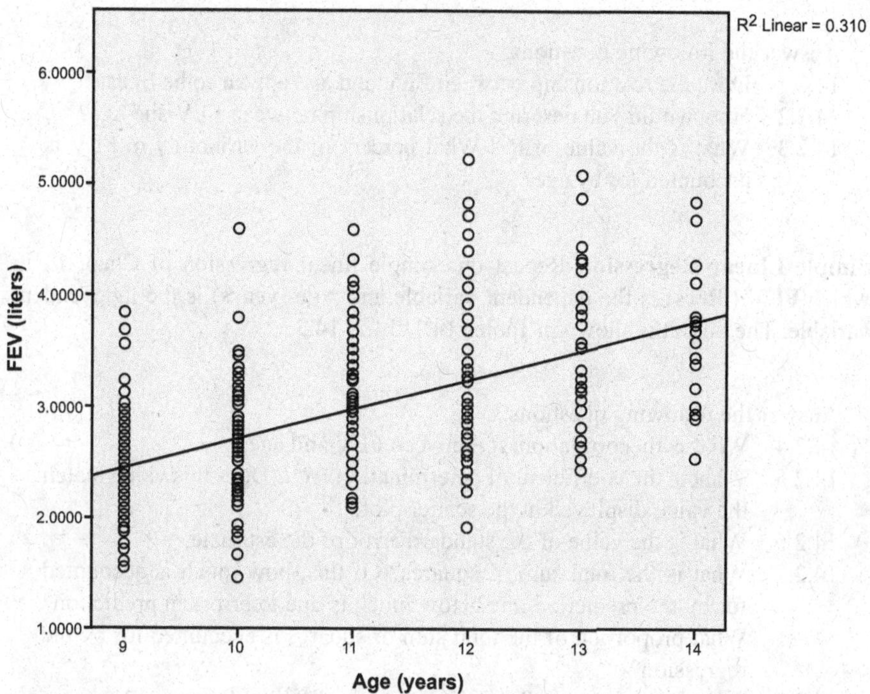

Fig. 14.1 Scatter plot of the relationship between forced expiratory volume (*FEV*) and age for 348 children who do not smoke

the independent and dependent variables we observed in our sample are indicative of those relationships within the population from which the sample was taken.

14.2 Assessing the Impact of a Single Predictor on Prediction Accuracy

We begin by revisiting our analyses of the relationship between FEV and age that we conducted in Chap. 13.

Scatter Plot Recall that the file, **FEV.sav** [1], consists of the following variables: **Age (years)** [*Age*] (variable 1), **FEV (liters)** [*FEV*] (variable 2), **Height (inches)** [*Height*] (variable 3), Sex [*Sex*] (variable 4; 0 = female, 1 = male), and **Smoking Status** [*Smoke*] (variable 5; 0 = nonsmoker, 1 = smoker). Following the instructions of the previous chapter, create a scatter plot with FEV (liters) on the *y*-axis and Age (years) on the *x*-axis, and then insert the best fitting straight line. As we did in Chap. 13, use **Data > Select Cases** to restrict your plot to nonsmokers who are between the ages of 9 and 14, inclusive.

The resulting scatter plot is displayed in Fig. 14.1. (We asked SPSS not to display the equation for the best fitting straight line.)

Answer the following questions:

14.2.1 Does the relationship between FEV and age appear to be linear?

14.2.2 How would you describe the relationship between FEV and age?

14.2.3 What is the value of R^2? What percent of the variability in FEV is accounted for by age?

Simple Linear Regression Repeat our simple linear regression of Chap. 13 in which **FEV (liters)** is the dependent variable and **Age (years)** is the independent variable. The output is shown in Tables 14.1, 14.2, 14.3.

Answer the following questions:

14.2.4 What is thecorrelation, *R*, between FEV and age?

14.2.5 What is the coefficient of determination, R^2 ? Does this value match the value displayed in the scatter plot?

14.2.6 What is the value of the standard error of the estimate, s ?

14.2.7 What is the total sum of squares? Of this, how much is accounted for by the prediction line? How much is due to errors in prediction? What proportion of the total sum of squares is accounted for by the regression?

14.2.8 What is the intercept? Is it significantly different from zero?

14.2.9 What is the unstandardized slope coefficient? Is it significantly different from zero?

14.2.10 The prediction equation for this analysis is of the form, $\hat{y} = a + b_1 x_1$. Compute by hand the number of liters we would expect would be forcefully exhaled by a 9-year-old.

Visualizing Prediction Accuracy You should have found that age accounts for 31 % of the variability in FEV and that we would expect a 9-year-old to exhale about 2.44 L. Before we go any further, let us try to visualize some of these findings. First, return to the *Linear Regression* dialog box and ask SPSS to generate unstandardized predicted values of FEV using age as the independent variable. After the predicted values have been generated, go to *Data View* and see if the predicted FEV of a 9-year-old you computed by hand matches the value computed by SPSS. While you are at *Data View,* compare the predicted value for a 9-year-old with the actual values of some of the 9-year-olds. A segment of those data is shown in Fig. 14.2.

There are 93 children in the data file who are 9 years old (and do not smoke). The predicted FEV for each of them is 2.44403. Notice though that the actual values are sometimes above the predicted value and sometimes below. This is in part because of random errors associated with the taking of an FEV and in part because FEV is a function of not only age but other factors as well. As a result, our predicted values are off the mark to some extent, sometimes underpredicting and sometimes overpredicting actual FEV values. Notice that the same can be said of other age groups. For example, the actual FEV values for 10-year-olds vary around their predicted value.

Table 14.1 Model summary for regression using age to predict forced expiratory volume

Model Summary

Model	R	R Square	Adjusted R Square	Std. Error of the Estimate
1	.557[a]	.310	.308	.5795303

a. Predictors: (Constant), Age (years)

Table 14.2 ANOVA table for regression using age to predict forced expiratory volume

ANOVA[a]

Model		Sum of Squares	df	Mean Square	F	Sig.
1	Regression	52.242	1	52.242	155.550	.000[b]
	Residual	116.206	346	.336		
	Total	168.448	347			

a. Dependent Variable: FEV (liters)
b. Predictors: (Constant), Age (years)

Table 14.3 Intercept and slope coefficient for the regression using age to predict forced expiratory volume

Coefficients[a]

Model		Unstandardized Coefficients		Standardized Coefficients		
		B	Std. Error	Beta	t	Sig.
1	(Constant)	.073	.229		.317	.751
	Age (years)	.264	.021	.557	12.472	.000

a. Dependent Variable: FEV (liters)

Another way to visualize our findings is to return to our scatter plot of the relationship between FEV and age that you created earlier. A version of the plot, borrowed from Chap. 13, is shown in Fig. 14.3. The points within the rectangle are the actual FEV values of our 93 9-year-old nonsmokers. The arrow indicates the predicted value of FEV for these 93 kids, about 2.44. Once again we see that our predicted value is too low for some of our 9-year-olds and too high for others.

A third way to visualize our data is to generate either a scatter plot of the actual values of FEV and the values of FEV predicted on the basis of age, or, as we did in Chap. 13, draw a residuals plot of the differences between the actual and predicted values. Those two plots are presented in Figs. 14.4 and 14.5, respectively. As Fig. 14.4 shows, small values of FEV predicted on the basis of age are associated with small actual values, moderate predicted values are associated with moderate

Age	FEV	Height	Sex	Smoke	filter_$	PRE_1
9	2.4870	64.0	Female	Nonsmoker	Selected	2.44403
9	1.5910	57.0	Female	Nonsmoker	Selected	2.44403
9	2.6880	59.5	Female	Nonsmoker	Selected	2.44403
9	1.5580	53.0	Male	Nonsmoker	Selected	2.44403
9	1.8950	57.0	Male	Nonsmoker	Selected	2.44403
9	2.3520	59.0	Male	Nonsmoker	Selected	2.44403
10	3.0860	62.0	Female	Nonsmoker	Selected	2.70753
10	2.5680	63.5	Female	Nonsmoker	Selected	2.70753
10	3.1320	59.5	Female	Nonsmoker	Selected	2.70753
10	2.3280	64.0	Male	Nonsmoker	Selected	2.70753
10	1.8110	57.0	Male	Nonsmoker	Selected	2.70753
10	2.5610	62.0	Male	Nonsmoker	Selected	2.70753

Fig. 14.2 Actual values of forced expiratory volume (*FEV*) and predicted values (*Pre_1*) based on each child's age

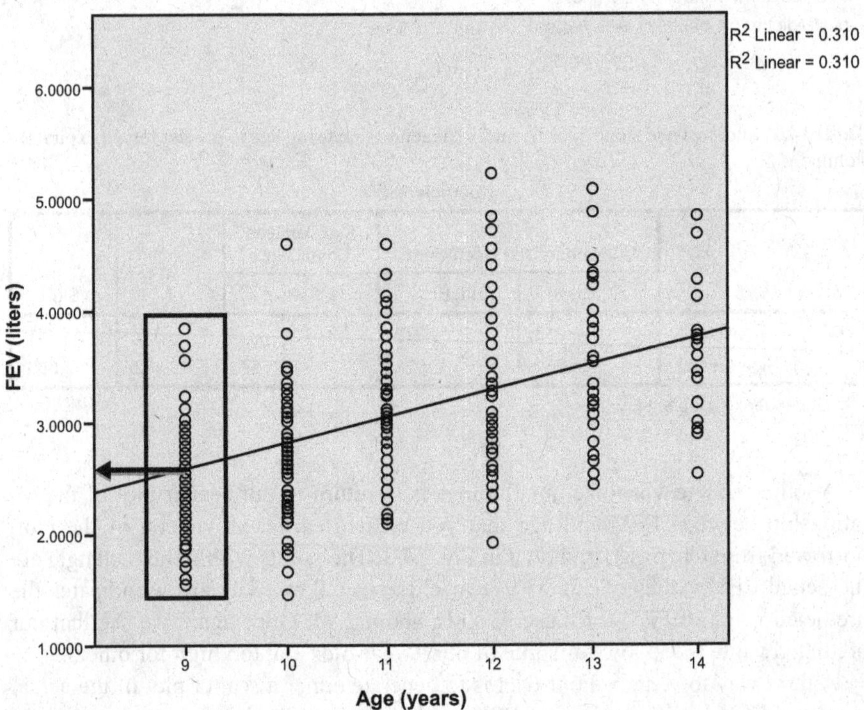

Fig. 14.3 Scatter plot highlighting the distribution of actual values of forced expiratory volume (*FEV*) of 9-year-olds around their predicted value

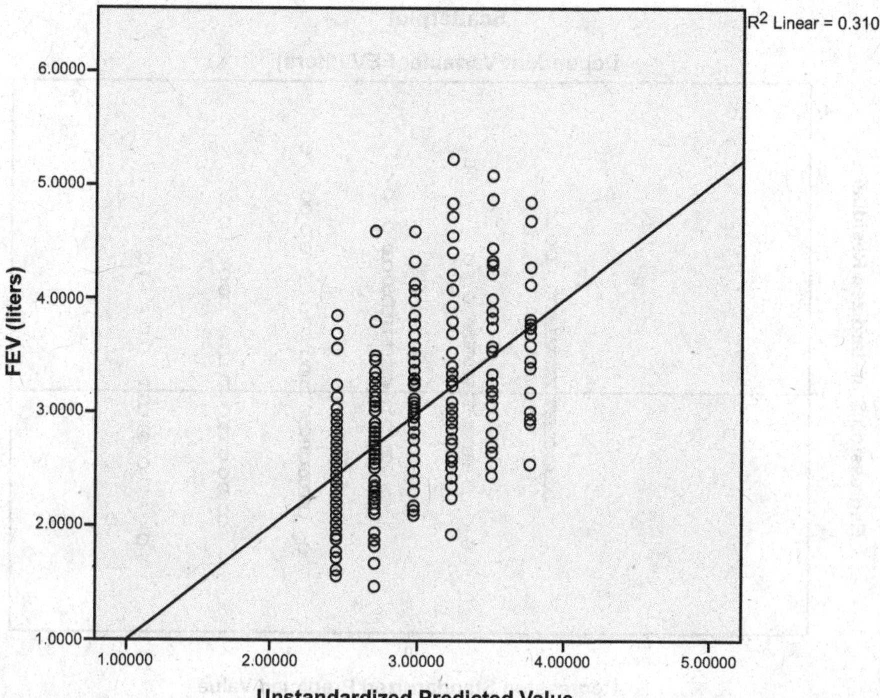

Fig. 14.4 Scatter plot of the relationship between the actual values of forced expiratory volume (*FEV*) and the unstandardized *FEV* values predicted on the basis of each child's age

actual values, and large predicted values are associated with large actual values. So it appears that predicting FEV on the basis of a child's age has merit. However, both plots show that our predictions are far from perfect. Clearly, if we want to predict a child's FEV more precisely, we need to do more than base predictions on the child's age.

14.3 Improving Prediction by Adding a Second Predictor

We have seen that knowing children's ages allows us to account for a portion of the variability in the volume of air they can forcefully exhale. In fact, the value of R^2 tells us that age accounts for 31 % of the variability in FEV for children between the ages of 9 and 14. This leaves 69 % of the variability unaccounted for. Let us see if adding a second independent variable improves prediction.

Each child's height is included in the data set. Do you think height should be included in our prediction equation? Height would seem to be a likely candidate for our second predictor if we can assume that taller children exhale more air than shorter children. However, the predictive value of independent variables is the

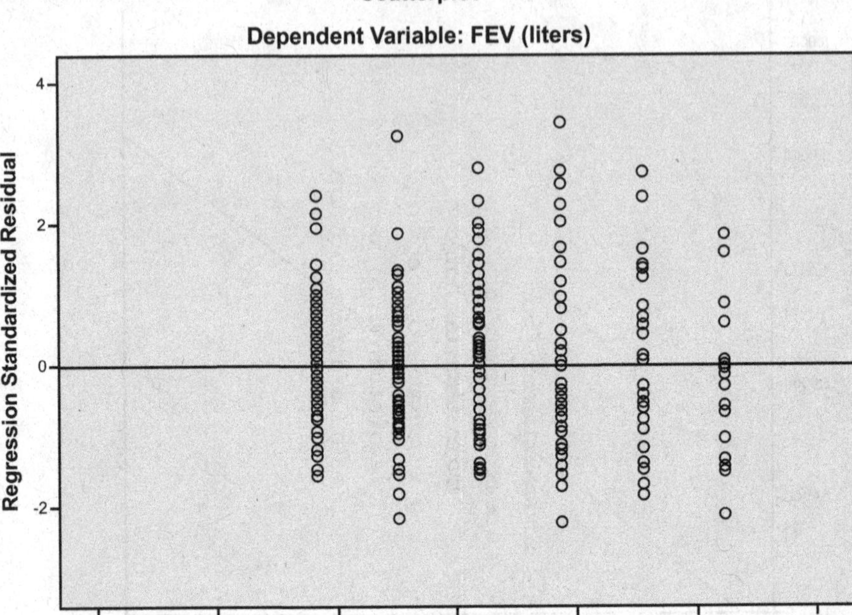

Fig. 14.5 Residuals plot of the differences between the actual values of forced expiratory volume (*FEV*) and the values of *FEV* predicted on the basis of each child's age

greatest when the variables are not only correlated with the dependent variable but are uncorrelated with one another. As children get older, they tend to get taller, so the heights and ages of the children in our sample are likely to be correlated. If the correlation between age and height is too high, knowledge of a child's height does not convey information about the child's FEV that was not already revealed by the child's age. So before we include height as our second independent variable, we should determine the extent to which it is correlated with FEV and with age. We can do this by selecting **Analyze** > **Correlate** > **Bivariate** to generate a correlation matrix that includes the variables **FEV (liters), Age (years),** and **Height (inches)**. The resulting correlation matrix is reproduced in Table 14.4.

Answer the following questions:

14.3.1 Is the correlation between FEV and age the same as the correlation you found in Sect. 14.2? It should be.

14.3.2 What is the correlation between FEV and height? Does this correlation suggest that including height in our prediction equation will improve the prediction?

14.3.3 Were age and height correlated? Does this correlation suggest that including height in our prediction equation will improve prediction?

Table 14.4 Matrix displaying correlations among forced expiratory volume, age, and height

Correlations

		FEV (liters)	Age (years)	Height (inches)
FEV (liters)	Pearson Correlation	1	.557**	.800**
	Sig. (2-tailed)		.000	.000
	N	348	348	348
Age (years)	Pearson Correlation	.557**	1	.545**
	Sig. (2-tailed)	.000		.000
	N	348	348	348
Height (inches)	Pearson Correlation	.800**	.545**	1
	Sig. (2-tailed)	.000	.000	
	N	348	348	348

**. Correlation is significant at the 0.01 level (2-tailed).

You should have found that height is indeed correlated with FEV. This finding suggests that including height in the prediction equation makes sense. However, you should have found that height is also correlated with age, so it remains to be seen whether predictions of FEV that are based on both a child's age and height will be more accurate than predictions based on the child's age alone. Let us conduct a multiple regression to find out.

Multiple Linear Regression Return to the *Linear Regression* dialog box and move **Height (inches)** into the *Independent(s):* window as shown in Fig. 14.6. Run the analysis and study the output.

Although our prediction equation now includes two predictors, the output will have a familiar look. Let us begin with the *Model Summary* table, shown in Table 14.5.

As before, R is the correlation between the predicted and actual values of the dependent variable, FEV. However, in a multiple regression analysis, R is called the *multiple correlation coefficient* to indicate that the predicted values are based on two (or more) independent variables. In our case, R is the correlation between actual values of FEV and values of FEV predicted on the basis of each child's age and height. As with simple linear regression, R^2 is the proportion of variability in FEV accounted for by our prediction equation. However, in multiple regression analysis, the equation has two (or more) independent variables. In our case, the prediction equation includes age and height, rather than just age alone, so R^2 is the proportion of variability in FEV accounted for when each child's age and height are considered.

Answer the following questions:

14.3.4 What is the correlation between actual and predicted values of FEV when predictions of FEV are based on each child's age and height? How does the multiple correlation coefficient compare to the value of R when our predictions of FEV were based only on each child's age?

14.3.5 What is the value of R^2 in our multiple regression analysis? How does this value compare to the value of R^2 when our predictions were based only on age?

14.3.6 Do predictions of FEV based on age and height seem to be more accurate than predictions based on age alone?

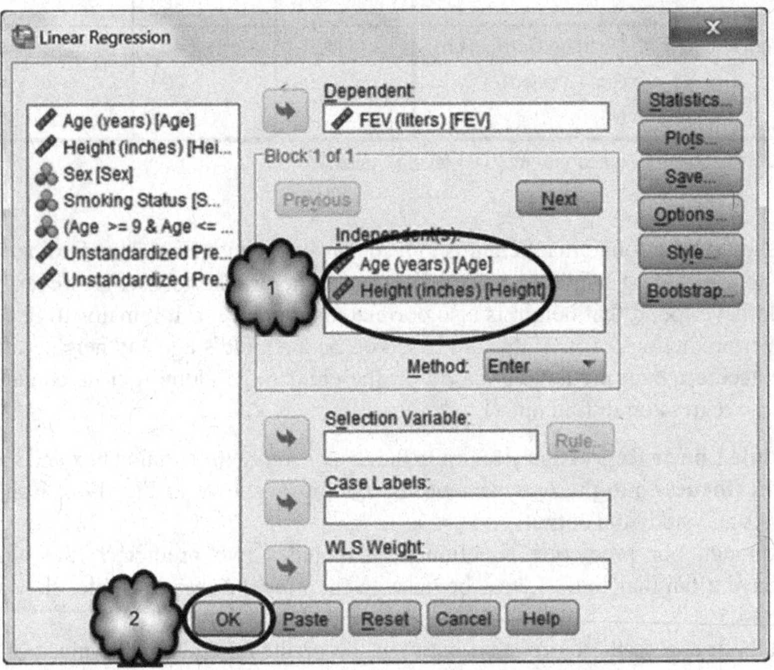

Fig. 14.6 Adding height to the regression

Table 14.5 Model summary of regression using age and height to predict forced expiratory volume

Model Summary

Model	R	R Square	Adjusted R Square	Std. Error of the Estimate
1	.813[a]	.661	.659	.4065937

a. Predictors: (Constant), Height (inches), Age (years)

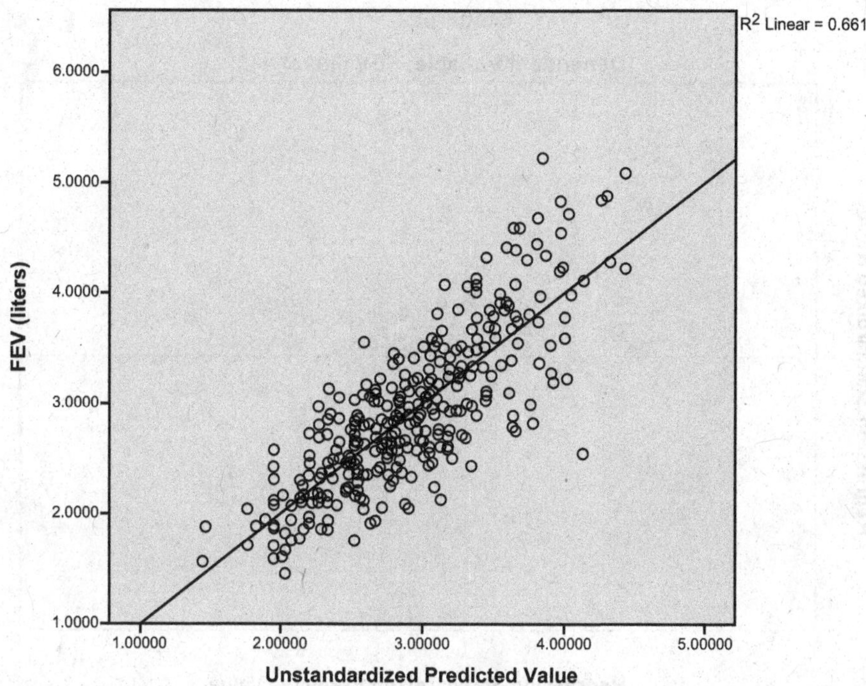

Fig. 14.7 Scatter plot of the relationship between the actual values of forced expiratory volume (*FEV*) and the values of *FEV* predicted on the basis of each child's age and height

Adjusted R^2 At this point, it seems clear that adding height to the prediction equation improved the prediction. However, any time an independent variable is added to the prediction equation, R^2 will always increase even if the added predictor has no predictive value. Therefore, it is necessary to adjust the value of R^2 to control for the number of predictors in the equation. This new value of R^2 is called *adjusted* R^2 and can be found in the *Model Summary* table. When comparing multiple regression models with a different number of independent variables, the adjusted R^2 should be used. Compare this value with the value of adjusted R^2 when we used age as our sole predictor.

14.3.7 Which regression model does a better job of predicting FEV?

Visualizing Prediction Accuracy In the next section, we will look at the prediction equation that we generated with our multiple regression analysis. But first let us look at a visual display of the goodness of fit of that equation. Fig. 14.7 displays a plot of the actual FEV values and predicted values of FEV based on age and height. The residuals plot is displayed in Fig. 14.8. Compare these plots with the

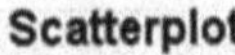

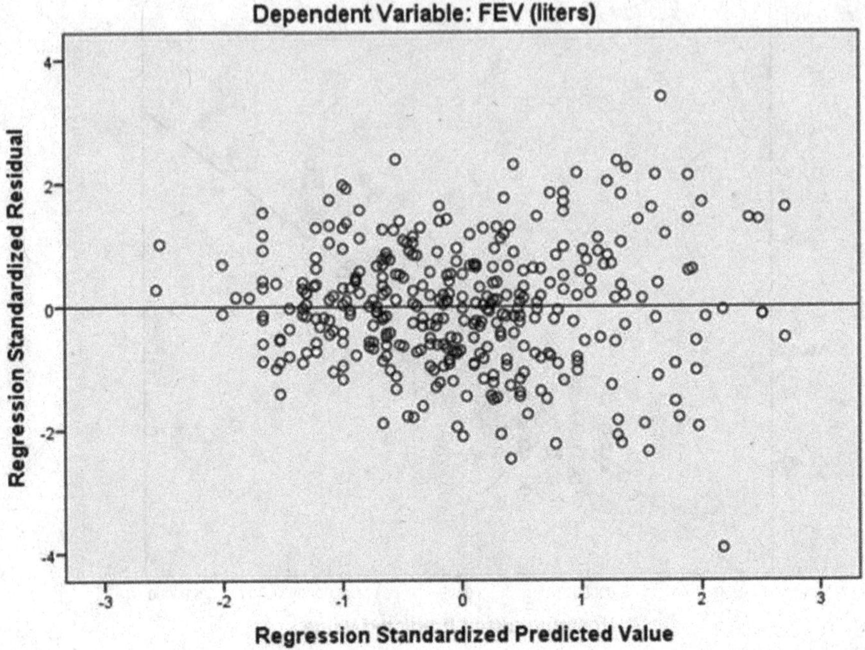

Fig. 14.8 Residuals plot of the differences between the actual values of forced expiratory volume (*FEV*) and the values of *FEV* predicted on the basis of each child's age and height

corresponding plots in which the predicted values are based on age alone (Figs. 14.4 and 14.5).

14.3.8 Which prediction equation fits the data better?

14.4 Interpreting Standardized and Unstandardized Slope Coefficients

As do simple regression analyses, multiple regressions generate *Coefficients* tables that include information about intercepts and slopes. Recall, however, that in a multiple regression, the prediction equation includes two or more independent variables. Therefore, the *Coefficients* table includes the unstandardized slope of each of the predictors. In our case, we have two independent variables, age and height, so the prediction equation takes the form,

$$\hat{y} = a + b_1x_1 + b_2x_2. \tag{14.2}$$

Table 14.6 Intercept and unstandardized slope coefficients for age and height

Coefficients[a]

Model		Unstandardized Coefficients		Standardized Coefficients		
		B	Std. Error	Beta	t	Sig.
1	(Constant)	-5.995	.359		-16.719	.000
	Age (years)	.081	.018	.171	4.587	.000
	Height (inches)	.127	.007	.707	18.919	.000

a. Dependent Variable: FEV (liters)

The values of the intercept (a) and the slopes (b_1, b_2) of the two predictors, age (x_1) and height (x_2) can be found in the *Coefficients* table reproduced in Table 14.6.

14.4.1 Specify the prediction equation for our multiple regression analysis by filling in the following blanks: Predicted values of FEV = ________ + ________ *(Age)* + ________ *(Height)*.

14.4.2 Imagine that you were about to measure the FEV of a 9-year-old child who is 53 inches tall and does not smoke. Compute by hand the number of liters you would expect the child to exhale.

14.4.3 Does the predicted value you calculated match the value that SPSS generated?

Unstandardized Slope Coefficients Let us take a closer look at the slope coefficients. The values of the coefficients take into account the degree to which the independent variables are related to the dependent variable and to one another, and whether those relationships are positive or negative. As was the case in simple regression, we must look at the results of the t-tests to determine whether or not the computed slope coefficient is statistically significantly different from zero. If a slope coefficient is statistically significantly different from zero, then the value of a slope assigned to a given independent variable tells us how much change in the dependent variable is associated on average with change in that independent variable above and beyond the impact of the other independent variables. Independent variables that either are not related to the dependent variable or do not tell us anything about the dependent variable that we do not already know from the other predictors will have slope coefficients that are not statistically significantly different from zero. A statistically significant positive slope tells us that increases in the independent variable are associated with increases in the dependent variable. A statistically significant negative slope tells us that increases in the independent variable are associated with decreases in the dependent variable.

As an example of how to interpret slopes, recall that the unstandardized slope coefficients generated by our multiple regression were 0.081 for age and 0.127 for height, and both of them were statistically significantly different from zero. Thus, each independent variable contributes to the prediction above and beyond the contribution of the other. This explains why predicted values based on age and height do a better job of accounting for the variability in FEV than do predicted values based on age alone. While knowing a child's age tells us something about what the child's FEV will be, knowing the child's height gives us additional information. When it comes to understanding FEV, apparently there is more to the story than just age.

Both coefficients are positive, telling us that increases in either age or height are associated with increases in FEV. The value of each of the unstandardized slopes tells us how much of an increase. Recall that FEV was measured in liters, age in years, and height in inches. The values of the slopes tell us that for children of a given height, FEV increases on average by 0.081 L for every one year increase in age, and that for children of a given age, FEV increases on average by 0.127 L for every one inch increase in height.

Standardized Coefficients We need to be a little careful about using the slopes to determine the relative importance of each of the independent variables. It might seem logical to assume that the larger the slope, the greater is the impact of the independent variable, indicating that the independent variable with the largest slope could be considered the most important predictor. However, the magnitude of unstandardized slopes is affected by the units of measurement associated with the independent and dependent variables, so comparing unstandardized slopes can be misleading. To be able to compare slopes meaningfully, it is necessary that they be calculated on the basis of variables that are expressed in terms of the same unit of measurement. This is accomplished by calculating slopes after the values of each independent and dependent variable have been transformed into *standardized scores*. A standardized score, also known as a *Z-score,* is the number of standard deviations the original score is above or below the mean of those scores. *Z-scores* have a mean of 0 and a standard deviation of 1.

As an example, consider the ages of the nonsmokers in the entire sample. The average age is 9.53 years with a standard deviation of 2.74 years. A 13-year-old within this sample is older than the average child by 3.47 years $(13-9.53)$ which is about 1.27 standard deviations above the mean $(3.47/2.741=1.27)$. A 3-year-old is 6.53 years younger than the average child or 2.38 standard deviations below the mean. Thus, the age of any child in the sample who is 13 years old can be expressed as a standardized score of 1.27 while the age of any 3-year-old can be expressed as a standardized score of -2.38.

If we transform the values of our independent and dependent variables into standardized scores, FEV will no longer be expressed in terms of feet, age in terms of years, or height in terms of inches. Instead, all of our variables will be expressed in terms of the same unit of measurement—the number of standard deviations above or below the mean. If we then calculate slope coefficients from standardized scores, the slopes will be expressed in terms of standard deviations rather than in terms of the original units of measurement. These slopes are called *standardized* or *beta*

Table 14.7 Standardized slope coefficients for age and height

Coefficients[a]

Model		Unstandardized Coefficients		Standardized Coefficients	t	Sig.
		B	Std. Error	Beta		
1	(Constant)	-5.995	.359		-16.719	.000
	Age (years)	.081	.018	.171	4.587	.000
	Height (inches)	.127	.007	.707	18.919	.000

a. Dependent Variable: FEV (liters)

coefficients and are displayed in the *Coefficients* table as shown in Table 14.7. You will notice that there is no value reported for the intercept. This is because the intercept is always equal to zero when the data are standardized. According to the table, a one standard deviation increase in age is associated with an increase in FEV scores of 0.171 standard deviation while a one standard deviation increase in height is associated with an increase in FEV scores of 0.707 standard deviation. Now that we have converted all of our variables to the same scale of measurement, we can meaningfully compare the two slopes. When we do so, we see that a one standard deviation change in height results in a much larger change in FEV, in standard deviation terms, than does age.

Use Caution When Interpreting Slope Coefficients When comparing slopes, it is important to remember that a slope coefficient for a given independent variable is sensitive to the presence of the other independent variables within the regression model. Standardized and unstandardized slopes can vary as independent variables are added or removed from the prediction equation. As an example, the unstandardized coefficient for height when age is included in the model is 0.081. However, we saw in Table 14.3 that the unstandardized slope coefficient for age when it was the only predictor was 0.264. We will see in the next section that this coefficient will change again when sex is added to the model. Because slope coefficients are dependent upon the set of independent variables that happen to be in the prediction equation, the results of a regression analysis do not indicate in some absolute sense the predictive, theoretical, or clinical importance of a given variable.

Slope coefficients can also be sensitive to the presence of outliers, especially when sample sizes are small. In addition, coefficients reflect the range of values of the independent variables of the sample. *Extrapolating* or making predictions using values that lie outside those upon which the prediction equation was fitted is risky. In our example, the slopes for age and height were based on kids between the ages of 9 and 14. There is no guarantee that our prediction equation would provide an equally good fit for people outside this age range. Finally, even if the values of the independent variables are within the range, the prediction equation may not generalize to populations different from the one from which the sample that generated the equation was taken. In our example, there is no guarantee that our prediction equation would be accurate in predicting the FEV of children who smoke.

Table 14.8 Model summary for regression using age, height, and sex to predict forced expiratory volume

Model Summary

Model	R	R Square	Adjusted R Square	Std. Error of the Estimate
1	.814[a]	.662	.660	.4065354

a. Predictors: (Constant), Sex, Age (years), Height (inches)

14.5 Using Categorical Predictors

Independent variables are often quantitative, but they can be categorical as well. In this section, we add gender to our prediction equation and see if knowing a child's sex as well as his or her age and height improves the prediction. In our sample of 9- to 14-year-olds, the boys, on average, are over 2 in. taller than the girls. Given that height and gender are related, do you think that including gender in our regression model will improve prediction?

Return to the *Linear Regression* dialog box and move **Sex** into the *Independents:* window. Run the analysis. The resulting *Model Summary* and *Coefficients* tables are displayed in Tables 14.8 and 14.9, respectively.

14.5.1 According to the *Model Summary* table, did the addition of sex seem to account for variability in FEV not accounted for by age and height? How can you tell?

14.5.2 Did including sex reduce s? How can you tell?

The *Coefficients* table now shows slope coefficients for three independent variables: age, height, and sex. The interpretation of the first two coefficients is similar to our interpretation of the slopes we have studied thus far, so see if you can answer the following questions:

14.5.3 After controlling for sex and height, does FEV increase or decrease on average as children get older? By how much per year?

14.5.4 After controlling for sex and age, what is the average impact on FEV of an increase of one standard deviation of height?

14.5.5 Did the slope coefficients for age and height differ in this analysis from their values generated in Sect. 14.4? Why or why not?

Table 14.9 Intercept and slope coefficients for regression using age, height, and sex to predict forced expiratory volume

Coefficients[a]

Model		Unstandardized Coefficients		Standardized Coefficients	t	Sig.
		B	Std. Error	Beta		
1	(Constant)	-5.892	.372		-15.853	.000
	Age (years)	.085	.018	.179	4.704	.000
	Height (inches)	.124	.007	.692	17.314	.000
	Sex	.049	.047	.035	1.048	.295

a. Dependent Variable: FEV (liters)

Age (years) and **Height (inches)** are quantitative variables. When we interpreted their slope coefficients, we took into account that the slopes were positive, and therefore, we knew that increases in the predictors were associated with increases in FEV. When a predictor is categorical, the slope is interpreted in terms of the numerical values assigned to the categories. Usually these values are 0 and 1. A positive slope means that changes from 0 to 1 are associated with increases in the dependent variable while a negative slope means that changes from 0 to 1 are associated with decreases in the dependent variable. In our analysis, we have a categorical variable, **Sex**. Its categories, female and male, were assigned the values of 0 and 1, respectively. Its unstandardized slope coefficient is 0.049. Although the slope coefficient is positive, it makes no sense to conclude that increases in sex were associated with an average increase of 0,049 L of FEV. However, we can conclude that changes from 0 to 1were associated with an average increase of 0.049 L of FEV. Because girls were assigned the value of 0 and boys the value of 1, we can conclude that after controlling for age and height, the boys in the sample had an average FEV that was 0.049 L greater than that of girls in the sample.

Including sex in the regression equation has the net effect that there are essentially two parallel regression lines with the regression line for boys being 0.049 L higher than that for girls. If it is suspected that the two lines may not be parallel, then one equation for boys and a separate one for girls will be fitted, or as we will discuss later in this chapter, an interaction variable will be added to the prediction equation.

Dummy Variables Sex is but one of many categorical variables that clinical researchers might include in regression analyses. For example, race (white versus nonwhite), marital status (married versus single), or smoking status (smoker versus nonsmoker) might be relevant predictors. When a categorical variable has more than two categories, however, it must be converted into a set of *dummy variables*. The number of dummy variables is equal to the number of categories minus 1. Each dummy variable represents a category and has two numerical values, 0 and 1.

For example, imagine a study of the effects of smoking on pulmonary function as measured by FEV. Patients are categorized as smokers, former smokers, or nonsmokers. As there are three categories, two dummy variables would be needed to represent the smoking status of each patient. One dummy variable would cor-

Table 14.10 Hypothetical unstandardized slope coefficients for two dummy variables (Smoker and Former Smoker) representing a categorical variable (smoking status) with three values

	Dummy variable		
Smoking status	Smoker	Former smoker	Coefficient
Smoker	1	0	−0.25
Former Smoker	0	1	−0.10
Nonsmoker (reference)	0	0	–

respond to one of the three categories, the other to one of the remaining two. In our example, we might name one of the dummy variables, **Smoker,** and use it to indicate whether each patient is a smoker or not. We might name the other dummy variable, **Former Smoker,** and use it to indicate whether each patient is a former smoker or not. As shown in Table 14.10, smokers would be assigned the value of 1 on the first dummy variable and a 0 on the second. Former smokers would be assigned a 0 on the first dummy variable and a 1 on the second. The category not represented by its own dummy variable is called the *reference* category. Cases falling into the reference category are assigned a 0 on each of the dummy variables. In our example, the reference category is nonsmokers. Nonsmokers, being neither smokers nor former smokers, would be assigned a 0 on both dummy variables. The decision as to which category will be the reference can be arbitrary, but often it represents a group that was not exposed to a health risk or to a treatment.

In order to create these dummy variables in SPSS, we would need to use **Transform > Recode into Different Variables** twice. We would create the variable **Smoker** by using it to give smokers a value of 1 and everyone else a value of 0. Then, we would use **Transform** a second time to create the variable **Former Smoker,** this time giving every former smoker a value of 1 and everyone else a value of 0.

Slope coefficients assigned to dummy variables are interpreted relative to the reference category. In our example, if the unstandardized slope coefficient for the dummy variable, **Smoker,** were −0.25, then we would know that the average FEV of smokers was 0.25 L less than that of the average nonsmoker. If the slope coefficient for the dummy variable **Former Smoker** was −0.10, then we would know that the average former smoker exhaled 0.10 L of air less than the average nonsmoker. You will have an opportunity to create dummy variables in one of the exercise questions.

Use Caution when Adding Predictor Variables In theory, researchers can keep adding predictors until they are satisfied that they have accounted for as much variability in the dependent variable as possible. However, when including additional predictors, researchers keep the following in mind. First, investigators prefer to use independent variables that are uncorrelated with one another so that each predictor provides maximum unique information about the dependent variable. The more the independent variables are correlated with one another, the more redundant they are with one another, and thus, the less useful they are collectively as predictors. In fact, independent variables that are too highly correlated with one another can have slope coefficients that are not statistically significantly different from zero despite the fact that they are correlated with the dependent variable. For this reason, when the correlation between two predictors is quite high, researchers consider using one or the other predictor, but not both.

Second, at some point adding more predictors is likely to capitalize on random variation present in the given sample and produce results that will not replicate across samples. To guard against generating unstable coefficients, it is often recommended that the sample be 10–20 times as large as the number of independent variables.

Third, blindly adding additional predictors may increase the value of adjusted R^2, but is unlikely to generate a prediction equation that makes theoretical sense. Finally, scientists prefer theories that are *parsimonious*. The theory that uses the least number of causal factors to explain an outcome is generally preferred. In terms of multiple regression analysis, the goal is to discover the prediction equation that accounts for the maximum amount of variability with the fewest number of independent variables.

14.6 Testing Model Coefficients

If the data can be considered to have been randomly drawn from a larger population, we will want to use our sample statistics to estimate corresponding population parameters. To do this, we follow procedures similar to those explained in the previous chapter for simple regression. However, in the case of multiple regression, we will have two or more predictors so that the population model becomes

$$y_i = \alpha + \beta_1 x_{1i} + \beta_2 x_{2i} + \ldots + \beta_k x_{ki} + \varepsilon_i, \tag{14.3}$$

where y_i is an actual value of y for the ith member of the population, α is the population y-intercept, $\beta_1, \beta_2, \ldots \beta_k$ are the population slopes for k predictors, $x_{1i}, x_{2i} \ldots x_{ki}$ are known, fixed values of each of the predictors, and ε_i is a random value that is assumed to have a normal distribution with a mean of 0 and a standard deviation of σ. Thus, the population parameters are α, $\beta_1, \beta_2, \ldots \beta_k$, and σ. Our estimator for α is the least squares value for the intercept, a. Our estimators for $\beta_1, \beta_2, \ldots \beta_k$ are the least squares values for the slopes $b_1, b_2 \ldots b_k$, respectively. Finally, σ is estimated by the standard error of the estimate, s, which in the case of multiple regression is calculated as follows:

$$s = \sqrt{\frac{1}{n-k-1}\sum (y_i - \hat{y}_i)^2}. \tag{14.4}$$

In this section, we see how to test hypotheses about population parameters and to generate their confidence intervals.

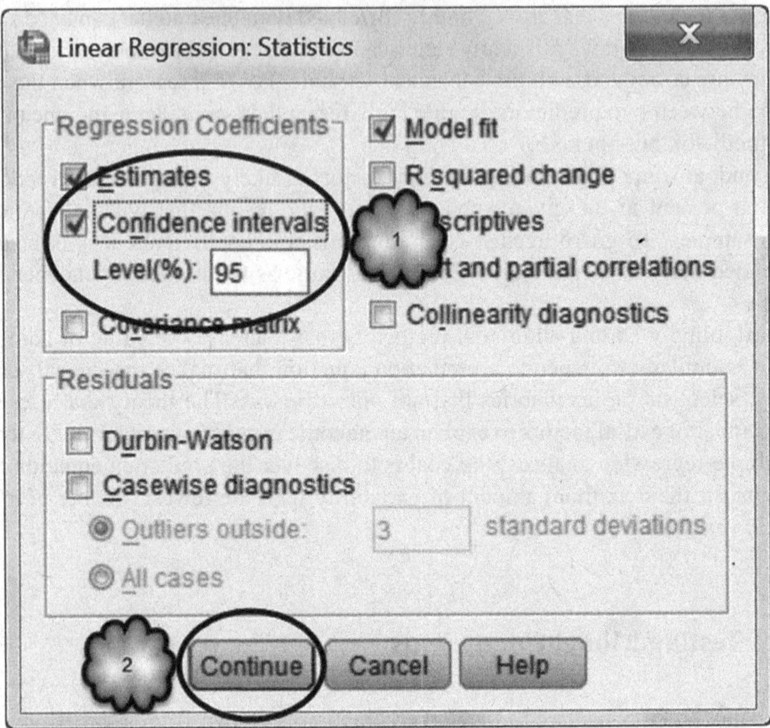

Fig. 14.9 Requesting 95 % confidence intervals for the intercept and slope coefficients

Confidence Intervals for Coefficients Return to the *Linear Regression* dialog box of our last analysis, choose *Statistics* and select *Confidence Intervals* in the *Regression Coefficients* area. In this example, we generate a 95 % confidence interval, so be sure that the correct level of confidence is displayed in the *Level (%)* window. When you are finished, the dialog box should be similar to the one shown in Fig. 14.9. Run the analysis.

The output is identical to that which we generated in Sect. 14.5 except that now the *Coefficients* table displayed in Table 14.9 include confidence intervals for our population parameters. These confidence intervals are shown in Table 14.11.

Study the confidence intervals and answer the following questions:

14.6.1 Which of the slope coefficients are significantly different from zero?

14.6.2 Can we be at least 95 % confident that in the population from which thechildrenofoursampleweredrawn,achild'ssexisassociatedwithFEV independent of the child's age and height?

14.6.3 What is the 95 % confidence interval for the slope for height? Why is it important to know whether the value of zero is included in this interval?

Table 14.11 Coefficients table displaying 95 % confidence intervals for the intercept and slope coefficients

Model		Unstandardized Coefficients		95.0% Confidence Interval for B	
		B	Std. Error	Lower Bound	Upper Bound
1	(Constant)	-5.892	.372	-6.623	-5.161
	Age (years)	.085	.018	.049	.120
	Height (inches)	.124	.007	.110	.138
	Sex	.049	.047	-.043	.141

Table 14.12 Testing the null hypothesis that all population slope coefficients are zero

ANOVA[a]

Model		Sum of Squares	df	Mean Square	F	Sig.
1	Regression	111.595	3	37.198	225.075	.000[b]
	Residual	56.853	344	.165		
	Total	168.448	347			

a. Dependent Variable: FEV (liters)
b. Predictors: (Constant), Sex, Age (years), Height (inches)

Testing Hypotheses About Coefficients The *ANOVA* table, shown in Table 14.12, displays the results of a test of the null hypothesis that all of the population slopes are equal to zero. In our example, we have three predictors, so the ANOVA tests the null hypothesis that

$$\beta_1 = \beta_2 = \beta_3 = 0. \tag{14.5}$$

The alternative hypothesis is that one or more population slopes are not equal to zero.

Before we see whether we can reject the null hypothesis, take a moment to note the values for regression, residual, and total sum of squares in Table 14.12. Now consult Table 14.13 to compare these values to those generated by our analysis in which the prediction equation used only **Age (years)** or used **Age (years)** and **Height (inches)**. The total sum of squares of the three analyses will of course be the same as the total is the variability in actual values of FEV. However, the regression and residual sum of squares differ across the three analyses.

Table 14.13 Effect of adding independent variables on regression and residual sum of squares

	Independent variable(s)		
	Age	Age and height	Age, height, and sex
Regression	52.242	111.413	111.595
Residual	116.206	57.035	56.853
Total	168.448	168.448	168.448

Study Table 14.13 and answer the following questions:

14.6.4 Which analysis has the greatest regression sum of squares? Why?

14.6.5 The analysis with the greatest regression sum of squares also has the lowest residual sum of squares? Why?

Returning to the null hypothesis that the population slope coefficients for age, height, and sex equal zero, the probability that the values of the sample slopes would be obtained if the null hypothesis is true can be found in the column labeled *Sig* of Table 14.12.

14.6.6 According to Table 14.12, should we accept or reject the null hypothesis?

14.6.7 Should we conclude that at least one of our three sample slopes is statistically significantly different from zero?

The results of our ANOVA told us that it is extremely unlikely that the population slopes are all equal to zero. To determine which of the slopes is significantly different from zero, *t*-tests are conducted on each sample slope. For each test, the null hypothesis is that the population slope is equal to zero. The alternative hypothesis is that the population slope is not equal to zero. A *t*-test on the intercept is also conducted to test the null hypothesis that the population intercept is equal to zero against the alternative hypothesis that the intercept is not equal to zero. As with a simple regression, the results of the *t*-tests are reported in the *Coefficients* table except this time the table displays *t*- and *p*-values for more than one slope. The table also contains confidence intervals for each of the parameters if confidence levels had been requested. Remember that the reported *p*-values are two-tailed. If the alternative hypothesis is either that the population parameter is greater than zero or that the population parameter is less than zero, the reported *p*-values need to be adjusted as explained in the previous chapter.

Refer back to Table 14.9, which displays the results of the *t*-tests of the slope coefficients for age, height, and sex, and answer the following question:

14.6.8 Are the three slope coefficients statistically significantly different from zero? If not, which one(s) is/are not? How do you know?

14.7 Interaction Effects

The regression models that we have been using assume that the relationship between a given independent variable and the dependent variable is the same across all levels of any other independent variables included in the prediction equation. When the relationship between an independent variable and a dependent variable is not the same across the values of another independent variable, statisticians say that there is an *interaction effect* between the two independent variables. The regression analyses that we have conducted thus far assume that there are no interaction effects. In this section, we see how to determine whether interaction effects are present.

Begin by setting up a regression analysis in which **FEV (liters)** is the dependent variable and **Age (years)** and **Sex** are the independent variables. Once you have set up the analysis, the *Linear Regression* dialog box should look similar to the one displayed in Fig. 14.10.

Click **OK** to generate the table of coefficients shown in Table 14.14.

These coefficients tell us that both the age and sex of the child contribute to FEV. FEV increases on average by 0.262 L for every one year increase in age, and boys on average have an FEV that is 0.337 L greater than girls.

This analysis assumes that the relationship between age and FEV is the same for both boys and girls. By assuming that there is no interaction effect between sex and age, the analysis leads to the conclusion that an increase in 1 year of age is associated with an increase of 0.262 L of FEV, regardless of whether the child is a boy or girl.

A common way to test the assumption that there is no interaction effect between two independent variables is to include in the prediction equation a variable that represents the interaction and determine whether the slope coefficient associated with this variable is significantly different from zero. In our example, the model becomes

$$y_i = \alpha + \beta_1 x_{1i} + \beta_{12} x_{1i} x_{2i} + \varepsilon_i, \tag{14.6}$$

where y_i is the actual value of FEV for the ith member of the population, α is the population y-intercept, x_{1i} is the age of the ith member of the population, x_{1i}, x_{2i} is the interaction between age and sex for the ith member of the population, and β_1 and β_{12} are the slope coefficients for age and the interaction between age and sex, respectively. As before, ε_i is a random value that is assumed to have a normal distribution with a mean of 0 and a standard deviation of σ. The presence of a significant interaction effect is then determined by testing the slope coefficient, β_{12}.

To conduct this analysis, we must first create a variable that represents the interaction between the two independent variables. To do this, we create a new variable that is equal to the product of the two independent variables. In our example, we are interested in knowing whether the relationship between age and FEV varies by sex, so we begin by multiplying age and sex together.

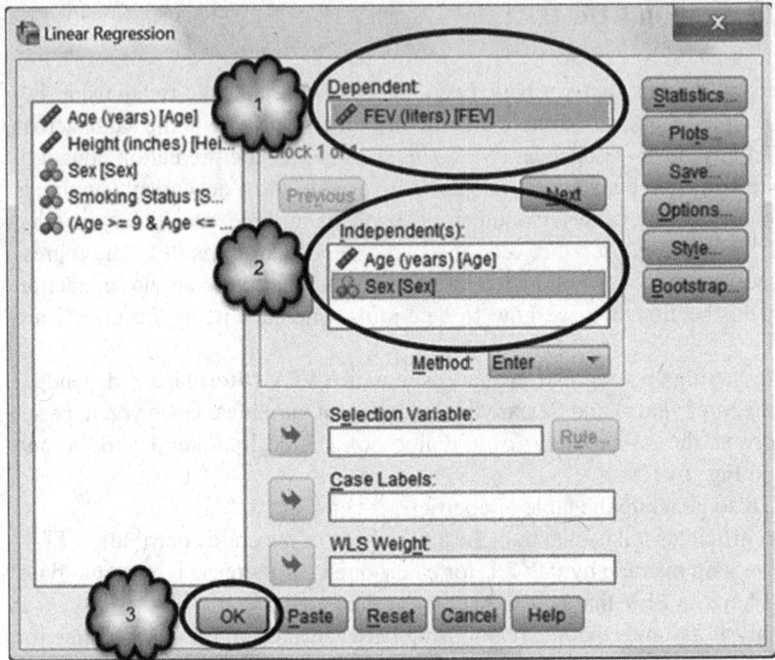

Fig. 14.10 Requesting a regression using age and sex to predict forced expiratory volume (*FEV*)

Table 14.14 Intercept and slope coefficients generated by regression using age and sex to predict forced expiratory volume

Coefficients[a]

Model		Unstandardized Coefficients		Standardized Coefficients		
		B	Std. Error	Beta	t	Sig.
1	(Constant)	-.100	.221		-.450	.653
	Age (years)	.262	.020	.555	12.959	.000
	Sex	.337	.060	.241	5.639	.000

a. Dependent Variable: FEV (liters)

Select **Transform > Compute Variable** to bring up the *Compute Variable* dialog box. Since we are multiplying one variable by the other, it would be common practice to call this variable, **Age*Sex**. Unfortunately, SPSS allows asterisks to be used in variable labels but not in variable names. Accordingly, enter *Age_Sex* in the *Target Variable box,* then after clicking ***Type & Label***, enter *Age*Sex* in the *Label* area. Click **Continue**. In the *Numeric Expression* area, instruct SPSS to multiply **Age (years)** and **Sex** together. Click **OK.** These steps are displayed in Figs. 14.11 and 14.12.

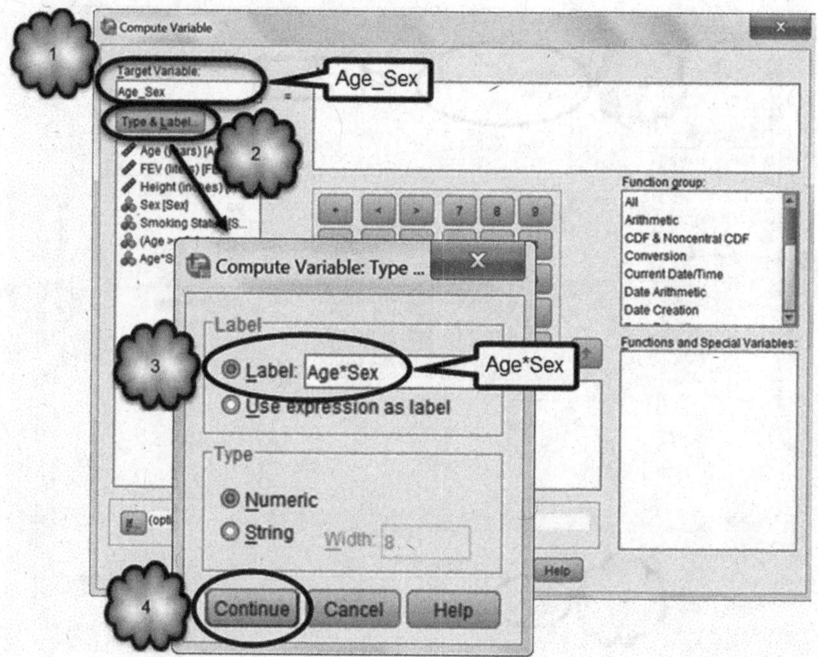

Fig. 14.11 Naming and labeling the variable representing the interaction effect between age and sex

Return to the *Linear Regression* dialog box. In the *Independent(s)* area, replace **Sex** with **Age*Sex.** The dialog box should now be similar to the one shown in Fig. 14.13. Click **OK**.

Study the resulting output, in particular the coefficients table, reproduced in Table 14.15.

We can see from the table that the slope coefficients for both **Age (years)** and the interaction between age and sex, **Age*Sex,** are significant. The significant slope for **Age (years)** tells us that overall, FEV is positively associated with age: For every 1 year increase in age, there is a 0.243 L increase in the FEV. The significant slope for the interaction effect however tells us that the slope that describes the relationship between FEV and age is not the same for boys and girls. We can also see this in the prediction equation.

According to the coefficients table, the prediction equation is as follows:

$$FEV = 0.092 + 0.243\,(Age) + 0.034\,(Age * Sex). \tag{14.7}$$

To interpret the equation, remember that sex was coded such that girls were assigned a 0 and boys a 1. For girls, the equation becomes:

$$FEV = 0.092 + \ 0.243\,(Age) + 0.034\,(Age * 0). \tag{14.8}$$

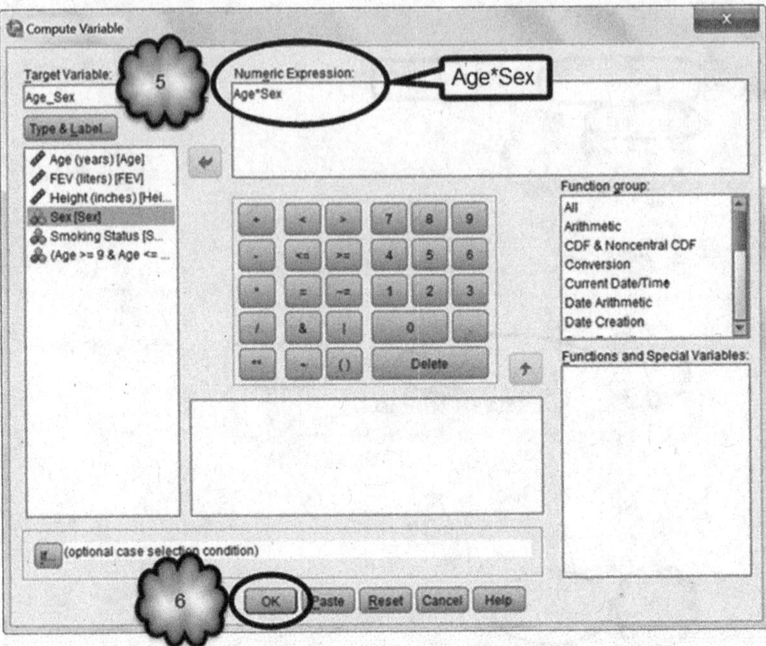

Fig. 14.12 Generating a variable representing the interaction effect between age and sex

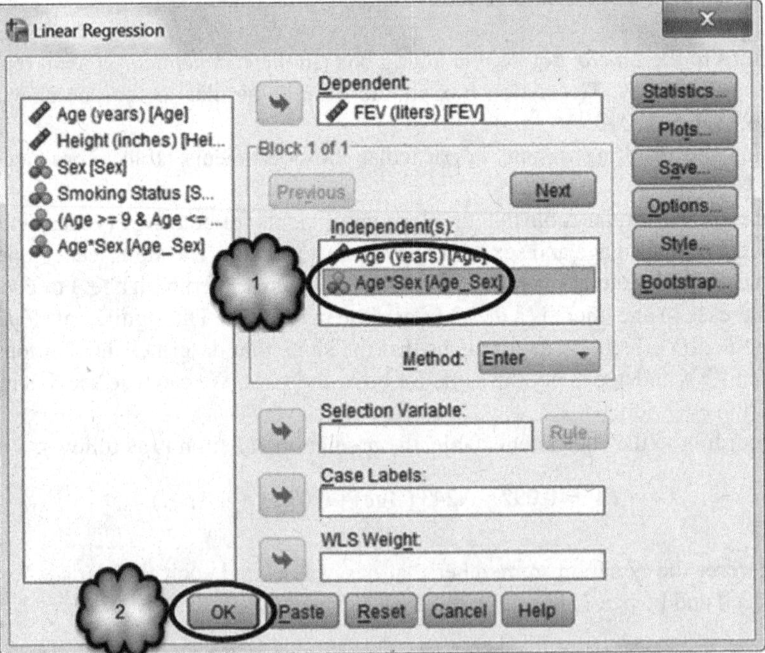

Fig. 14.13 Generating a regression analysis to test for the presence of an interaction effect between age and sex

Table 14.15 Intercept and slope coefficients generated by regressing the forced expiratory volume on age and the interaction effect between age and sex

Coefficients[a]

Model		Unstandardized Coefficients		Standardized Coefficients	t	Sig.
		B	Std. Error	Beta		
1	(Constant)	.092	.217		.426	.670
	Age (years)	.243	.020	.513	11.954	.000
	Age*Sex	.034	.005	.268	6.245	.000

a. Dependent Variable: FEV (liters)

Because the value of **Sex** for girls is zero, the prediction equation for girls simplifies to:

$$FEV = 0.092 + 0.243\,(Age). \tag{14.9}$$

For boys, the prediction equation is as follows:

$$FEV = 0.092 + 0.243\,(Age) + 0.034\,(Age * 1). \tag{14.10}$$

Because the value of **Sex** for boys is 1, the prediction equation becomes:

$$FEV = 0.092 + 0.243\,(Age) + 0.034\,(Age). \tag{14.11}$$

This in turn becomes:

$$FEV = 0.092 + 0.277\,(Age). \tag{14.12}$$

Thus, for both boys and girls, FEV is positively associated with age, but the increase is significantly greater for boys (slope of 0.277) than it is for girls (slope of 0.243).

14.8 Exercise Questions

1. Conduct a simple linear regression analysis on the **FEV (liters)** of children between the ages of 9 and 14, inclusive, using **Smoking Status** as the predictor.

   a. Complete the following prediction equation:

   FEV = __________ + __________ (*Smoking Status*).

   b. What is the proportion of variability in the FEV that is accounted for by the children's smoking status?

c. On average, what is the difference in the FEV between kids who smoked and kids who did not? _________ liter.
d. According to your analysis, which group had the larger average FEV—smokers or nonsmokers? Does this finding make sense? Why or why not?

2. Add **Age (years)** to **Smoking Status** and run the multiple regression analysis.
   a. Complete the following prediction equation:

   $FEV =$ _________ + _________ $(Smoking\ Status) +$ _________ (Age)

   b. After taking into account age, what is the average difference in the FEV between kids who smoked and kids who did not? _________ liter.
   c. After adjusting for age, which group had the larger average FEV—smokers or nonsmokers? Does this finding make sense? Why or why not?
   d. Given the results of your multiple regression analysis, what might explain the slope coefficient for *Smoking Status* in the simple linear regression of Question 1?
   e. What is the value of adjusted R^2? How does it compare to the corresponding value of the simple linear regression of Question 1? Does including age improve prediction?

3. Curious about the fitness and exercise habits of male and female volunteer firefighters, a physician assistant student asked firefighters to report anonymously their sex, age, height, weight, and the number of days per week they exercised. She then converted height and weight into the body mass index (BMI). The data can be found in **Firefighters.sav** [2] as **Sex** [*Sex*] (variable 1; 0=M, 1=F), **Age** [*Age*] (variable 2; 1=18 to 29, 2=30 to 40, 3=41 to 50, and 4=over 50), **Frequency of Exercise** [*TimesPerWeek*] (variable 6), and **Body Mass Index** [*BMI*] (variable 7). Conduct a multiple regression analysis in which **Body Mass Index** is the dependent variable and **Sex** and **Frequency of Exercise** are the independent variables.
   a. Report below the unstandardized slope coefficient for each of the two predictors.
      Sex: _________
      Frequency of Exercise: _________
   b. Based on her own experience as a firefighter, the researcher expected that the BMI of the average male firefighter who does not exercise would be above the normal range, that is, above 25. According to the results of your regression analysis, was she correct? How can you tell?
   c. The researcher predicted that the BMI is negatively related to the frequency of exercise. In terms of slope coefficients, what is the null hypothesis associated with this expectation? What is the alternative hypothesis? Should the test of hypothesis be one- or two-tailed? Why?
   d. Regarding the slope coefficient associated with the exercise hypothesis stated in 3c, should we accept or reject the null hypothesis? Why or why not?

Table 14.16 Coefficients table for question 5: regression of forced expiratory volume on age for children aged 10 years or younger

Coefficients[a]

Model		Unstandardized Coefficients		Standardized Coefficients		
		B	Std. Error	Beta	t	Sig.
1	(Constant)	.278	.106		2.628	.009
	Age (years)	.232	.013	.668	17.233	.000
	Age*Sex	.007	.005	.051	1.309	.191

a. Dependent Variable: FEV (liters)

Table 14.17 Coefficients table for question 5: regression of forced expiratory volume on age for children older than 10 years

Coefficients[a]

Model		Unstandardized Coefficients		Standardized Coefficients		
		B	Std. Error	Beta	t	Sig.
1	(Constant)	1.305	.284		4.603	.000
	Age (years)	.130	.023	.310	5.646	.000
	Age*Sex	.059	.006	.503	9.151	.000

a. Dependent Variable: FEV (liters)

e. Which of the two predictors was more strongly related to the BMI? How do you know?
f. Using the unstandardized slope coefficient, describe in words the relationship between BMI and frequency of exercise.
g. In words, reexpress the relationship between BMI and frequency of exercise in terms of the standardized slope coefficient.

4. Repeat the regression analysis of Question 3, but this time include in the regression model dummy variables that will allow you to determine whether the average BMI of firefighters between the ages of 18 and 29 is significantly different from the average BMI of each of the remaining three age groups.

   a. Given the number of independent variables, is the sample sufficiently large to justify conducting the analysis? Why or why not?
   b. Does including age improve goodness of fit? How do you know?
   c. According to this analysis, what is the average difference in the BMI between the two youngest age groups after adjusting for the other independent variables? Between the youngest and the oldest? Is either of these differences statistically significant?

5. Imagine that an investigator used the FEV data set to test the hypothesis that for children who do not smoke and who are 10 years old or younger, FEV increases with age at the same rate for boys and girls, but that for children who do not smoke but are over the age of 10, the rate of increase is greater for boys (**SEX** = 1) than for girls (**SEX** = 0). To test the hypothesis, the researcher conducted a multiple linear regression for each of the two age groups of children who do not smoke. The resulting coefficients tables are displayed in Tables 14.16 and 14.17.

   a. What is the prediction equation for children who are older than 10 years of age?

      FEV= ________ + ________ *(Age)* + ________ *(Age*Sex)*.

   b. What is the slope coefficient for age for boys who are older than 10 years of age?
   c. Was the researcher's hypothesis supported by the analysis? Why or why not?

Data Sets and References

1. FEV.sav obtained from: Rosner, B.: Fundamentals of Biostatistics. 6th ed. Thomson Brooks/Cole, Belmont, CA (2006). With the kind permission of Professor Bernard Rosner. For context, see Tager, I.B., Weiss, S.T., Rosner, B., Speizer, F.E.: Effect of parental cigarette smoking on pulmonary function in children. Am. J. Epidemiol. 110, 15–26 (1979)
2. Firefighters.sav obtained from: Marlow, C.E., Cappelletti, E.M., Holmes, W.H.: Relationship between availability of exercise equipment and BMI among volunteer firefighters. Unpublished data, Le Moyne College, Syracuse (2006)

Chapter 15
Logistic Regression

Abstract This chapter deals with predicting a categorical response variable that has two categories. The chapter begins with using a single independent variable to make this prediction. It moves on to discuss the case where there are two categorical independent variables. Next comes a discussion of making predictions with a mixture of quantitative and categorical independent variables. Finally, adjusted odds ratios are considered followed by testing for an interaction effect between the independent variables.

15.1 Overview

In Chap. 13, we considered predicting a quantitative response variable using simple linear regression with a single independent variable. In Chap. 14, we expanded those ideas to multiple regression where two or more independent variables were used to predict the value of a quantitative response variable. There are occasions, however, where the response variable may be categorical. For example, we may be interested in the relationship, if any, between a patient's age and whether or not the patient has coronary heart disease. In such a case, the response variable could consist of two values, 0 if the patient does not have coronary heart disease, and 1 if the patient does have coronary heart disease. Fitting a simple linear regression line of the form

$$y = a + bx, \tag{15.1}$$

where b represents the slope (the change in y for a one unit increase in x) and a represents the y-intercept (the value of y when x equals 0) to these data presents some difficulties. For instance, if the predicted value of y is not equal to 0 or 1, how do we know whether to predict that the patient has coronary heart disease or not? One possible fix is not to use the presence or absence of coronary heart disease as the predicted response variable, but rather the *probability* that the patient will have coronary heart disease. If we let p be the probability of having coronary heart disease, then the simple regression equation would be of the form.

$$p = a + bx. \tag{15.2}$$

W. H. Holmes, W. C. Rinaman, *Statistical Literacy for Clinical Practitioners*,
DOI 10.1007/978-3-319-12550-3_15

One problem with this approach is that it can generate values of p that are greater than 1 or less than 0. Since the probability of having coronary heart disease can neither exceed 1 nor be negative, we need to predict a dependent variable that can take on any positive or negative value, but from which we can derive probabilities. The solution is twofold. First, the regression equation is used to predict the *odds* that the patient has coronary heart disease. Recall from Chap. 6 that a probability can be expressed as odds through the following transformation:

$$\text{ODDS} = \frac{p}{1-p}. \tag{15.3}$$

For example, if the probability that a patient has coronary heart disease is 0.20, the odds that she has the disease are 0.20 to 0.80 or 0.25. This means that the probability that she has the disease is one-fourth the probability that she does not have the disease. Recall also that the odds can be greater than 1. For example, if the probability that a second patient has coronary heart disease is 0.80, the odds that she has the disease are 0.80 to 0.20 or 4. The probability that she has the disease is four times the probability that she does not have the disease.

Using the odds as the dependent variable allows us to predict values greater than 1. Unfortunately, odds cannot be negative, but their *natural logarithms* can. So the second step of our two-step solution is to use the regression equation to predict the natural logarithm of the odds that the patient has coronary heart disease. The natural logarithm of a number a is the power of the number e (approximately equal to 2.71828) that gives a. For example, the natural logarithm of 10 is about 2.303 because $2.71828^{2.303} = 10$. Natural logarithms can be positive or negative. If the odds of disease are 4, for example, the natural logarithm of those odds would be 1.386. If the odds of disease are 0.25, the natural logarithm of those odds would be -1.386.

The natural logarithm of the odds is called the *logit*. It is the logit that will be predicted by the regression equation. Therefore, the resulting model will be

$$\ln\left(\frac{p}{1-p}\right) = a + bx. \tag{15.4}$$

The symbol *ln* stands for the natural logarithm. Once we have the equation of this line, we can use it to make predictions of the logit for any value of the independent variable, x. Once we have the logit for a given value of x, we can convert it to the odds' original units to get the odds that a patient with a given value of x has the coronary heart disease. From those odds, we can derive the probability that the patient has the disease with the following:

$$p = \frac{\text{ODDS}}{1+\text{ODDS}}. \tag{15.5}$$

Alternatively, we can use the following equation to derive the probability directly from the logit:

$$p = \frac{e^{a+bx}}{1+e^{a+bx}}. \tag{15.6}$$

That is, to get p, we raise e to the power equal to a+bx (in other words, to the power equal to the logit), then divide by 1+e to the power equal to a+bx.

Raising e to a given power can be easily done with the exponential function, e^x, found on any scientific calculator. The *Windows* operating system also includes a scientific calculator. The function raises the number e to any power specified by the user. In this case, that power would be equal to the logit.

Once we have the predicted value of p, we can decide whether to classify the patient as having or not having coronary heart disease. Typically, if the predicted value of p is greater than 0.5, we would predict that the patient has coronary heart disease, and if the predicted value of p is not greater than 0.5, we would predict that the patient does not have coronary heart disease.

For technical reasons, the slope and intercept in the equation using the independent variable to predict the logit cannot be obtained using the method of least squares that was used in simple and multiple linear regression. Another method, known as *maximum likelihood,* must be used. This method essentially uses trial-and-error to obtain a solution. SPSS uses this method to obtain estimates of the slope and intercept coefficients.

15.2 Logistic Regression with One Predictor

In this section, we will see how logistic regression is used to study the relationship between probability of disease and a single predictor. The disease will be coronary heart disease and the predictor will be the patient's age.

Load the data file **Coronary Heart Disease.sav** [1] into SPSS. Our goal is to use **Age** [*Age*] (variable 3) to predict **Coronary Heart Disease** [*CHD*] (variable 4). **Age** contains a patient's age in years, and **Coronary Heart Disease** contains a value of 0 if the patient does not have coronary heart disease and a value of 1 if the patient does have the coronary heart disease. This coding scheme is typical of medical research. Risk factors are coded such that higher numbers reflect more of the factor, and the disease is coded such that its absence is assigned a 0 and its presence a 1. To conduct a logistic regression, select **Analyze > Regression > Binary Logistic** as shown in Fig. 15.1 to bring up the dialog box shown in Fig. 15.2. The term *binary* simply means that the categorical response variable has only two categories.

Place the quantitative independent variable (**Age**) in the *Covariates* box and the categorical dependent variable in the *Dependent* box. The resulting dialog box should look like the one shown in Fig. 15.2. Click **OK** to run the logistic regression. Output like that shown below will appear in an output window.

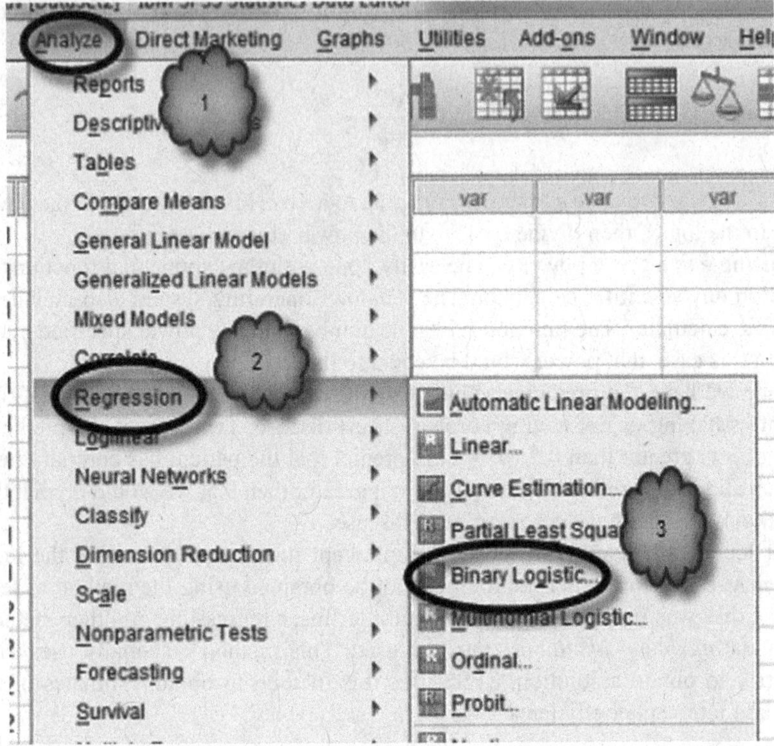

Fig. 15.1 Requesting a binary logistic regression

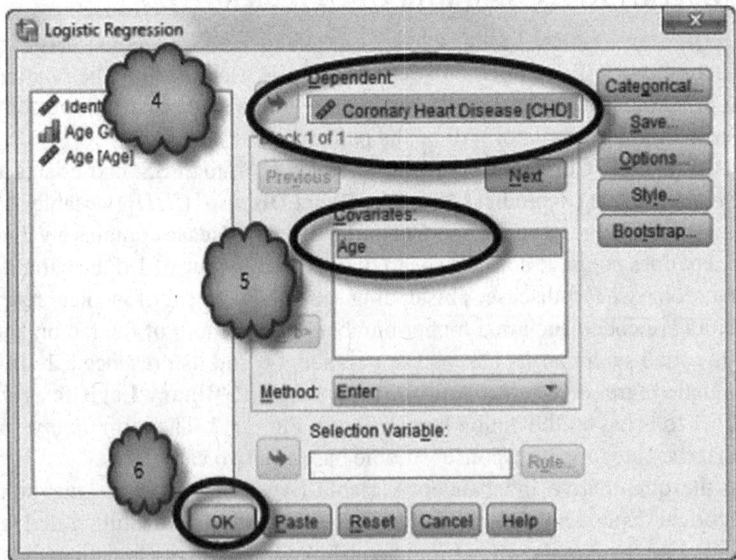

Fig. 15.2 Performing the logistic regression

Table 15.1 Case processing summary

Case Processing Summary

Unweighted Cases[a]		N	Percent
Selected Cases	Included in Analysis	100	100.0
	Missing Cases	0	.0
	Total	100	100.0
Unselected Cases		0	.0
Total		100	100.0

a. If weight is in effect, see classification table for the total number of cases.

Table 15.2 The model with no predictors

Block 0: Beginning Block

Classification Table[a,b]

Observed			Predicted		
			Coronary Heart Disease		Percentage Correct
			No	Yes	
Step 0	Coronary Heart Disease	No	57	0	100.0
		Yes	43	0	.0
	Overall Percentage				57.0

a. Constant is included in the model.
b. The cut value is .500

The Table 15.1 summarizes the number of cases in the study.

SPSS runs two models. The first contains no independent variables. This is called the *beginning block*. Three tables summarize the results of this model, the first of which is of interest to us and is displayed in Table 15.2.

The *classification table* shown in Table 15.2 tells us how accurately we can categorize our patients as having or not having coronary heart disease when we ignore the independent variable. We can see from the table that the majority of the patients (57 out of 100) did not have coronary heart disease. Consequently, if we were to ignore the age of each patient, we would most often be correct in classifying our patients if we categorize all 100 as being free of the disease. This would allow us to correctly categorize 57 % of our patients. Later in the output, we will see if taking age into account increases the accuracy.

The second model contains all of the independent variables. This is called *Block 1*.

Table 15.3 Omnibus tests of model coefficients

Omnibus Tests of Model Coefficients

		Chi-square	df	Sig.
Step 1	Step	29.310	1	.000
	Block	29.310	1	.000
	Model	29.310	1	.000

Table 15.4 Model summary

Model Summary

Step	-2 Log likelihood	Cox & Snell R Square	Nagelkerke R Square
1	107.353[a]	.254	.341

a. Estimation terminated at iteration number 5 because parameter estimates changed by less than .001.

The Table 15.3 gives the results of testing that all of the population slope coefficients are 0. This is analogous to the ANOVA *F*-test in linear regressions. The null hypothesis is that all slope coefficients are 0, and the alternative hypothesis is that at least one slope coefficient is not equal to 0. The degrees of freedom are equal to the number of independent variables.

- The *model summary* shown in Table 15.4 includes an entry called −2 *log likelihood.* This value has to do with the maximum likelihood estimation process and is not very informative.
- Logistic regression does not have a quantity that is analogous to R^2 in linear regression. A number of quantities, called pseudo-R-squares, have been proposed to create such a quantity. The *model summary* gives two of the more popular ones. None of them is very reliable.

The classification table shown in Table 15.5 shows how well the logistic regression correctly classifies a subject as to whether or not he or she has coronary heart disease when the independent variable is taken into account. Comparing this classification table with the one in Block 0, we see that by taking the patients' ages into account, the percentage of correct classifications increased from 57 to 74 %. The 74 % value is found by adding the number of patients that were correctly classified (45 + 29 = 74), dividing that sum by the total number of patients classified (100) and multiplying that result by 100. The cut value footnote indicates that patients were

Table 15.5 Final classification table

Classification Table[a]

Observed			Predicted		
			Coronary Heart Disease		Percentage Correct
			No	Yes	
Step 1	Coronary Heart Disease	No	45	12	78.9
		Yes	14	29	67.4
	Overall Percentage				74.0

a. The cut value is .500

Table 15.6 Variables in the equation

Variables in the Equation

		B	S.E.	Wald	df	Sig.	Exp(B)
Step 1[a]	Age	.111	.024	21.254	1	.000	1.117
	Constant	-5.309	1.134	21.935	1	.000	.005

a. Variable(s) entered on step 1: Age.

classified as having coronary heart disease if their predicted values for p were above 0.5.

Table 15.6 shows the variables in the equation and is analogous to the *coefficients* table in linear regression.

- The value in the *B* column in the row for the independent variable is the slope coefficient.
- The value in the *B* column in the row labeled *Constant* is the intercept.
- The values in the *S.E.* column are the standard errors for the slope and intercept coefficients, respectively.
- The values in the *Wald* column are the square of the *B* coefficient divided by the standard error. It is analogous to the individual t-test in simple and multiple regression. The null hypothesis is that the population coefficient is equal to 0, and the alternative hypothesis is that the coefficient does not equal to 0.
- The *df* column shows that there is 1 degree of freedom associated with each *Wald* statistic.
- The *Sig.* column gives the p-value for each Wald test. The p-values are interpreted in the usual way.
- The *Exp(B)* gives the value of e raised to the power of the *B* coefficient. For the independent variable, the entry is the odds ratio and indicates the change in the odds for a 1-unit increase in the independent variable. The entry for the intercept are the odds (not the odds ratio) for patients for whom the independent variable is coded as 0. In our example, the intercept coefficient is not useful as age cannot be 0.

Study the output of *Block 1* and answer the following questions:

15.2.1 What is the logistic regression equation?

15.2.2 What percentage of the patients is correctly classified as to whether or not they have coronary heart disease using this equation?

15.2.3 Is the patient's age useful information?

15.2.4 What is the change in the odds ratio for a one year increase in a patient's age?

15.2.5 What is the log of the odds that a 60-year-old patient will have coronary heart disease?

Predicted Probabilities and Confidence Intervals for Odds Ratios You should have found that the log of the odds that a 60-year-old patient will have coronary heart disease is −5.309+0.111(60) or 1.351. This is the logit for a 60-year-old patient. As we explained earlier, we could then derive the model's predicted probability that a 60-year-old patient will have coronary heart disease by raising *e* to the power of 1.351 to get the odds expressed in its original units (the odds would be about 3.8) and then calculate the probability from those odds. Alternatively, we could derive the predicted probability directly by raising *e* to the power of the logit and dividing the result by 1+e raised to the power of the logit. Yet another option is to instruct SPSS to generate the predicted probabilities for us. In this section, we will see how. We will also see how to get confidence intervals for the odds ratios.

To get each patient's predicted probability of having coronary heart disease, first set up the logistic regression in the usual manner. Then click **Save.** In the resulting dialog box shown in Fig. 15.3, choose *Probabilities*. Click **Continue.**

To get the confidence intervals, click **Options** to bring up the dialog box shown in Fig. 15.4. Now check *CI for exp(B)* and enter the desired confidence level in percent in the *%* box. In this example, enter *95%* if it is not already there. Click **Continue** followed by **OK**.

The predicted probabilities generated by the prediction equation will appear in the last column of the data file, a section of which is shown in Fig. 15.5. We saw earlier that the log of the odds that a 60-year-old patient will have coronary heart disease is 1.351. We can see from the column labeled **PRE_1** that this value of the logit corresponds to a probability of 0.79344. Thus, the prediction equation predicts that a 60-year-old patient has about a 79% chance of having coronary heart disease.

15.2.6 According to the prediction model, what are the chances that a 69-year-old patient would have coronary heart disease?

The confidence interval of the odds ratio will be appended to the *Variables in the Equation* table as shown Table 15.7.

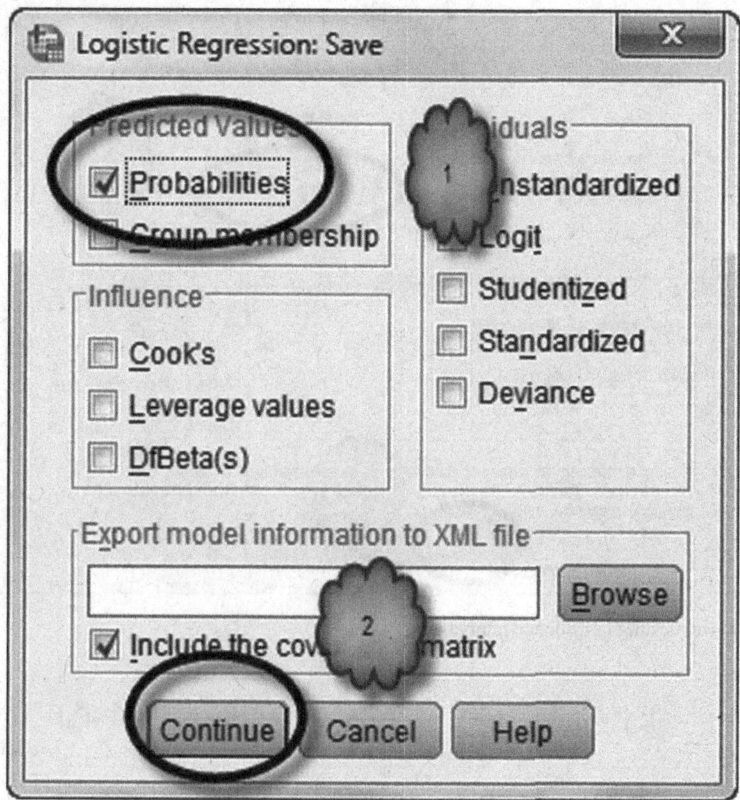

Fig. 15.3 Requesting probabilities

15.2.7 According to this output, what is the 95 % confidence interval for the odds ratio associated with age?

15.3 Logistic Regression with Two Categorical Predictors

Our logistic regression consisted of a single predictor, and the predictor was quantitative. However, a logistic regression can include two or more independent variables and the independent variables can be categorical. In this section, we will look at an example of a logistic regression in which we have two categorical independent variables. In the next section, we will look at an example that includes both categorical and quantitative variables. If the categorical variable has only two categories, such as gender, then *Exp(B)* gives the change in the odds for going from one category to the next. If the categorical variable has three or more categories,

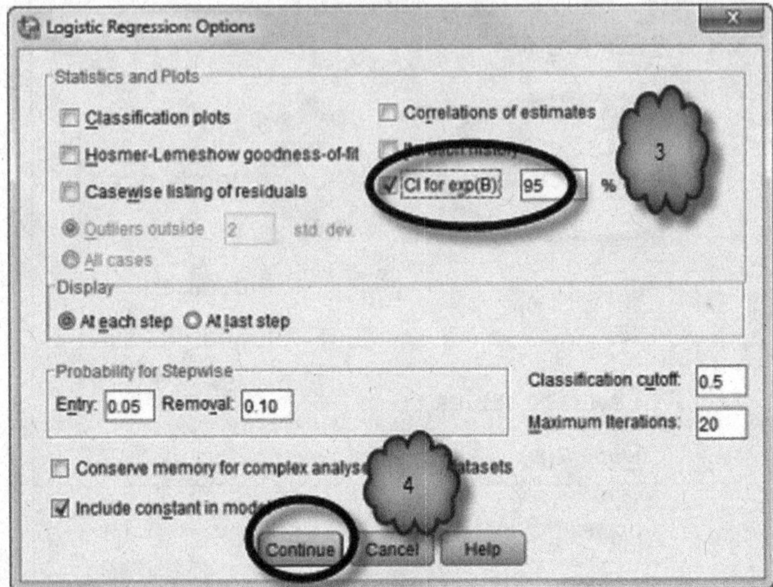

Fig. 15.4 Requesting confidence intervals

	ID	AGRP	Age	CHD	PRE_1
87	87	7	58	1	.75472
88	88	7	58	1	.75472
89	89	7	59	1	.77467
90	90	7	59	1	.77467
91	91	8	60	0	.79344
92	92	8	60	1	.79344
93	93	8	61	1	.81103
94	94	8	62	1	.82745
95	95	8	62	1	.82745

Fig. 15.5 Data file displaying predicted probabilities

Table 15.7 Confidence interval for the odds ratio

Variables in the Equation

		B	S.E.	Wald	df	Sig.	Exp(B)	95% C.I. for EXP(B)	
								Lower	Upper
Step 1[a]	Age	.111	.024	21.254	1	.000	1.117	1.066	1.171
	Constant	-5.309	1.134	21.935	1	.000	.005		

a. Variable(s) entered on step 1: Age.

then things get a little bit trickier. In this section, we will stick to categorical variables with two categories.

Load the data file, **Diabetes.sav** [2]. This file was compiled by physician assistant students who interviewed patients at a clinic for the uninsured in order to document the prevalence of diabetes mellitus type 2 and its risk factors among patients who have no health insurance. The dependent variable is **Diabetes Status** [*Diabetes*] (variable 8). It has two values. Following standard practice, a 0 was assigned if the patient reported that he or she did not have diabetes and a 1 if he or she did. Several risk factors were assessed. In our example, we will focus on two: **Family History** [*Family*] of diabetes (variable 9) and **Hypertension** [*Hypertension*] (variable 10). As is usually the case with research on risk factors, a 0 indicates the absence of the factor while a 1 represents its presence.

To run the regression, select **Analyze > Regression > Binary Logistic** to bring up the *Logistic Regression* dialog box. Enter the categorical dependent variable (**Diabetes Status**) in the *Dependent* box. Enter the two independent variables (**Family History** and **Hypertension**) in the *Covariates* box. The dialog box should now be similar to the one shown in Fig. 15.6.

Next we have to declare that the two predictors are categorical. To do this, click **Categorical** as shown in Fig. 15.6 to bring up the *Define Categorical Variables* dialog box. Move the two categorical variables to the *Categorical Covariates* area. For each variable, select whether the reference category will be the lowest numbered category (*First*) or the highest numbered category (*Last*). *Last* is the default choice.

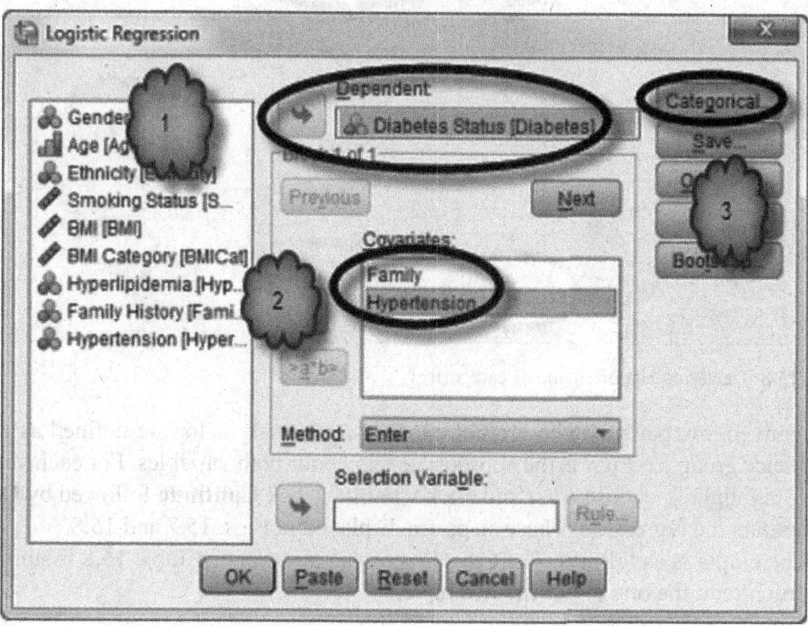

Fig. 15.6 Declaring categorical predictors

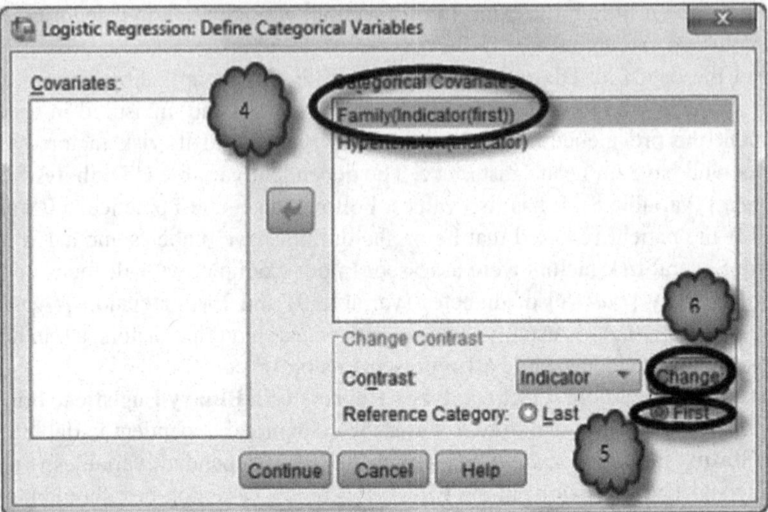

Fig. 15.7 Declaring Family as categorical

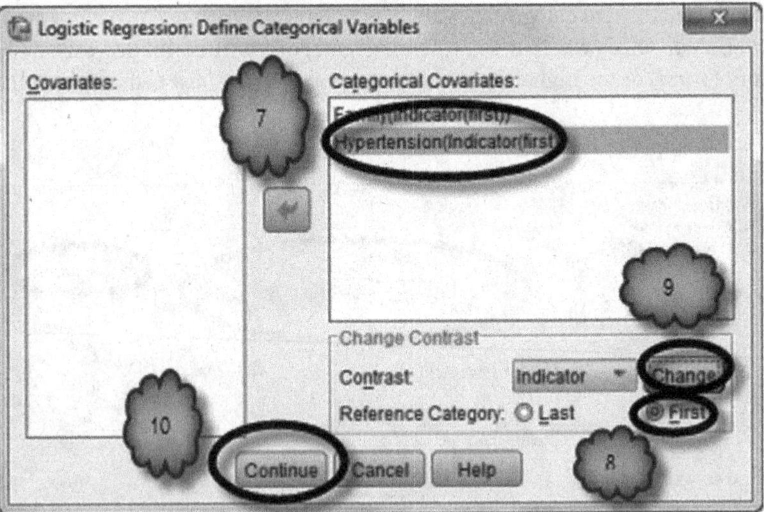

Fig. 15.8 Declaring Hypertension as categorical

By convention, patients who are not exposed to the risk factor are defined as the reference group, so *First* is the appropriate choice for both variables. For each variable, highlight it, choose *First* and click **Change**. Click **Continue** followed by **OK** to conduct the regression. These steps are displayed in Figs. 15.7 and 15.8.

The output is as follows. The *Case Processing Summary* in Table 15.8 is similar in structure to the one in our first example.

Table 15.8 Case processing summary

Case Processing Summary

Unweighted Cases[a]		N	Percent
Selected Cases	Included in Analysis	131	100.0
	Missing Cases	0	.0
	Total	131	100.0
Unselected Cases		0	.0
Total		131	100.0

a. If weight is in effect, see classification table for the total number of cases.

Table 15.9 Information on the variables in the model

Dependent Variable Encoding

Original Value	Internal Value
No	0
Yes	1

Categorical Variables Codings

		Frequency	Parameter coding (1)
Hypertension	No	67	.000
	Yes	64	1.000
Family History	No	79	.000
	Yes	52	1.000

Table 15.9 displays the output that explains the codes assigned by SPSS to the dependent variable and to the categorical independent variables.

- Tables 15.10 and 15.11 are the similar in structure to those in the first example. Notice in the *Classification Table* that when we ignore the independent variables, we can accurately categorize 72.5 % of the patients as to whether or not they had diabetes. The accuracy rate is as high as it is because the bulk of the subjects in the study do not have diabetes.

Table 15.10 Predictions in the empty model

Block 0: Beginning Block

Classification Table[a,b]

Observed			Predicted		
			Diabetes Status		Percentage Correct
			No	Yes	
Step 0	Diabetes Status	No	95	0	100.0
		Yes	36	0	.0
	Overall Percentage				72.5

a. Constant is included in the model.
b. The cut value is .500

Table 15.11 Wald test for the empty model

Variables in the Equation

		B	S.E.	Wald	df	Sig.	Exp(B)
Step 0	Constant	-.970	.196	24.582	1	.000	.379

Table 15.12 Tests on variables not in the model

Variables not in the Equation

			Score	df	Sig.
Step 0	Variables	Family(1)	12.139	1	.000
		Hypertension(1)	13.581	1	.000
	Overall Statistics		25.251	2	.000

- Table 15.12 shows whether or not each independent variable would be significant if it were entered in the model.
- Tables 15.13, 15.14, and 15.15 give the same type of information as in the first example.
- As in the first example, Table 15.16 displays the slope coefficients, their standard errors, the results of the test statistic, and the exponents of the slope coefficients. For family history of diabetes, we see that the slope coefficient is 1.554. The exponent of this (that is, $e^{1.554}$) is the odds ratio, 4.731. The odds of having diabetes for a patient who has a family history of diabetes is about 4.7 times greater than those who do not have a family history of the disease. The *p*-value tells us that the odds ratio is significantly different from 1.

Table 15.13 Omnibus test of the model

Omnibus Tests of Model Coefficients

		Chi-square	df	Sig.
Step 1	Step	27.031	2	.000
	Block	27.031	2	.000
	Model	27.031	2	.000

Table 15.14 Model summary

Model Summary

Step	-2 Log likelihood	Cox & Snell R Square	Nagelkerke R Square
1	127.021[a]	.186	.270

a. Estimation terminated at iteration number 5 because parameter estimates changed by less than .001.

Table 15.15 Final classification table

Classification Table[a]

Observed			Predicted: Diabetes Status No	Predicted: Diabetes Status Yes	Percentage Correct
Step 1	Diabetes Status	No	84	11	88.4
		Yes	21	15	41.7
	Overall Percentage				75.6

a. The cut value is .500

Table 15.16 Results for variables in the model

Variables in the Equation

		B	S.E.	Wald	df	Sig.	Exp(B)
Step 1[a]	Family(1)	1.554	.449	11.997	1	.001	4.731
	Hypertension(1)	1.700	.470	13.069	1	.000	5.472
	Constant	-2.680	.475	31.834	1	.000	.069

a. Variable(s) entered on step 1: Family, Hypertension.

- The entry for hypertension shows that the odds ratio for the second predictor is also significantly different from 1, and that the odds of having diabetes for a patient who has hypertension is about 5.5 times greater than those who do not have hypertension.
- The entry for *Constant* gives the odds for cases for whom all values of the independent variables are 0. In research on risk factors, the cases not exposed to any of the risk factors are assigned a 0 for each factor. Consequently, the information in this row tells us the odds that a patient has diabetes if he or she has neither a family history of diabetes nor hypertension. These odds are sometimes referred to as the *baseline odds*. In our example, the log of the baseline odds is −2.68, while the baseline odds are 0.069. If we were to convert the baseline odds into a probability, we would see that the chances that a patient from this population would have diabetes if he or she does not have a family history of diabetes and is not hypertensive is about 6.5% (0.069/1.069=0.0645).

Using Odds Ratios and Baseline Odds to Estimate Odds of Disease Once the odds ratio for each risk factor has been determined, the extent to which the exposure to various combinations of those factors increases the odds of disease can also be determined by multiplying together the odd ratios in question. For instance, according to our example data, amongst patients who are uninsured, the odds of having diabetes increase almost five fold for those who have a family history of diabetes and over five times for those who are hypertensive. By how much do the odds increase for patients who are unfortunate enough to have been exposed to both risk factors? To find out, we multiply the two sets of odds ratios together and see that if patients have a family history of diabetes and are hypertensive, their odds of having diabetes increase by almost a factor of 26 ($4.731 \times 5.472 = 25.888$).

The odds ratios can be combined with baseline odds to predict the odds of disease for cases exposed to various risk factors and combinations of risk factors. This is done by multiplying the baseline odds by the odds ratios in question. For instance, in our example, the baseline odds are the odds of diabetes for patients who have no family history of diabetes and are not hypertensive. If we multiply those odds (0.069) by the odds ratio for family history (4.731), we see that the predicted odds of disease for patients who have a family history, but are not hypertensive are 0.3264, a value that corresponds to a probability of about 0.25. If we multiply the baseline odds by the odds ratio for hypertension, we would get the odds of disease for patients who are hypertensive, but do not have a family history of diabetes.

Answer the following question:

15.3.1 What would be the odds of disease for patients who have a family history of diabetes *and* are hypertensive?

15.4 Logistic Regression with Quantitative and Categorical Predictors

In this section, we will conduct another logistic regression. This time though we will use one quantitative and two categorical independent variables, and one of the categorical variables will have more than two categories. In the example, we will try to predict whether or not a patient died after having been admitted to an intensive care unit (the dependent variable) based on one quantitative and two categorical independent variables: the patient's age (quantitative), the type of admission (categorical), and the patient's level of consciousness at admission (categorical).

When using a categorical variable that has more than two categories, one of those categories must be selected as a reference category. In research on risk factors, the reference category is usually the one that represents the absence of the risk factor. Otherwise, it is usually the category that is most frequent in the data. The SPSS will calculate *B* coefficients for each of the other categories for a change from the reference category to that category. This means that *Exp(B)* will give the change in the odds for going from the reference category to the other category. The ratio of the *Exp(B)* values of two non-reference categories yields the change in the odds between two non-reference categories.

Load the data file **ICU.sav** [3] into SPSS. The file contains data on patients in an intensive care unit. The variable **Vital Status** [*STA*] (variable 2) contains a 0 if the patient survived and a 1 if the patient died. The variable, **Age** [*AGE*] (variable 3), contains the patient's age in years. The variable, **Type of Admission** [*TYP*] (variable 14), indicates the type of admission to the intensive care unit. A value of 0 indicates that the admission was elective, and a value of 1 indicates that the admission was an emergency. The variable, **Level of Consciousness** [*LOC*] (variable 21), gives the level of consciousness when the patient was admitted to the intensive care unit. A value of 0 represents no coma or stupor, a value of 1 represents a patient in a deep stupor, and a value of 2 represents a patient in a coma. We wish to use **Age**, **Type of Admission** and **Level of Consciousness** to predict whether or not a particular patient survived.

To run the regression, open the *Logistic Regression* dialog box, enter the categorical dependent variable (**Vital Status**) in the *Dependent* box, and the three independent variables (**Age**, **Type of Admission** and **Level of Consciousness**) in the *Covariates* box, as shown in Fig. 15.9.

To declare that **Type of Admission** and **Level of Consciousness** are categorical, click **Categorical** to bring up the *Define Categorical Variables* dialog box. Move the two categorical variables to the *Categorical Covariates* area. For each variable, select whether the reference category will be the lowest numbered category (*First*) or the highest numbered category (*Last*).

As we saw in the previous section, *Last* is the default choice. Since most patients come to an intensive care unit on an emergency basis, *Last* is the appropriate choice for **Type of Admission**. However, since most patients come to an intensive care unit conscious, choose *First* for **Level of Consciousness** and click **Change**. Click **Continue** followed by **OK** to conduct the regression. This is displayed in Fig. 15.10.

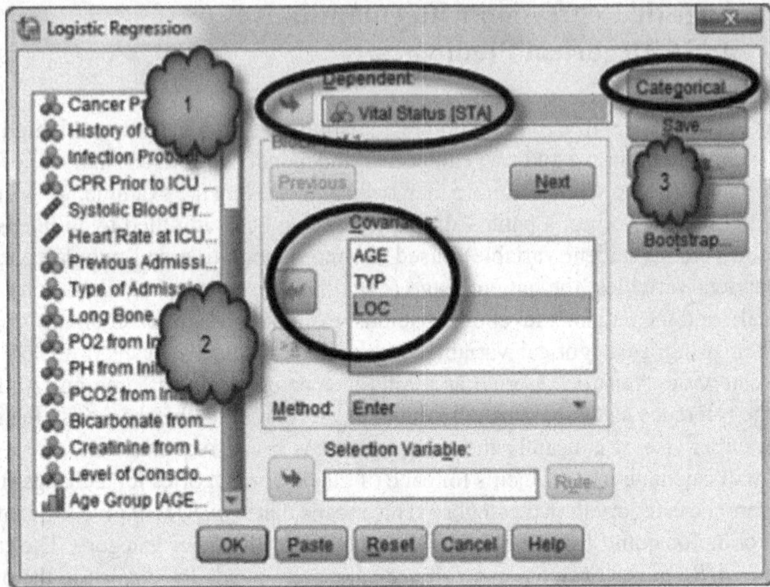

Fig. 15.9 Selecting the variables in the model

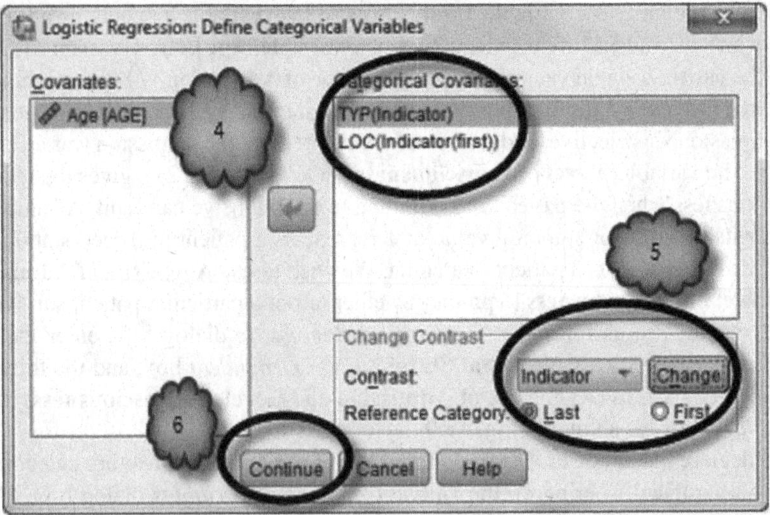

Fig. 15.10 Declaring the categorical variables in the model

A portion of the output is shown below. Interpretation of Tables 15.17 and 15.18 of the output is similar to our previous example.

As in the previous example, the table displaying the codes of the categorical variables in Table 15.19 depicts the codes assigned by SPSS to the categorical variables.

Table 15.17 Case processing summary

Case Processing Summary

Unweighted Cases[a]		N	Percent
Selected Cases	Included in Analysis	199	99.5
	Missing Cases	1	.5
	Total	200	100.0
Unselected Cases		0	.0
Total		200	100.0

a. If weight is in effect, see classification table for the total number of cases.

Table 15.18 Values of the dependent variable

Dependent Variable Encoding

Original Value	Internal Value
Lived	0
Died	1

Table 15.19 Encoding for the categorical predictors

Categorical Variables Codings

		Frequency	Parameter coding (1)	(2)
Level of Consciousness	No Coma or Stupor	185	.000	.000
	Deep Stupor	5	1.000	.000
	Coma	9	.000	1.000
Type of Admission	Elective	52	1.000	
	Emergency	147	.000	

For a categorical variable with only two categories, the reference category is given a value of 0, and the other category is given a value of 1. For a categorical variable with three categories, SPSS creates two internal variables called *dummy variables*, each of which takes on either a 0 or a 1. For patients in the reference category, the SPSS sets both dummy variables to 0. The other categories get a value of 0 in one dummy variable and a value of 1 in the other. For categorical variables with more than three categories, the pattern is similar. For *k* categories, SPSS creates *k*-1 dummy variables. The reference category always receives a value of 0 for all of the dummy variables. The other categories receive a value of 1 for one of the dummy variables and a value of 0 in all of the other dummy variables. The logic of creating dummy variables is similar to the logic we used in Chap. 14 on multiple linear

Table 15.20 Classification table for the empty model

Block 0: Beginning Block

Classification Table[a,b]

Observed			Predicted		
			Vital Status		Percentage Correct
			Lived	Died	
Step 0	Vital Status	Lived	159	0	100.0
		Died	40	0	.0
	Overall Percentage				79.9

a. Constant is included in the model.
b. The cut value is .500

Table 15.21 Test of the empty model

Variables in the Equation

		B	S.E.	Wald	df	Sig.	Exp(B)
Step 0	Constant	-1.380	.177	60.866	1	.000	.252

Table 15.22 Tests of variables not in the model

Variables not in the Equation

			Score	df	Sig.
Step 0	Variables	AGE	6.918	1	.009
		TYP(1)	11.580	1	.001
		LOC	41.357	2	.000
		LOC(1)	20.387	1	.000
		LOC(2)	19.525	1	.000
	Overall Statistics		56.404	4	.000

regression except that there we would have had to create the dummy variables ourselves by using **Transform > Recode into Different Variables**. Here SPSS creates the dummy variables automatically.

- The interpretation of Tables 15.20 and 15.21 is similar to the previous example.
- Table 15.22 shows whether or not each independent variable would be significant if entered in the model. Whether or not the dummy variable for its corresponding

Table 15.23 Test of final model

Omnibus Tests of Model Coefficients

		Chi-square	df	Sig.
Step 1	Step	55.101	4	.000
	Block	55.101	4	.000
	Model	55.101	4	.000

Table 15.24 Final model summary

Model Summary

Step	-2 Log likelihood	Cox & Snell R Square	Nagelkerke R Square
1	144.612[a]	.242	.382

a. Estimation terminated at iteration number 20 because maximum iterations has been reached. Final solution cannot be found.

Table 15.25 Final classification table

Classification Table[a]

Observed			Predicted		
			Vital Status		Percentage Correct
			Lived	Died	
Step 1	Vital Status	Lived	157	2	98.7
		Died	28	12	30.0
	Overall Percentage				84.9

a. The cut value is .500

category would be significant if entered in the model is provided by the *LOC(1)* and *LOC(2)* entries.

- Tables 15.23, 15.24, and 15.25 give the same type of information as in the previous examples.
- From Table 15.26 we see that for every additional year in the age of a patient, the logit increases by 0.033, resulting in odds ratio of 1.034. The entry for the type of admission tells us that the odds of dying for patients who chose to be admitted are 0.06 of those for patients who were of emergency admissions.

Table 15.26 Tests of the individual variables in the equation

Variables in the Equation

		B	S.E.	Wald	df	Sig.	Exp(B)
Step 1[a]	AGE	.033	.012	8.008	1	.005	1.034
	TYP(1)	-2.815	1.038	7.349	1	.007	.060
	LOC			8.245	2	.016	
	LOC(1)	23.577	16716.083	.000	1	.999	1.735E+10
	LOC(2)	2.423	.844	8.245	1	.004	11.280
	Constant	-3.348	.776	18.591	1	.000	.035

a. Variable(s) entered on step 1: AGE, TYP, LOC.

- The entry for *LOC* shows that, overall, the level of consciousness is a significant variable. There is no slope coefficient or an odds ratio because the variable has been replaced by the dummy variables in the model.
- *LOC(1)* and *LOC(2)* represent the difference between the reference category and the other two categories. *LOC(1)* is for deep stupor and *LOC(2)* is for coma. We see that the slope for *LOC(1)* is not significantly different from 0. This means that the odds ratio is not significantly different from 1, and not the extremely high value (1.735×10^{10}) that is shown in the output. Thus, the odds of dying for a patient who is in a deep stupor are the same as for a patient who is neither in a stupor nor in a coma. However, the slope coefficient for *LOC(2)* is significantly different from 0, indicating that the odds of dying for a patient who is admitted in a coma are 11.28 times as high as for a patient with no coma or stupor.
- If you wanted the odds ratio for a patient arriving in a coma compared to a person arriving in a deep stupor, you would divide the odds ratio for a patient arriving in a coma by the odds ratio for a patient arriving in a deep stupor. In this case, since the odds ratio for a patient arriving in a deep stupor compared to a patient arriving in neither a deep stupor nor a coma is 1, the odds ratio comparing the odds of the coma patient against the odds of the patient in a deep stupor works out again to 11.28, indicating that a person in a coma is 11.28 times more likely to die than is a patient arriving in a deep stupor.
- The entry for *Constant* gives the odds for a patient for whom all values of the independent variable are 0. Since in this example a patient's age cannot be 0, this value is uninteresting.

15.5 Adjusted Odds Ratios

Logistic regression models often include several independent variables. One reason for this is to improve the fit of the model to the data. Another is to determine the relationship between a dependent variable and a given independent variable after controlling for the presence of other independent variables. In either case, the resulting odds ratios are referred to as *adjusted odds ratios*, as their values take into

Table 15.27 Variables in the equation table with type of admission removed

Variables in the Equation

		B	S.E.	Wald	df	Sig.	Exp(B)
Step 1[a]	AGE	.028	.012	5.310	1	.021	1.028
	LOC			11.699	2	.003	
	LOC(1)	22.948	17882.024	.000	1	.999	9249041421
	LOC(2)	2.860	.836	11.699	1	.001	17.464
	Constant	-3.403	.794	18.362	1	.000	.033

a. Variable(s) entered on step 1: AGE, LOC.

account or adjust for the relationships among the independent variables included in the model. As a consequence, the adjusted odds ratio for a given predictor may change as independent variables are added to or removed from the model. This is analogous to the way in which the slope coefficients in mutilple regression change as independent variables are added or removed. In order to see this, remove **Type of Admission** from our previous analysis of Sect. 15.4, and run the regression.

The *Variables in the Equation* table you generated in *Block 1* should match the one shown in Table 15.27. Compare this table to Table 15.26.

Answer the following questions:

15.5.1 Did the adjusted odds ratio for **Age** change?

15.5.2 How about the dummy variables for **Level of Consciousness**?

15.6 Testing for an Interaction Effect

As with multiple regression, logistic regression assumes that the effect of an independent variable is constant across the values of the other independent variables in the model, that is, there are no *interaction effects*. This assumption can be tested in a logistic regression in the same way it is tested in a multiple regression. First, a new variable representing the interaction between the two independent variables of interest is created by multiplying the two independent variables together. The resulting variable is then added to the model. If the slope coefficient associated with the interaction term is significant, then we would have evidence that the effect of one of the independent variables depends on the value of the other. For example, a logistic regression investigating the effects of age and sex on vital status would assume that the effect of age is the same for both men and women. To test this assumption, we would multiply age by sex to obtain a variable that represents the interaction between these two predictors, replace the independent variable **Sex** with this interaction term, and run the analysis. If the slope coefficient for the interaction is significant, we would have evidence that the relationship between age and survival depends on the sex of the patient.

As was the case in Chap. 14, **Transform>Compute Variable** would be used to create the interaction variable. In our example, the interaction variable might be called **Age*Sex.** The logistic regression would then be conducted in which **Age** and **Age*Sex** would be the independent variables and **Vital Status** the dependent variable. You will get a chance to do this in the exercises.

15.7 Exercise Questions

1. This exercise question uses the intensive care unit (ICU) data set.
   a. Use **Analyze>Descriptive Statistics>Crosstabs** to create a contingency table comparing **Vital Status** [*STA*] (variable 2; 0=Lived, 1=Died) with **History of Chronic Renal Failure** [*CRN*] (variable 8; 0=No, 1=Yes). Calculate by hand the odds of a patient with a history of chronic renal failure dying. Calculate by hand the odds of a patient with no history of chronic renal failure dying. Divide the odds of a patient with a history of chronic renal failure dying by the odds of a patient of a person with no history of chronic renal failure dying. What is the resulting odds ratio?
   b. Conduct a binary logistic regression using the categorical variable **History of Chronic Renal Failure** as the independent variable and **Vital Status** as the dependent variable. What is the odds ratio for chronic renal failure? How does it compare with your answer from Question 1a? What does this odds ratio tell you about the likelihood of survival of patients with a history of renal failure compared to patients with no history of renal failure?
2. This exercise question continues using the ICU data set.
   a. Repeat the logistic regression of the previous question, but add **Age**, **Sex**, and **Level of Consciousness** as independent variables. Report the odds ratio for renal failure.
   b. Compare the odds ratio you just reported with that of Question 1. How do they compare? Explain any difference that you see.
   c. What is the 95 % confidence interval of the odds ratio for renal failure?
   d. What is the predicted probability of death for a 69-year-old man who has a history of renal failure and arrives at the ICU in a coma?
3. Conduct a logistic regression on the ICU data using *Age* and the interaction between age and sex as the independent variables.
   a. What is the slope coefficient for the interaction term?
   b. What is the *p*-value for the interaction term?
   c. According to the analysis, does the relationship between age and likelihood of survival depend on the sex of the patient? Why or why not?
4. A team of physician assistant students wanted to know whether the lack of flexibility is a risk factor for lower extremity injuries among male collegiate athletes [4].

Table 15.28 Output for Question 4

Variables in the Equation

		B	S.E.	Wald	df	Sig.	Exp(B)
Step 1[a]	Flexibiity			4.122	2	.127	
	Flexibiity(1)	.350	.527	.442	1	.506	1.419
	Flexibiity(2)	1.027	.515	3.986	1	.046	2.794
	Constant	-1.587	.366	18.817	1	.000	.205

a. Variable(s) entered on step 1: Flexibiity.

To find out, the research team measured the flexibility of male Division III athletes at the beginning of the fall of season. Flexibility was measured by asking the athletes to reach towards their toes as far as possible while sitting on the floor with their legs outstretched in front of them. The distance each athlete was able to reach served as the measure of flexibility. The researchers then classified each athlete into one of three categories of flexibility: low (coded as 2), moderate (1), and high (0). At the end of the season, the team recorded the number of practice and game days that each athlete had missed during the season due to a lower extremity injury. Athletes who missed at least 1 day were classified as having been injured. The team conducted a logistic regression in which injury status was the dependent variable, and the level of flexibility was the independent variable. A fragment of output is below. The high flexibility category was the reference group. Study the output shown in Table 15.28 and then complete the following sentences.

a. The *log of the odds* (or the logit) of injury for an athlete who is highly flexible is _________ while the *log of the odds* (or the logit) of injury for an athlete who is low in flexibility is _________.
b. The *odds* of injury for an athlete who is low in flexibility are _________ times the *odds* of injury for an athlete who is high in flexibility.
c. The *odds* of injury for an athlete who is low in flexibility are _________ while the *odds* of injury for an athlete who is high in flexibility are _________.
d. The *probability* of injury for an athlete who is low in flexibility is _________ while the *probability* of injury for an athlete who is high in flexibility is _________.
e. One of the findings of this study tests the null/alternative (choose one) hypothesis that athletes who are *moderate* in flexibility are no more likely to be injured than the athletes who are high in flexibility. This hypothesis should be accepted/rejected (choose one).

Data Sets and References

1. Coronary Heart Disease.sav obtained from: Hosmer, D.W., Lemeshow, S.: Applied Logistic Regression. Wiley, New York (1989). (With the kind permission of Professors David W. Hosmer and Stanley Lemeshow)

2. Diabetes.sav obtained from: Cassel, S., Mahoney, G., Troia, L., Volles, A., Henry, N.J., Holmes, W.H.: Prevalence of Risk Factors for Type 2 Diabetes Mellitus in a Population Served by a Health Clinic for the Uninsured. Unpublished data, Le Moyne College, Syracuse, New York (2010)
3. ICU.sav obtained from: Hosmer, D.W., Lemeshow, S.: Applied Logistic Regression. Wiley, New York (1989). (With the Kind Permission of John Wiley and Sons, and Professors David W. Hosmer and Stanley Lemeshow)
4. Barker, S., Jerome, J., Woods, D., Zaika, C., Brown, R.G., Holmes, W.H.: The Sit and Reach Test as a Measure of Flexibility for Predicting Lower Extremity Injury in Division III Athletes. Unpublished data, Le Moyne College, Syracuse, New York (2010)

Chapter 16
Survival Analysis

Abstract This chapter reviews the analysis of time to event data. Following a discussion of censored observations, the Kaplan–Meier estimator of the survival function, median and mean survival times, and comparing two survival functions with the log-rank test are reviewed. A second method of comparing survival functions is then introduced—Cox proportional hazards model. Topics include hazard and cumulative hazard functions, interpreting a hazard ratio, Cox regression, and testing for interactions among the covariates.

16.1 Overview

In Chap. 13 we considered predicting a quantitative response variable using simple linear regression with a single independent variable. In Chap. 14 we expanded those ideas to multiple regression where two or more independent variables were used to predict the value of a quantitative response variable. Chapter 15 considered the models where the dependent variable was a categorical variable having two categories. In this chapter we will consider a very different situation which will give rise to a different kind of regression—survival analysis. Survival analysis is used in longitudinal studies to assess the impact of factors on the amount of time that passes between a patient's entry into the study and the occurrence of a specified critical event. For example, survival analysis is used to study factors that affect the recurrence of a tumor following treatment, the length of hospital stay following surgery, or survival time following diagnosis.

Consider a hypothetical study that is interested in the survival time of patients having a certain type of cancer. Suppose the study ran from January 1, 2005 through December 31, 2010. After a patient had a confirmed diagnosis of having cancer, the patient would have been followed until death due to this type of cancer, until the end of the study, or until the patient was lost to follow-up (i.e., left the area, died due to some other cause, etc.). There would be a number of possible independent variables. Some might be age, alcohol use, and smoking.

The dependent variable in our hypothetical example is the time until death or *survival time*. However, measuring survival time (and more generally, time to event) can be somewhat complicated. Time is measured as the time from entry in

W. H. Holmes, W. C. Rinaman, *Statistical Literacy for Clinical Practitioners*,
DOI 10.1007/978-3-319-12550-3_16

the study until either death, termination of the study, or the patient leaves the study. The complication is that while we will know the time of death, and thus the survival times of patients who die while the study is ongoing, we will not know the time of death of patients who are still alive at the end of the study or who leave the study while still alive. Because the time variable is not the actual time to death for every patient, we cannot use the descriptive methods we studied in the previous chapters that summarize quantitative data, and we cannot use multiple linear regression to determine the effect of various independent variables on survival time.

When the time to event for a patient is not known, that patient's time measurements are said to be *censored*. An observation that is censored is not to be confused with one that is missing. If an observation is missing for a particular patient, the variable of interest was not measured for that patient, and we have no information about the patient for that variable. With censored data, the variable of interest was measured, but only until the time the patient left the study while still not having experience the event, or until the study ended. Consequently, that patient's data are not so much missing as they are incomplete. For example, in a survival time study, we would not know the survival time of a patient who left the study after 2 years of observation. However, we would know that the patient lived for at least 2 years. In this chapter, we will investigate descriptive and regression methods that have been designed for the analysis of censored time to event data.

16.2 Kaplan–Meier Estimator of the Survival Function

To begin, we shall consider what is known as the *survival function*. Simply stated, the survival function, *S(t)*, is the probability that a patient will survive longer than t time periods. We will consider what is known as the *Kaplan–Meier* estimator of the survival function. This estimator has the advantage that it accounts for the possible effect of censored patients on the probability of survival. It goes as follows:

a. Let n_i = the number of patients known to be at risk at time period *i*.
b. Let d_i = the number of patients who die at time period *i*.
c. Then for patients that are alive at the start of time period *i*, the estimated probability of surviving time period *i* given that d_i dies during time period *i* is

$$p_i = \frac{n_i - d_i}{n_i}. \tag{16.1}$$

d. Then the estimated probability that a patient survives the first t time periods is

$$\hat{S}(t) = p_1 \times p_2 \times \cdots \times p_t. \tag{16.2}$$

Table 16.1 Survival times of five hypothetical cancer patients

Patient	Survival time	Censored?
1	10	No
2	4	No
3	7	No
4	6	Yes
5	5	No

To illustrate, consider the following simple example. Suppose we have five patients who are diagnosed as having cancer. Table 16.1 gives their survival times and whether or not each time measurement is censored.

Since each patient is still alive until time period 4,

$$p_1 = p_2 = p_3 = \frac{5-0}{5} = 1. \tag{16.3}$$

So, for $t = 1$, 2, and 3,

$$S(t) = 1. \tag{16.4}$$

During the time period 4, there are five patients in the study and one of them (Patient 2) dies. Therefore,

$$p_4 = \frac{5-1}{5} = 0.8. \tag{16.5}$$

Consequently,

$$S(4) = 1 \times 1 \times 1 \times 0.8 = 0.8. \tag{16.6}$$

Now there are four patients in the study. During the time period 5, a second patient (Patient 5) dies, giving

$$p_5 = \frac{4-1}{4} = 0.75, \tag{16.7}$$

and

$$S(5) = 0.8 \times 0.75 = 0.6. \tag{16.8}$$

Now there are three patients remaining. During the time period 6, Patient 4 leaves the study, leaving two patients in the study. Therefore,

$$p_6 = \frac{2-0}{2} = 1, \tag{16.9}$$

Table 16.2 Survival table of five hypothetical cancer patients

Survival Table

	Time	Status	Cumulative Proportion Surviving at the Time		N of Cumulative Events	N of Remaining Cases
			Estimate	Std. Error		
1	4.000	No	.800	.179	1	4
2	5.000	No	.600	.219	2	3
3	6.000	Yes	.	.	2	2
4	7.000	No	.300	.239	3	1
5	10.000	No	.000	.000	4	0

and

$$S(6) = 0.6 \times 1 = 0.6. \tag{16.10}$$

During time period 7, another patient (Patient 3) dies, giving

$$p_7 = \frac{2-1}{2} = 0.5, \tag{16.11}$$

and

$$S(7) = 0.6 \times 0.5 = 0.3. \tag{16.12}$$

There is one patient left in the study up until time period 10. Therefore,

$$S(8) = S(9) = 0.3. \tag{16.13}$$

Finally, that patient dies during time period 10, giving

$$p_{10} = \frac{1-1}{1} = 0, \tag{16.14}$$

and

$$S(10) = 0.3 \times 0 = 0. \tag{16.15}$$

The Kaplan–Meier estimator of the survival function can be displayed in a *survival table* or as a graph. Both as generated by SPSS for the above five patients are presented in Table 16.2 and Fig. 16.1, respectively. Let us look at the table first.

In Table 16.2, the outcome (death or censored) for each patient is indicated in the order in which it occurred. The first column lists the numerical order, the second column the time period in which the event occurred, and the third whether the event was censored. For example, the first two events occurred during time periods 4 and 5, respectively, and were deaths. The third event occurred during time period 6 and

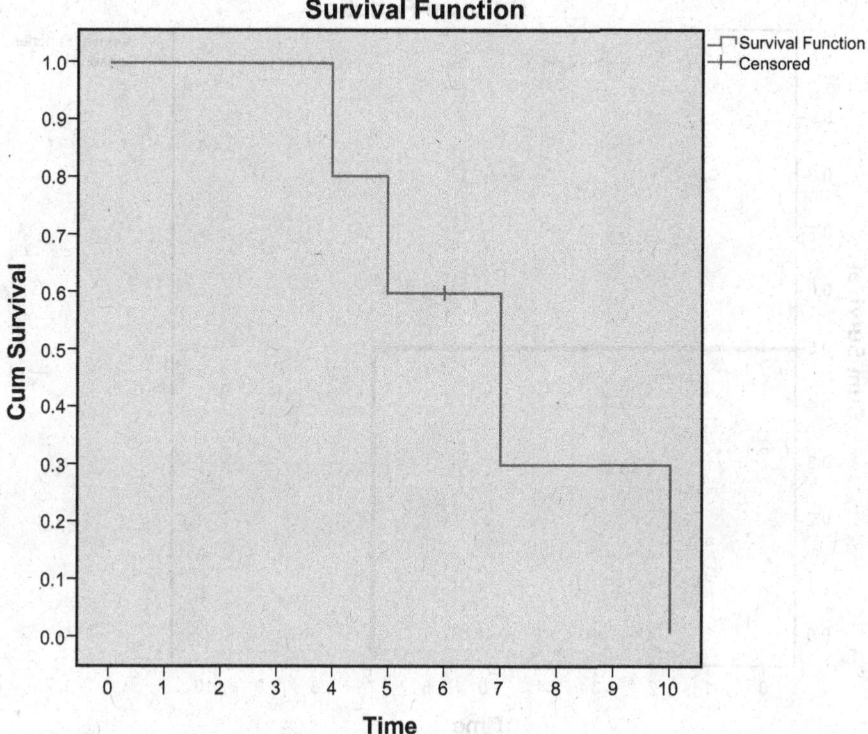

Fig. 16.1 Survival function of five hypothetical cancer patients

was the departure of a patient from the study. The fourth column presents the cumulative proportion of the five patients who survived through the corresponding time period. For example, at the end of the time period 7, 0.30 or 30 % of the original five patients were still alive. These cumulative proportions constitute the estimated survival function, that is, Kaplan–Meier estimates of the probability of surviving over time. The fifth column presents each estimate's standard error—a measure of the extent to which the estimate would vary across a large number of samples. The last two columns display running totals of patients who died and patients who remained in the study. Note that the fate of each patient is listed in the table. For this reason, the survival tables can be quite lengthy in studies of large numbers of patients.

Now let us look at the graphical display of the survival function, presented in Fig. 16.1. This plots the cumulative proportion of patients surviving at each time period and depicts a series of steps. The height of a step reflects the proportion of all patients enrolled in the study who survived to the end of the corresponding time period. Whenever a patient dies, the height of the step decreases. It is common practice to illustrate the censoring of a patient's outcome with a cross at the time of censoring occurred.

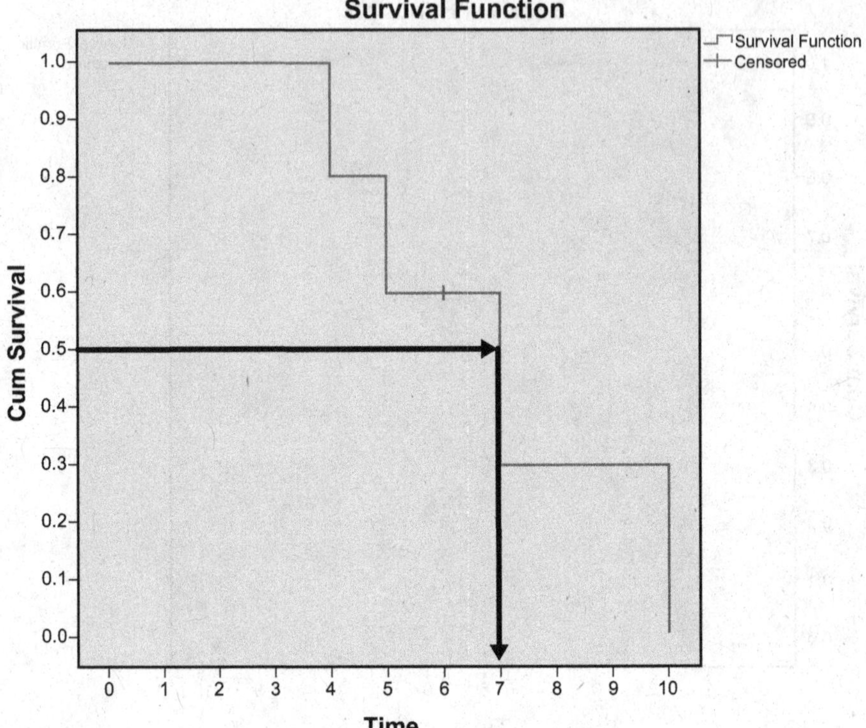

Fig. 16.2 Median survival time: point in time at which the cumulative survival is 0.5. In this example, the median is 7 years.

Median and Mean Survival Times The Kaplan–Meier survival function can be used to estimate mean and median survival times. The median survival time is the time period at the end of which 50 % of the patients enrolled have survived. As you can see in Fig. 16.2, the median survival time for our hypothetical data would be estimated to be 7 years. The estimate of the mean survival time is more complicated. It is found by calculating what is known as the "area under the curve," that is, the total area under the steps of the graph of the survival function. The area under each step is the area of the rectangle that is formed. In our hypothetical example shown in Fig. 16.3, the leftmost rectangle has a height of 1 with a base of 4; the next rectangle has a height of 0.8 with a base of 1; the third rectangle has a height of 0.6 with a base of 2; and the rightmost rectangle has a height of 0.3 with a base of 3. The area under the curve is the sum of the areas of these four rectangles or 6.9 years.

Another Example with Real Data Now that we have studied a hypothetical example of a survival function, let us look at a real one: the survival function of 481 male and female patients from the Worcester Heart Attack Study who had experienced one or more myocardial infarctions. The patients were observed following their most recent heart attack for an average of about 5 years. The file containing

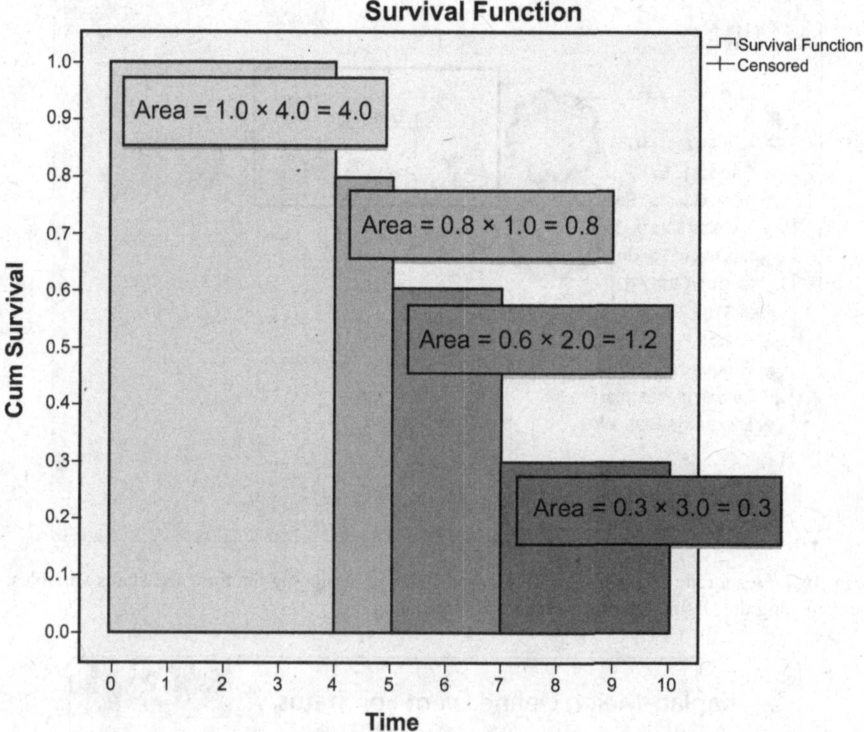

Fig. 16.3 Mean survival time: total area under the survival function. In this example, the mean equals 4.0+0.8+1.2+0.9 or 6.9 years.

these data is called **WHAS.sav** [1], and it consists of the following variables. **Total Length of Follow-up from Hospital Admission (days)** [*LENFOL*] (variable 13) gives the time in days from the date a patient entered the study until the end of the patient's follow-up time. **Status as of Last Follow-up** [*FSTAT*] (variable 14) contains a 1 if the patient died and a 0 if the patient was alive at the end of the follow-up. Our goal is to compute and graph the Kaplan–Meier estimator for the survival function and to calculate the mean and median survival times.

Load the data file. Select **Analyze>Survival>Kaplan–Meier.** In the dialog box that opens, enter the survival time variable, **Total Length of Follow-up from Hospital Admission (days)**, in the *Time* box. Enter the variable that indicates whether the value for time is censored or not, **Status as of Last Follow-up**, in the *Status* box. Click **Define Event.** In the resulting dialog box, enter the value that indicates that the subject died (a value of **1**) into the *Single value* box. Click **Continue**. These steps are displayed in Figs. 16.4 and 16.5.

Back in the Kaplan–Meier dialog, notice that *FSTAT(?)* has been replaced by *FSTAT(1)* in the *Status* box. This change can be seen in Fig. 16.6. Now click **Options.** In the resulting dialog, select *Mean and median survival* in the *Statistics* area if it is not already checked, and select *Survival* in the *Plots* area. So as not to

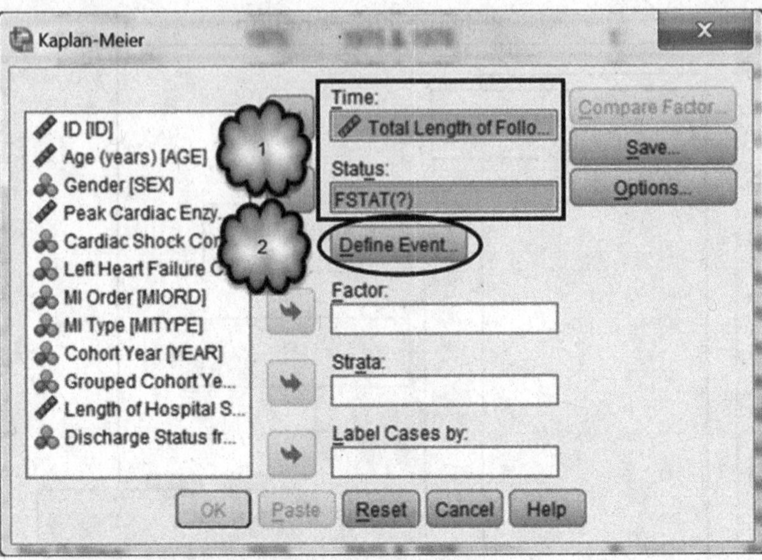

Fig. 16.4 Generating a Kaplan–Meier survival function: assigning the time and status variables, and opening the Define Event for Status Variable dialog

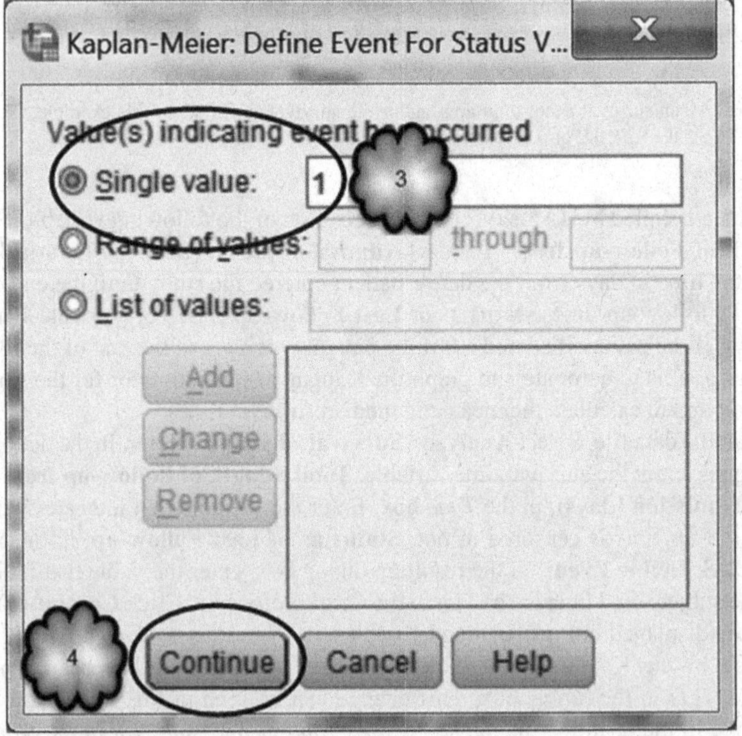

Fig. 16.5 Generating a Kaplan–Meier survival function: defining the event value

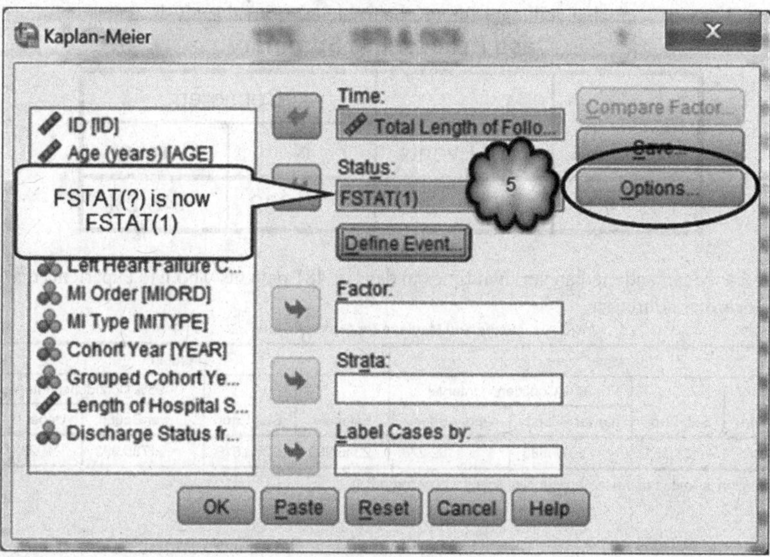

Fig. 16.6 Generating a Kaplan–Meier survival function: opening the Options dialog

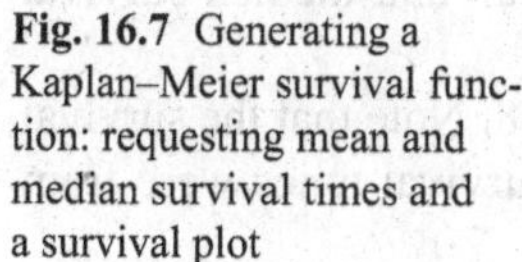

Fig. 16.7 Generating a Kaplan–Meier survival function: requesting mean and median survival times and a survival plot

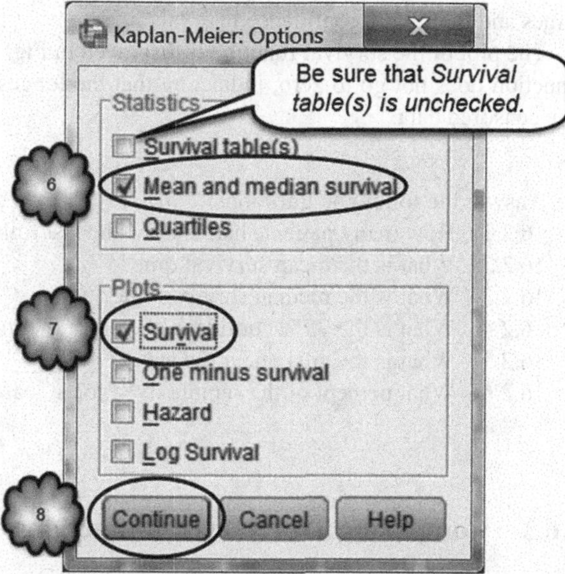

generate a lengthy survival table, uncheck *Survival table(s)* in the *Statistics* area. When you have finished, the dialog box should look similar to the one in Fig. 16.7. Now click **Continue** followed by **OK**.

The output will consist of two tables and a plot of the survival function. The first table is the *Case Processing Summary*, shown in Table 16.3. The first column reports the sample size. The second column displays the number of patients who died.

Table 16.3 Case processing summary for a Kaplan–Meier survival analysis

Case Processing Summary

Total N	N of Events	Censored	
		N	Percent
481	249	232	48.2%

Table 16.4 Mean and median survival times in days of 481 patients who had experienced at least one myocardial infarction

Means and Medians for Survival Time

Mean[a]				Median			
		95% Confidence Interval				95% Confidence Interval	
Estimate	Std. Error	Lower Bound	Upper Bound	Estimate	Std. Error	Lower Bound	Upper Bound
2916.981	125.151	2671.685	3162.278	2335.000	305.616	1735.993	2934.007

a. Estimation is limited to the largest survival time if it is censored.

The last two columns report the number and percentage of patients who were alive at the last follow-up observation.

The second table, shown in Table 16.4, reports the mean and median survival times and their 95 % confidence intervals.

The plot of the survival function is displayed in Fig. 16.8. Note that the survival function does not go to zero, indicating that the longest survival times were from the censored data.

Answer the following questions:

16.2.1 How many patients had died by the last follow-up observation?

16.2.2 What is the mean survival time?

16.2.3 What is the median survival time?

16.2.4 What is the 95 % confidence level for the median?

16.2.5 What is the area under the curve? __________ days.

16.2.6 What percent of the sample lived for at least 2335 days? __________%.

16.3 Comparing Two Survival Functions

In clinical research, the survival functions of two groups of patients are often compared. As an example, we will compare the survival times of patients whose myocardial infarctions (MIs) were their first (first MI group) to the survival times of patients with a history of MIs (recurrent MI group).

Select **Analyze > Survival > Kaplan–Meier** to open the dialog box shown in Fig. 16.9. Enter the group identifying the variable, **MI Order** [*MIORD*] (variable 7), in the *Factor* box. To determine whether the survival functions of the two groups

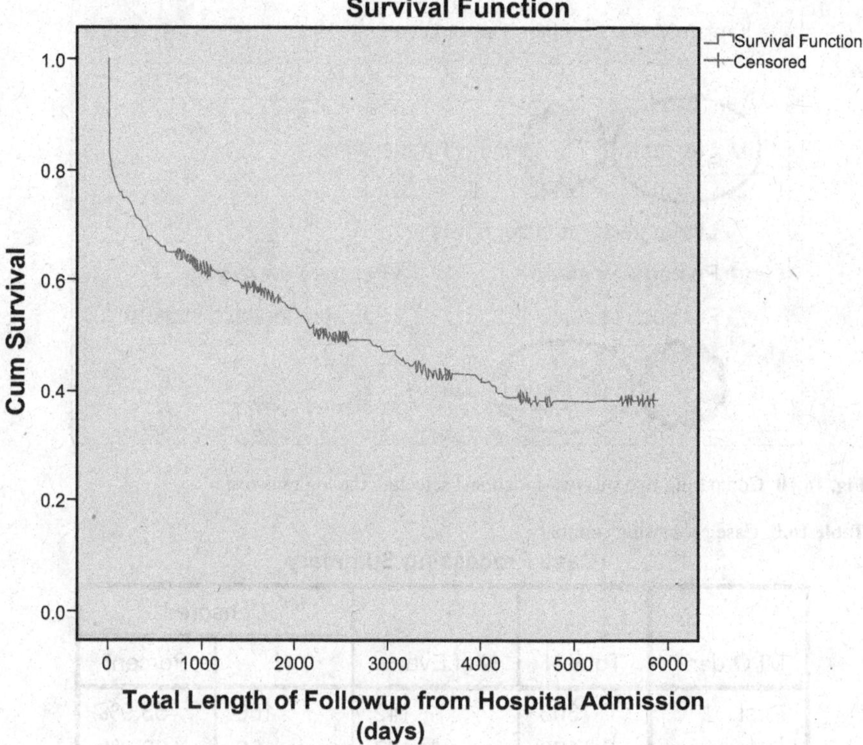

Fig. 16.8 Survival function of 481 Patients who had experienced at least one myocardial infarction

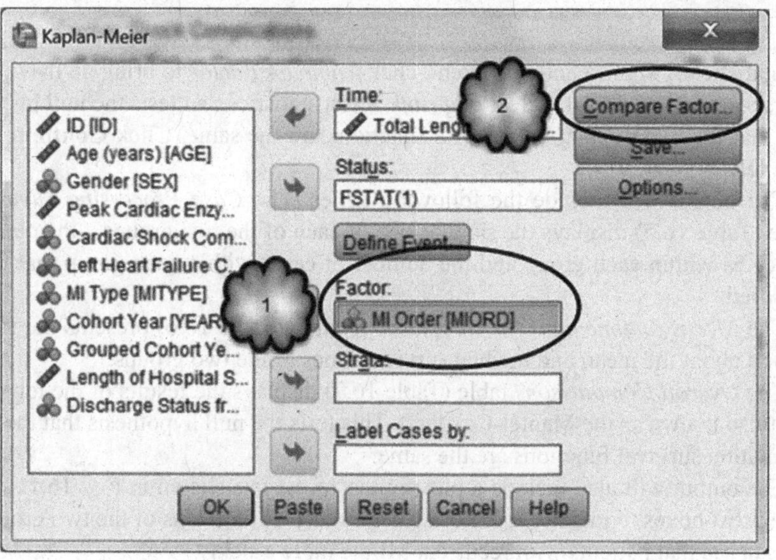

Fig. 16.9 Comparing two survival functions: assigning a group identifying variable or factor, and opening the Compare Factor dialog

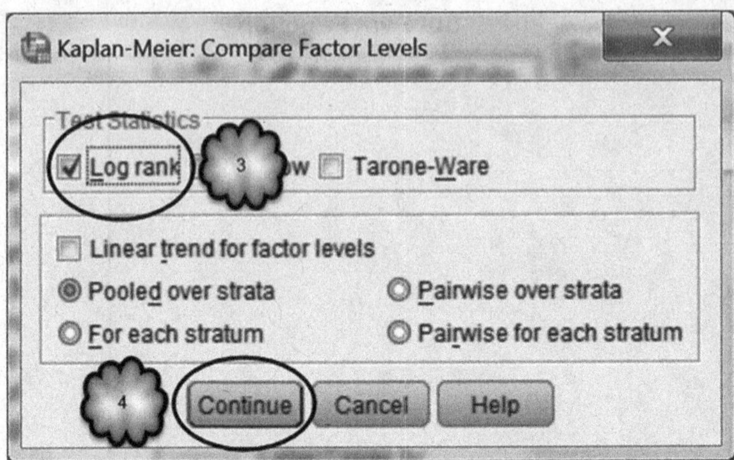

Fig. 16.10 Comparing two survival functions: selecting the log rank test

Table 16.5 Case processing summary

Case Processing Summary

MI Order	Total N	N of Events	Censored	
			N	Percent
First	308	142	166	53.9%
Recurrent	173	107	66	38.2%
Overall	481	249	232	48.2%

are statistically significantly different, click *Compare Factor* to bring up the dialog box shown in Fig. 16.10. Select *Log rank,* a test statistics that tests the null hypothesis that the two population survival functions are the same. Click **Continue** and then **OK**.

The output will include the following tables. The *Case Processing Summary* table (Table 16.5) displays the sample size of each of the two groups—the number of deaths within each group and the number of cases within each group that were censored.

The *Means and medians for survival time* table (Table 16.6) presents the information about the mean and median survival times of the two groups.

The *Overall Comparisons* table (Table 16.7) displays the results of the log rank test (also known as the Mantel-Cox test). This tests the null hypothesis that the two population survival functions are the same.

The output will also include a plot similar to the one shown in Fig. 16.11. (We added text boxes to identify more clearly the survival functions of the two groups.) We can see that patients with recurrent MI die more quickly.

Table 16.6 Mean and median survival times of first and recurrent MI patients

Means and Medians for Survival Time

	Mean[a]				Median			
			95% Confidence Interval				95% Confidence Interval	
MI Order	Estimate	Std. Error	Lower Bound	Upper Bound	Estimate	Std. Error	Lower Bound	Upper Bound
First	3215.980	156.319	2909.594	3522.366	3171.000	548.935	2095.088	4246.912
Recurrent	2388.059	202.967	1990.244	2785.874	879.000	503.804	.000	1866.456
Overall	2916.981	125.151	2671.685	3162.278	2335.000	305.616	1735.993	2934.007

a. Estimation is limited to the largest survival time if it is censored.

Table 16.7 Results of the log rank test

Overall Comparisons

	Chi-Square	df	Sig.
Log Rank (Mantel-Cox)	12.358	1	.000

Test of equality of survival distributions for the different levels of MI Order.

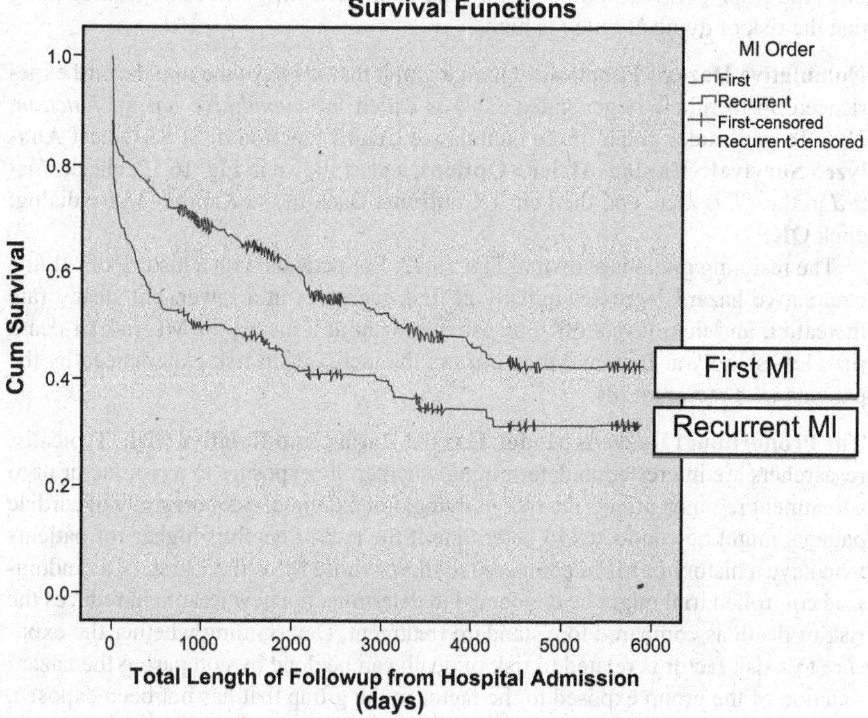

Fig. 16.11 Survival functions of First MI and Recurrent MI patients. (*MI* myocardial infarction)

16.3.1 What are the mean and median survival times for a patient with no history of myocardial infarction?
16.3.2 For a patient with recurrent MI?
16.3.3 Do the two survival functions significantly differ?

16.4 Hazard Functions, the Proportional Hazards Model, and Relative Risk

We now turn to the estimation of relative risk. This begins with the introduction of what is known as a *hazard function.*

Hazard Functions Generally speaking, the hazard function, *h(t),* is the instantaneous rate at which patients are dying at time *t.* The connection with the survival function goes as follows. If at time *t* no one has died, then at that point in time the graph of *S(t)* will be flat and *h(t)* will equal to 0. This means that there is no risk of dying at time *t.* On the other hand, if at time *t* many people die, then at that point in time, the graph of *S(t)* will drop rapidly and the value of *h(t)* will be large, indicating that the risk of dying at time *t* is high.

Cumulative Hazard Functions Often a graph that displays the total hazard experienced up to time *t* is generated. This is called the *cumulative hazard function, H(t).* To generate a graph of the cumulative hazard function in SPSS, select **Analyze>Survival>Kaplan–Meier>Options,** and as shown in Fig. 16.12, check *Hazard* in the *Plots* area, and then click **Continue**. Back in the *Kaplan–Meier* dialog, click **OK.**

The resulting graph is shown in Fig. 16.13. For patients with a history of MI, the cumulative hazard increases quickly at first, increases at a lower, but steady rate thereafter, and then levels off. For patients without a history of MI, risk of death rises less sharply at first, and then mirrors the increases in risk experienced by the patients with recurrent MI.

The Proportional Hazards Model, Hazard Ratios, and Relative Risk Typically, researchers are interested in determining whether the exposure to a risk factor or to a treatment regimen affects the risk of dying. For example, a cohort study of cardiac patients might be conducted to determine if the risk of death is higher for patients who have a history of MI as compared to those whose MI is their first, or a randomized controlled trial might be conducted to determine if a new treatment reduces the risk of death as compared to a standard treatment. Determining whether the exposure to a risk factor is related to risk of death can be done by comparing the hazard function of the group exposed to the factor to the group that has not been exposed. Similarly, assessing the efficacy of a new treatment can be done by comparing the hazard function of patients exposed to a new treatment to a control group that has received the standard treatment.

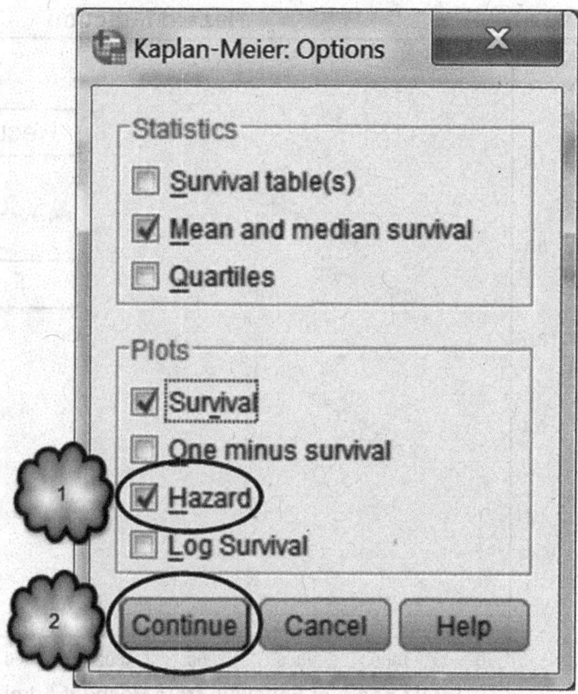

Fig. 16.12 Requesting a cumulative hazard function

The simplest model for comparing hazard functions is known as the *proportional hazards model.* If $h_1(t)$ is the hazard function of the nonexposed or control group, then this model assumes that $h_1(t)$ is proportional to $h_0(t)$ for all *t,* or

$$\frac{h_1(t)}{h_0(t)} = k, \tag{16.16}$$

for all *t.* In our example of cardiac patients, the exposed group would be those patients with a history of MI, and their hazard function would be $h_1(t)$. The non-exposed group would be those patients with no history of MI, and their hazard function would be $h_0(t)$. If we were to assume proportional hazards, then we would assume that the ratio of the hazard functions of the two groups of cardiac patients is the same over time.

The simplest proportional hazards model is one that only makes use of the fact that a patient is in either the exposed group or the control group. As applied to our example, the model looks like the following. Let $h_0(t)$ be the hazard function for patients with no history of MI. Let $x_i = 1$ if the *i*th patient has a history of MI and 0 if not. Then the proportional hazards model will be

$$h_i(t) = h_0(t)e^{\beta x_i}, \tag{16.17}$$

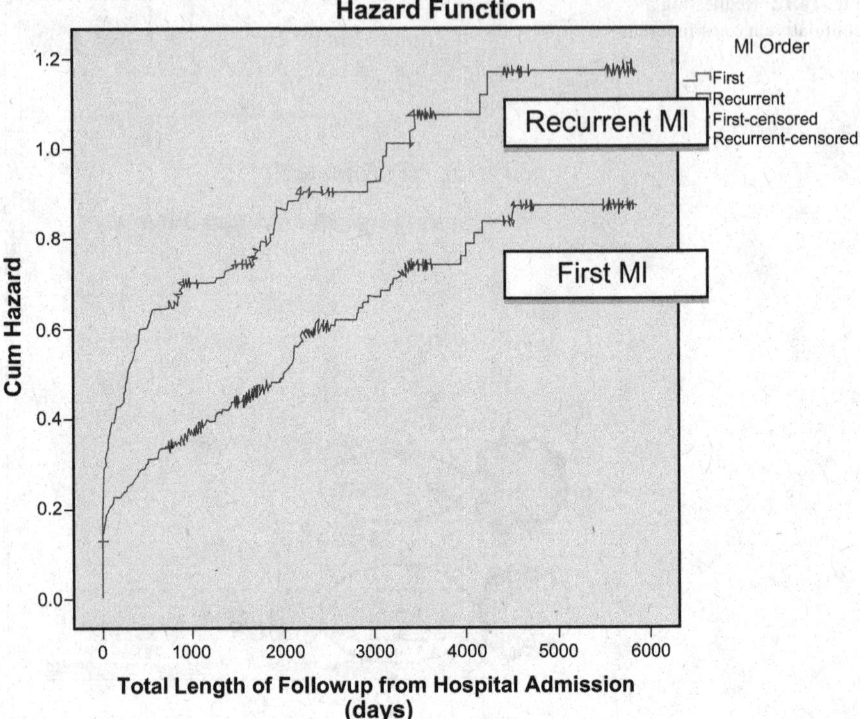

Fig. 16.13 Cumulative hazard functions of first and recurrent MI patients

where e is a constant approximately equal to 2.71828 and β is an unknown parameter that needs to be estimated. Let us take a closer look at this equation.

Note that if the ith patient has a history of MI, then the equation becomes

$$h_i(t) = h_0(t)e^{\beta}. \tag{16.18}$$

If we divide both sides of the equation by $h_0(t)$, then

$$\frac{h_i(t)}{h_0(t)} = e^{\beta}. \tag{16.19}$$

The quantity e^{β} is the ratio of the hazard associated with the patients with recurrent MI to the hazard associated with the patients with their first MI. This ratio is called the *hazard ratio*. A hazard ratio greater than 1 indicates that the exposure is associated with increased risk, while a hazard ratio less than 1 indicates that exposure is associated with decreased risk. In this situation, it turns out that the hazard ratio is also the relative risk of the exposed group compared to the control group.

This model was developed by David Cox in 1972, and it is commonly referred to as the *Cox proportional hazards model.* You may have recognized that *e* is the base of the natural logarithm and e^{β} is an antilog or exponent. According to the Cox model, we obtain the hazard ratio or relative risk by first estimating the value of β and then raising the base of the natural logarithm by this value. β is a population slope coefficient. The process of estimating it is commonly referred to as *Cox regression.*

16.5 Cox Regression with One Covariate

In this section, we will see how Cox regression is used to estimate the value of β by investigating the risk of death for cardiac patients who have a history of MI relative to the risk of death for cardiac patients who have experienced their first MI. In the next section, we will again estimate the relative risk, but after taking into account each patient's age.

Select **Analyze>Survival>Cox Regression** to bring up the dialog box shown in Fig. 16.14. Enter the survival time variable, **Total Length of Follow-up from Hospital Admission (days)**, in the *Time* box. Enter the censoring variable, **Status**

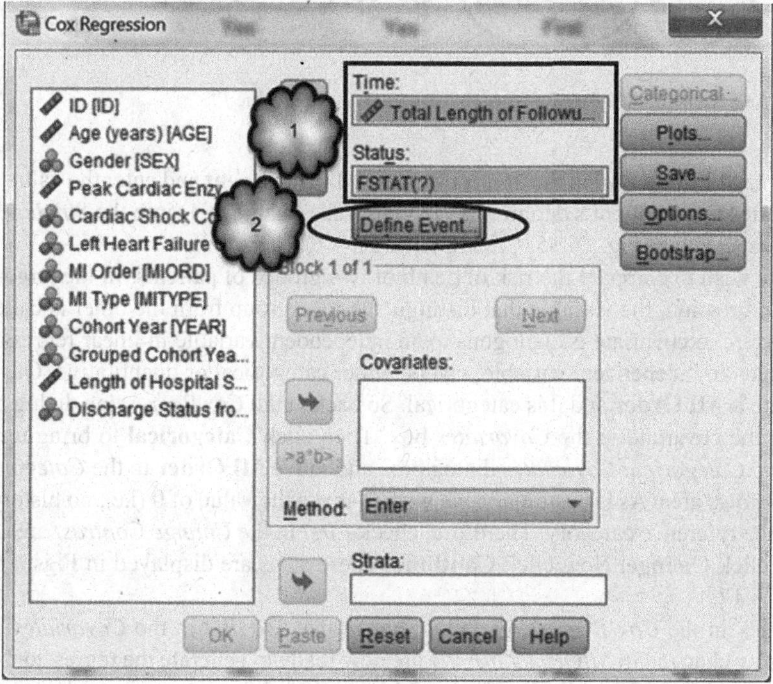

Fig. 16.14 Generating a Cox regression: assigning the time and status variables, and opening the Define Event for Status Variable dialog

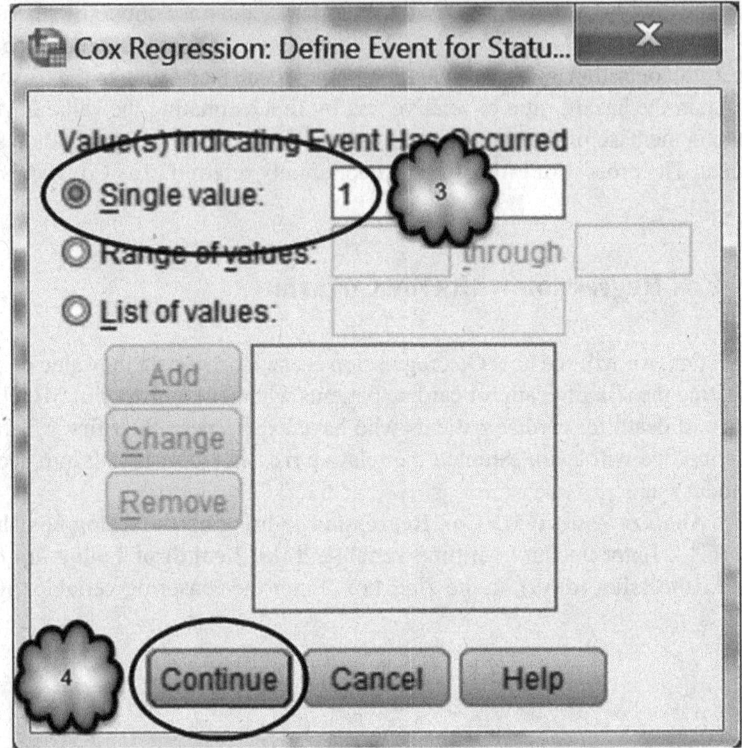

Fig. 16.15 Generating a Cox Regression: defining the event value

as of Last Follow-up, in the *Status* box. Click **Define Event** and enter the value that indicates that a patient's datum was not censored (a value of **1**) into the *Single value* box, as shown in Fig. 16.15. Click **Continue**.

We wish to compare the risk of death of two groups of patients. In the jargon of Cox regression, the variable that distinguishes one group from the other is called a *covariate*. A covariate is analogous to an independent variable in linear regression, and like an independent variable, can be either categorical or quantitative. Our covariate is **MI Order** and it is categorical. So back at the *Cox Regression* dialog box, enter the covariate in the *Covariates* box. Then click **Categorical** to bring up the *Define Categorical Covariates* dialog box, and move **MI Order** to the *Categorical Covariates* area. As is customary, we wish to make the value of 0 (i.e., no history of MI) the reference category. Therefore, check *First* in the *Change Contrast* area and then click **Change**. Now click **Continue**. These steps are displayed in Figs. 16.16 and 16.17.

Back in the *Cox Regression* dialog, notice that *MIORD* in the *Covariates* area has now changed to *MIORD(Cat)*. We are now ready to generate the regression. But first let us ask SPSS to display the confidence interval for the relative risk estimate. Click **Options** and select *CI for exp(B)*. The confidence level can be set to 90, 95,

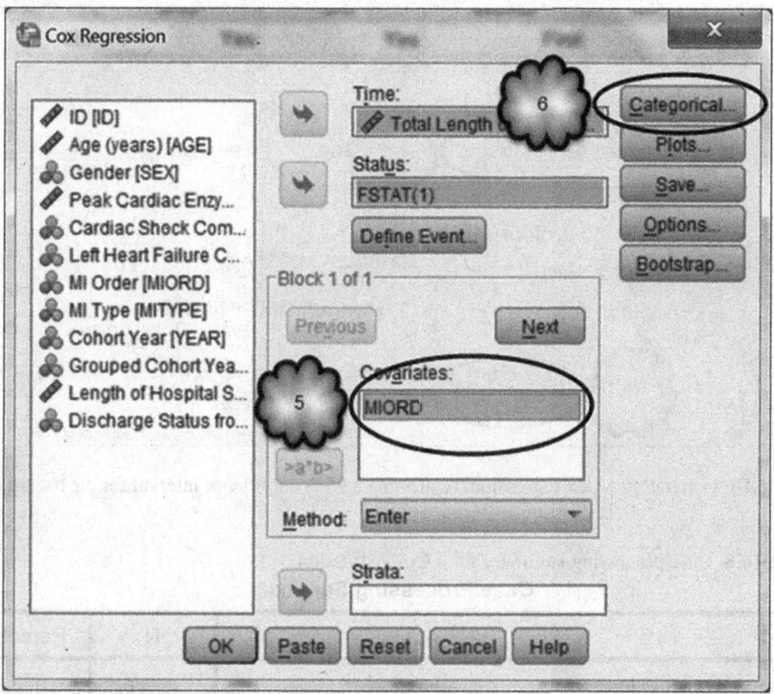

Fig. 16.16 Generating a Cox Regression: identifying the predictor variable and opening the Define Categorical Covariates dialog

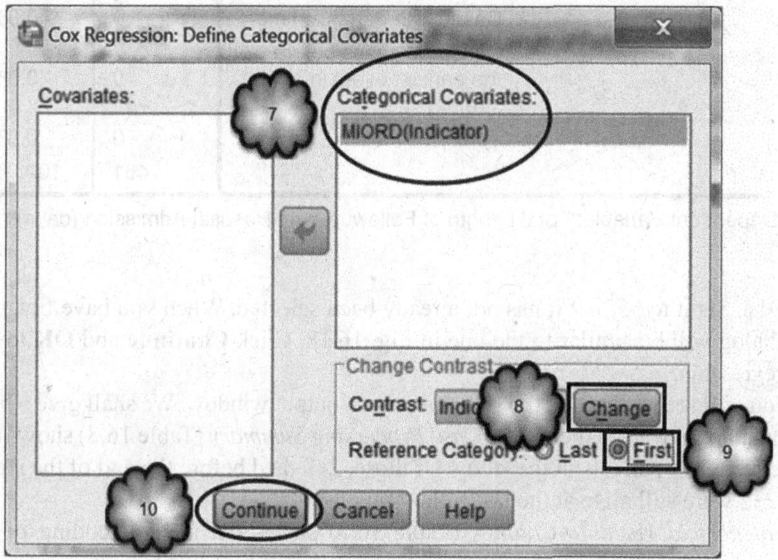

Fig. 16.17 Generating a Cox Regression: identifying the categorical variable and reference category

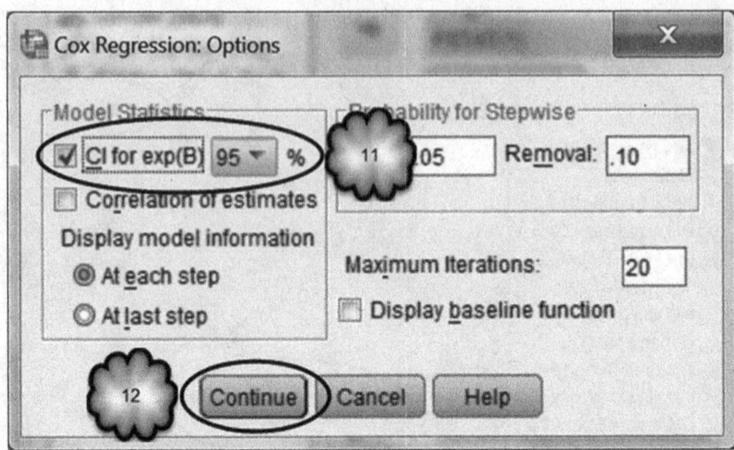

Fig. 16.18 Generating a Cox regression: requesting a 95 % confidence interval for the hazard ratio

Table 16.8 Case processing summary for a Cox regression

Case Processing Summary

		N	Percent
Cases available in analysis	Event[a]	249	51.8%
	Censored	232	48.2%
	Total	481	100.0%
Cases dropped	Cases with missing values	0	0.0%
	Cases with negative time	0	0.0%
	Censored cases before the earliest event in a stratum	0	0.0%
	Total	0	0.0%
Total		481	100.0%

a. Dependent Variable: Total Length of Followup from Hospital Admission (days)

or 99 %. Set it to 95 % if it has not already been selected. When you have finished, the dialog will be similar to the one in Fig. 16.18. Click **Continue** and **OK** to run the regression.

You will see results like the following in an output window. We shall give a brief explanation of what is there. The *Case Processing Summary* (Table 16.8) shows that there were 481 patients in the study. Of those, 249 died before the end of the study, and 232 were still alive at the last follow-up observation.

Categorical Variable Codings (Table 16.9) shows the internal coding of the group identifying variable.

Table 16.9 Categorical variable codings for a Cox regression in which the categorical variable is myocardial infarction order (MIORD)

Categorical Variable Codings[a]

		Frequency	(1)
MIORD[b]	0=First	308	0
	1=Recurrent	173	1

a. Category variable: MIORD (MI Order)
b. Indicator Parameter Coding

Table 16.10 Omnibus tests of model coefficients for a Cox regression at Block 0

Block 0: Beginning Block

Omnibus Tests of Model Coefficients

-2 Log Likelihood
2841.217

Table 16.11 Omnibus tests of model coefficients for a Cox regression at block 1

Block 1: Method = Enter

Omnibus Tests of Model Coefficients[a]

-2 Log Likelihood	Overall (score)			Change From Previous Step			Change From Previous Block		
	Chi-square	df	Sig.	Chi-square	df	Sig.	Chi-square	df	Sig.
2829.460	12.295	1	.000	11.756	1	.001	11.756	1	.001

a. Beginning Block Number 1. Method = Enter

Estimation is done by an iterative method known as maximum likelihood. This is the same method that was mentioned in the chapter on logistic regression. The *Omnibus Tests of Model Coefficients* table for the beginning block (Table 16.10) shows the starting value for the process.

Table 16.11 displays the *Omnibus Tests of Model Coefficients* at Block 1. This version of the table is analogous to the ANOVA table in regression. A small p-value for the *Overall (score)* portion of the table indicates that the population slope coefficient is not zero.

The *Variables in the Equation* table (Table 16.12) is analogous to the *Coefficients* table in the regression.

Table 16.12 Variables in the equation for a Cox regression

Variables in the Equation

	B	SE	Wald	df	Sig.	Exp(B)	95.0% CI for Exp(B)	
							Lower	Upper
MIORD	.446	.128	12.095	1	.001	1.562	1.215	2.008

Table 16.13 Mean of covariate predictor in a Cox regression

Covariate Means

	Mean
MIORD	.360

- *B* is the estimate of the parameter β, and is 0.446 with a standard error (*SE*) of 0.128.
- The *Wald* statistics is like that in logistic regression. It is the square of *B/SE*, and it has a chi-square distribution with 1 degree of freedom. The null hypothesis is that $\beta = 0$, and the alternative hypothesis is that $\beta \neq 0$.
- The *p*-value (*Sig.*) indicates that there is strong evidence that $\beta \neq 0$.
- *Exp(B)* = 1.562. This is the relative risk. This shows that a patient with a history of MI is about 1.6 times more likely to die than a patient with no history of MI.
- The 95% confidence interval for the relative risk ranges from 1.215 to 2.008.

Covariate Means (Table 16.13) gives the sample mean of the independent variable. This quantity is of little interest to us.

16.6 Cox Regression with Two Covariates

We now turn to a discussion of the inclusion of more than one covariate in the model. Specifically, we will see what happens in our running example if we include in the model the age of the patient on entry in the study. The patients' ages can be found in **Age (years)** [*AGE*] (variable 2). The new model will be

$$h_i(t) = h_0(t)e^{\beta_1 x_i + \beta_2 (age)}. \tag{16.20}$$

Return to the *Cox Regression* dialog box and move **Age (years)** to the *Covariates* box. The resulting dialog box should look like the one shown in Fig. 16.19. Click **OK** to run the regression.

The resulting output is pretty much the same as that shown in Sect. 16.5. The main difference is in the *Variables in the Equation* table. It is shown in Table 16.14.

- Note that the value of *B* for **MI Order** changed from 0.446 to 0.422. As was the case in multiple regression and logistic regression, each *B* coefficient is sensitive to the presence of the other covariates. Thus, once the contribution of **Age**

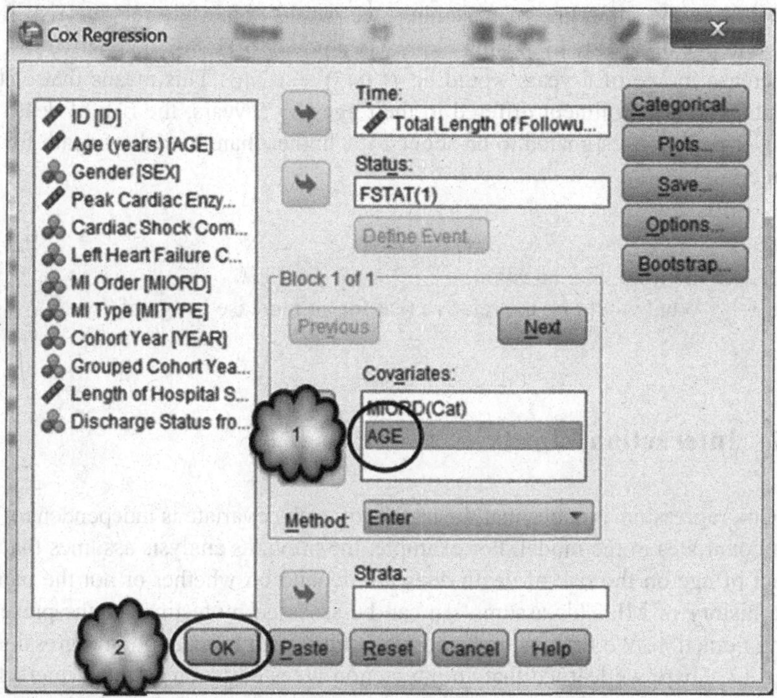

Fig. 16.19 Adding a second predictor to a Cox regression

Table 16.14 Variables in the equation for a Cox regression with two predictors

Variables in the Equation

	B	SE	Wald	df	Sig.	Exp(B)	95.0% CI for Exp(B)	
							Lower	Upper
MIORD	.422	.128	10.819	1	.001	1.525	1.186	1.961
AGE	.044	.005	67.445	1	.000	1.045	1.034	1.056

(years) is accounted for, the risk of dying for an MI patient with a history of MI relative to that of an MI patient with no such history decreases to $e^{0.422}$ or 1.525.

- The value of *B* for the patient's age is 0.044. The Wald test shows that this value is significantly different from 0. In addition, *Exp(B)* is 1.045, indicating that the relative risk of dying increases by a factor of 1.045 for every additional year in the age of the patient at the time of entry into the study. Note that *Exp(B)* is the estimate of e^{β} in the proportional hazards model. The value of *Exp(B)* can be used to obtain the relative risk for, say, a change in age of 2 years. This works as follows.

$$\frac{\text{Risk at year 2}}{\text{Risk at year 0}} = \frac{\text{Risk at year 2}}{\text{Risk at year 1}} \times \frac{\text{Risk at year 1}}{\text{Risk at year 0}} = e^{\beta}e^{\beta} = \left(e^{\beta}\right)^2. \quad (16.21)$$

If we follow the same line of reasoning, we would obtain the relative risk for a change in age of 5 years by raising *Exp(B)* to a power of 5. So, the relative risk for an increase in age of 5 years would be $(1.045)^5 = 1.246$. This means that of two patients who at enrollment differed in their ages by 5 years, the risk of death for the older patient is estimated to be about 25 % higher than the risk of death for the younger.

Answer the following question.
16.6.1 What would be the relative risk for an increase in age of 7 years?

16.7 Interaction Effects

The Cox regression assumes that the impact of each covariate is independent of the other covariates in the model. For example, the previous analysis assumes that the impact of age on the risk of death does not depend on whether or not the patient has a history of MI. This assumption can be assessed by testing for the presence of an interaction. We first encountered the notion of an interaction in regression in Chap. 14. There we learned that an interaction is tested by creating an interaction variable that is the product of the two variables of interest, entering the interaction variable into the regression model as a predictor, and determining if its slope coefficient is significantly different from zero. In this section, we will test for the presence of an interaction between age and history of MI.

Select **Transform>Compute Variable** to bring up the *Compute Variable* dialog box. Enter *Age_MIOrder* in the *Target Variable* box, and then click **Type & Label.** Give the new variable a label of **Age*MI Order** and click **Continue.** Back in the *Compute Variable* dialog, enter **Age*MI Order** in the *Numeric Expression* box. Click **OK** to create the interaction variable. These steps are shown in Figs. 16.20, 16.21 and 16.22.

Select **Analyze>Survival>Cox Regression**. Set up the regression as in Sect. 16.6 with the exception that **MI Order** is replaced by **Age*MI Order**. The resulting dialog box should look like the one shown in Fig. 16.23. Click **OK** to run the regression.

We will focus on the *Variables in the Equation* table, shown in Table 16.15.

From the *p*-values, we see that both **Age (years)** and **Age*MI Order** have the slope coefficients that are highly significantly different from zero. The interpretation of the slope coefficients goes as follows. The equation is

$$0.042 * Age + 0.006 * Age * MI\ Order. \tag{16.22}$$

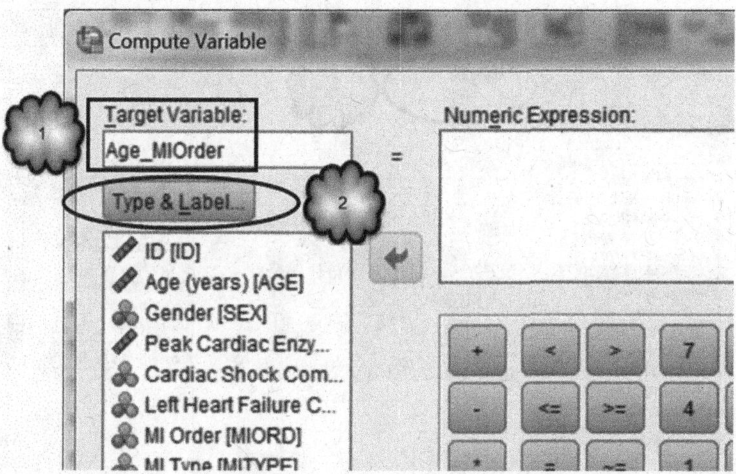

Fig. 16.20 Fragment of the Compute Variable dialog: naming the interaction variable

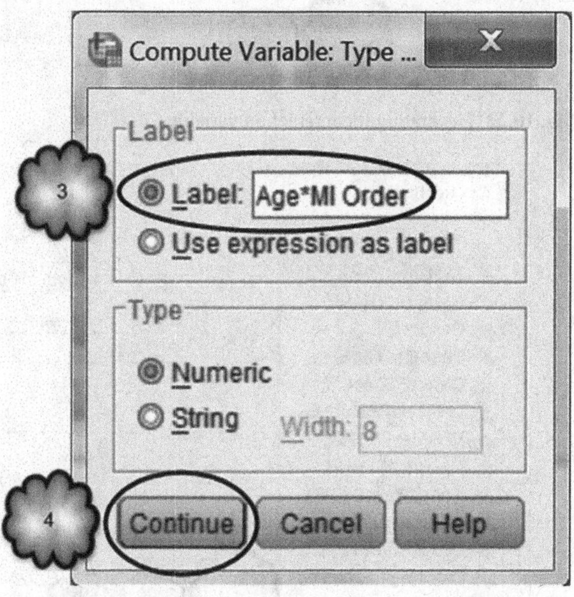

Fig. 16.21 Labeling the interaction variable

Recall that *MI Order* was coded 0 for a cardiac patient with no history of MI, and 1 for a cardiac patient having a history of MI. So for a patient with no history of MI, the equation becomes

$$0.042 * Age. \tag{16.23}$$

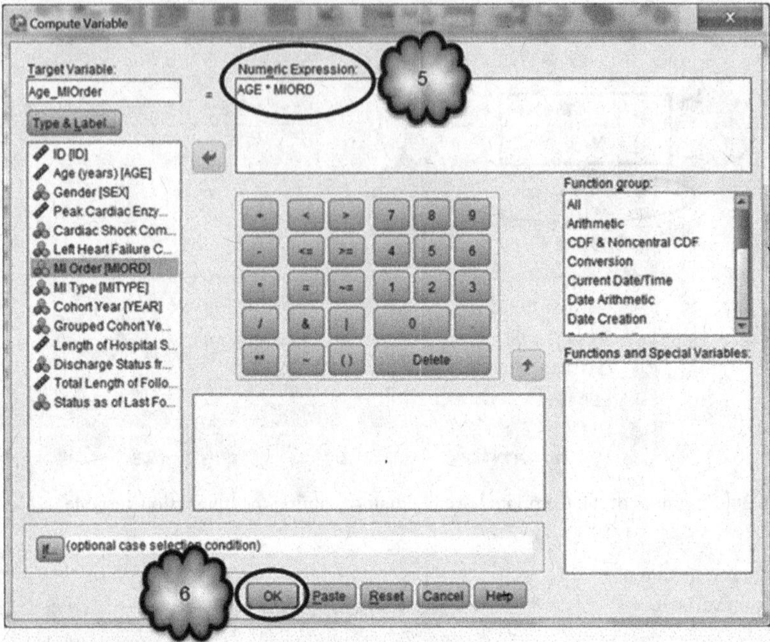

Fig. 16.22 Generating the interaction variable

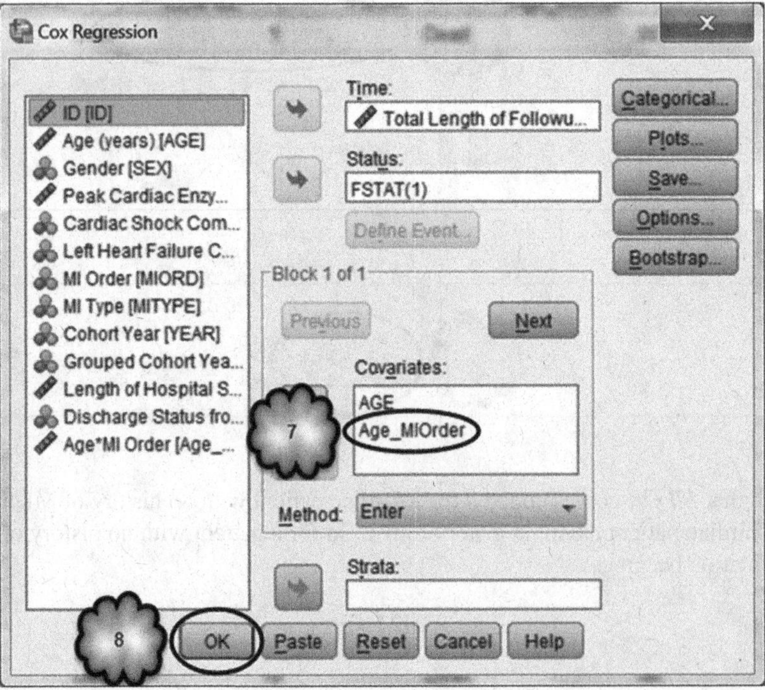

Fig. 16.23 Adding an interaction variable to a Cox regression

Table 16.15 Variables in the equation table for a Cox regression testing for the presence of an interaction

Variables in the Equation

	B	SE	Wald	df	Sig.	Exp(B)
AGE	.042	.005	60.342	1	.000	1.043
Age_MIOrder	.006	.002	11.070	1	.001	1.006

Since *Exp(B)* = 1.043, the relative risk is 1.043 for every additional year in the age of a patient with no history of MI.

For a patient with a history of MI, the equation becomes

$$0.042 * Age + 0.006 * Age = 0.048 * Age. \tag{16.24}$$

For a patient with a history MI, the value of *Exp(0.048)* is the product of the *Exp(B)* values given in the table, or (1.043)(1.006) = 1.049. This means that the relative risk for a patient with a history of MI is 1.049 for every additional year in age.

16.8 Exercise Questions

These exercise questions use the Framingham Heart Study data set, **Framingham.sav** [2]. The variables in the data set include:

- **Gender** [*sex*] (variable 1; 0 = Male, 1 = Female).
- **Serum Cholesterol** [*scl*] (variable 4).
- **Coronary Heart Disease** [*chdfate*] (variable 5; 1 = Yes, 0 = No). This is the censoring variable for the event, coronary heart disease.
- **Follow-up in Days** [*followup*] (variable 6). This is the time to event variable.
- **Body Mass Index** [*bmi*] (variable 8).

1. Open the data file and draw the Kaplan–Meier estimator survival function comparing the survival times (or in this context, the times to event) of males against females. There are over 4000 subjects in this study. So, avoid producing the survival table by unchecking *Survival table(s)* in the *Statistics* area of the *Options* dialog box. Include in the analysis a test of the null hypothesis that the two population survival (time to event) functions are equal.
   a. Describe the survival (time to event) function.
   b. Do men and women significantly differ in the distribution of their survival times? How do you know?
   c. What are the mean and median survival times for male patients?
2. Use Cox regression to determine the risk of a man developing coronary heart disease relative to the risk of a woman developing coronary heart disease. How

Table 16.16 Output for Question 4

Variables in the Equation

	B	SE	Wald	df	Sig.	Exp(B)
age	.066	.003	419.685	1	.000	1.069
Age_Gender	-.014	.001	164.960	1	.000	.986

much more likely is it for a man to develop coronary heart disease relative to a woman?

3. Use Cox regression with **Gender**, **Serum Cholesterol**, and **Body Mass Index** as predictors of follow-up time.
   a. Are the *B* coefficients for each of these covariates significantly different from zero?
   b. What is the risk of a male subject developing coronary heart disease relative to that of a female subject?
   c. What is the change in risk for a one unit increase in BMI?
   d. What is the change in risk for a one point increase in serum cholesterol?
   e. What is the change in risk for a 10-point increase in serum cholesterol?

4. Using the Framingham data, a researcher found an interaction between **Age (in years)** and **Gender**. The results of the analysis are included in Table 16.16.
   a. How did the researcher create the variable, Age_Gender?
   b. What is the relative risk for each additional year in the age of a male?
   c. What is the relative risk for each additional year in the age of a female?

Data Sets and References

1. WHAS.sav obtained from: Hosmer, D.W., Lemeshow, S.: Applied Survival Analysis. Wiley, New York (1999). (With the kind permission of John Wiley and Sons, and Professors David W. Hosmer and Stanley Lemeshow)
2. Framingham.sav obtained from: Dupont, W.D.: Statistical Modeling for Biomedical Researchers. 2nd ed. Cambridge University Press, New York (2009). (With the kind permission of Sean Coady, National Heart, Blood, and Lung Institute)*MI* myocardial infarction

Chapter 17
Regression Analysis of Count Data

Abstract This chapter reviews negative binomial regression. Often used to document incidence and mortality rates, this form of regression generates a rate ratio to assess the degree of relationship between a predictor variable and the frequency with which an event occurs over a given period of time. The chapter begins with a discussion of the case of a single predictor variable, and then moves on to a discussion of two or more predictors, and of testing for the presence of interactions. As an example of the difference between cumulative incidence and incidence rate, the concept of person-years, and the use of an offset variable, the chapter concludes with an application of negative binomial regression to count data collected over unequal follow-up times.

17.1 Overview

In Chap. 13 we considered predicting a quantitative response variable using simple linear regression with a single independent variable. In Chap. 14, we expanded those ideas to multiple regression where two or more independent variables were used to predict the value of a quantitative dependent variable. Chapter 15 considered logistic regression models where the dependent variable was a categorical variable having two categories, and Chap. 16 applied Cox regression to survival data. In this chapter, we will consider a kind of regression that is appropriate when the dependent variable consists of count data. The number of doctor-visits made by patients during a 2-week period or the number of new cases of coronary heart disease that occur in a year are examples of count data. Because the response variable is the frequency with which an outcome occurs per some unit of time, this kind of regression is useful for studying the *rate* at which an outcome occurs, such as the annual incidence of a given disease.

Several regression models can be used when the dependent variable is a count taken over a fixed period of time. The one we will consider in this chapter is known as *negative binomial regression*. This kind of regression is so named because it is based on the assumption that the count variable is distributed as a random variable known as a *negative binomial*. There is an important special case of negative binomial regression that is applicable in a situation when it is possible to safely assume

W. H. Holmes, W. C. Rinaman, *Statistical Literacy for Clinical Practitioners*,
DOI 10.1007/978-3-319-12550-3_17

that the mean and variance of the frequency of the outcome variable are equal. In such a case, the count variable can be assumed to be distributed as a *Poisson random variable*, and a technique known as *Poisson regression* can be used. The steps in conducting a Poisson regression and the manner in which its output are interpreted are very similar to those employed with negative binomial regression, so we will not discuss Poisson regression in this chapter.

Let the observed count for patient *i* be denoted by y_i. We assume that there are *k* predictors, $x_{1i}, x_{2i}, \ldots, x_{ki}$ that are observed for patient *i*. The negative binomial regression model fits the following equation:

$$\ln(y_i) = \beta_0 + \beta_1 x_{1i} + \beta_2 x_{2i} + \cdots + \beta_k x_{ki} \tag{17.1}$$

The $\ln(y_i)$ term is the natural logarithm of the count. We first encountered the use of the natural logarithm in regression in Chap. 15. There we learned that logistic regression is used to predict the logit, the natural logarithm of the odds of a binary event, such as the log of the odds that a patient has coronary heart disease. The reason why the predicted outcome in negative binary regression is the log of the actual count is similar to the reason that the logit is the predicted outcome in the logistic regression. Taking the log of the counts produces values which can be any real number. This eliminates the issue of how to handle predicted counts that are negative.

As in logistic regression, the parameters in a negative binomial regression are βs, that is, the population intercept coefficient and the population slope coefficients associated with each of the independent variables. The goal of negative binomial regression is to use sample data to obtain estimates of the βs. As is the case in logistic regression, an iterative procedure known as the *method of maximum likelihood* is used to obtain these estimates. However, in logistic regression, the exponents of predicted outcome variables and intercepts are odds, and the exponents of slope coefficients are odds ratios. In negative binomial regression, the exponents of predicted outcome variables and intercepts are *rates*, and the exponents of slope coefficients are *rate ratios*.

17.2 Negative Binomial Regression with One Predictor

In this section, we will conduct a negative binomial regression to determine if the rate at which Australian patients visit their doctors is related to the patients' general health. The data come from a study of 5190 adult Australians on whom information about several health-related factors was collected, including the number of times they each had visited a doctor in a 2-week period.

Calculating a Rate Before we conduct the regression, it might be helpful to first take a closer look at what a rate is. In medical research, a rate usually refers to the number of times an outcome of some kind occurs over a given unit of time. In our example, the outcome is the number of visits to the doctor and the unit of time is

Table 17.1 Frequency distribution of doctor visits

Number of consultations with a doctor or specialist in the past 2 weeks

		Frequency	Percent	Valid Percent	Cumulative Percent
Valid	0	4141	79.8	79.8	79.8
	1	782	15.1	15.1	94.9
	2	174	3.4	3.4	98.2
	3	30	.6	.6	98.8
	4	24	.5	.5	99.2
	5	9	.2	.2	99.4
	6	12	.2	.2	99.7
	7	12	.2	.2	99.9
	8	5	.1	.1	100.0
	9	1	.0	.0	100.0
	Total	5190	100.0	100.0	

2 weeks (or as Australians might put it—a fortnight). The rate can be expressed in terms of a single patient (e.g., the number of visits per patient per fortnight) or, if the rate is small, in terms of some multiple of patients (e.g., the number of doctor-visits per 1000 patients per fortnight). If the outcome in question is a disease, the rate is called the *incidence rate.* If the event is death, the rate is called the *mortality rate.*

Table 17.1 is a frequency distribution of the number of doctor visits made by our sample of 5190 Australians over a fortnight. We can see from the frequency distribution that during the 2-week interval, most of the samples did not visit their doctors at all. But we can also see that 782 patients each visited their doctors once. Another 174 individuals saw their doctors twice, resulting in a total of 348 visits. Thirty patients each saw their doctors three times, for a total of 90 visits, 24 patients made a total of 96 visits, nine a total of 45 visits, and so on. If we were to count up the total number of visits made by the entire sample, we would see that over a fortnight the 5190 patients as a group made a total of 1566 visits. If we divide the total number of visits by the total number of patients, we get a rate of 0.3017 visits per patient (1566 visits/5190 patients = 0.3017 visits/patient) per fortnight. If we multiply the numerator and denominator of our rate by 1000, we get a 2-week rate of 301.7 visits per 1000 patients. This latter rate means that we can expect that in every fortnight, a 1000 adult Australians will make about 300 doctor-visits.

Conducting a Negative Binomial Regression You may have noticed from our calculation of the rate of doctor visits that a rate is the average number of times an outcome occurs per person over a single unit of time. In our example, the rate of 0.3017 is the average number of visits made per patient over a fortnight. As with all averages, a rate summarizes what is true of a group of patients as a whole, but does not necessarily equal the rate of any given patient within that group. For example, our frequency analysis makes clear that our rate of 0.3017 visits per person overestimates the frequency of visits for those 4141 patients who made zero visits and underestimates it for the remainder of the patients. Our next step then is to conduct a negative binomial regression to uncover those factors that explain or account for the variation we observed across patients in their frequency of visits. Possible explanatory factors might be the general health of the patient, the patient's sex and age, the number of illnesses the patient had experienced during the 2-week period, and so on.

The file, **Doctor Visits.sav** [1], contains the number of doctor visits made in a fortnight by our sample of 5190 Australian patients. The number of doctor visits is in the variable, **Number of consultations with a doctor or specialist in the past 2 weeks** [*doctorco*] (variable 13). This will be the count response. The file also contains a number of possible predictors. We will begin by using the patient scores on a general health questionnaire to predict their number of doctor visits. The questionnaire scores are in the variable, **General health questionnaire score** [*hscore*] (variable 10). This will be the predictor. In the data set, this score varies from 0 to 12. The higher the score, the *poorer* was the patient's general health.

Open the data file and select **Analyze > Generalized Linear Models > Generalized Linear Models**. Select the *Type of Model* tab if it is not selected to open the dialog box shown in Fig. 17.1. Check *Negative binomial with log link.* (Note that if we wished to conduct a Poisson regression, we would choose *Poisson log linear* instead. The remaining steps for setting up the regression are the same for both negative binomial and Poisson.)

Select the *Response* tab to open the dialog box shown in Fig. 17.2. Enter **Number of consultations with a doctor or specialist in the past 2 weeks** in the *Dependent Variable* box.

Click the *Predictors* tab to open the dialog box shown in Fig. 17.3. The categorical predictors are called *Factors* in the dialog box, and quantitative predictors are called *Covariates*. Health questionnaire scores are quantitative, so enter **General health questionnaire score** in the *Covariates* box.

Click the *Model* tab to open the dialog box shown in Fig. 17.4. Select ***General health questionnaire score*** in the *Factors and Covariates* boxes and place it in the *Model* box. Make sure that *Main effects* is selected for the *Type* button in the *Build Term(s)* area.

We want the output to include the exponents of the intercept and slope coefficients, so click the *Statistics* tab to open the dialog box shown in Fig. 17.5, and check *Include exponential parameter estimates* in the *Print* area.

If you wish to have SPSS generate the predicted number of doctor visits for each patient, click the *Save* tab to bring up the dialog box shown in Fig. 17.6. Check *Predicted value of mean of response.* This will generate a new variable called **Predicted Value of Mean of Response** [*MeanPredicted*] that will store for each patient his or her predicted number of visits based on the regression model. By default, SPSS sets the number of decimal places for this variable to zero and displays its

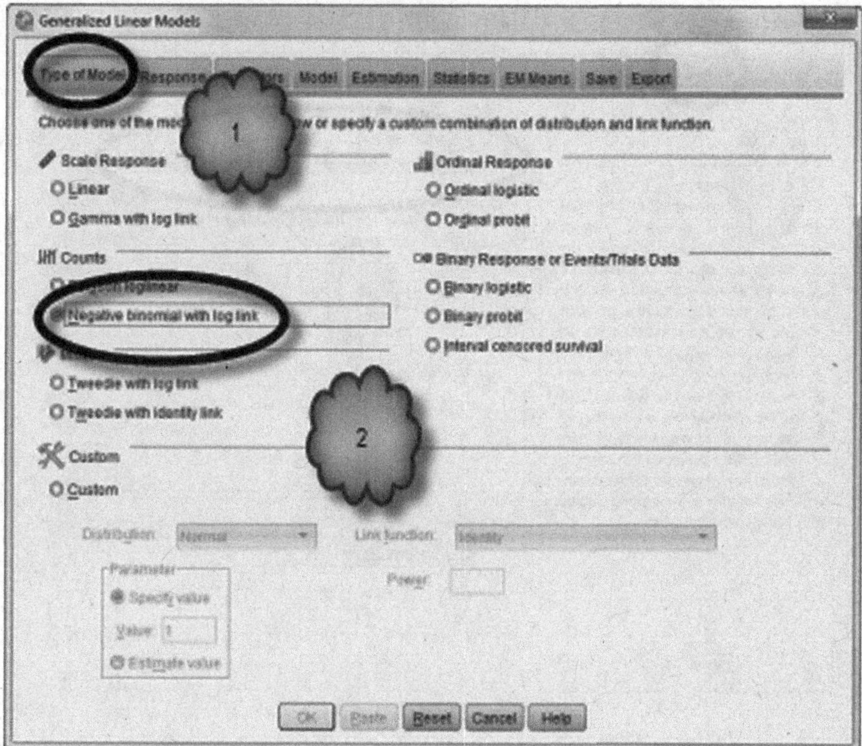

Fig. 17.1 Selecting negative binomial regression

values to the nearest whole number. To see more exact values, go to *Variable View* after the variable has been created and change its *Decimals* setting.

The values stored in **Predicted Value of Mean of Response** are the exponents of the original log values generated by the prediction equation. If you wish to see these log values, check in the *Save* tab *Predicted value of linear predictor*. This will result in the creation of a new variable called **Predicted Value of Linear Predictor** [*XBPredicted*] whose values will be displayed to the third decimal place.

Click **OK** to run the regression. As was the case with logistic and Cox regressions, there are a number of items in the output. We shall go through them pointing out the ones that are relevant.

- The dependent variable entry in the *Model Information* table (Table 17.2) states that the response variable is the number of doctor visits in a 2-week period.
- The probability distribution entry in Table 17.2 shows that this is a negative binomial regression.
- The link function entry in the table shows that the link function is a natural logarithm.

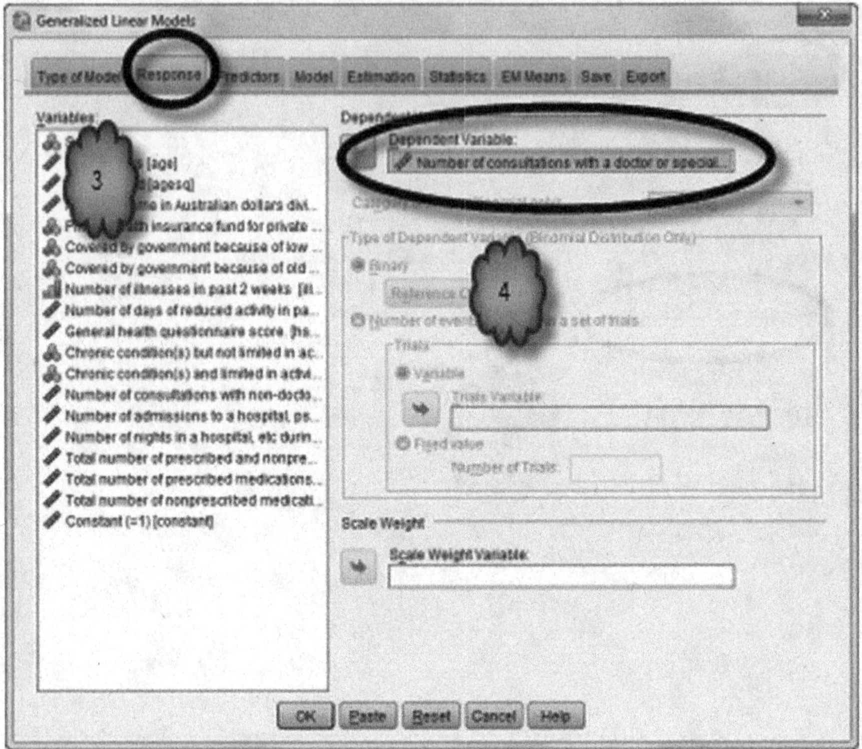

Fig. 17.2 Selecting the response variable

- The *Case Processing Summary* table shows that all of the 5190 cases were used in the analysis (Table 17.3).
- The *Continuous Variable Information* table (Table 17.4) gives the sample size, minimum observed value, maximum observed value, the mean, and the standard deviation for each quantitative variable that was used in the current model. As we shall see later, there is a separate table for categorical variables.
- Notice in Table 17.4 that the mean of the dependent variable is 0.30. This is the rate rounded off to the second decimal place of doctor visits per patient over a 2-week period.
- The *Goodness of Fit* table (Table 17.5) contains a number of statistics that are used to assess the degree to which the negative binomial regression correctly predicts the number of doctor visits for each patient. These can be considered to be very roughly similar to R^2 in linear regressions. They are used to compare different models when trying to find the best set of predictor variables. For these measures, with the exception of *Log Likelihood,* the smaller is the better.

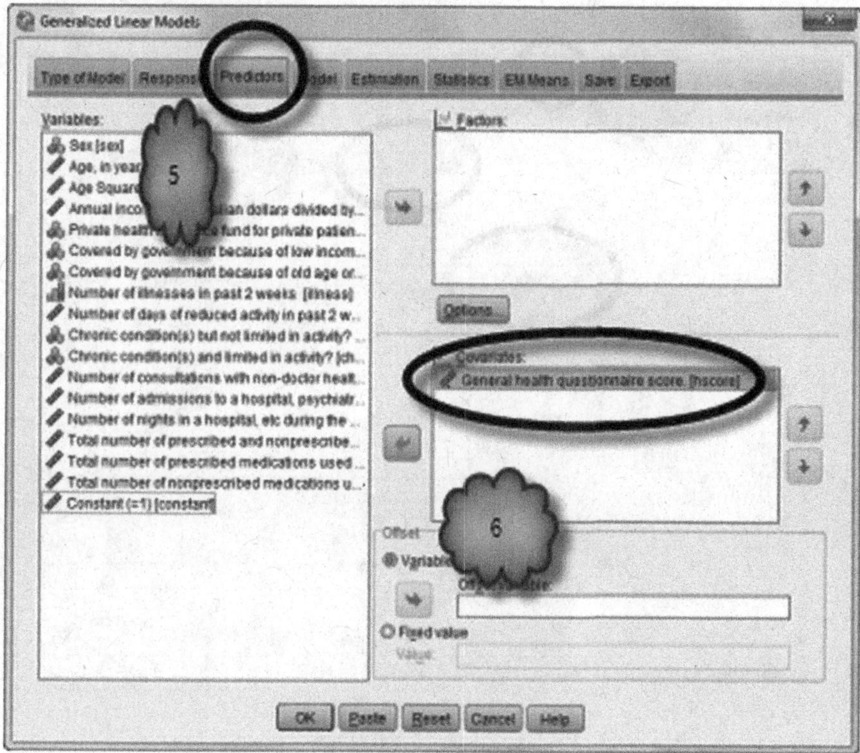

Fig. 17.3 Selecting the predictor variable

- The *Omnibus Test* table (Table 17.6) contains the results of testing the null hypothesis that the population slope coefficients for all of the predictor variables are 0 against the alternative hypothesis that at least one of them is not. This is analogous to the ANOVA *F*-test in the linear regression. This result shows that the population slope coefficient for **General health questionnaire score** is not 0.
- The *Tests of Model Effects* table (Table 17.7) reproduces the same information that appears in Table 17.8.
- The *Parameter Estimates* table (Table 17.8) is analogous to the *Coefficients* table in linear regression. The *(Intercept)* row shows that the population intercept, *B*, is estimated to be −1.479. The standard error is used to calculate the Wald test statistics and the confidence interval. The confidence interval shows that we are 95 % confident that the population intercept is between −1.549 and −1.409. The *Hypothesis Test* area gives the results of testing the null hypothesis that the population intercept is 0 against the alternative hypothesis that the population intercept is not 0. The *p*-value (*Sig.*) shows that we can safely reject the null hypothesis.
- Recall that the intercept (−1.479 in this case) is a natural logarithm. The *Exp(B)* entry on the *(Intercept)* row of Table 17.8 displays the exponent of the intercept.

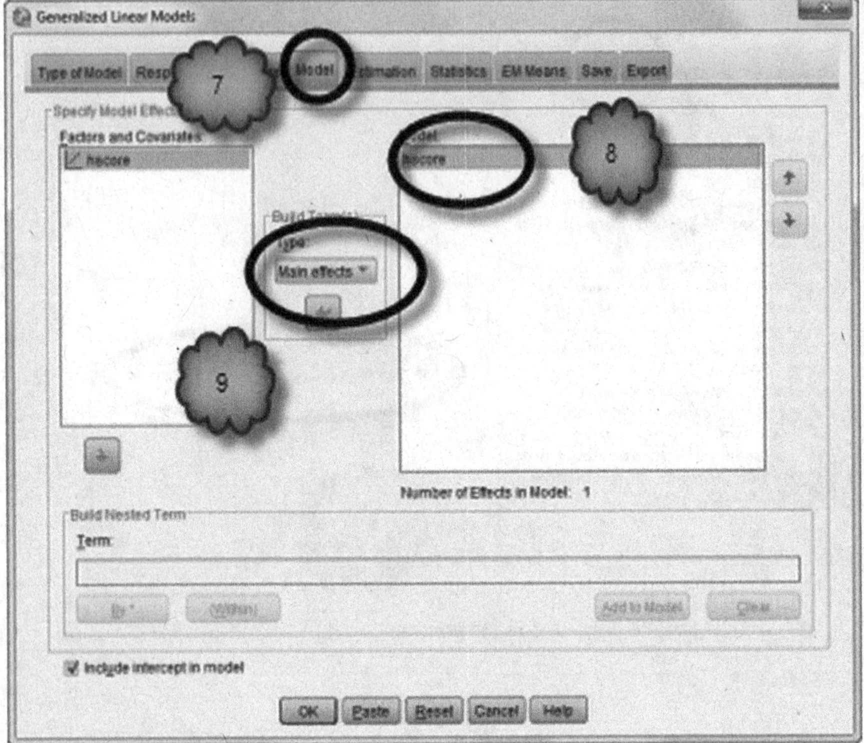

Fig. 17.4 Selecting the model

The exponent of the intercept is the rate of the outcome under investigation for patients whose value on the predictor variable is zero. In our example, the exponent of the intercept is 0.228 ($e^{-1.479} = 0.228$). Our regression model estimates that the population rate of doctor visits for patients with a health questionnaire score of 0 is 0.228 visits per patient per fortnight. The confidence interval for the exponent tells us that we are 95 % confident that the population rate for patients with a health score of 0 is between 0.212 and 0.244.

- The *hscore* row of Table 17.8 shows that the slope coefficient for the health questionnaire scores is estimated to be 0.166. We can be 95 % confident that the true slope is between 0.145 and 0.188. The Wald test of the null hypothesis that the slope coefficient is 0 against the alternative hypothesis that it is not 0 tells us that the null can be safely rejected.
- Recall that slope coefficients are natural logarithms. The *Exp(B)* entry on the *hscore* row displays the exponent of the *hscore* slope coefficient. The exponent of the slope coefficient is a rate ratio and indicates the extent to which the rate changes for every one unit increase in the predictor variable. A rate ratio equal to 1 indicates that the predictor variable is unrelated to the rate under investigation. In our example, the exponent is 1.181. Our regression model estimates that the

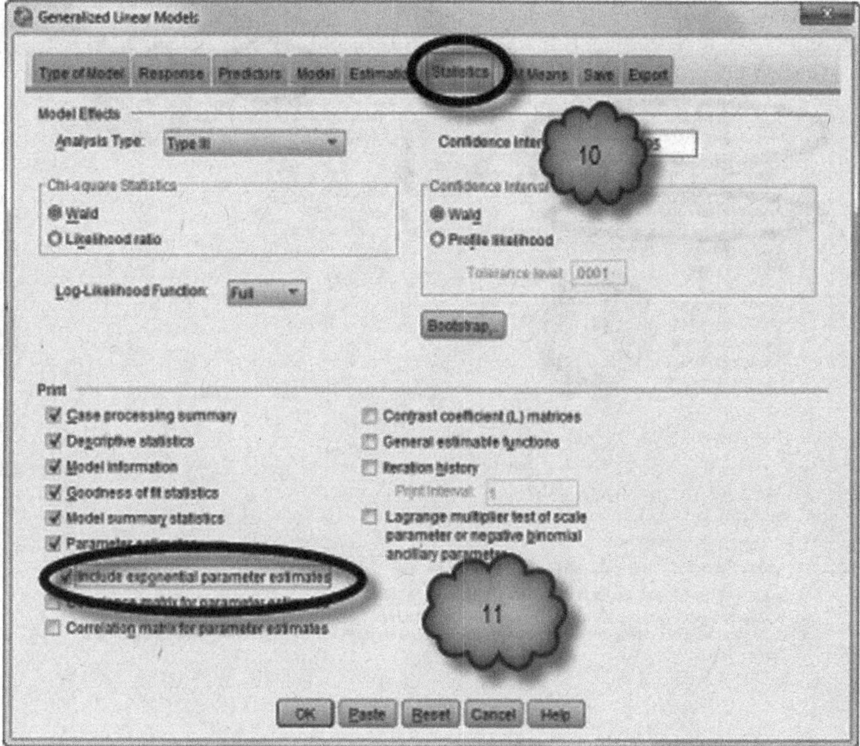

Fig. 17.5 Requesting exponential parameter estimates

rate of doctor visits increases by a ratio of 1.181 for every one unit increase in the health score. Put another way, the rate at which Australian patients visit their doctors increases by about 18 % for every one unit increase in their general health scores (remember, higher scores on the health questionnaire used in this study reflect poorer health). The confidence interval tells us that we are 95 % confident that the population rate ratio is between 1.156 and 1.207. Recall that the *p*-value in the (*Sig.*) column allows us to confidently reject the null hypothesis that the slope coefficient (0.166) is equal to zero. This also means that we can confidently reject the null hypothesis that the population rate ratio is equal to 1.

- The entry for *(Scale)* in Table 17.8 is of no interest.

Answer the following questions about the negative binomial regression we just conducted.

17.2.1 What are the missing values in the following prediction equation? Predicted log of the rate of doctor visits = __________ + __________ (*hscore*).

17.2.2 Using the prediction equation in Question 17.2.1, calculate by hand the log of the rate of doctor-visits for a patient with a health score of 10.

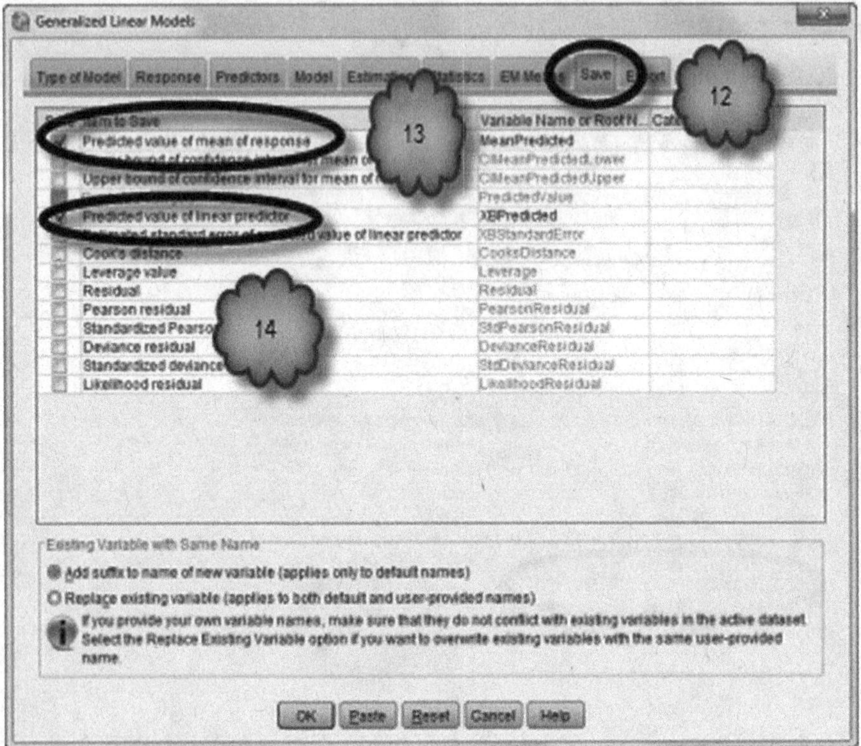

Fig. 17.6 Saving predictions

Table 17.2 Model information

Model Information

Dependent Variable	Number of consultations with a doctor or specialist in the past 2 weeks.
Probability Distribution	Negative binomial (1)
Link Function	Log

17.2.3 What is the predicted number of visits for a patient with a health score of 10?

17.2.4 The *p*-value in the *Parameter Estimates* table told us that we can reject the null hypothesis that the population rate ratio is equal to 1. The 95 % confidence interval for the rate ratio also tells us that we can reject the null hypothesis. How can we tell from the confidence interval that the null hypothesis can be rejected?

Table 17.3 Case processing summary

Case Processing Summary

	N	Percent
Included	5190	100.0%
Excluded	0	0.0%
Total	5190	100.0%

Table 17.4 Information about the predictor variable

Continuous Variable Information

		N	Minimum	Maximum	Mean	Std. Deviation
Dependent Variable	Number of consultations with a doctor or specialist in the past 2 weeks	5190	0	9	.30	.798
Covariate	General health questionnaire score	5190	0	12	1.22	2.124

Table 17.5 Goodness of fit test results

Goodness of Fit[a]

	Value	df	Value/df
Deviance	3776.544	5188	.728
Scaled Deviance	3776.544	5188	
Pearson Chi-Square	7675.801	5188	1.480
Scaled Pearson Chi-Square	7675.801	5188	
Log Likelihood[b]	-3546.042		
Akaike's Information Criterion (AIC)	7096.083		
Finite Sample Corrected AIC (AICC)	7096.085		
Bayesian Information Criterion (BIC)	7109.192		
Consistent AIC (CAIC)	7111.192		

Dependent Variable: Number of consultations with a doctor or specialist in the past 2 weeks.
Model: (Intercept), hscore
a. Information criteria are in smaller-is-better form.
b. The full log likelihood function is displayed and used in computing information criteria.

Table 17.6 Test of the overall model

Omnibus Test[a]

Likelihood Ratio Chi-Square	df	Sig.
223.786	1	.000

Dependent Variable: Number of consultations with a doctor or specialist in the past 2 weeks.
Model: (Intercept), hscore
a. Compares the fitted model against the intercept-only model.

Table 17.7 Tests of the slope and intercept coefficients

Tests of Model Effects

	Type III		
Source	Wald Chi-Square	df	Sig.
(Intercept)	1706.478	1	.000
hscore	227.325	1	.000

Dependent Variable: Number of consultations with a doctor or specialist in the past 2 weeks.
Model: (Intercept), hscore

Table 17.8 Parameter estimates

Parameter Estimates

			95% Wald Confidence Interval		Hypothesis Test				95% Wald Confidence Interval for Exp(B)	
Parameter	B	Std. Error	Lower	Upper	Wald Chi-Square	df	Sig.	Exp(B)	Lower	Upper
(Intercept)	-1.479	.0358	-1.549	-1.409	1706.478	1	.000	.228	.212	.244
hscore	.166	.0110	.145	.188	227.325	1	.000	1.181	1.156	1.207
(Scale)	1[a]									
(Negative binomial)	1[a]									

Dependent Variable: Number of consultations with a doctor or specialist in the past 2 weeks.
Model: (Intercept), hscore
a. Fixed at the displayed value.

17.3 Testing Two or More Predictors

As was the case with the other regression models we have considered, it is possible to use multiple predictors. The predictors may be either categorical or quantitative. Recall that we said earlier that categorical predictors in this setting are called *factors* and quantitative predictors are called *covariates*. As an example, we will add to

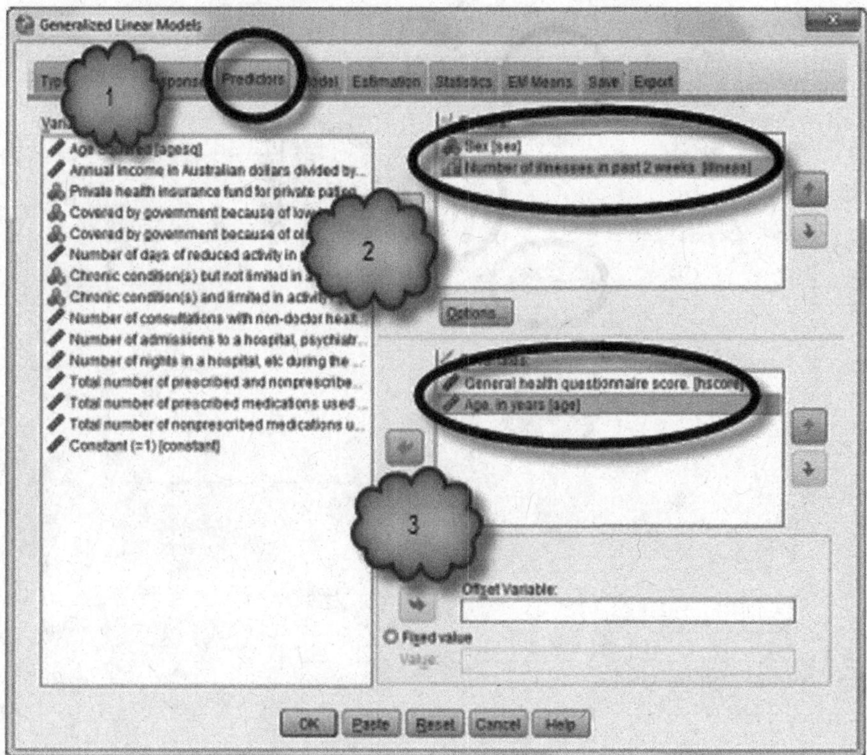

Fig. 17.7 Adding the new predictors

our regression model the patient's sex and age as well as the number of illnesses the patient had experienced during the 2-week period.

Select **Analyze>Generalized Linear Models>Generalized Linear Models**. Set up the dialog boxes for the *Type of Model* and *Response* tabs as was done in Sect. 7.2. Then click the *Predictors* tab to open the dialog box shown in Fig. 17.7. Place the two categorical variables **Sex** [*sex*] (variable 1; 0=Male; 1=Female) and **Number of illnesses in past 2 weeks** [*illness*] (variable 8, 0=0, 1=1…5=5 or more) in the *Factors* box. Place the two quantitative variables **General health questionnaire score** [*hscore*] and **Age in years** [*age*] (variable 2) in the *Covariates* box.

Click the *Model* tab to open the dialog box shown in Fig. 17.8, Place all of the variables from the *Factors and Covariates* boxes into the *Model* box. Make sure that *Main Effects* is selected for the *Type* button in the *Build Term(s)* area.

Be sure that *Include exponential parameter estimates* has been checked in the *Statistics* tab. Now click **OK** to run the regression. The regression output is shown in Tables 17.9, 17.10, 17.11, 17.12, 17.13, 17.14, 17.15 and 17.16.

- Tables 17.9 and 17.10 are identical to the earlier example.
- The *Categorical Variable Information* shown in Table 17.11 lists each categorical variable used in the regression. For each one, it shows a frequency table for

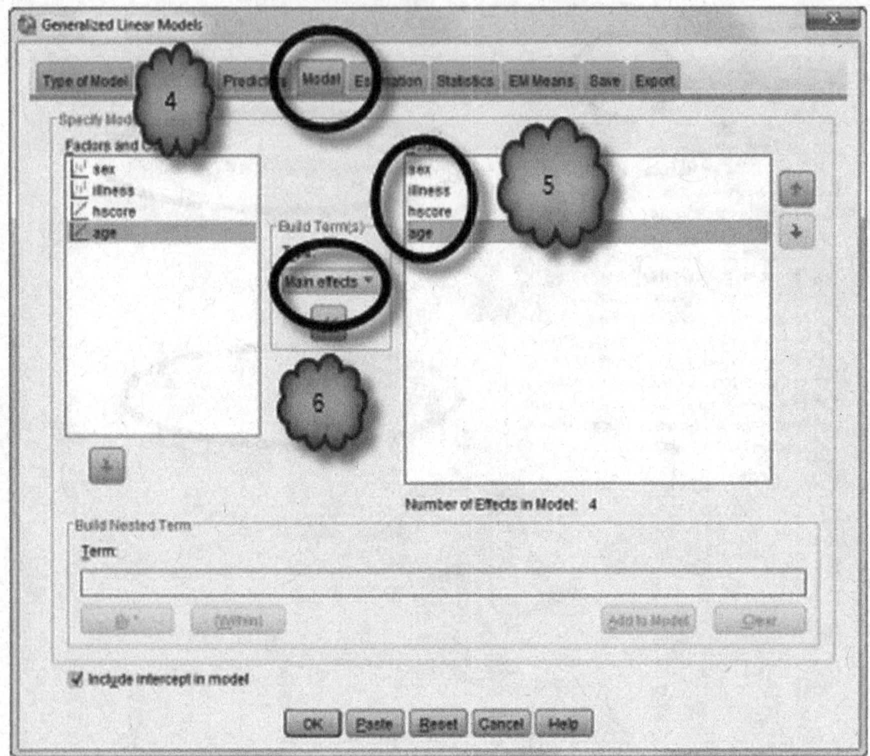

Fig. 17.8 Creating the new model

Table 17.9 Model information

Model Information

Dependent Variable	Number of consultations with a doctor or specialist in the past 2 weeks.
Probability Distribution	Negative binomial (1)
Link Function	Log

Table 17.10 Case processing summary

Case Processing Summary

	N	Percent
Included	5190	100.0%
Excluded	0	0.0%
Total	5190	100.0%

Table 17.11 Information on the categorical predictors

Categorical Variable Information

			N	Percent
Factor	Sex	Male	2488	47.9%
		Female	2702	52.1%
		Total	5190	100.0%
	Number of illnesses in past 2 weeks	0	1554	29.9%
		1	1638	31.6%
		2	946	18.2%
		3	542	10.4%
		4	274	5.3%
		5 or more	236	4.5%
		Total	5190	100.0%

Table 17.12 Information on the quantitative predictors

Continuous Variable Information

		N	Minimum	Maximum	Mean	Std. Deviation
Dependent Variable	Number of consultations with a doctor or specialist in the past 2 weeks	5190	0	9	.30	.798
Covariate	General health questionnaire score	5190	0	12	1.22	2.124
	Age, in years	5190	19	72	40.64	20.478

each of the possible categories. For example, it shows that 47.9 % of the patients were male and 52.1 % were female.

- As in the first example, the *continuous variable information* table shown in Table 17.12 gives the sample size, minimum, maximum, mean, and standard deviation for each quantitative variable used in the regression.
- The *Goodness of Fit* table shown in Table 17.13 gives the same goodness of fit measures as in the first example. Compare the values with those there. Notice that, with the exception of *Log Likelihood,* the values here are smaller than the earlier ones. This shows that using multiple predictors does a better job of predicting the log of the counts than just using **General health questionnaire score**.
- Again, the *Omnibus Test* table shown in Table 17.14 gives the results of testing that the slope coefficients for all of the predictors are simultaneously 0 against the alternative hypothesis that at least one is not 0. As before, we can safely conclude that at least one predictor has a non-zero population slope coefficient.
- As before, the *Tests of Model Effects* table shown in Table 17.15 gives results that are duplicated in the next table.

Table 17.13 Goodness of fit test results

Goodness of Fit[a]

	Value	df	Value/df
Deviance	3383.332	5181	.653
Scaled Deviance	3383.332	5181	
Pearson Chi-Square	6810.524	5181	1.315
Scaled Pearson Chi-Square	6810.524	5181	
Log Likelihood[b]	-3349.435		
Akaike's Information Criterion (AIC)	6716.871		
Finite Sample Corrected AIC (AICC)	6716.905		
Bayesian Information Criterion (BIC)	6775.861		
Consistent AIC (CAIC)	6784.861		

Dependent Variable: Number of consultations with a doctor or specialist in the past 2 weeks.
Model: (Intercept), sex, illness, hscore, age
a. Information criteria are in smaller-is-better form.
b. The full log likelihood function is displayed and used in computing information criteria.

Table 17.14 Overall model test

Omnibus Test[a]

Likelihood Ratio Chi-Square	df	Sig.
616.998	8	.000

Dependent Variable: Number of consultations with a doctor or specialist in the past 2 weeks.
Model: (Intercept), sex, illness, hscore, age
a. Compares the fitted model against the intercept-only model.

- Again, Table 17.16 is analogous to the *Coefficients* table in a linear regression. For each predictor and the intercept, it gives the estimated β coefficient, its standard error, a 95 % confidence interval for the actual value, the results of a test of the null hypothesis that the β coefficient is 0 against the alternative hypothesis that it is not 0, and the exponent and its 95 % confidence interval. We shall discuss the results for **Sex, Number of illnesses in past 2 weeks,** and **General health questionnaire score**.

Table 17.15 Test of individual predictors

Tests of Model Effects

Source	Type III		
	Wald Chi-Square	df	Sig.
(Intercept)	440.261	1	.000
sex	8.849	1	.003
illness	213.648	5	.000
hscore	77.330	1	.000
age	46.083	1	.000

Dependent Variable: Number of consultations with a doctor or specialist in the past 2 weeks.
Model: (Intercept), sex, illness, hscore, age

Table 17.16 Results for individual predictors

Parameter Estimates

			95% Wald Confidence Interval		Hypothesis Test				95% Wald Confidence Interval for Exp(B)	
Parameter	B	Std. Error	Lower	Upper	Wald Chi-Square	df	Sig.	Exp(B)	Lower	Upper
(Intercept)	-1.126	.1457	-1.411	-.840	59.748	1	.000	.324	.244	.432
[sex=0]	-.189	.0636	-.314	-.065	8.849	1	.003	.828	.730	.937
[sex=1]	0[a]	.	.	.	.	.	.	1	.	.
[illness=0]	-1.790	.1440	-2.072	-1.508	154.445	1	.000	.167	.126	.221
[illness=1]	-.559	.1182	-.791	-.327	22.347	1	.000	.572	.454	.721
[illness=2]	-.346	.1202	-.581	-.110	8.260	1	.004	.708	.559	.896
[illness=3]	-.391	.1294	-.645	-.138	9.145	1	.002	.676	.525	.871
[illness=4]	-.170	.1425	-.449	.109	1.424	1	.233	.844	.638	1.115
[illness=5]	0[a]	.	.	.	.	.	.	1	.	.
hscore	.104	.0119	.081	.128	77.330	1	.000	1.110	1.085	1.136
age	.010	.0015	.007	.013	46.083	1	.000	1.010	1.007	1.013
(Scale)	1[b]									
(Negative binomial)	1[b]									

Dependent Variable: Number of consultations with a doctor or specialist in the past 2 weeks.
Model: (Intercept), sex, illness, hscore, age
a. Set to zero because this parameter is redundant.
b. Fixed at the displayed value.

- For **Sex**, there are two entries, one for a value of 0 (male) and one for a value of 1 (female). For a categorical variable with just two categories, the category with the higher numerical value is by default the reference group. Consequently, women are the reference group. The entry in the *B* column for sex=0 is −0.189, meaning that the population slope coefficient for males is estimated to be −0.189. That is, on an average, the log of the number of doctor visits for a male patient is -0.189 less than for a female patient, although the 95 % confidence interval tells us that we can be 95 % confident that the average difference between men and women in the population may be as large as −0.314 or as small as −0.065. The results of the Wald test shows that there is a p-value of 0.003, meaning that there is moderately strong evidence that the true slope coefficient for **Sex** is not 0. The exponent is the rate ratio for sex and is equal to 0.828, indicating that the number of visits made by men is about 0.83 of those made by women. We can be 95 % confident that the population rate ratio is between 0.730 and 0.937.

- For **Number of illnesses in past 2 weeks**, there are six categories. So, SPSS estimates a slope coefficient for each category, again with the highest numbered category being the reference group. The Wald tests indicate that the slope coefficients for 0 through 3 illnesses are not 0. However, we must accept the null hypothesis that the slope coefficient for 4 illnesses is zero. The exponents and their confidence intervals refer to the rate ratios. For example, the rate ratio for 0 illnesses is 0.167, indicating that the number of visits made in a 2-week period by patients who had no illnesses during those 2 weeks is about 17 % of the number of visits made by patients who had 5 or more illnesses, although we are 95 % confident that the true rate ratio could be as low as 0.126 or as high as 0.221. The rate ratios for patients with 0 to 3 illnesses are significantly different from 1, indicating that we can be confident that in the population of Australian adults, patients with 3 illnesses or less visit their doctors less often than patients with 5 or more illnesses. However, the rate ratio for patients with 4 illnesses is not significantly different from 1, so we cannot be confident that the Australian patients with 4 illnesses see their doctors less often than do the Australian patients with 5 or more illnesses.
- For **General health questionnaire score**, we see that the slope coefficient is estimated to be 0.104. The Wald test has a p-value less than 0.001, giving strong evidence that the population slope coefficient is not 0. Compare the B value for this variable with the first example (Table 17.8). They are not the same. As was the case in the other types of regression we have studied, the slope coefficients give the change in the response variable for a one unit increase in the predictor *in the presence of the other predictors.* Notice also that the two intercept coefficients are not the same.

Answer the following questions:
17.3.1 Is the slope coefficient for **Age** significantly different from 0?
17.3.2 What is the rate ratio for **Age**? Is it significantly different from 1?

Changing the Reference Category In the previous analysis, the category with the highest numerical value was by default the reference category for each categorical variable. If you wish the reference groups to be the categories with the lowest numerical values, click the *Predictors* tab to open the dialog shown in Fig. 17.3, and then click **Options** to open the *Generalized Linear Models: Options* dialog shown in Fig. 17.9. Select *Descending* in the *Category Order for Factors* area followed by **Continue**.

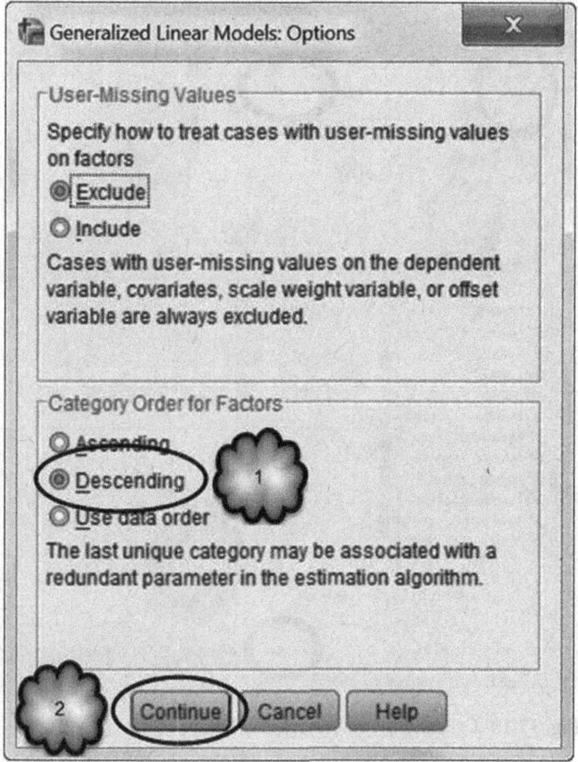

Fig. 17.9 Defining the reference category as the category with the lowest numerical value

17.4 Testing for an Interaction Effect

As with the other forms of regression we have studied, interaction effects among predictors can be tested in a negative binomial regression. In this section, we will investigate the possible interaction between a patient's age and gender. We proceed in a similar manner as was introduced in Chap. 14 by creating an interaction variable that is the product of age and gender, and then including the new variable in the regression model.

Select **Transform>Compute Variable** to open the dialog box shown in Fig. 17.10. Give the target variable a name of *age_sex* and a label of **Age*Sex**. In the numeric expression box enter *age*sex* and click **OK** to create the interaction variable.

Select **Analyze>Generalized Linear Models>Generalized Linear Models** and set up the dialog boxes for the *Type of Model* and *Response* tabs as before. Set up the dialog box in the *Predictors* tab so that **Age** and **Age*Sex** are in the *Covariates* box. In the dialog box for the *Model* tab, move both **Age** and **Age*Sex** to the *Model* box. In the *Build Term(s)* area, make sure that *Type* is set to *Main Effects*. Be sure that *Predicted value of mean of response* has been checked in the dialog box of the *Save* tab. Finally, click **OK** to run the regression.

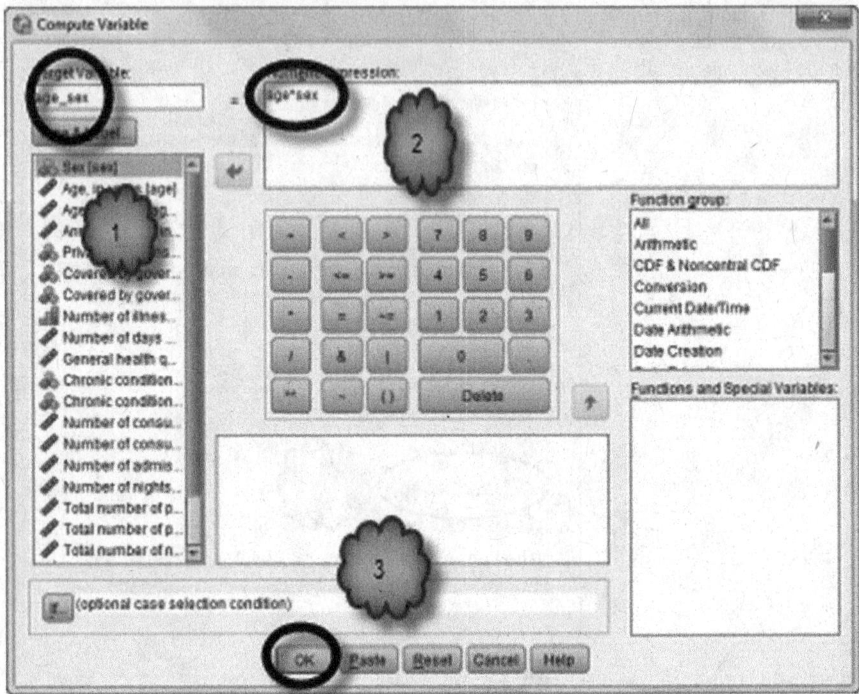

Fig. 17.10 Creating the interaction variable

Table 17.17 Information for the model with an interaction term

Parameter Estimates

Parameter	B	Std. Error	95% Wald Confidence Interval Lower	Upper	Hypothesis Test Wald Chi-Square	df	Sig.	Exp(B)	95% Wald Confidence Interval for Exp(B) Lower	Upper
(Intercept)	-1.846	.0714	-1.986	-1.706	669.103	1	.000	.158	.137	.182
age	.013	.0018	.009	.016	51.405	1	.000	1.013	1.009	1.017
age_sex	.003	.0013	.000	.005	5.032	1	.025	1.003	1.000	1.005
(Scale)	1[a]									
(Negative binomial)	1[a]									

Dependent Variable: Number of consultations with a doctor or specialist in the past 2 weeks
Model: (Intercept), age, age_sex
a. Fixed at the displayed value.

Examine the output for the regression. We will concentrate on the *Parameter Estimates* table shown in Table 17.17.

The Wald tests for the intercept and slope coefficient for **Age** show that there is very strong evidence that they are different from 0. The Wald test for the slope coefficient for the interaction term shows that there is some evidence that there is an interaction between **Age** and **Sex**. The resulting regression equation is

$$\begin{aligned} \ln(y_i) &= -1.846 + 0.013Age + 0.003AGE * SEX \\ &= -1.846 + (0.013 + 0.003SEX)AGE. \end{aligned} \tag{17.2}$$

Sex equals to 0 for a male patient and 1 for a female patient. Accordingly, for a male patient the regression equation is

$$\ln(y_i) = -1.846 + 0.013AGE. \tag{17.3}$$

The exponent of 0.013 is 1.013, as shown in the *Parameter Estimates* table (Table 17.17). This means that for every additional year in the age of a male patient, the average number of doctor visits in a 2-week period increases by a factor of 1.013, or by 1.3 %.

For a female patient the regression equation is

$$\ln(y_i) = -1.846 + 0.016AGE. \tag{17.4}$$

Using a scientific calculator, we find that the exponent of 0.016 is 1.016. This means that for every additional year in the age of a female patient, the average number of doctor visits in a 2-week period increases by a factor of 1.016, or by 1.6 %.

An alternative method for computing the exponent for female patients is to multiply the two rate ratios displayed in the *Parameter Estimates* table—1.013 (the rate ratio for age) times 1.003 (the rate ratio for the interaction) equals 1.6 %. The rate of increase in the number of doctor visits per fortnight for every 1 year increase in age is 0.3 % greater for female patients.

17.5 Regression with Unequal Follow-up Times

So far we have been analyzing the data from a study in which the interval of time across which counts were made was constant across all patients. For each patient, the time frame was always 2 weeks. However, in medical studies, the interval of time across which the counts are made often varies from one patient to the next. For example, in studies of disease incidence, patients who are free of the disease are followed from the time they are enrolled into the study until the time they develop the disease, withdraw from the study or the study is ended, whichever comes first. This results in unequal time intervals or *follow-up times* across patients. For example, the disease might appear in some patients 1 year following enrollment, but not in others until 5 years after enrollment. Among patients who remain disease-free, some might leave the study 6 months after enrollment while others might not leave until years later. If we want to know how often on an average the disease appears each year, we need to take into account each patient's follow-up time.

Calculating Rates When Follow-up Times Are Unequal When follow-up times are unequal, the number of times the event under investigation occurred across all patients who had enrolled in the study is divided by the total follow-up times of all of the patients. Often follow-up times are measured in terms of years, but any convenient unit of time can be used, such as days, weeks, months, and so on. If the time interval is expressed in terms of years, then the total follow-up time is expressed in terms of *person-years*, and the resulting rate is expressed in terms of the number of events that occurred per person-year. As one person-year of follow-up is equivalent to observing one person for 1 year, the resulting rate tells us the number of times the event occurs per person per year.

For example, the data set, **Framingham.sav** [2], contains observations from a cohort study of the heart health of 4699 men and women with varying cholesterol levels. Of these patients, 1473 or about 31 % developed coronary heart disease during follow-up. The remaining patients were believed to be disease-free either at the time the data set was created or at the time the patients were lost to follow-up. The 31 % figure is the *cumulative incidence* of the disease, the number of patients who at some point during follow-up developed the disease compared to the total number of enrolled patients. To calculate an incidence rate, that is, the number of incidents of heart disease that occur each year, we need to take into account each patient's follow-up time.

Each patient was followed on an average for roughly 22 years with individual follow-up times varying from 18 days (about 0.05 year) to 32 years. If we wish to calculate the annual incidence rate of heart disease, we would compare the number of patients who developed heart disease (1473) to the total number of *person-years* during which the entire sample of 4699 patients was observed. Adding up the number of years each patient was observed, we discover that those 4699 patients were followed for a total of about 103,710 person-years. We now divide the number of cases of heart disease (1473) by the number of person-years of follow-up (103,710) and find that the incidence rate is about 0.0142 per person-year. If we multiply the rate by 1000, the rate becomes 14.2 new cases of heart disease per 1000 person-years. One thousand person-years is equivalent to observing 1000 patients for 1 year, so the rate of 0.0142 per person-year is equivalent to a rate of 14.2 new cases of heart disease per 1000 patients per year. Based on these data, we would expect that on an average, about 14 out of every 1000 patients would develop heart disease over the course of a year.

Negative Binomial Regression with Unequal Follow-ups When follow-up times are unequal, a negative binomial regression must take into account the follow-up time of each patient. This is done by including in the regression analysis an *offset variable* that stores the natural logarithm of the follow-up times. Using the offset variable, the analysis generates the parameter estimates after controlling for the length of the follow-up time of each patient. For example, using an offset variable that stores the natural logarithm of the number of years each patient in the Framingham data set was followed, we could determine whether the annual rate of heart disease is related to sex and cholesterol level.

Open the data file, **Framingham.sav.** In this file, the follow-up times are stored in the variable, **Follow-up in Days** [*followup*] (variable 6). This variable will be the basis of our offset variable. However, in order that we can express our findings in terms of person-years, we will first transform each patient's days of follow-up into years of follow-up, and then take the natural log of the result to create the offset

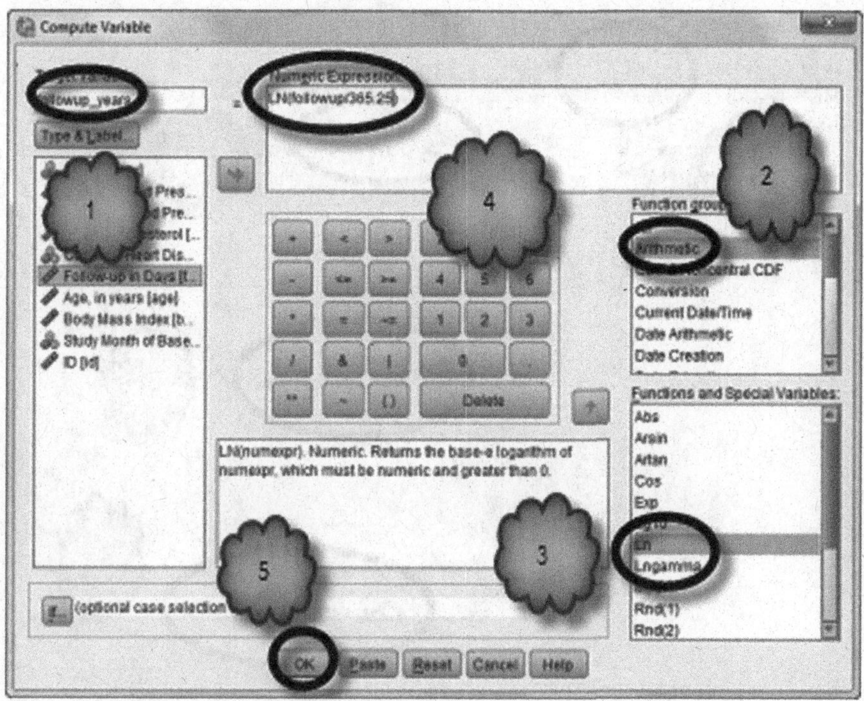

Fig. 17.11 Creating the offset variable

variable. In order to take leap years into account, we will define a year as 365.25 days. Open **Transform > Compute Variable,** and as shown in the dialog box of Fig. 17.11, name the target variable *followup_years*, and enter into the *Numeric Expression* window the following:

$$\ln(\mathit{followup}\,/\,365.25\,). \qquad (17.5)$$

If you wish, you can give the new variable a label, such as, **Follow-up Years**.

The natural logarithm function can be found in the *Arithmetic* group. When you have finished, click **OK.** This is shown in Fig. 17.11.

Now we are ready to set up the regression. Open the *Generalized Linear Models* dialog box and select *Negative binomial with log-link* in the dialog box of the *Type of Model* tab. In the dialog box of the *Response* tab, move **Coronary Heart Disease** [*chdfate*] (variable 5) to the *Dependent Variable* window. Click the *Predictors* tab, and as shown in the dialog box of Fig. 17.12, move **Gender** [*sex*] (variable 1; 0 = Male, 1 = Female) to the *Factors* window and **Serum Cholesterol** [*scl*] (variable 4) to the *Covariates* window. Now move the offset variable, *followup_years*, to the *Offset Variable* window.

In the dialog box of the *Model* tab, move the two predictors to the *Model* window, and in *Statistics,* check *Include exponential parameter estimates.* Click **OK**.

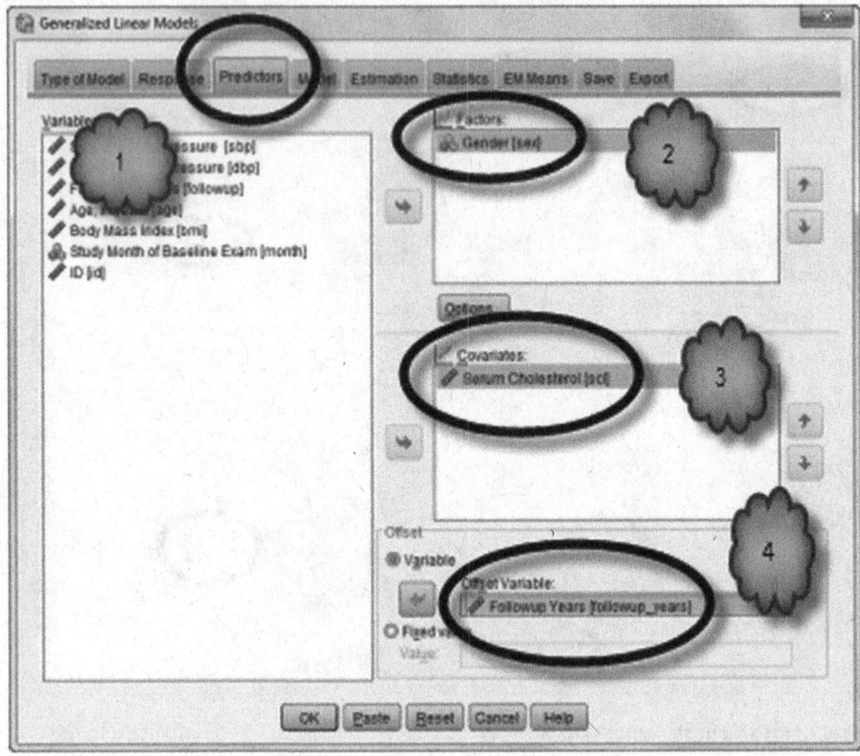

Fig. 17.12 Selecting the predictor and offset variables

Table 17.18 Information on the quantitative variables in the model

Continuous Variable Information

		N	Minimum	Maximum	Mean	Std. Deviation
Dependent Variable	Coronary Heart Disease	4666	0	1	.31	.464
Covariate	Serum Cholesterol	4666	115	568	228.29	44.543
Offset	Follow-up Years	4666	-3.01	3.47	2.9138	.73350

The output will be very similar in form to the output we have reviewed earlier, and it is interpreted in the same manner. We will focus on the *Continuous Variable Information* and *Parameter Estimates* tables.

As before, the *Continuous Variable Information* table (Table 17.18) displays descriptive statistics for the dependent variable and any covariates. It also displays descriptive statistics for the offset variable, which in our case is the natural log of the follow-up times measured in years. Consulting the exponent function of any scientific calculator, we can tell that the follow-up times ranged from 0.05 years (0.05 is the exponent of −3.01, the minimum value of the offset) to 32.14 years (32.14 is the exponent of 3.47, the maximum value), with a mean of 18.43 years (the exponent of 2.9138). Notice that the number of patients in this analysis (4666) is 33 less than the total sample size. This is because cholesterol levels were missing for 33 patients.

Table 17.19 Estimates of the parameters in the model

Parameter Estimates

Parameter	B	Std. Error	95% Wald Confidence Interval Lower	Upper	Hypothesis Test Wald Chi-Square	df	Sig.	Exp(B)
(Intercept)	-6.481	.1686	-6.811	-6.150	1478.332	1	.000	.002
[sex=0]	.706	.0626	.584	.829	127.283	1	.000	2.027
[sex=1]	0[a]	.	.	.	.	.	.	1
scl	.009	.0007	.007	.010	162.931	1	.000	1.009
(Scale)	1[b]							
(Negative binomial)	1[b]							

Dependent Variable: Coronary Heart Disease
Model: (Intercept), sex, scl, offset = Followup_years
a. Set to zero because this parameter is redundant.
b. Fixed at the displayed value.

Note also that the mean for coronary heart disease is 0.31. This is equivalent to the cumulative incidence of heart disease for the 4666 patients.

The *Parameter Estimates* table, a fragment of which is shown in Table 17.19, is interpreted in the same manner as before.

Study the table and answer the following questions.

17.5.1 What are the missing values in the following prediction equation for a male patient with a cholesterol level of 200?
ln (rate of coronary heart disease) = ________ + ________ + ________ (200).

17.5.2 The exponent of the log rate of coronary heart disease for a male with a cholesterol level of 200 is about 0.019. According to these results, how many new cases of coronary heart disease each year can we expect for every 1000 men with a cholesterol level of 200?

17.5.3 According to these data, the rate of coronary heart disease for men is ________ times the rate for women.

17.5.4 Do the results allow us to conclude that in the population from which the Framingham patients were drawn, the rate of coronary heart disease is greater in men than in women? Why or why not?

17.6 Exercise Questions

The first three exercise questions use the Centers for Disease Control and Prevention (CDC) data set, **CDC BRFSS.sav** [3]. Open the file. This file contains the responses of New York state residents to a telephone survey conducted in 2005 by the CDC. Respondents were asked to report the number of days during the past month in which their physical health was not good. These data are contained in **NUMBER**

OF DAYS PHYSICAL HEALTH NOT GOOD [*PHYSHLTH*] (variable 4). The CDC coded a response of 0 days as 88 to signify "none." The CDC also asked respondents to report their sex and to categorize their general health. These responses are located in the variables **SEX** [*SEX*] (variable 32; 1 = Male, 2 = Female), and **GENERAL HEALTH** [*GENHLTH*] (variable 3; 1 = Excellent, 2 = Very Good, 3 = Good, 4 = Fair, and 5 = Poor). The respondents reported their height and weight as well. From these responses the CDC calculated each respondent's **BODY MASS INDEX** [*BMI*] (variable 107).

Recode (**Transform > Recode into Different Variables**) **NUMBER OF DAYS PHYSICAL HEALTH NOT GOOD** into a new variable called **NEW PHYSICAL HEALTH** [*NEWPHYSHLTH*] so that all instances of 88 are recoded as 0. Then in *Variable View* declare all instances of 77 and 99 in the new variable as missing. Be sure that for **GENERAL HEALTH**, values of 7 and 9 have been declared as missing.

1. Conduct a negative binomial regression using **BODY MASS INDEX** as a predictor and **NEW PHYSICAL HEALTH** as the response.
   a. Is BMI a significant predictor of the number of days a New Yorker's health is not good? How do you know?
   b. What is the slope coefficient for **BODY MASS INDEX**?
   c. What is the rate ratio for **BODY MASS INDEX**?
   d. Is the rate ratio significantly different from 1? How do you know?
   e. Complete the following sentence: The number of days per month during which the physical health of New Yorkers is not good increases by ________ % for every 1 unit of increase in BMI.

2. Conduct a negative binomial regression using **SEX, GENERAL HEALTH** and **BODY MASS INDEX** as predictors and **NEW PHYSICAL HEALTH** as the response.
   a. What are the slope coefficient and its *p*-value for **SEX**?
   b. On average, which sex experienced significantly more days during which their physical health was not good?
   c. Was the respondents' general health significantly related to the number of days during which their physical health was not good? Describe the relationship.
   d. In what way, if any, does the relationship between **BODY MASS INDEX** and the response variable change when **SEX** and **GENERAL HEALTH** are included as predictors?

3. Table 17.20 shows the output from a negative binomial regression in which **BODY MASS INDEX** and an interaction variable between **SEX** and **BODY MASS INDEX (SEX_BMI)** were the predictors and **NEW PHYSICAL HEALTH** was the response.
   a. What is the slope coefficient for the interaction term?
   b. What is the BMI slope coefficient for men? And for women?
   c. Which of the following conclusions is supported by the data, at least as of 2005? For residents of New York state,

Table 17.20 Output for Question 3

Parameter Estimates

Parameter	B	Std. Error	95% Wald Confidence Interval Lower	Upper	Hypothesis Test Wald Chi-Square	df	Sig.	Exp(B)
(Intercept)	.337	.0632	.213	.460	28.423	1	.000	1.400
BMI	.029	.0027	.024	.035	115.298	1	.000	1.030
SEX_BMI	.005	.0010	.003	.006	21.422	1	.000	1.005
(Scale)	1[a]							
(Negative binomial)	1[a]							

Dependent Variable: NEW PHYSICAL HEALTH
Model: (Intercept), BMI, SEX_BMI
a. Fixed at the displayed value.

i. BMI is equally related to the response variable for men and women.
ii. BMI is more strongly related to the response variable for men than for women.
iii. BMI is more strongly related to the response variable for women than for men.

4. Open the file, **Caerphilly.sav** [4]. This file contains data from a study of the incidence of myocardial infarction (MI) or stroke among a cohort of 2398 Welsh men who were followed for an average of about 9.5 person-years. The follow-up times are recorded in the variable, **Person-years at Risk** [*pyar*] (variable 5). At enrollment, each patient's smoking status was recorded and is stored in the variable, **Smoking Status** [*Smoking Status*] (variable 4; 0=Never Smoked, 1=Former Smokers, 2=Mild Smokers, 3= Moderate or Heavy Smokers). Body mass index, **BMI** [*BMI*] (variable 2), was also recorded and used to create the variable, **BMI Category** [*BMI_group*] (variable 3; 1=Underweight, 2=Normal, 3=Overweight, 4=Obese). The variable, **Non-fatal MI** or **Stroke** [*CVD*] (variable 7), stores the outcomes experienced by the patients during follow-up. Patients were assigned the value of 1 if during follow-up they either experienced an MI or a stroke; otherwise, they were assigned a 0. Conduct a negative binomial regression in which the dependent variable is **Non-fatal MI** or **Stroke** and the predictor variable is **Smoking Status.** In the analysis, assign patients who never smoked to the reference category.

   a. What percentage of these 2398 men either suffered an MI or a stroke during the follow-up?
   b. What is the log of the rate of MI or stroke for men who never smoked?
   c. Complete the following sentence: According to the prediction equation, the rate of MI or stroke for men who are moderate or heavy smokers is ________ times that of men who never smoked.
   d. According to the regression analysis, how many new cases of MI or stroke on average will occur each year among 1000 Welsh men who are moderate or heavy smokers?

Table 17.21 Output for Question 5

Parameter Estimates

Parameter	B	Std. Error	95% Wald Confidence Interval Lower	Upper	Hypothesis Test Wald Chi-Square	df	Sig.	Exp(B)
(Intercept)	-6.309	.4473	-7.186	-5.433	198.979	1	.000	.002
[SmokingStatus=3]	.714	.1986	.325	1.103	12.930	1	.000	2.042
[SmokingStatus=2]	.815	.1840	.455	1.176	19.644	1	.000	2.260
[SmokingStatus=1]	.507	.1757	.163	.851	8.326	1	.004	1.660
[SmokingStatus=0]	0[a]	.	.	.	.	.	.	1
BMI	.040	.0154	.009	.070	6.606	1	.010	1.040
(Scale)	1[b]							
(Negative binomial)	1[b]							

Dependent Variable: Non-fatal MI or Stroke
Model: (Intercept), SmokingStatus, BMI, offset = Offset
a. Set to zero because this parameter is redundant.
b. Fixed at the displayed value.

5. Table 17.21 displays output from a negative binomial regression of the **Caerphilly.sav** data described in Question 4. In the analysis, the predictor variables are **Smoking Status** and **BMI**.

   a. The offset variable was equal to the natural logarithm of which of the following?

      i. **Person-years at Risk**
      ii. **Smoking Status**
      iii. **BMI**
      iv. **Non-fatal MI or Stroke**

   b. Complete the following sentence: According to the output in Table 17.21, the rate of MI or stroke increases by _____ % for every 1 unit increase in the BMI.
   c. Using a calculator and the data displayed in the output in Table 17.21, compute and report the average number of new cases of MI or stroke that are expected to occur each year among every 1000 Welsh men who have a BMI of 30 and are moderate or heavy smokers.
   d. The rate you computed in 5c should be ________ times the rate of new cases of MI or stroke that are expected to occur each year among 1000 Welsh men who have a BMI of 30 but have never smoked.

Data Sets and References

1. Doctor Visits.sav obtained from: Cameron, A.C., Trivedi, P.K.: Regression Analysis of Count Data. 2nd ed. Econometric Society Monograph No. 53. Cambridge University Press, Cambridge (2013). (With the kind permission of Professor A. Colin Cameron)

2. Framingham.sav obtained from: Dupont, W.D.: Statistical Modeling for Biomedical Researchers, 2nd ed. Cambridge University Press, New York (2009). (With the kind permission of Sean Coady, National Heart, Blood, and Lung Institute)
3. CDC BRFSS.sav obtained from: Centers for Disease Control and Prevention (CDC). Behavioral Risk Factor Surveillance System Survey Data. Atlanta, Georgia: US Department of Health and Human Services, Centers for Disease Control and Prevention (2005). Public domain. For more information about the BRFSS, visit http://www.cdc.gov/brfss/. Accessed 16 Nov 2014
4. Caerphilly.sav obtained from: Caerphilly Prospective Study. With the kind permission of the Caerphilly Prospective Study Steering Committee, Professor Yoav Ben-Shlomo, Secretary. For more information about the Caerphilly Prospective Study, consult the Caerphilly Prospective Study website at http://www.bris.ac.uk/social-community-medicine/projects/caerphilly/about/.

Index

A
Analysis of variance, 11
    One-way analysis of variance, 252, 259–263, 304–308
    Repeated measures analysis of variance, 284–285, 288–298
    Two-way analysis of variance, 303
        With one independent groups factor and one repeated measures factor, 327–336
        With two independent groups factors, 308–318
        With two repeated measures factors, 318–327
Arm (parallel group trial), 10
Assessing screening and diagnostic tests
    accuracy, 209
    criterion standard, 205
    cutoff value, 217, 223
    diagnostic test, 205
    Fagan's nomogram, 216
    false negative, 208, 209
    false negative rate, 210, 211
    false positive, 208, 209
    false positive rate, 210, 211
    gold standard, 205
    likelihood ratio, 212–216, 222
    likelihood ratio for a negative result, 216
    negative predictive value, 206
    negative test result, 206
    positive predictive value, 206
    positive test result, 206
    posterior odds, 215
    posterior or posttest probability, 215
    prior odds, 212, 215
    prior or pretest probability, 214
    receiver operating characteristic (ROC) curve, 217–226
        area under the curve, 224
        comparing two or more tests, 225–226
    screening test, 205
    sensitivity, 211–212
    specificity, 211–212
    true negative, 208
    true negative rate, 209
    true positive, 208
    true positive rate, 209

B
Blinding, 10

C
Carryover effects, 12
Categorical variable
    nominal, 36, 59
    ordinal, 36, 59
Censored data, 424
Chart builder
    creating a bar chart, 67–69
    creating a box plot, 98–101
    creating a clustered bar chart, 101–103
    creating a histogram, 107
    creating a scatter plot, 234
Chart editor
    adding a chart title, 65
    adding text within the body of a chart, 65–66
    adding the best fitting straight line to a scatter plot, 234–235
    changing a chart's background color and frame, 65
    changing the location of data labels, 64, 65

W. H. Holmes, W. C. Rinaman, *Statistical Literacy for Clinical Practitioners*,
DOI 10.1007/978-3-319-12550-3

editing *X*- or *Y*-axis labels, 65
editing *Y*-axis numerical entries, 65
exploding a pie chart, 67
transposing the axes of a bar chart, 67
Chi-square test, 187
Conditional logistic regression, 7
Confidence intervals, 6
for the difference between two independent means, 258
for the difference between two proportions, 155
for a hazard ratio, 444
for an intercept
from a linear regression, 355
from a logistic regression, 404
from a negative binomial regression, 458
for a mean, 90, 128–132
for mean and median survival times, 432
for an odds ratio, 174, 404
for a Pearson correlation coefficient, 242–243
for a proportion, 150–153
for a rate ratio, 459
for a relative risk, 169
for a slope coefficient
from a linear regression, 355
from a logistic regression, 404
from a negative binomial regression, 458
Confounder, confounding factor, confounding variable, 2, 3
Contingency table, 179–184
Contrast analysis, 274–277
Controlling confounding variables
experimental control, 368
matching, 7
randomization, 10
random assignment, 10
random sequencing, 12
statistical control, 368
stratification, 7
Copying SPSS charts into Word, 73
Cox regression, 17
proportional hazards model, 439
slope coefficient, 444
exponent, 444
with one covariate, 439–444
with two covariates, 444–446
Cramér's *V*, 2, 193–198
Critical value, 129, 150
Cross-tabulation, 165
Cumulative incidence, 472, 475
Curvilinear relationship
monotonic, 244
non-monotonic, 244

D

Data, 1
Data editor, 26
Data view, 27, 31–37
Degrees of freedom
independent-samples *t*-test, 258
linear regression, 354
logistic regression, 402, 403
one sample *t*-test, 135
one-way analysis of variance, 262–263, 266
repeated measures analysis of variance, 291
robust tests of equality of means (Welch and Brown-Forsythe), 262–263
Two-way analysis of variance, 311, 323
Wald statistic, 403, 444
Demonstrating causality, 3
Dependent variable, 341, 342
Descriptive statistics, *see* Measures of spread; Measures of central tendency
Difference between means, 19
Differential attrition, 12
Distribution of a variable, 60, 87
kurtosis, 93
normal distribution, 93, 136
skewness, 93
Dummy variable, 383–384, 415–416
reference category, 384, 415, 468

E

Effect size, 14, 253, 263–268, *see also* Partial eta squared
Explanatory variable, 180, 233
Exponent of a logarithm, 108, 112–113

F

Frequencies and frequency tables, 60–64
Functions of statistics, 1–2

G

Gamma, 2, 199–200
Generalizability, 13
Goodness of fit, 349, 377, 456
Graphical techniques
bar chart, 64–67
box plot, 87, 94–96
clustered bar chart, 184

cumulative hazard function, *see* Hazard function, cumulative hazard function
detrended normal Q-Q plot, 139
forest plot, 14–15
histogram, 93–94
interaction plot, 310, 315–317, 322, 325–327, 332
means plot, 292–294, 305, 311, 322, 323, 332
normal probability plot of residuals, 361
normal Q-Q plot, 136–139
pie chart, 67
residual plot, 360–361
scatter plot, 179, 233–238
best fitting straight line, 234–236
stem-and-leaf plot, 87, 94
survival function, *see* Survival analysis

H
Hazard function, 436
cumulative hazard function, 436
Hazard ratio, 2, 9, 438

I
Importing an Excel spreadsheet, 26
Incidence, 18, 149
Incidence rate, 453, 472
Inclusion/exclusion eligibility criteria, 10
Independent variable, 341, 342
Inferential statistics, 2, 19, 127
Intention-to-treat analysis, 13
Interaction effect
in analysis of variance, 309, 313–318, 325–327, 332
in regression analysis, 389–393, 419–420, 446–449, 469–471

L
Labeling SPSS output, 51–52
Least squares method, 341, 345
Levene's test, 256–257, 269
Linear regression
coefficient of determination or *R* squared, 348–350
intercept, 341
least squares regression line, 345
prediction intervals, 355–359
residual analysis, 359–362
slope coefficient, 341
standardized, 380–381
unstandardized, 347, 378–380
standard error of the estimate, 352
sum of squares
regression sum of squares, 348, 388
residual or error sum of squares, 348, 388
total sum of squares, 348, 388
Linear relationship, 234, 342
negative, 234, 342
positive, 234, 342
strength of relationship, 234, 342
Logistic regression
adjusted odds ratio, 418–419
baseline odds, 412
classification table, 401, 402
converting odds to probabilities, 398
converting probabilities to odds, 398
intercept, 403
exponent, 403
logit, 398
predicted probabilities, 404
slope coefficient, 397, 403, 410
exponent, 410
with one predictor, 399–405
with quantitative and categorical predictors, 413–418
with two categorical predictors, 405–412

M
Masking, 10
Mauchly's test of sphericity, 290–291
Maximum likelihood method, 399, 443, 452
Measures of association
between categorical variables, *see* Chi-square test; Cramér's *V*; Gamma
between quantitative variables, *see* Pearson correlation coefficient; Spearman's rho coefficient
Measures of central tendency
arithmetic mean, 88
geometric mean, 113, 117
median, 92
trimmed mean, 92
Measures of spread
interquartile range, 93
range, 92
standard deviation, 92
variance, 92
Mortality rate, 2, 453

N
Negative binomial regression
intercept, 454, 457
exponent, 454, 457–458, 466
slope coefficient, 452, 454, 458, 466–468
exponent, 459

with one predictor, 452–462
with two or more predictors, 462–469
with unequal follow-up times, 471–475
offset variable, 472
person-years, 472
Nonparametric test, 140
Wilcoxon signed ranks test, 140–142

O

Odds, 6, 150, 170, 398
Odds ratio, 2, 6, 162, 170–174, 403,410, 412, 418
Opening SPSS data files, 26
Outliers, 87, 96

P

Paired comparisons analysis, 251, 283
Pairwise comparisons, 11, 294
Partial eta squared, 264–268
Pasting SPSS output into Word, 53
Pearson correlation coefficient, 238–243
correlation matrix, 239
Fisher's *Z* transformation, 242
Percentages, 60–64
cumulative percent, 64
valid percent, 64
Poisson regression, 9, 452, 454
Population parameter, 96, 127, 128
Post hoc comparisons, 271–274
Predictor variable, 19, 36, 458
Prevalence, 18, 149
Printing SPSS output, 53
Probability, 150, 398
Protective factor, 6, 9

Q

Quantitative or scale variable, 36, 59

R

R squared, 236–238
Adjusted *R* squared, 377
Random measurement error, 5, 7
Random sample, 128, 134, 140
Random sampling variability, 2, 5, 6, 9, 10, 124
Rate ratio, 2, 9, 11, 452, 458, 468
Relative risk, 2, 9, 150, 161, 162–170, 438, 444, 445–446
Repeated measures analysis, 283, 284–285
Replication, 13
Residual confounding, 8
Response variable, 180, 233, 234
Risk, 162
Risk factor, 6, 9, 150

S

Sample versus population, 2
Sample statistic, 128, 133, 150, 153
Saving an SPSS data file
as an Excel file, 40
as an SPSS file, 38
Saving SPSS output
as an Excel or PDF file, 55
as an SPSS file, 55
Scripts, 151
Selecting cases
all cases, 44
by category, 41–44
by more than one condition, 49–51
by range of responses, 49
Sorting a dialog box variable list, 51
Spearman's rho, 2, 244–247
Sphericity, 290–291
Splitting a file, 155
Standard error of the mean, 96–97, 133
Standardized score (*Z*-score), 380
Statistical power, 142–143
Statistical significance, 133–136
alpha level, 134
contrasted with clinical significance, 143
significance level, 134, 143, 189
p-value, 12, 133–134, 189
Type I error, 189
Structure of SPSS data files
column width, 35
data type, 28
missing values, 33–35
number of decimal places, 31
value labels, 32
values alignment, 36
variable label, 31–32
variable measure, 36
variable name, 28
variable role, 36
variable width, 30
Study designs
case report, 4–5
case series, 4–5
case-control study, 5–8, 17, 161–162
cohort study, 8–10, 16–18, 161
prospective cohort study, 16–17
retrospective cohort study, 16–17
cross-sectional study, 18, 162
meta-analysis, 14–15

randomized controlled trial, 10–13
crossover trial, 11–12
parallel group trial, 10–11
systematic review, 14–15
Survival analysis
survival function, 424, 427
Kaplan-Meier estimator, 424–432
comparing two survival functions, 432–436
survival table, 426–427
survival time, 423–424
mean survival time, 428, 432
median survival time, 428, 432

T
Test of hypotheses, 132–136
alternative hypothesis, 132–133
one-tailed or one-sided, 132
two-tailed or two-sided, 132
null hypothesis, 132–133
robust test, 140
testing a mean, *see* *t*-test, one sample *t*-test
testing a median, *see* Nonparametric test, Wilcoxon signed ranks test
testing a Pearson correlation coefficient, 241–243
testing a single proportion, 153–155
testing a slope coefficient
from a Cox regression, 444
from a linear regression, 352, 354, 387–388
from a logistic regression, 403, 410, 417–418
from a negative binomial regression, 458–459, 466–468
testing an intercept
from a linear regression, 353
from a logistic regression, 403
from a negative binomial regression, 457, 466
testing for the presence of sphericity, *see* Mauchly's test of sphericity
testing the equality of two proportions, 158–160
testing the equality of two survival functions, *see* Survival analysis, Kaplan-Meier estimator
testing the equality (homogeneity) of variances, *see* Levene's test
testing whether two categorical variables are related, *see* Chi-square test
Test of normality, 136–139
Test statistic, 19, 133, 135, 140, 153, 241, 265, 352, 410
Brown-Forsythe, 262–263
chi-square, 19, 187
F, 19, 261, 265, 354
t, 19, 135, 352
Wald, 19, 403, 444
Welch, 262–263
Z, 19, 140, 155, 160
Time to event, 19, 423
Transforming variables, 70–73
log transformation, 106–107
to change the shape of a distribution, 106–110
to create an interaction variable for a regression, 390
to create a dummy variable, 384
to create an offset variable, 472–473
to create a quantitative variable, 104–106
to equalize variability across groups, 110–111
to recode a categorical variable into another categorical variable, 72–73
to recode a quantitative variable into a categorical variable, 70–71
to reverse the coding of a variable, 163–164
Treatment effectiveness, 13
Treatment efficacy, 13
t-test
paired-samples *t*-test, 18, 252, 284, 285–288
one sample *t*-test, 134–136
independent-samples *t*-test, 17, 253–258

V
Variable view, 28–37
Viewer window, 41
contents pane, 64
outline pane, 64

W
Washout period, 11
Weighting cases, 172

Printed in the United States
By Bookmasters